Outcomes Management

Applications to Clinical Practice

www.mosby.com

OUTCOMES MANAGEMENT

Applications to Clinical Practice

ANNE W. WOJNER, PhD(c), MSN, RN, CCRN

President
Health Outcomes Institute, Inc.
The Woodlands, Texas

Assistant Research Professor, Neurology
University of Texas—Houston, Stroke Treatment Team
Houston, Texas

With 49 illustrations

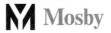 Mosby

A Harcourt Health Sciences Company

St. Louis   London   Philadelphia   Sydney   Toronto

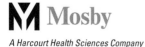

A Harcourt Health Sciences Company

Vice President, Nursing Editorial Director: Sally Schrefer
Editor: Yvonne Alexopoulos
Developmental Editor: Kimberly A. Netterville
Project Manager: Catherine Jackson
Production Editor: Marc P. Syp
Designer: Judi Lang

Copyright (c) 2001 by Mosby, Inc.

Mosby, Inc.
A Harcourt Health Sciences Company
11830 Westline Industrial Drive
St. Louis, Missouri 63146

Printed in the United States of America

ISBN 1-55664-411-6

01   02   03   04   05 CL/MV 9   8   7   6   5   4   3   2   1

Contributors

Thomas S. Ahrens, DNSc, RN, CCRN, CS
Research Scientist
Nursing Department
Barnes-Jewish Hospital
St. Louis, Missouri

Andrei V. Alexandrov, MD
Assistant Professor of Neurology and
   Radiology
Director, Cerebrovascular Ultrasound
Stroke Treatment Team
University of Texas
Houston, Texas

Kathleen M. Griffin, PhD
President and CEO
Valley Consultants, Inc.
Scottsdale, Arizona

Timothy Kight, BA, M.Div.
President
Management Resource Group
Fallbrook, California

Mark A. MacCutcheon, MHSA
Senior Consultant
Health Dimensions Consulting Group
Benedictine Health System
Scottsdale, Arizona

Leslie H. Nicoll, PhD, MBA, RN
Associate Research Professor
College of Nursing and Health
   Professions
University of Southern Maine
Portland, Maine

Linda H. Yoder, RN, MBA, PhD, AOCN
Colonel, United States Army Nurse
   Corps
Deputy Commander of Nursing
McDonald Army Community Hospital
Fort Eustis, Virginia

Reviewers

Jackie Birmingham, MS, BSN, RN, A-CCC, CMAC
Executive Director
Continuum Care Services
Suffield, Connecticut

Ruth A. Burnett, RN, BSN, CRRN, CCM, CDMS, ABDA
Medical Process Owner
CIGNA Group Insurance
Philadelphia, Pennsylvania

Jane Campbell, RN, MSN, CNA
Associate Professor
Department of Nursing
Northern Michigan University
Marquette, Michigan

Nancy E. Fredrich RN, AA, BSN
Infection Control Nurse/Staff Development/Supervisor
Cooper County Memorial Hospital
Boonville, Missouri

Betty Kuiper, RN, BSN, CEN
Case Manager
ED and Outpatient Services
Western Baptist Hospital
Paducah, Kentucky

June Morrison, RN, BSN
Senior Investigator
Enforcement Department
Virginia Department of Health Professions
Virginia Beach, Virginia

Anna M. Smith, RN, MSN
Director
Emergency Services
University of Louisville Hospital
Louisville, Kentucky

Preface

Today's society has high expectations of the health care system. Regardless of disease state, etiology, co-morbid characteristics or general demographic makeup, the general public approaches practitioners and organizations with an expectation of caring, competent, efficient, and high quality health care services. Practitioners and health care organizations have shown an increasing interest in performance measurement and benchmarking to drive improvement in the quality of care. At the core of this phenomenon lies a growing need for the measurement and management of health care outcomes.

Outcomes Management: Application to Clinical Practice is the culmination of years of worldwide practice, exploration, innovation, and engineering of health care practices and systems across a variety of settings from prehospital to postacute. This text provides the reader with insight into the process of implementing an outcomes management program, along with the challenges and pitfalls of the process, as well as tried and true methods. It is rich with examples, tools, formulas, templates and figures to promote a thorough understanding of outcomes measurement and management.

Outcomes Management: Application to Clinical Practice was written with a broad appeal for clinical quality and accreditation. Practitioners in all disciplines and settings, graduate health science students, payers, legislators and administrative personnel will find this text is a source that supports science-based improvement and continuous refinement of health care services.

The text is organized in a manner that promotes a logical approach to the successful implementation and refinement of an outcomes management initiative. **Part I: Getting Started in Outcomes Measurement and Management** provides a framework for outcomes management, details methods for environmental assessment, identifies key leadership personnel, and includes an introduction to research design. **Part II: Project Implementation: Driving Change to Improve Outcomes** presents concepts related to use of scientific method, implementation strategies, statistical analyses, and meaningful data presentation. This section explores methods of using standardized practices for outcomes measurement, technology assessment applications, successful program implementation, and staff education. It also addresses implications related to the expanding role of health informatics, and outcomes/quality program integration. **Part III: Looking Ahead: Complementary Next Steps** introduces the concept of disease management, showcases successful strategies for bridging continuum-based outcomes measurement and management, and highlights methods to grow and enhance organizational culture through an outcomes-based initiative.

At a time when outcomes are a focus for improving practice, *Outcomes Management: Application to Clinical Practice* provides a framework to support the measurement and improvement of health care services in a variety of settings. The only other necessary ingredient is commitment on the part of the user of this text to begin the journey of exploration associated with outcomes management. While the trip can be challenging, the rewards associated with the implementation of outcomes management and science-driven care improvement is a rewarding one. The authors of this text hope its readers will step up to the challenge of exploring uncharted territory, view hurdles and obstacles as predictable, strategically implement successful partnerships in practice transformation, and become inspired along the way. Tomorrow's health care leaders will be those that embrace critical self-analysis today and strive to create services that enhance societal health outcomes. To that end, bon voyage and best wishes as you pioneer health care improvement through outcomes management.

Anne W. Wojner

Brief Contents

Contents

PART III

Looking Ahead: Complementary Next Steps   *167*

Outcomes Management

Applications to Clinical Practice

PART I

Getting Started
in Outcomes
Measurement
and
Management

CHAPTER 1

An Introduction to Outcomes Management

INTRODUCTION

Health care is undergoing a challenging and painful transition, as providers learn to redefine patient care by new rules and values. Until the 1980s, the rising cost of U.S. health care was not a concern of the general public. During this era, health care providers leaned heavily on their own value systems to drive the development of new technologies, pharmaceuticals, and practices aimed at reducing mortality associated with disease and injury. The concept of consumer-driven health care was yet to be born.

A dramatic shift in values has occurred that has affected the U.S. health care system in ways like never before. This migration of values has its roots in consumer-driven health services, redirecting care delivery in ways that were unforeseeable 20 years ago. There are many consumers of health services, each reflecting special interests and concerns for system improvement. Outcomes of interest to this diverse group include cost, length of stay (LOS), recidivism, patient satisfaction, and a variety of physiologic and psychosocial outcomes that serve as markers for quality of life, resource utilization, and functional status.

It is likely that U.S. health care will continue to evolve into a consumer-driven system over the next 10 years. But as the system continues to evolve, health service consumers themselves must rise to a level of involvement for which they have been poorly prepared to accept. In the new paradigm, consumers will likely be held accountable for their care decisions, for behaviors that contribute to illness, and for making use of the resources made available to them to promote wellness. Health care providers must partner with consumers to facilitate the evolution and continuous improvement of this emerging delivery model, to ensure that needs are satisfied, and to enhance quality of life.

THE CALL FOR OUTCOMES MEASUREMENT

In 1917, a physician by the name of Ernest A. Codman called for implementation of a program that he titled the *End-Result Idea*. Codman advocated the measurement and publication of physiologic and psychosocial end results or outcomes, as well as determination of the cause of all untoward outcomes. He radically suggested that hospitals use this information to improve the practice of their medical staff.[1]

Unfortunately, Codman's *End-Result Idea* was scoffed by his peers, who viewed measurement and possible public knowledge of health outcomes as detrimental to the advancement of medical practice. Codman was labeled an eccentric for recommending publicly that hospitals should be bent on improvement, know their results, compare their results with those of other hospitals, and promote members of the medical staff based on what they accomplish for their patients.[2] In the epilogue of his last publication, Codman spoke of the *End-Result Idea:* "Who knows but that some day a copy [of this book] may be dusted off in a library and shown to some lonely hospital trustee . . . I am convinced that if a single great general hospital did this thoroughly, the others would have to follow."[2]

Scientific researchers have valued the measurement of "results" or "outcomes" since the dawn of empirical reasoning. Empirical theory is an expression of what is known, which is developed and tested through scientific research efforts that generate factual descriptions, explanations, or predictions supported by subjective or objective data. Research designs used to generate and test empirical theory include both descriptive and analytical methods (e.g., case control, cohort, and experimental designs). Health care providers dedicated to improving health outcomes have, rightfully so, based decisions about the treatment of specific disorders on the findings of rigorous scientific research.

Interest in the measurement of health outcomes among populations of patients has grown significantly over the past 10 years among payers, managed care organizations, health care administrators, the federal government, and health service providers. Issues such as universal health care coverage, improved consumer access, preventative services, futile care, cost, and consumer-defined quality improvement have brought Codman's *End-Result Idea* to life within the practice arena, challenging providers to prove what they claim about their services.

Today, the measurement, analysis, and publication of health outcomes is common. Some of the challenges that must be overcome as we learn and explore the science of outcomes measurement include issues related to study design, methodology, measurement principles, the use of appropriate analyses, and acknowledgment of limitations to our findings. As a young science that is undergoing rapid dissemination, we must consciously look with caution at our results to avoid errors in interpretation, which may cause us to change otherwise successful delivery models and interdisciplinary practices. Skepticism and replication will be essential tools as we work toward a better understanding of outcomes measurement and management processes.

Clinical researchers must take an active role in shaping the methods used to determine results of health care interventions. Prerequisites for leadership in outcomes measurement should include masters or doctoral education, active clinical practice expertise, research mastery, and a value system that supports lifelong learning and interdisciplinary collaborative practice. Decisions effecting changes in practice and delivery models, as well as the addition or elimination of specific health services or personnel should be made by these leaders in collaboration with each discipline involved in producing care. In turn, administrators must support providers in the search for superior practices by assuming a servant-leader role that empowers those delivering care to meet the holistic needs of patients and families.

| OUTCOMES MANAGEMENT

Outcomes management (OM) is "the enhancement of physiologic and psychosocial patient outcomes through development and implementation of exemplary health practices and services, driven by outcomes assessment."[3] As illustrated in Figure 1–1, OM is a research-based process that consists of a never-ending cycle of measurement and continuous quality improvement (CQI) of clinical practice. OM facilitates dissemination of health outcomes information to appropriate decision makers, namely patients, providers, and payers of health services.

OM gained attention in the late 1980s by advocating the measurement of health outcomes among disease-specific patient populations and utilizing these data to drive improvement of patient care. OM

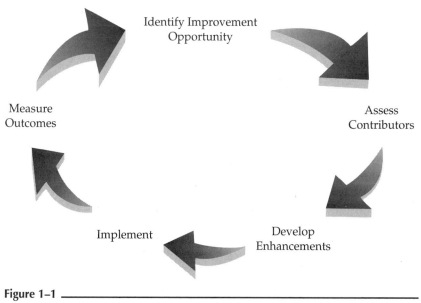

Identify Improvement
Opportunity

Measure
Outcomes

Assess
Contributors

Implement

Develop
Enhancements

Figure 1–1 _____
Continuous quality improvement of clinical practice.

acknowledges that interdisciplinary practices, physiologic and psychosocial factors, and characteristics of health service delivery systems and providers all contribute to the production of health outcomes.

Creation of a new health care paradigm must be driven by research that measures the outcomes, or byproducts, of care, continuously comparing actual findings against desired results. Outcomes measurement is powerful. It enables patients to choose among treatment options through predictive modeling and sharing of outcomes data, which facilitates a level of informed consent that is not yet experienced in most health care centers. Outcomes measurement also identifies opportunities for building and modifying health services along a continuum of illness to wellness. The identification of opportunities to improve health services continuously is also facilitated through outcomes measurement. Through targeted systematic improvement, enhancement of provider practice naturally evolves toward achievement of *best practice*. Finally, outcomes measurement and management reduces financial risk for providers, patients, and payers through reduction of costly complications, enhanced service efficiency, appropriate health resource utilization, and provider practice revision that is grounded in science.[4]

Models for OM are derived from the work of Paul Ellwood, who in 1988 suggested that clinical quality measurement should be driven by outcomes analysis. According to Ellwood, OM is a "technology of patient experience designed to help patients, payers, and providers make rational medical care-related choices based on better insight into the effect of these choices on patient life."[5]

Ellwood suggested four essential principles for inclusion in an OM program:

1. An emphasis on standards that providers can use to select appropriate interventions;
2. The measurement of patient functional status and well-being, along with disease-specific clinical outcomes;
3. A pooling of outcome data on a massive scale; and
4. The analysis and dissemination of the database to appropriate decision makers.[5]

| OUTCOMES RESEARCH

A strong research arm is integral to the success of an OM program. Outcomes research quantifies the byproducts of care for defined patient cohorts and supports evaluation and continuous improvement of a variety of care practices and services.

Outcomes are considered the "end result" of specific processes. Favorable outcomes include the achievement of defined goals.[6] As part of the initiation of an OM program, health care providers must set goals that serve as benchmarks for health outcomes achievement. By establishing benchmarks, health care providers can test the effects of interventions on goal attainment. Both descriptive and analytical research methods complement an OM initiative. Chapters 4 and 5 provide information supporting outcomes research methodology.

A MODEL FOR OUTCOMES MANAGEMENT

A model can be used to define the series of phases that drive the process of OM (Figure 1–2). As a research-based initiative, OM is guided by steps that promote systematic clinical inquiry within a cohort of patients. The process begins in Phase I, with the identification of desired patient outcomes and the construction of a database to support ongoing analysis of patient experience. In Phases II through IV, interventions are developed, implemented, and tested toward outcomes achievement. Consistent with CQI philosophy, the process returns to Phase II repeatedly when outcomes measurement in Phase IV identifies room for further refinement of interventions or when the need for new processes to enhance patient outcomes arises.[3]

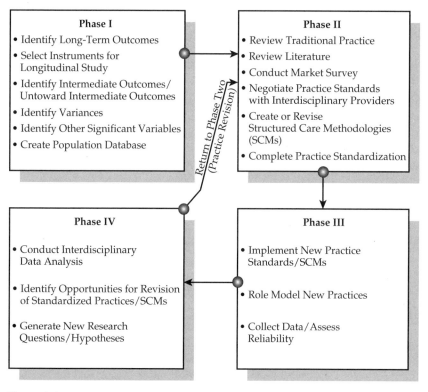

Figure 1–2 _____

Outcomes management model.

Phase I: Describing the Population

In Phase I, a population for study is selected from the practice arena. Interdisciplinary providers generate questions for the cohort that are designed to elicit descriptive data of the cohort's characteristics and outcomes. Desired intermediate and long-term outcomes are identified for measurement within the cohort. Both intermediate and long-term outcomes represent the occurrence of specific physiologic or psychosocial "results."

Long-term outcomes are measured distally, or longitudinally, at specified points following a health care intervention (e.g., 3, 6, 12, and 24 months following discharge or release from provider management). Long-term outcomes are typically assessed through use of instruments that measure quality of life, resource utilization, functional status, and/or satisfaction.

Intermediate outcomes are measured proximally; that is, at the time of discharge from a specific level of care (e.g., hospital, subacute unit, skilled nursing facility, rehabilitation program, home care services). The attainment of intermediate outcomes is measured directly, through documentation of outcomes attainment and also the identification of untoward intermediate outcomes (UIOs) and variances. UIOs are undesired physiologic and psychosocial occurrences, which are measured in the cohort upon completion of a phase of care. Variances are processes; they include inefficient systems or provider practices that occur among the cohort during a phase of care delivery.[4]

The capture of UIOs and system/provider variances provides rich data for practitioners by identifying untoward occurrences that may be amenable to resolution through the use of new interventions. A rigorous definition must support each UIO or variance to ensure the validity and reliability of the data retrieved. Box 1–1 provides an example of some undefined UIOs and system/provider variances for patients undergoing inpatient rehabilitation following stroke.

Once outcome targets have been set and definitions have been written, interdisciplinary team members begin development of an outcomes data repository (ODR), a database that will support study of the questions generated by the interdisciplinary team. Chapter 7 discusses the development and maintenance of ODRs. Data elements that might be included to support the study of a research question aimed at identifying risk factors for postoperative mediastinitis among a cardiac surgery cohort are listed in Box 1–2. This form of descriptive research identifies opportunities for improvement of clinical practice but falls short of defining a cause-and-effect relationship. Interdisciplinary providers may create and employ new interventions directed at improving patient outcomes in Phase II.

Phase II: Practice Standardization for Analytic Research

Phase II involves the development of interdisciplinary practice standards for the achievement of a specified outcome. Five steps are taken during this phase of the OM process: (1) traditional practice patterns are analyzed, (2) literature is reviewed, (3) a market survey is com-

---

BOX 1–1   *Undefined Untoward Intermediate Outcomes and Variances Occurring in the Rehabilitation Phase of Stroke Management*

Untoward Intermediate Outcomes (UIOs)
Aspiration pneumonia
Patient fall, with or without injury
Activity intolerance
New neurologic deficit
Skin breakdown
Poststroke depression
Incontinence

Variances
Provider failure to order nutrition
Delay in test completion over holiday or weekend
Delay in insurance verification of home care coverage

Note: This list represents a small sample of variables for inclusion in this cohort of patients. UIOs reflect physiologic or psychosocial events that prohibit attainment of desired intermediate outcomes; variances reflect deviation from accepted standard practice. A rigorous definition must support each UIO and variance to ensure tracking of valid and reliable information.

---

pleted to determine alternative practice options, (4) the addition of new practices is negotiated, and (5) standardization of practice occurs.[3]

Structured care methodologies (SCMs), which represent the new intervention(s) to be tested for outcome achievement, are developed during Phase II. Four different categories of SCMs support the use of a new interdisciplinary standard or intervention within the cohort: pathways, algorithms, protocols, and order sets. Each type of SCM varies in both specificity and degree of provider practice flexibility. SCMs should be derived from a combination of research, successful existing practices, published guidelines, and expert opinion. In keeping with the CQI process illustrated in the OM model (see Figure 1–2), SCMs are dynamic —not static—and never represent a final product; SCMs are always in a state of evaluation and ongoing enhancement. Chapter 6 details the process of the development and utilization of SCMs, while Appendix B provides numerous examples of SCMs from a variety of practice settings.

Phase III: Process Implementation
During Phase III of the OM process, implementation of the new practice standards and interventions developed in Phase II occurs. Interdisciplinary provider education and credentialing is undertaken and the new

---

| **Box 1–2** | *Variables for a Database Supporting the Study of the Risk Factors for Postoperative Mediastinitis in a Cardiac Surgery Cohort* |

- Age
- Time on cardiopulmonary bypass
- Comorbidities:
  - Diabetes mellitus (i.e., blood glucose control)
  - Chronic obstructive pulmonary disease (i.e., pulmonary function)
- Cigarette pack/day smoking history
- Emergency vs. elective case
- Nutritional status (e.g., prealbumin level)
- Surgical team
- Specific cardiac procedure (e.g., coronary artery bypass graft, cardiac valve replacement)

Note: This list represents a small sample of variables for inclusion in a database for the study of risk factors for mediastinitis within a cardiac surgery cohort. Definitions must accompany each variable on the list to ensure validity and reliability.

---

processes are piloted and subsequently implemented. As with any new process, ongoing assessment of provider reliability must be conducted. Once reliability has been established, data collection begins and continues over a predefined period of time to document whether the use of the new intervention(s) made a difference in the targeted patient outcome.

Phase IV: Interdisciplinary Analysis

Phase IV involves data analysis and the reporting of study findings to all stakeholders. This phase facilitates the identification of additional opportunities for practice enhancement and stimulates members of the interdisciplinary team to generate new research questions and hypotheses. The process then returns to Phase II, in which practice standards are renegotiated and new SCMs are generated for implementation.

| CASE MANAGEMENT VERSUS OUTCOMES MANAGEMENT

OM is often confused with case management (CM), but these two processes differ significantly. CM was first used by psychiatric social workers. In the early 1980s, CM reemerged as a method to restructure nursing care toward the provision of cost efficient, timely health service. In fact, early nursing CM models were referred to as "second generation primary nursing," which depicts the accountability and autonomy of the primary nurse prototype as the basis upon which to build a new, fiscally-conscious dimension of patient care.[4]

CM, in the purest sense, is concerned with the case-by-case delivery of patient care by providers; commonly CM is combined with processes such as utilization review/management, discharge planning, the orchestration of individualized care for select patient cases, and cost containment.[4] Given the importance of these CM duties, all providers, regardless of discipline, should be held accountable and act as case managers for their assigned patients.

OM is a research-based process that works in concert with CM. The combination of OM- and CM-driven care enables providers to improve clinical practice and individual performance by highlighting opportunities to enhance care, stimulating the use of science-based interventions, and conducting systematic evaluation of overall program effectiveness. Outcomes measurement facilitates OM, which is imparted on a patient-by-patient basis through CM.[4]

Within an OM program, an advanced practice nurse (APN) with either a masters or doctoral degree and clinical expertise in a specific practice area is often used to facilitate the research process for an interdisciplinary group of providers. These APNs, or "outcomes managers," work collaboratively with case managers and other members of an interdisciplinary team. Outcomes managers are interested in the aggregate health experience of the cohort. Case managers, on the other hand, concern themselves with the case-by-case details of patient movement across the health care continuum.[7] Chapters 2, 3, and 9 detail the roles and relationships of interdisciplinary providers such as case managers and outcomes managers.

| SUMMARY

Today, health care providers are challenged to produce both high quality and cost-efficient care in an environment with new rules that no longer support traditional practice patterns. As new practice paradigms are explored, it is essential to let scientific findings guide the change process.

The use of an OM model enables health care practitioners to undertake an endless quest for best practice. The OM process is utilized to its fullest when, through the patient's eyes, untoward physiologic and psychosocial problems that limit the attainment of desired health outcomes are identified and eliminated through practice redesign.

Finally, measurement of health outcomes has come of age. Codman would be pleased to see that outcomes data are valued today as a major vehicle driving change in interdisciplinary practice. As providers embark on the quest for best practice, Codman's *End-Result Idea* will grow in significance. OM provides a mechanism to turn Codman's vision into reality, while fostering the development of a system designed to meet the holistic needs of patients and their families.

References

1. Codman EA: The value of case records in hospitals, *Modern Hospitals* 9:426-428, 1917.
2. Codman EA: *The shoulder: rupture of the supraspinatus tendon and other lesions in or about the subacromial bursa*, Brooklyn, 1934, G. Miller.
3. Wojner AW: Outcomes management: from theory to practice, *Crit Care Nurs Quarterly*, 19(4):1-15, 1997.
4. Wojner AW: Widening the scope: from case management to outcomes management, *Case Manager* 8(2):77-82, 1997.
5. Ellwood PM: Outcomes management: a technology of patient experience, *N Engl J Med* 318:1549-1556, 1988.
6. Davies AR et al: Outcomes assessment in clinical settings: a consensus statement on principles and best practices in project management, *Jt Comm J Qual Improv* 20:6-16, 1994.
7. Wojner AW, Kite-Powell D: Outcomes manager: a role for the advanced practice nurse, *Crit Care Nurs Quarterly* 19(4):16-24, 1997.

CHAPTER 2

Environmental Assessment: Orchestrating Effective Change

| INTRODUCTION

Today's payer-driven system challenges providers to move patients across the health care continuum in a timely, productive fashion. The delivery of efficient, effective health services requires interdisciplinary teamwork supported by open lines of communication and a collaborative framework. Outcomes management (OM) is an interdisciplinary process that provides data-driven continuous quality improvement (CQI), facilitating movement toward a *best practice* model. Teams of interdisciplinary providers implement OM, identifying standardized practices for testing, analyzing the effectiveness of these interventions, and continuously improving care to enhance patient outcomes.

This chapter focuses on the assessment and management of organizational readiness for an OM initiative, including the identification of organizational strengths and challenges, strategies for successfully initiating organizational change, and the concept of shared leadership through collaborative patient management.

| SWOT ANALYSIS

Before implementing widespread organizational change, health care institutions should assess their readiness for action through a systematic process such as SWOT analysis. SWOT analysis is a process used to identify Strengths, Weaknesses, Opportunities, and Threats to an organization on the threshold of change; it assists stakeholders in the establishment of an action plan for project implementation that is tailored to the institution's unique internal and external characteristics.

As a grassroots, interdisciplinary process, OM implementation should be guided by a SWOT analysis that provides input from a variety of positions throughout the health care institution. Participants involved in this type of readiness assessment should consider not only internal organizational characteristics but also external contributors that may pose as strengths, weaknesses, opportunities, or threats to the success of the initiative. Table 2–1 provides an example of criteria that should be assessed using SWOT analysis.

TABLE 2–1

Strengths, Weaknesses, Opportunities, and Threats (SWOT) Analysis Criteria

Criteria	S	W	O	T
I. Internal Assessment: Clinical Sphere				
1. The contributions of interdisciplinary providers are valued by all members of the health care team.				
2. Changes in practice are based on current research.				
3. Care processes are driven by the needs of patients, not providers.				
4. Resources are used prudently and effectively.				
5. Interdisciplinary care practices are standardized throughout the institution.				
6. Institutional systems work efficiently.				
7. Patient flow through the system is logical and well orchestrated; providers and patients are not burdened by inefficient patient flow.				
8. Employees of the organization consider their workplace to be a "center of excellence" in the provision of health services to three or more populations of patients.				
9. The organization provides specialized and/or high-tech services, which have fostered its ability to capture the market for these services within the surrounding community.				
10. Automated information systems are used to document care delivery, use of resources, patient assessments, patient movement through the system, cost, care variances, and patient outcomes.				
11. Advanced practice nurses (APNs) (with masters or doctoral degrees) are used to guide practice improvement and research initiatives.				
12. An active institutional review board exists to support a program of research.				
13. Case management (utilization review/discharge planning) is conducted.				
14. Ancillary service providers (e.g., physical therapists, social workers, dietitians) move along the in-house continuum of care with their patient populations.				
15. There is physician support for the project.				
16. A physician leader has been identified to spearhead each population-based team.				
17. There is no evidence of territoriality; shared ownership and collegial relationships are evident.				
18. The organization endorses risk taking, valuing mistakes as part of the learning and growing process.				
19. Team spirit and pride is evident throughout the organization.				

Continued

TABLE 2–1 ━━━━━━━━━━━━━━━━━━━━━━━━━━━━━━━━━━━━━━━

Strengths, Weaknesses, Opportunities, and Threats (SWOT) Analysis Criteria—cont'd

Criteria	S	W	O	T
20. Research and statistical support resources are available to assist with the project as needed.				
21. Computer hardware and software are accessible to each population-based project team.				
22. A commitment to continuous quality improvement and health outcomes measurement is evident across all disciplines and services.				
II. Internal Assessment: Business Sphere				
1. Service line structures have been established to support the business and clinical analyses of programs in population management.				
2. Service line definitions have been written using diagnosis-related groups (DRGs) or international classification of disease (ICD-9) codes.				
3. Key marketing and business support personnel have been identified for the program.				
4. Avenues for internal and external program marketing exist within the institution.				
5. Administrators have prioritized populations to be targeted.				
6. Mechanisms for confidential sharing of cost data with population team leaders have been established.				
7. Business-related data (cost and length of stay) are available to clinical leaders without administrative approval.				
8. Mechanisms that ensure regular communication between business and clinical spheres have been established.				
III. External Assessment				
1. A continuum of health care services exists to support the institution in the movement of specified patient populations.				
2. A relationship exists between the institution and transferring institutions across the continuum, enabling practice standardization and longitudinal outcomes measurement.				
3. A mechanism for community health education and health support groups exists and is tied to the institution.				
4. The institution is recognized by the community at large as a center of excellence in the delivery of specific health services.				
5. Legislative representatives acknowledge the institution as a source for health policy advisement and community service excellence.				
6. Payers view the institution as one that provides superior-quality, cost-efficient services.				
7. Academic institutions value the privilege to provide health science students with clinical rotations within the organization.				

Copyright Health Outcomes Institute, The Woodlands, Texas.

Internal Assessment

Internal assessment of an organization may be divided into several broad categories: personnel, environment, technology, and culture. Personnel assessment should include an inventory of the positions within major divisions of the institution that are likely to be affected by an outcomes initiative. Personnel assessment should be undertaken to determine the distribution of responsibilities, projected workload, project support, and opportunities for position redesign.

The environmental assessment should focus on current patient and provider flow through the system, the potential for enhancement, opportunities to create new services within existing spaces, and system constraints not amenable to simple redesign. The technology assessment evaluates the organization's use of computerized information systems, including existing hardware and software. Specialized medical services made possible through the use of available technology—internal or external to the system—should be noted. Finally, culture should be assessed continuously throughout a SWOT analysis. Organizational "sacred cows"—those traditions or services that are valued most highly and defended at all costs—should be assessed carefully and objectively. The presence and degree of interdisciplinary collaboration, *esprit de corps* or team spirit, flexibility, perceived power bases, territoriality, perceived commitment to CQI, ability to effectively institute and manage change, and endorsement of risk taking should be noted.

External Assessment

The external assessment of an organization should focus on the existence of continuum-based services within the community and the relationship between the organization and these other providers. Assessment should identify opportunities for the development of coordinated patient services that may expedite patient movement, enhance quality of care delivery, and facilitate longitudinal outcomes measurement through the use of a consistent standard of care. The ability to avoid the duplication of services and enhance the sharing of both technology- and personnel-related resources should be considered.

The organization's participation in ensuring community health should also be assessed during this phase of SWOT analysis. Opportunities for development and implementation of community awareness and health education should be identified as they pertain to the populations identified for OM. Additionally, the organization should evaluate and critically examine their recognition within the community as a center of excellence in the delivery of specific health service products. Consumers of health care, as well as providers and academic centers, should all be considered when assessing organizational reputation within the community. A reputation as a center of excellence also depends on the organization's ability to influence health policy with state and national legislators. Finally, relationships with payers should be examined critically to identify opportunities to market and improve services.

TABLE 2–2

Action Plan Format

Action Issue	Expected Outcomes	Action Steps	Responsible Parties	Expected Completion Date
Action issues identified in the SWOT analysis are listed in this column. Monthly or quarterly status reports should be completed that reflect the project's ongoing status.	Measurable expected outcomes are listed in this column. The outcomes identified should be the product of the defined action steps. Outcomes achievement should reflect the resolution of specified action issues.	Action steps are processes that will be implemented to achieve expected outcomes. The steps should be logically ordered and build upon previous processes.	The names and positions of the responsible parties for each defined action step are listed in this column. These individuals accept accountability for the completion of their assigned processes.	The expected date for the completion of all of the action steps and indicators of the achievement of expected outcomes are listed in this column. The date selected should be realistic but encourage a steady work pace among project managers.

Constructing an Action Plan

Once a thorough SWOT analysis has been conducted, stakeholders should write an action plan that specifies the processes that will be used to improve or further enhance their readiness for implementation of an OM program. During the writing of an action plan, key elements identified in the SWOT analysis are targeted as action issues. Expected outcomes, action steps, and target dates are negotiated. Parties that will be held accountable for completing their assigned action steps are identified. Progress made toward the resolution of action issues should be reported regularly and barriers to progress should be identified along the way. Table 2–2 provides an example of an action plan format that may be used to guide the implementation of OM based on SWOT analysis findings.

COMMANDEERING INSTITUTIONAL CHANGE

As is evident in the OM model (see Figure 1–2), OM evokes change, which fosters movement away from traditional practice. Discomfort during the change process is usually evident. In fact, what should be labeled a "fear of the unknown" is the typical human response to change.

Practice traditions are comfortable, predictable, and not stressful. Many providers reveal their complacency with traditions through statements such as "we've always done it this way"; "that's the way we do things here"; or "our patients are different; that wouldn't work here." However, many of the practices used today by interdisciplinary providers are outdated or not supported by scientific evidence as *best practice*.[1]

A health care provider's response to change commonly reflects an attempt to work toward an acceptance of the "death" of much valued practice traditions and rituals.[2] Interestingly, this acceptance may follow closely the phases of mourning identified by Kubler-Ross[1]:

Stage 1: Denial (e.g., refusal to participate: "This *fad* will pass.")

Stage 2: Anger (e.g., dramatic, often intimidating, strategically-placed threats and outbursts)

Stage 3: Depression (e.g., strong-armed participation; resigned but still coming to work)

Stage 4: Acceptance (e.g., active participation)

Stage 5: Process Zeal (e.g., championing the cause, recruiting others to participate)

Three strategies have been proposed to facilitate change acceptance. The empirical rationale strategy assumes that when a proposed change is in an individual's best interest, acceptance is guaranteed. When effective, this strategy is capable of producing swift, long-lasting change.[3] The use of the empirical rational strategy to produce change in provider practice can be illustrated by the onset of capitated payment plans. Providers paid under capitated agreements are very likely to consider new practices secondary to financial incentives.[1] But, capitation still remains far-off in the future for many providers, making the empirical rationale strategy currently unrealistic in many health centers.

The use of force or power has also been suggested as a mechanism to promote acceptance of a proposed change. The results of forced change are swift, but commitment to the process is minimized.[3] The individual using forceful change tactics must be empowered with the authority to mandate immediate change, rendering this change strategy unrealistic in most health care settings. Forced change destroys collaboration and should be discouraged unless immediate change is necessary to prevent patient harm.[1]

The normative reeducative strategy assumes that sociocultural norms drive the acceptance of change. This strategy suggests that measures should be taken to alter preconceived attitudes and improve knowledge to facilitate the acceptance of a proposed change.[3] This model for change acceptance requires an investment over time to demonstrate results and increase comfort among participants, but when effective, the normative reeducative strategy produces strong group commitment. The use of data from an outcomes measurement initiative facilitates change using the normative reeducative model. A body of data provides

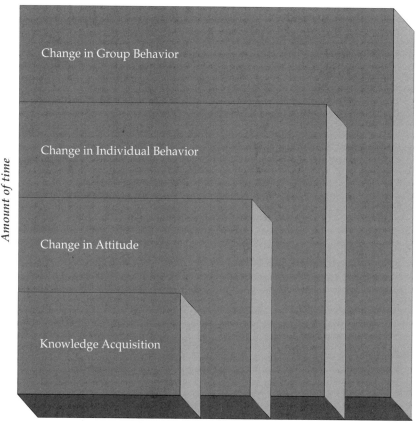

Figure 2–1
Hershey's model—Phases of change: the time investment and degree of difficulty incurred in change achievement. *(Adapted from Hershey P, Blanchard KH, Johnson D:* Management of organizational behavior: utilizing human resources, *ed 8, Englewood Cliffs, NJ, 2001, Prentice Hall. Reprinted with permission from the Center for Leadership Studies, Escondido, Calif.)*

concrete evidence that practice change is necessary and serves as a catalyst for swaying consensus towards practice redesign.[1]

Three important principles support the use of the normative re-educative change strategy. Principle One suggests that change is a time-consuming process.[1] This principle is illustrated in the work of Hershey (Figure 2–1), who identified a hierarchy of change stages within groups: knowledge; attitude; individual; and, lastly, group change. The achievement of the knowledge necessary for a change is relatively easy and requires a minimal time investment; altering attitudes associated with the proposed change takes longer and is more difficult. Changing individual behaviors is even more challenging and labor intensive, and achieving group change may take several years or may never occur.[3]

Principle Two suggests that the strongest negative attitude and reaction to a proposed change typically comes from the group that is most empowered in the system status quo. There is a direct relationship

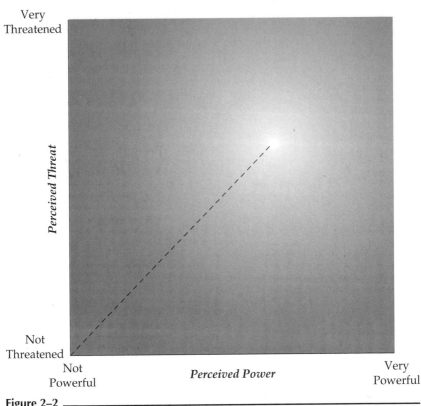

Figure 2–2 ——————————————————————————

Perceived power vs. perceived threat in the use of force strategy. *(Redrawn from Grady GF, Wojner AW: Collaborative practice teams: the infrastructure of outcomes management,* AACN Clinical Issues *7(1):153-158, 1996.)*

between perceived power and the degree of threat produced by practice redesign. As illustrated in Figure 2–2, feelings of threat related to a proposed change rise according to perceived power.[1]

Shared ownership for the change project must be fostered within the *power group* to ensure success. Power group *champions*, or those possessing a collaborative practice philosophy, should be sought out for one-on-one discussion and strategic planning of the change initiative. Once planning is complete, the champions should carry the change message to their peer groups so that it is viewed as a proposal generated and owned by the power group.[1]

Principle Three suggests that the attitudes that individuals possess towards change are normally distributed. Using the normal curve to illustrate this principle (Figure 2–3), most individuals are uncertain about newly proposed practice changes, favoring a "wait and see" attitude, which is a politically safe position among their peer group. However, a few individuals always emerge that are strongly "in favor" or "opposed to" the proposed change.[1]

The tail of the normal curve with those in favor of a change is characterized by the champions, described previously. New processes should be

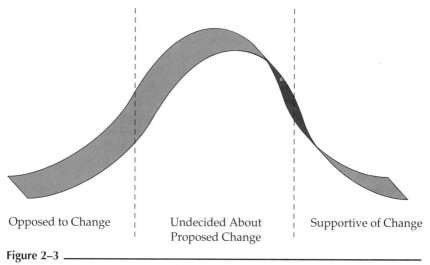

| Opposed to Change | Undecided About Proposed Change | Supportive of Change |

Figure 2–3

Attitudes towards change are normally distributed. *(Redrawn from Luquire R, Huston S, Wojner AW:* Outcomes management: a user's guide, *Houston, Tex, 1994, St Luke's Hospital.)*

implemented within this group; once refined, sharing positive outcomes related to the newly implemented processes generally sways participation among the ranks of the undecided, skewing the shape of the curve[1] (normative reeducative strategy).

It is important to note that it may never be possible to sway a strongly opposed group to participate in a change project; in such cases, the change agent's energy should not be wasted in attempts to encourage this group's participation. As Hershey's model demonstrates, the attainment of 100% group change is nearly impossible to accomplish. Outcomes can still be enhanced without total group support for a change project.[1]

Administrators must understand normal human responses to change and prepare to support their project personnel accordingly. Unfortunately, when this understanding is lacking, administrators may "slam on the brakes" when the first wave of negative reactions comes rolling in, blaming project coordinators for unsuccessful implementation strategies. When change projects are terminated in this sudden fashion, a powerful message is sent to the opposition group: "Flamboyant outbursts and threats successfully halt change." Successful practice redesign will only occur when administrators support their change agents adequately and avoid responses that engender coercive, intimidating, and controlling behaviors in the opposition group.[4]

Furthermore, administrators must sanction outcomes measurement among all patient groups selected for project implementation, regardless of individual provider endorsement and involvement in the OM effort. If OM is to provide CQI that enables the achievement of *best practice* paradigms, all patients within a select diagnostic group admitted to a facility or practice must be included in the project. Using a quasiexperimental design, patient cases that are managed using a new intervention may be enrolled in a study group and compared against cases managed by providers not endorsing the use of the new intervention (i.e., the control group). By sanctioning outcomes measurement across all patient cases, regardless of provider endorsement of a proposed practice change, administrators and caregivers are able to draw causal inferences about potential *best practice* models through the use of analytic research designs.

BUILDING A COLLABORATIVE PRACTICE PHILOSOPHY

The benefits of interdisciplinary collaborative practice to patients and health care providers are well described in the literature. The relationship between interdisciplinary collaboration and patient outcomes is so positive that collaborative planning and delivery of health services is mandated by both the Health Care Finance Administration (HCFA) and the Joint Commission on Accreditation of Health Care Organizations (JCAHO). However, despite the known benefits of collaboration, this practice philosophy is not uniformly valued by all provider disciplines.[1]

Our former provider-driven system proved itself unable to meet consumers' holistic health needs. Now, payer-driven health care appears to be following the same, fruitless path. A shift toward patient-driven care is long overdue, challenging providers to develop collaborative, synergistic work relationships aimed at satisfying the holistic needs of patients and their families.

The *American Heritage Dictionary* defines collaboration as the ability to "work together, especially in a joint intellectual effort."[5] Effective collaboration is born of a bond rich in trust, shared wisdom, and expertise; it occurs when individuals recognize the value of each team member's contribution. Collaborative relationships do not form magically; they result from mutual respect and collegial relations that develop through continuous interaction between team members.[1]

Research findings indicate that collaborative practice is related to a number of positive outcomes. Intensive care unit (ICU) physician and nurse collaboration has been associated with decreased patient mortality.[6-8] Significant decreases in complication incidence and ICU readmission are shown to be related to the provision of health care within a collaborative framework.[6,8] Patients have reported increased levels of care satisfaction when hospitalized in units with an interdisciplinary collaborative practice philosophy.[8] The synergy achieved through collaborative care delivery cannot be duplicated by singular provider efforts.

Within an OM program, collaboration is the key to successful patient outcomes; however, unfortunately the changing health care environment poses so many threats to providers that often competition, instead of collaboration, is the norm. The *American Heritage Dictionary* captures this concept in its second definition for collaboration: "To cooperate treasonably, as with an enemy occupying one's country."[5]

Change theory and the strategies recommended for enhancing acceptance of change should assist providers in moving toward a collaborative practice philosophy. Champions should be identified within each discipline and collaborative relationships should be built. Collaboration is contagious when a spirit of respect and trust is evident. Over time, a collaborative infrastructure is built that supports team growth and *esprit de corps*, facilitating the team's ability to meet and respond to the needs of health care consumers.

| ORGANIZING A SERVICE LINE MODEL

Service line organization was adopted from the business sector as a method of segmenting and organizing the clinical and financial work of health care institutions. Service line organization shifts the focus away from departmental function to an entire episode of care, enabling administrators to view the health care institution as a collection of strategic business units.[4] Box 2–1 provides a list of service lines for a health care organization providing acute care, outpatient clinics, and home care services. To achieve specific objectives that contribute to overall organizational performance, each service line within an organization should be empowered and held accountable.

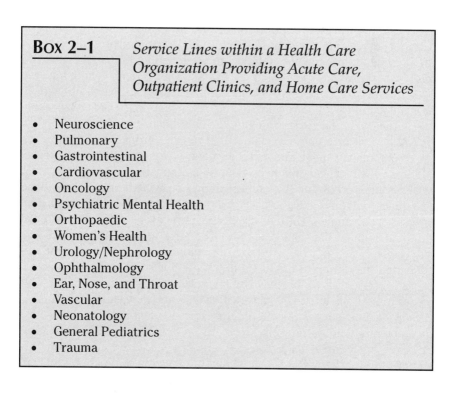

BOX 2–1 *Service Lines within a Health Care Organization Providing Acute Care, Outpatient Clinics, and Home Care Services*

- Neuroscience
- Pulmonary
- Gastrointestinal
- Cardiovascular
- Oncology
- Psychiatric Mental Health
- Orthopaedic
- Women's Health
- Urology/Nephrology
- Ophthalmology
- Ear, Nose, and Throat
- Vascular
- Neonatology
- General Pediatrics
- Trauma

TABLE 2–3

Diagnosis-Related Groups (DRGs) Used to Define A General Pediatric Service Line

DRG	Description
026	Seizure Disorders
033	Concussion
067	Epiglottitis
081	Respiratory Infections and Inflammations
091	Simple Pneumonia and Pleurisy
098	Bronchitis and Asthma
163	Hernia Procedures
164-167	Appendectomy
295	Diabetes
343	Circumcision
417	Septicemia
422	Viral Illness and Fever of Unknown Origin
451	Poisoning and Toxic Effects of Drugs

Distinct boundaries must be drawn between populations within a service line. Often, the use of diagnosis-related groups (DRGs) or international classification of disease (ICD-9) codes are used to define patient populations or procedures that fall into a particular service line. The use of DRGs or ICD-9 codes to define service line boundaries enables the quantification of both financial and clinical outcomes related to a specialty practice area and defines both patients and providers within the service realm. Specific patient populations can be targeted for OM after assessing variables such as population volume, length of stay (LOS), ventilator days, cost, readmission, intensive care unit utilization, mortality, and complication incidence. As an example, DRGs used to define a general pediatric service line are listed in Table 2–3.

Within a service line model, a structure can be organized that allows for direct management and measurement of two distinct, but parallel spheres—the business sphere and the clinical sphere. These spheres must work synergistically for the orchestration of population-based strategic and quality initiatives (Figure 2–4). Complementary business and clinical processes culminate in the delivery of research-based, cutting-edge clinical care and optimal financial outcomes. The separation of the service line into two spheres promotes the use of personnel based on the talent and education they bring to the institution. Therefore business-related activities are conducted by business or financial strategists and clinical outcomes measurement and management is conducted by expert clinicians.[4]

Service line successes should be used in negotiations with third party payers when attempting to increase business for the institution or carve out contracts for the delivery of specialized care. A key assumption underlying OM is that clinical CQI yields optimal patient out-

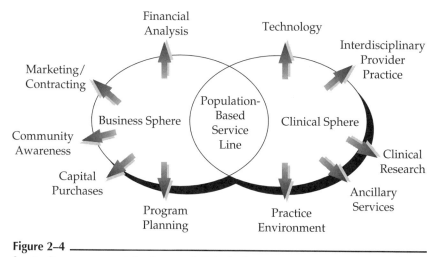

Figure 2–4

Service line management: business and clinical spheres.

comes, which, because of reductions in complications and improved functional status, drives down the cost of health care. The bottom line is that enhanced clinical outcomes drive enhanced financial outcomes, which is appealing to patients, providers, and consumers.

The Business Sphere

The business sphere within a service line is responsible for the development and implementation of a population-based business plan. A service line manager should be appointed to coordinate and communicate business sphere activities with the clinical sphere leadership team. Specific functions within the business sphere include program development, marketing products and provider services, developing and measuring attainment of program goals, and conducting financial analyses of service line performance.[4]

As populations are targeted for OM, service line objectives are developed collaboratively by business and clinical sphere leaders, determining the strategic initiatives that the service line manager uses to develop services and acquire technology for the support and enhancement of care for the population. Opportunities for the marketing of health services for the specified population to providers, the community-at-large, and payers should be identified by the service line manager. As results are measured that confirm optimal patient outcomes, the service line manager incorporates these data with the help of the research team into meaningful marketing material.

Financial reporting is an ongoing business sphere activity. Service line and provider-specific report cards have become a popular way to reflect both performance enhancement and opportunities for improvement graphically within targeted patient populations (see Chapter 7). While financial results are driven by clinical outcomes, financial reporting should be integrated into clinical reports cautiously, because OM is not driven solely by financial incentives.[4]

The Clinical Sphere

The clinical sphere of a service line takes responsibility for initiating the process of OM for a defined population of patients. Once a population has been targeted for OM, collaborative practice teams (CPTs) are organized, consisting of an interdisciplinary group of providers that are involved in producing the care for the selected group of patients. It is within the framework of a population-based CPT that the OM model (see Figure 1–2) is implemented; a key group of individuals forms the backbone for all OM endeavors—creating the database, identifying outcomes, developing and testing interventions, and building a body of scientific evidence in an effort to deliver best practice.

The providers selected to serve on a CPT vary according to the diagnoses to be managed and the scope of the continuum that will be addressed by the team. Box 2–2 provides an example of the health care disciplines represented on a pediatric CPT working with the diagnosis of asthma within the health care institution previously profiled in Box 2–1

Box 2–2   *CPT Membership in a General Pediatric OM Initiative for the Pediatric Asthma Population*

- Pediatrician(s)
- Advanced practice pediatric nurse
- Staff nurse representative (one from each practice setting targeted)
- Pediatric nurse manager
- Pediatric case manager
- Home care coordinator
- Outpatient clinic coordinator
- Pediatric service line manager
- Pulmonologist
- Immunologist
- Emergency services physician
- Pharmacist
- Dietitian
- Respiratory therapist
- Child life coordinator
- Occupational therapist
- Laboratory representative
- Radiology representative
- Community school district representative

---

and Table 2–3. As the OM process branches out across the continuum, other providers may be added to the CPT to reflect care delivery within each specific setting. Ad hoc members should also be considered for inclusion. These members may not need to attend all meetings but should be actively involved when the discussion concerns care delivery in their clinical domain.

The process of OM is challenging; providers attempting to manage more than one population at a time initially will quickly admit defeat. Because OM involves the research process, the need to limit the number of initial populations managed by each CPT is clear; the initiation of more than one research study at a time is simply impossible for a newly formed CPT. Later, as the CPT meets with success and CPT members become more skilled at OM, other populations may be added.

The leadership requirements within a CPT may vary according to the needs of the group. Leadership may rotate annually from discipline to discipline, or an outcomes manager and physician may co-chair the group. Outcomes managers act as clinical researchers and should remain in positions that oversee CPT progress, keeping the group focused and organized.[9] The success of a CPT in reaching population goals is dependent upon the contributions of each team member; the loss of one team member's participation affects the team's performance as a whole.

Table 2–4 lists the developmental stages of a CPT and strategies for building team spirit among members. It is imperative that all activities of the CPT be conducted with a shared leadership philosophy. Peter Drucker's "management by objective (MBO)"[10] model provides a framework for organizing and leading CPTs toward the achievement of clinical CQI. Consistent with the OM model (see Figure 1–2), MBO directs each role and position within a CPT toward the achievement of a defined population objective. Excellence in individual workmanship and shared ownership is stressed, promoting pride among CPT members in team accomplishments.

As mentioned previously, trust and collaborative/collegial relations do not develop overnight among CPT members. Newly formed CPTs should be expected to mature and achieve synergy over time when placed in the hands of a highly skilled change agent. Through continuous interaction, clinical consultation, group problem solving, and the achievement of improved patient outcomes, valued relationships develop, stimulating the interest and enthusiasm to tackle new challenges. Collaboration is the offspring of the recognition and celebration among professionals of their ability to positively affect patient outcomes.

Successes should be credited to teams, not individuals, and should be celebrated and widely publicized throughout the institution. Positive publicity is a powerful stimulus for increased involvement in OM activities across all disciplines. Newly enlisted members should be skillfully nurtured to develop ownership and subsequent shared success in CPT projects.

TABLE 2–4

Developmental Stages of a Collaborative Practice Team (CPT)

Developmental Stage	Task	Characteristics and Accomplishments
Forming	Establishment of member commitment to CPT objectives, structure, and mission	• Sharing of each member's clinical experience, expertise, and interests, as well as educational preparation • Clarification of group mission and objectives • Negotiation of meeting times and place • Agreement on group "norms" or ground rules for participation.
Storming	Acceptance of conflict as a healthy stimulus; agreement to disagree, while staying committed to the group's mission; possible negotiation of objectives and strategies	• Off-line discussion and discontent among subgroups of CPT members • Power plays • Attempts to modify the objectives originally established by the CPT, viewed positively or negatively by varying polarized members • Uncertainty about conflict and disagreement related to the established ground rules and "norms" • Challenge to accept differences in member opinion
Norming	Actively working as a team toward achievement of CPT mission and objectives	• Acceptance and valuing of member differences in opinion • Exploring deeper team commitment • Beginning to use interdisciplinary team members to actively collaborate on management of clinical practice issues
Performing	Establishment of an interdependent relationship among CPT members	• Members possessing initiative to see projects through to completion • Striving toward achievement of clinical practice excellence • Evidence of collaboration and collegiality among team members • *Esprit de corps* • Practice synergy

Adapted from Tuckerman BE: Developmental sequence in small groups, *Psychological Bulletin*, 63:384-399, 1965.

| SUMMARY

The successful development and implementation of an OM program requires a concerted team effort. The process should begin with an objective evaluation of organizational readiness, highlighting opportunities for the enhancement of clinical services for defined patient populations. Interdisciplinary CPTs, which serve as vehicles for the implementation of OM, provide a powerful foundation that not only supports movement toward best practice but also fosters collegial, patient-focused provider relationships. Complemented by the strengths of a business sphere, CPTs work toward improving patient outcomes while promoting market leadership for their organizations.

References

1. Grady GF, Wojner AW: Collaborative practice teams: the infrastructure of outcomes management, *AACN Clinical Issues* 7(1):153-158, 1996.
2. Kubler-Ross E: *On death and dying*, New York, 1969, Macmillan.
3. Lancaster J, Lancaster W: *Concepts for advanced nursing practice: the nurse as a change agent*, St Louis, 1982, Mosby.
4. Wojner AW, Rauch P, Mokracek M: Collaborative ventures in outcomes management: roles and responsibilities in a service line model, *Crit Care Nurs Quart* 19(4):25-41, 1997.
5. American Heritage: *American Heritage Dictionary*, ed 2, Boston, 1992, Houghton Mifflin Company.
6. Baggs JG et al: The association between interdisciplinary collaboration and patient outcomes in a medical intensive care unit, *Heart & Lung* 21:18-24, 1992.
7. Knaus WA et al: An evaluation of outcomes from intensive care in major medical centers, *Ann Intern Med* 104:410-418, 1986.
8. Mitchell PH et al: American Association of Critical-Care Nurses Demonstration Project: profile of excellence in critical care nursing, *Heart & Lung* 18:219-237, 1989.
9. Wojner AW, Kite-Powell D: Outcomes manager: a role for the advanced practice nurse, *Crit Care Nurs Quart* 19(4):16-24, 1997.
10. Drucker P: *Management: tasks, responsibilities and practice*, New York, 1993, Harper Business.

CHAPTER 3

Project Leadership

INTRODUCTION

As an interdisciplinary research initiative, outcomes management (OM) requires strong leadership to facilitate ongoing practice assessment, produce change effectively, and work toward building shared ownership among all collaborative practice team (CPT) members. Project leaders must possess exemplary interpersonal skills, a shared leadership philosophy, and an ability to generate enthusiasm and interest in the OM project. This chapter examines the key leadership roles in an OM program, namely advanced practice nurse (APN) outcomes managers, physician leaders, and service line managers. Essential role components are examined and performance criteria for each role are highlighted.

INTERDISCIPLINARY LEADERSHIP

Successful OM is largely dependent on the quality of the clinical and business leaders in the program. Clinical leaders must have a sound understanding of interdisciplinary research-based practice and must be capable of managing a patient population. Clinical and business leaders must have a manner that respectfully supports and empowers interdisciplinary ownership of the process, thereby constructively maneuvering practice changes for the good of patients and families.[1] These important characteristics describe the overall responsibility of APN outcomes managers, principal physician leaders, and service line managers, which are all continuum-based positions that hold accountability for the research-driven, continuous quality improvement (CQI) of clinical practice for a population of patients.

The APN Outcomes Manager

An APN is a nurse who has completed a minimum of graduate, masters-level nursing education in one of a variety of roles, including clinical nurse specialist (CNS), nurse practitioner (NP), nurse midwife, and nurse anesthetist. While each APN role is valuable, CNSs and NPs are particularly well prepared to assume the role of outcomes manager

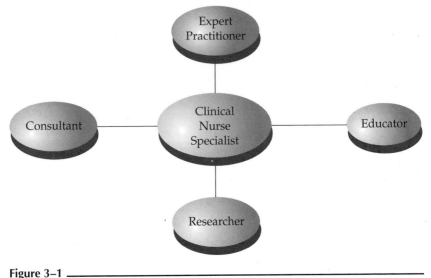

Figure 3–1 _____
The traditional clinical nurse specialist role.

for a population of patients. These highly educated nurses provide the necessary support for an outcomes initiative, acting in concert with a physician leader to implement the OM model within a CPT framework.[2]

The Clinical Nurse Specialist

The CNS role is attained through graduate study in nursing within a clinical specialty, APN licensure, and professional certification. CNSs provide expert care and oversee care delivery to patients within their area of practice specialization. Traditionally, the CNS position encompasses four subroles: Expert practice, education, consultation, and research (Figure 3–1). The success of the CNS has been defined by the individual's ability to integrate these four sub-roles in practice.[3]

Until recently, the CNS role met with mixed reviews from both nursing and hospital administrators. These expert clinicians had often been misused by their employers as project managers and staff development educators, removing these valuable practitioners from the bedside where the talents of an expert practitioner are best used. Today, many CNSs are finally being used in a manner conducive to their education and clinical expertise. Those empowered as outcomes managers have redefined their roles to be driven primarily by clinical inquiry/research and clinical practice; the other subroles of the CNS are reorganized into a hierarchical configuration driven by practice and research (Figure 3–2). This redesigned CNS role provides a powerful basis for affecting patient outcomes through expert nursing practice and research, which has caused a resurgence of the CNS role in both practice settings and academic curricula.[2]

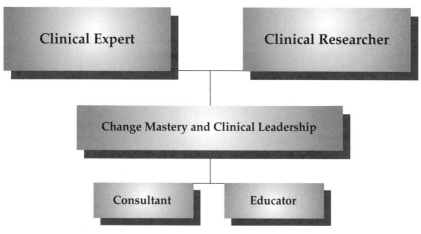

Figure 3–2
Hierarchy of advanced practice nursing roles supporting the outcomes manager position.

Nurse Practitioner

The NP role dates to 1965, when the pediatric nurse practitioner role was developed at the University of Colorado as a mechanism to bridge the gap between child health care needs and the family's ability to access affordable health care. Similar to the CNS role, NP status is attained through graduate nursing education, licensure as an APN, and professional certification.[4]

The NP role differs from the CNS role in that the primary focus has always been provision of care as an expert clinical practitioner, with an emphasis on patient education in health restoration, health maintenance, and illness prevention. Graduate preparation in the NP role provides a foundation in research.[5,6] However, as primarily practice-oriented providers, some NPs, while interested in research, have difficulty integrating a program of clinical inquiry/research into their practice. This difficulty must be overcome through negotiation with practice peers if the NP is to assume a leadership position as an APN outcomes manager for an OM program.[2]

The Outcomes Manager

Educational preparation as an APN provides a sound basis for orchestrating research-based, state-of-the-art, interdisciplinary clinical practice within an OM framework. But other essential professional and personal qualifications for the position of outcomes manager should include[2,7]:

- Hands-on clinical expertise
- Leadership skills
- Change mastery
- Talent as an educator/consultant

- Clinical research experience
- Collaborative practice philosophy
- Perseverance
- Finesse
- Maturity
- Willingness to take appropriate risks

The outcomes manager role differs from that of the nurse case manager, which was described by Zander in 1985 as a second-generation primary nurse.[8] Outcomes managers function as "attending nurses" for populations of patients. These APNs work synergistically with multiple disciplines to optimize patient care delivery and health outcomes. A second difference between outcomes managers and case managers is the relative levels of academic preparation. Outcomes managers must be educated at the masters or doctoral nursing level, because of the research component of the role, while today's nurse case managers vary in their academic preparation—some have earned baccalaureate and/or masters degrees and some have not.[2]

Further distinction can be drawn between the case and outcomes manager roles through an examination of the primary functions that have historically comprised nursing case management, namely utilization review/management, implementation of cost control measures, and discharge planning. The outcomes manager role differs substantially in that it is supported by an APN practice model (see Figure 3–2). Use of APNs to perform utilization review/management and discharge planning is a costly waste of clinical and research talent, substituting low-level tasks such as insurance verification for expert practice assessment, intervention testing, and outcomes measurement. More traditional case management tasks should be managed by team members under the clinical direction of an APN outcomes manager, who provides research-based direction for case-by-case interdisciplinary care across the continuum.[2,7]

Within an acute care setting, outcomes manager positions should be continuum-based, unrestricted by geographic boundaries, and free to move with their population through a variety of settings, including the emergency department, intensive care units, intermediate and general care, surgery, and interventional radiology laboratories.[2] As parts of the postacute continuum are added to the program, outcomes managers should consider enlarging their scope or teaming up with other APNs to meet the needs of their population as they move through rehabilitation centers, physician offices, clinics, subacute facilities, skilled nursing care, and home care settings. This extends the APN outcomes manager's ability to measure longitudinal outcomes and manipulate practice settings to assess the effects on the population's health care experience.

Two primary role domains support the outcomes manager position: Expert clinical practitioner and clinical inquiry/researcher (see Figure 3–2).

EXPERT CLINICAL PRACTITIONER.   Within the clinical domain, outcomes managers act as attending nurses overseeing delivery of interdisciplinary patient care for specific populations. Outcomes managers collaborate and consult with interdisciplinary providers; act as role models in expert nursing practice; troubleshoot complex patient care issues; provide impromptu education for patients, family members, and interdisciplinary staff; and continuously assess the results of clinical interventions from a researcher's perspective (Figure 3–3).[2] Table 3–1 lists performance criteria specific to the clinical realm of the outcomes manager role.

The outcomes manager role requires true hands-on clinical expertise; this is not a role that can be handled by a clinical impostor. Outcomes managers should spend approximately 60% to 70% of their time in clinical practice, working toward the development of relationships with bedside providers that will later facilitate their ability to manipulate the practice environment. Being a role model in expert clinical practice ensures not only credibility but also respect for the outcomes manager. It also makes a strong statement that the OM process supports quality patient care through research-based clinical enhancements.[2,7]

OM is founded on a premise that suggests that high quality clinical care improves patient outcomes, which in turn reduces cost and length of stay (LOS). Outcomes managers, therefore, should be held accountable for the financial outcomes incurred by the quality of clinical practice. Financial accountability is one of the most powerful aspects of the APN outcomes manager position, reinforcing the importance of APN-led OM to the enhancement of institutional financial viability.[2,7]

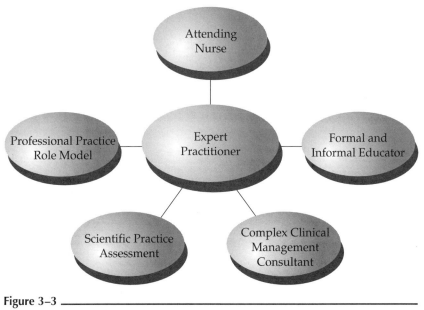

Figure 3–3
The clinical domain of the outcomes manager.

TABLE 3–1

Outcomes Manager Performance Criteria: The Clinical Domain

The role of expert clinical practice—To analyze practice and design interdisciplinary interventions for testing and implementation within an assigned patient population.

Effective (10)	Exceeds Effective (15)	Highly Effective (20)
1. Demonstrates and communicates clinical expertise in an assigned patient population and is a role model in the application of clinical practice standards. 2. Responds to interdisciplinary requests for evaluation and management of complex patients as they move across the continuum. 3. Analyzes factors contributing to variable cost, making recommendations for change in clinical practice to facilitate cost-effective, quality care. 4. Provides informal education to interdisciplinary providers and consumers as indicated by patient outcomes.	1. Supports the development of business and marketing plans for the assigned patient population. 2. Provides formal educational programs to interdisciplinary providers and/or consumers. 3. Practices beyond the boundaries of his/her assigned patient population, as requested, to enhance quality and financial outcomes. 4. Mentors graduate nursing students in the provision of expert, research-based clinical care. 5. Supports the ongoing professional growth of his or her collaborative practice team (CPT).	1. Demonstrates increased efficiency and quality in clinical practice. 2. Affects community wellness through the development and implementation of continuum-based services. 3. Achieves a balance between clinical quality and financial outcomes that positively affects the institution's bottom line. 4. Develops service and divisional policy and procedures as driven by outcomes measurement.

Reprinted with permission from the Health Outcomes Institute, The Woodlands, Texas.

Traditional staff development responsibilities, such as provision of routine inservice educational programs, should not be considered part of the outcomes manager role. Instead, education provided by outcomes managers should reflect research findings for the populations of interest. When findings suggest a need for a new practice standard and additional staff education, outcomes managers should take responsibility for constructing the new standard in concert with other provider disciplines and be actively involved in disseminating staff education. Outcomes managers may also spend a considerable amount of time imparting education to patients and families in their role as attending nurses.[2,7]

TABLE 3–2

Outcomes Manager Performance Criteria in the Research Domain

The role of clinical inquiry and research—To facilitate enrichment of the body of scientific and research-based care, leading to the identification of best practice for the assigned patient population.

Effective (10)	Exceeds Effective (15)	Highly Effective (20)
1. Facilitates development, implementation, and ongoing revision of structured care methodologies, based on scientific evidence. 2. Establishes outcomes measures and methods for data collection. 3. Builds an OM database to describe quality and efficiency of care. 4. Participates in the development of descriptive research. 5. Engages members of the interdisciplinary team in the generation of research questions or hypotheses for study within the population of interest. 6. Shares findings from the OM database with interdisciplinary grassroots providers.	1. Participates as a coinvestigator in the development of research proposals suitable for submission to the internal review board (IRB). 2. Implements well-conducted observational studies related to the assigned population. 3. Implements a research-based change in practice that results in improved patient outcomes. 4. Provides formal education regarding the research process to interdisciplinary providers. 5. Coordinates a service-based journal club that is charged with research utilization for the assigned patient population.	1. Serves as a principal investigator in the development of research proposals. 2. Implements well-conducted, randomized, controlled trials or cohort studies. 3. Serves as an administrator for funded research projects. 4. Submits grant proposals for funding of proposed research studies. 5. Publishes original research in peer-reviewed journals. 6. Mentors inter-disciplinary providers in the process of research proposal development.

Reprinted with permission from the Health Outcomes Institute, The Woodlands, Texas.

CLINICAL INQUIRY/RESEARCHER.   The use of APN outcomes managers fosters an ability to conduct ongoing outcomes research for defined patient populations, enabling changes in clinical practice guided by science. The primary function of the clinical inquiry/research realm of the outcomes manager role is to facilitate interdisciplinary movement toward the discovery and implementation of best practice through the process of outcomes measurement.[2,7] Table 3–2 identifies performance criteria for outcomes managers within the research domain.

Outcomes managers must be familiar with current practice literature, assessing the quality of published research findings, identifying conceptual difficulties in research, and recognizing the implications of interdisciplinary practice and opportunities for the implementation of new research findings. The significant concentration of time spent in the clinical practice domain by outcomes managers enhances their ability to generate clinically significant, interdisciplinary research questions or hypotheses, as well as identify opportunities for intervention development and testing.[2]

Outcomes managers with nursing education at the masters level should enlist the support of a doctorally-prepared research mentor to assist them with building a program of research for their defined patient population.[2] The "ideal" research mentor is a health science researcher with a similar clinical background and interest in the target population who has remained current with the constructs of expert clinical practice. Mentors may come from a variety of disciplines, functioning as nurses, physicians, epidemiologists, or other health science professionals. The degree and need for research mentorship varies according to the experience of the outcomes manager and may lessen over time as research ability develops. Doctorally-educated outcomes managers should function as independent researchers in collaboration with the other disciplines represented on the CPT.

Within the clinical inquiry and research domain, outcomes managers act as consultants and educators regarding the research process, inviting CPT ownership, sharing study results in an easily understandable format, and facilitating involvement of CPT members in the design of interventions for testing toward achievement of best practice. The interdisciplinary team's clinical inquiry endeavors are more likely to be successful when practicing within an institution that values clinical research. By focusing on scientifically-guided clinical improvement, outcomes managers and their interdisciplinary teams are able to steer grassroots providers toward delivery of care that is designed to enhance population outcomes, thereby achieving institutional goals for cost reduction through the prevention of untoward patient experiences.[2]

Physician Leadership for OM

Physician leaders of an OM endeavor must embody specific personal and professional characteristics to be successful as project leaders. Physicians accepting the responsibility of OM leadership should be viewed as advocates for interdisciplinary collaborative practice, bringing to life practice philosophies that value the contributions of providers from a variety of health disciplines. Interest and, if possible, expertise in the research process are essential; physicians who question practice, utilize research findings, and investigate clinical problems and strategies for outcomes enhancement make powerful leaders of an OM initiative.[1]

While financial outcomes should not drive an OM program, they are a direct reflection of one aspect of the quality of the OM initiative. Physicians selected for OM leadership should display an ability to work collaboratively with administrative leaders—specifically the service line manager—toward the achievement of targeted financial outcomes through enhanced clinical performance. A willingness to review cost data objectively and an acceptance of the contribution of clinical practice to institutional financial integrity is mandatory. Physician leaders should assess the readiness of their peer group to review financial data and act as advisors to service line managers to determine the timing and format for financial presentations that will promote success.

Finally, physician leaders of an OM process must be comfortable pushing for changes in clinical practice and possess an ability to inspire strong interest and involvement in the project among their physician peer group. Since outcomes findings may challenge the continued use of valued practice traditions, physician leaders must be savvy change agents, using a variety of strategies that promote interest in proposed practice revisions.

Similar to the APN outcomes manager, the clinical practice and clinical inquiry and research realms drive performance for the physician leader of an OM initiative. Box 3–1 highlights performance criteria for physicians providing OM leadership. Regardless of whether the selected physician leaders are in private practice or serve as institution employees, performance should be critiqued against a set of criteria specific to the needs of the institution on a regular basis. Given the resources allocated by an institution to an OM initiative, this requirement is both realistic and essential.

The Service Line Manager

Service line managers within an OM initiative are concerned with the "business" of population management. Prerequisites for service line leadership include an understanding of overall hospital operations, departmental relationships, and financial and business principles, as well as a commitment to CQI of health care services. Clinical experience is not necessary because of the abundance of clinical resources within the clinical sphere.[1]

The primary responsibility of service line managers is the coordination of a team of individuals to develop and facilitate achievement of service line goals. Team membership for a service line should include representatives from the clinical sphere, including the APN outcomes manager, OM physician leader, and other clinical leaders; as well as representatives from sectors of the business sphere, namely marketing, corporate communications, and finance/accounting. Service line managers use the collective talents of their team to assess, develop, and improve the delivery of institutional services for defined populations, marketing initiatives strategically within and outside the organization to consumers, providers, and payers of health care.[1]

Service line managers must develop strong, collaborative relationships with their clinical counterparts, the OM physician leader and the APN outcomes manager. The service line manager must acknowledge and use the respective clinical and technical expertise of the physician

---

BOX 3–1   *Performance Criteria for Physician Leaders of OM*

Clinical Practitioner
- Acts as a role model in clinical expertise and has a collaborative practice philosophy in the provision of care to the patient population of interest.
- Supports the ongoing professional growth of his or her collaborative practice team (CPT).
- Provides formal and informal education to interdisciplinary providers, consumers, and administrators related to the population of interest.
- Supports the development of business and marketing plans for the assigned patient population.
- Demonstrates increased efficiency and quality in clinical practice.
- Affects community wellness through the development and implementation of continuum-based services.
- Achieves a balance between clinical quality and financial outcomes that positively affects the institution's bottom line.

Clinical Researcher
- Facilitates development, implementation, and ongoing revision of structured care methodologies (SCMs) based on scientific evidence.
- Provides leadership for the development of an OM database to support ongoing study of the assigned population.
- Engages members of the interdisciplinary team in the generation of research questions or hypotheses for study within the population of interest.
- Participates as a principal or mutual investigator of population-centered research initiatives.
- Shares findings from outcomes studies with his or her peer group, facilitating discussions of the effectiveness of current or proposed practice standards.
- Implements research-based changes in practice that result in improved patient outcomes.

Reprinted with permission from the Health Outcomes Institute, The Woodlands, Texas.

---

and outcomes manager to identify new program ventures and opportunities for marketing clinical services. Similarly, the physician and outcomes manager must respect the business savvy of the service line manager, turning over control for capital equipment acquisition, program development, and marketing of their clinical products.[1]

Box 3–2   *Service Line Manager*
Performance Criteria

- Coordinates and leads the service line team.
- Serves as both an internal and external advocate for the service line.
- Leads the process of service-wide goal development.
- Uses resources wisely; demonstrates efficiency, effectiveness, and quality in service-wide initiatives.
- Develops and manages budgeting and demonstrates profitability for service line products.
- Conducts business and financial analyses to support the development and evaluation of initiatives.
- Ensures that regulatory and licensing requirements are met by the institution.
- Keeps abreast of community and national practice standards and emerging technology.
- Develops initiatives that promote the institution and service line as a center of excellence—locally, regionally, and nationally.
- Provides evidence of a patient-first philosophy throughout the service line.
- Effectively represents institution and departmental interests.
- Exhibits a collaborative philosophy in interactions with interdisciplinary providers.

Reprinted with permission from the Health Outcomes Institute, The Woodlands, Texas.

Service line managers are accountable for overall financial and quality performance of the population products within their service lines. Accountability provides the service line manager with the authority to implement service-wide changes across departmental lines (i.e., nursing, medicine, ancillary services) and enhances both internal and external communication regarding service line initiatives. Both clinical and financial criteria may be used to evaluate the effectiveness of a service line manager.[1] Box 3–2 provides an example of role performance criteria used to evaluate service line managers.

MATRIX REPORTING

Within an OM program, both the business and clinical spheres take responsibility for reporting the results of specific population-based initiatives. While duplicate reporting may appear on the surface to be a waste of time and energy, the simultaneous reporting of outcomes increases the visibility of an OM program within an institution, highlighting the synergism of collaborative, complementary processes (Figure 3–4).

Clinical and business sphere reports should follow a consistent format to represent program accomplishments to stakeholders, though differences may exist in report detail depending upon the sphere of interest. For example, a business sphere report may emphasize fiscal accomplishments through a detailed representation of financial analyses, while a clinical sphere report for the same population may highlight specific clinical research findings. Service line managers, physician leaders, and APN outcomes managers should collaborate on the development of each sphere's report, ensuring that both clinical and business outcomes are appropriately represented to stakeholders.

Within the clinical sphere, population outcomes should be reported throughout all provider departments furnishing care to the population of interest. Since providers from each of these disciplines are represented

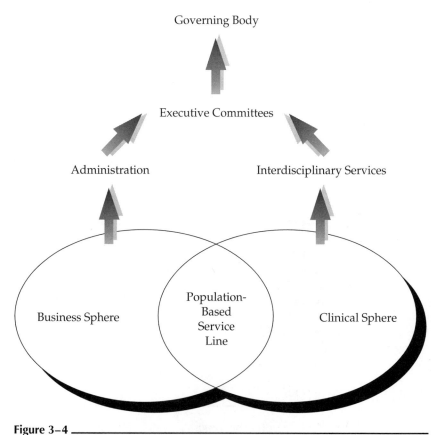

Figure 3–4

Matrix reporting: clinical and business spheres.

on the CPT, each CPT member should be empowered by the outcomes manager and physician leader to present team reports to their clinical practice peer group. Within the business sphere, the service line manager reports program outcomes directly to institutional administrators.

Regardless of the sphere, OM reports should be considered part of an institution's quality program. Matrix reporting ensures communication of quality improvement measures among all levels of the organization, thereby enhancing the facility's ability to understand interdisciplinary collaborative practice measures as the driving force behind clinical CQI. It also inspires pride among members of population-based CPTs and service line teams, who are recognized throughout the institution for their accomplishments in patient outcomes improvement.

| SUMMARY

OM offers leadership opportunities to APNs, physicians, and business leaders within an organization, enabling the construction and refinement of health care services across the continuum of care. Within an OM framework, leaders are challenged to facilitate shared ownership among interdisciplinary team members, promote changes in practice, and create a practice environment that enables grassroots providers to meet the needs of patients and families.

References

1. Wojner AW, Rauch P, Mokracek M: Collaborative ventures in outcomes management, *Crit Care Nurs Quart* 19(4):25-41, 1997.
2. Wojner AW, Kite-Powell D: Outcomes manager: a role for the advanced practice nurse, *Crit Care Nurs Quart* 19(4):16-24, 1997.
3. Hamric AB, Spross JA: *The clinical nurse specialist in theory and practice*, ed 2, Philadelphia, 1989, WB Saunders.
4. Brush BL, Capezuti EA: Point of view—revisiting "a nurse for all setting": the nurse practitioner movement, 1965-1995, *J Am Acad Nurse Pract* 8(1):5-11, 1996.
5. Forbes et al: The clinical nurse specialist and nurse practitioner: core curriculum survey results, *Clinical Nurse Specialist* 4(2):63-66, 1990.
6. Fenton MV, Brykszynski KA: Qualitative distinctions and similarities in the practice of clinical nurse specialist and nurse practitioners, *J Prof Nurs* 9(6):313-326, 1993.
7. Wojner AW: Outcomes management: an interdisciplinary search for best practice, *AACN Clinical Issues* 7(1):133-145, 1996.
8. Zander K: Second generation primary nursing. *J Nurs Admin* 15(3):18-24, 1985.

CHAPTER 4

Outcomes Measurement for Outcomes Management

INTRODUCTION

Success in today's health care environment is dependent on the ability to deliver quality health care services that result in positive outcomes. Regardless of the setting, measuring outcomes is an essential part of continuous quality improvement (CQI) in health care. Future health care systems will be more reliant on outcomes data or "hard evidence" to support new initiatives and reimbursement schedules. Increasingly, systems with outcomes data will drive health care process improvement and practice standardization. Health care organizations that can provide outcomes data verifying best practice at low cost will be in the best position to compete for market share.

Scarce data, combined with increasing demand, has made clinical outcomes information a "hot commodity."[1] It will be years before nationally-linked databases are able to provide reliable, understandable, severity-adjusted data. Without this "ideal" data set, health care providers and organizations must provide accurate information from their own practice settings. Providers must be proactive in using data to verify and document the extent of their practice successes, so they can compare themselves to competitors (e.g., benchmark) and identify areas of inefficient or ineffective practice.

In 1980, Donabedian introduced the "structure, process, and outcome" triad into the quality assurance process.[2] Structure and process monitoring are still alive and well in health care systems; process measurement, in particular, has become an area of expertise among health care providers. Yet few in practice today demonstrate expertise in outcomes measurement, a skill that is paramount to documenting effectiveness.

As defined in Chapter 1, health outcomes are "end results" of specific care processes.[3] Donabedian's work defined outcomes among individual cases as a "change in a patient's current and future health status that can be attributed to antecedent health care."[2] In 1988, Lohr described outcomes in negative terms, as the "five D's: Death, disease, disability, discomfort, and dissatisfaction."[4]

Hegyvary divided the measurement of outcomes into three levels: (1) micro level outcomes (i.e., individual patient results), (2) meso level outcomes (e.g., results of a group of patients or "sample"); and (3) macro level outcomes (e.g., results of a whole population).[5] Hegyvary's work can be applied to case management, outcomes management (OM), and disease management strategies. Micro level outcomes are outcomes of interest within case management; meso level outcomes are outcomes measured by OM processes; macro level outcomes are outcomes of disease management across an entire population. Today, the ability to measure macro level outcomes is limited by several factors, including a lack of consistent indicators and measurement methods across diagnoses, the need for widespread use of informatics systems in all health care settings across the continuum, and the need to bridge databases for longitudinal study.

Regardless of level, the business of outcomes measurement and management has been called both "tricky [and] dangerous,"[6] in that the inference of cause and effect implied by the term "outcome" requires rigorous study controls and precise measurement. Data-driven decision making in health care requires a systematic approach to study design, with an emphasis on cautious data collection, analysis, interpretation, and utilization, which are often lacking. Clearly "practice makes perfect" and builds expertise in the process of outcomes measurement and management.

Outcomes are inherently tied to processes; without understanding of the process, outcomes are useless bits of information. Similarly, processes need outcomes to guide clinical decision making and determination of best practice. Outcomes that have been identified for measurement must then be placed in the context of a research question that focuses on a particular process. Additionally, outcomes should be selected by interdisciplinary practitioners with clinical expertise in the management of the patient population of interest to ensure their relevance and appropriateness. Outcomes measurement in the hands of nonclinicians, unguided by a sound research framework, is not only useless but also potentially dangerous. Box 4–1 lists seven domains of outcomes identified by Lang and Marek[7] that should be considered by clinicians for analysis.

THE CYCLE OF RESEARCH

Research consists of three phases: knowledge generation, dissemination of findings, and utilization of findings in practice. Research generation is the process of increasing knowledge with specific scientific findings. Dissemination is the widespread review and critique of research findings by potential users and fellow researchers. Lastly, utilization is the process of changing practice to reflect the new knowledge generated by research methods. These three steps should be used by health care providers to bring to life best practice.

The past four decades have seen an explosion in health science research generation and dissemination. Best practice has been clearly

> **BOX 4–1**   *The Seven Domains of Outcomes*
>
> Physiologic outcomes
> Psychosocial outcomes
> Functional status
> Knowledge
> Symptom control
> Patient satisfaction
> Cost and resource utilization
>
> From Lang NM, Marek KD: Outcomes that reflect clinical practice, *Patient outcomes research: examining the effectiveness of nursing practice,* Washington, D.C., 1992, U.S. Department of Health and Human Services, NIH Publication No. 93-3411.

delineated in some areas where research replication has revealed consistent findings. However, many questions remain unanswered and much terrain is unexplored. Interestingly, problems with research utilization are prevalent in health care. Health care practitioners across all disciplines tend to be traditionalists. Guided by a belief that their patients are different (e.g., older, sicker), they may hold on tightly to inherited customs and practices, in some instances dating themselves to what was taught when they embarked upon their careers 20 or more years ago. However, the ability to provide effective and efficient health care is best accomplished when the three phases of the research cycle are used in practice.

When beginning the OM process, interdisciplinary providers must first understand the characteristics, risk factors, high-risk subgroups, and untoward outcomes that may exist within the population of interest. This initial step is often overlooked but is critical in determining targets for practice improvement. Once practice targets have been identified, a thorough review of the literature often directs providers toward either research generation or utilization strategies.

PURPOSE: RESEARCH QUESTIONS AND HYPOTHESES

The design of an outcomes study should be guided by a clear and distinct purpose. Purpose provides focus, clarifying methods for study design. The purpose may be stated as a broad statement, for example: "The purpose of this study is to examine the relationship between the social support of patients undergoing bone marrow transplants and their rates of recovery." Often the purpose is presented in the form of a *research question* as follows: "What is the relationship between the level of social support of patients undergoing bone marrow transplants and their rates of recovery?" Questions invite an answer, helping to identify the data that must be collected, and directing methods for data analysis.

A *hypothesis* is a tentative prediction or explanation of the relationship between two or more variables. For example, a research hypothesis could be: "Patients undergoing bone marrow transplants who have greater social support also have shorter periods of recovery." Hypotheses should be based on *theory*, in that theory provides both a foundation and direction for study. Theories selected for study support may derive from a domain such as the physiologic, psychologic, social, or spiritual. The use of theory enables speculation about study findings and the ability to suggest possible explanations for results.

In the hypothesis presented above, a negative relationship is suspected. In other words, as social support increases, the recovery period is expected to be shortened. When a prediction is not supported by study findings, the study limitations, theoretical framework, and related literature must be reevaluated critically to determine alternative explanations for the findings.

| RESEARCH DESIGN

The selection of a research design is tied closely to the questions or hypotheses proposed. While some argue that outcomes research is a new research typology, others insist that dependent variables, or "outcomes," have been in use since the dawn of scientific method. Outcomes research is a term that has gained favor among both researchers and nonresearchers as a method for documenting the effectiveness of health care interventions. Since effectiveness is best measured through the use of scientific method, this book favors defining outcomes research within the realms of epidemiologic research typology. Chapter 5 provides an in-depth examination of outcomes research design.

| DEPENDENT AND INDEPENDENT VARIABLES

After defining the research purpose and generating research questions or hypotheses, the investigators should consider the variables that will need to be measured to answer the study question. The terms *dependent variable* and *independent variable* are used to describe a study's variables of interest. The dependent variable is the outcome under study. Independent variables are conditions or characteristics that may influence the outcome (i.e., dependent) variable.

In nonexperimental research, the independent variable is sometimes referred to as the *predictor variable* or *risk factor*. Using the sample research question (i.e., "What is the relationship between the level of social support of patients undergoing bone marrow transplants and their rates of recovery?"), the rate of recovery is the outcome or dependent variable of interest and the level of social support is the independent variable that may or may not influence the specified outcome.

Variables must be clearly defined and an *operational definition* must be written for each. A review of the literature can guide the development of valid and reliable definitions, as well as point to the methods for measurement of each discreet variable.

For example, rate of recovery requires an agreed-upon definition and methods for measurement; depending upon the scope of the study and the investigators' interests, it can be defined as inpatient length of stay (LOS), self-reported return to recovery time, or results of specific laboratory tests. Investigators need to agree upon a definition and then identify *when, where,* and *how* recovery data will be collected. Similarly, social support also needs to be defined and measured objectively. When possible, the use of standardized instruments with established validity and reliability should be considered for the measurement of variables.

DATA COLLECTION INSTRUMENTS

Choosing the right instruments for data collection is essential to outcomes measurement. Once team members have decided on the outcomes to be measured, the literature must be reviewed for valid and reliable instruments that will be used to measure the variables of interest. While numerous instruments exist for variables such as functional status, quality of life, symptom distress, and patient satisfaction, other data collection tools must be created by the interdisciplinary team to collect additional variables of interest. For example, a study concerned with the dependent variable "skin breakdown in skilled nursing facility residents" could use a standardized instrument to measure and grade the outcome variable, such as the Braden Scale. However, the investigators would need to create an additional data collection tool that would assist them in understanding risk factors for the occurrence of skin breakdown; such a tool might include variables of interest such as prealbumin level and other nutritional indicators, age, type of turning surface, or comorbidities. When data collection tools are created, a review of the literature often points to important variables that may influence the dependent variable.

The selection of standardized instruments for longitudinal measurement of health outcomes should begin with a review of the variables measured by each tool. Using "functional status" as an example, instruments vary greatly in their ability to measure characteristics that relate to overall "functional" performance. Some instruments, such as the Barthal Index, use the narrow definition of functional status as the degree of independence in performing common activities of daily living

(ADLs) such as toileting, dressing, and feeding. The Medical Outcomes Study Short Form 36 Items (MOS SF-36), in contrast, defines functional status in a broad manner, including a variety of performance measures such as physical functioning, role limitations owing to both physical health and emotional problems, bodily pain, social functioning, and mental health.[8] Other considerations for the selection of an instrument should include the tool's psychometric properties (i.e., validity, reliability, responsiveness), the tool's appropriateness for the population of interest, the methods used to develop the tool, the availability of benchmark data, the methods for data collection required by the tool, and the skills and time needed to complete the tool.[9–11]

Differences between health care facilities must be considered when outcomes benchmarking is planned. DesHarnais, McMahon, and Wroblewski identify the following contributors to differences in outcomes[12]:

- Differences in the mix of patient diagnoses
- Differences in patient severity and complexity
- Differences in patient social and financial status
- Differences in patient health behavior

Differences such as these have caused many outcomes investigators to incorporate the use of severity measures into their data collection processes. Instruments that measure disease severity are useful in adjusting for *a priori* risks of poor outcome. Severity scores provide a glimpse at a patient's clinical trajectory, in that changes in severity are closely tied to a number of patient outcomes.[13] The adjustment of outcomes data for severity allows investigators to "compare apples to apples"; it quantifies the degree of physiologic complexity, enabling the comparison of like cases and the identification of high-risk subgroups within the sample that may benefit from a different standard of care. What severity scales do not measure, however, is whether the disease severity reflects the failure to respond to appropriate therapies or whether the severity reflects inappropriate medical management.

Many different severity instruments and computerized indexing systems are available for use in an outcomes measurement program and are discussed in greater detail in Chapter 7. Disease-specific instruments that may be incorporated into the data collection process, such as the National Institutes of Health Stroke Scale Score or the Hunt and Hess Score, provide a valid and reliable mechanism to measure and adjust data. Additionally, most disease-specific instruments can be used for severity measurement at minimal to no cost, as compared to the often hefty price tag associated with computerized severity index systems.

Most computerized severity indexing systems assign a numeric rating to patients based on clinical information abstracted from the medical record that is independent of patient diagnoses. The coded abstract data serves as the primary or sole source of data used to determine disease severity in many of these systems.

The use of this type of severity system has its advantages. Data are available in electronic format and benchmarking with large national and statewide databases is possible, because data elements consistently reflect the information found in the medical record discharge abstract. The disadvantages of using these types of systems primarily involve the quality of the data used to determine severity. The purpose of collecting medical record discharge abstract data is for billing, not research; reliability is questionable and valid data may be missing that can contribute to the determination of severity. Additionally, the timing of adverse occurrences is unclear.[14]

Most health care facilities engaged in the OM process use a variety of instruments for data collection. Data obtained from these instruments are funneled into outcomes data repositories (ODRs), which are used to study populations of interest. ODRs are archives of patient information, including demographics, important characteristics and comorbidities, laboratory values or other test results, process variances, and, of course, a variety of outcomes (see Chapter 7). The data categories identified in Phase I of the OM model provide an organizational framework for development of an ODR (see Figure 1–2). Ideally, in the future, standard data sets with uniform definitions and collection methods will be established across a wide variety of diagnoses, providing a sound foundation for the benchmarking of results and expedient determination of best practice.

Data Collection Procedures

Once instruments have been identified and/or created, data collection procedures must be determined. Specifically, who will collect the data? Will one person collect all the data, or will various team members collect data that is specific to their area of expertise? For example, the validity and reliability of data may be enhanced when the interdisciplinary team's dietitian is used as the sole collector of nutritional data. The number of data collectors should be kept to an absolute minimum; in programs where all staff members that interact with a patient are charged with data collection, the reliability and validity of findings are questionable. Additionally, routine reliability checks should be conducted at least monthly to ensure that responsible and accurate data collection methods are in place.

The interval that will be used for data collection must also be considered. Investigators need to determine if data will be collected daily, or at specific treatment milestones or intervals that can be accepted as a standard for the patient population. Most commonly, a decision is made to collect data once the medical record has been closed after discharge. Waiting until the end of the patient stay may pose problems, however, because of lost data elements (i.e., missing information). Unfortunately, "If it's not written in the chart—did it or did it not occur?" becomes a question that cannot be answered with great accuracy. Data integrity is greatly increased when data collection methods are used concurrently with patient outcomes.

Data Entry

Before statistical methods are applied to analyze the data, each variable must be formatted in a quantitative manner. All data must be assigned a numerical code if it is not a naturally occurring numerical variable, such as age, LOS, or number of ventilator days. Variables such as gender, race, and the presence or absence of a nosocomial infection require a method of coding and number assignment. Box 4–2 provides an example of numerical codes applied to a list of racial classification variables.

Coding processes should remain consistent throughout a database. Variables that are entered as "present" or "absent" in the cohort should be assigned numbers consistently; for example, an assignment of "1" would always represent the variable being present, while the assignment of "0" would always represent the variable being absent. A method for entering missing data elements must also be determined and adhered to consistently. Most statistical programs allow for a code assignment within a field that designates data as "missing."

A code book or data diary should be maintained after the data fields have been created for each discrete data element. Most statistical programs have commands that allow for the creation of a code book after the data fields are created. The code book should be maintained and used as a reference by data entry personnel. Table 4–1 provides an example of variables from a statistical software code book.

Data entry can be labor intensive work. Identifying the amount of data that will be entered and the skill level necessary for data entry personnel is important. Complicating the process is the demanding pace and quick turnaround times required to bring about data-driven change in clinical practice. Personnel assigned this role must be well trained in data entry methods and processes for ensuring reliability of their work. Since data entry can be a tedious and boring task, it is crucial to provide appropriate break times to lessen the monotony of the work.

Computer data entry may also be facilitated through the use of "bubble sheets" developed for data collection. A number of computer programs are available for use in the development and scanning of tools to facilitate data entry. Typically a batch scanner or a flatbed scanner is

---

BOX 4–2   *Numerical Coding of Racial Classification*

Caucasian	1
African American	2
Hispanic/Latino	3
Asian	4
Native American	5
Other	6

TABLE 4–1

Statistical Software Code Book Variables

List of Variables in Working File:

Variable Name	Position in Field
GENDER - Respondent's Gender	1
Print Format: F1	
Write Format: F8.2	
Missing Values: 9	
Value Label	
1 Male	
2 Female	
RACE - Respondent's Racial Class	2
Print Format: F1	
Write Format: F8.2	
Value Label	
1 Caucasian	
2 African American	
3 Hispanic/Latino	
4 Asian	
5 Native American	
6 Other	

used to enter the data into a computer program. The data are stored in program files and can subsequently be imported into spreadsheets or statistical software for analysis. Positions supporting the use of this type of equipment include personnel for form development and the scanning and cleaning of data. Although additional hardware and software are needed to support this type of data entry, the use of these systems may result in monetary savings through reduced man-hours.

As the use of clinical information systems increases in health care facilities, mechanisms for pulling data from archived or real-time patient files are becoming more accessible. Data fields from any number of documentation forms, or direct online sources, may be copied into ODRs. It is essential, however, that the validity and reliability of data be assessed and maintained when any number of people throughout a health care facility contribute to the total volume of data logged within a medical record, which will subsequently be loaded into an outcomes database. The larger and more complex the data collection process, the more difficult quality control maintenance becomes. The reliability of recorded data elements and the data entry process should be assessed at least monthly to ensure the accuracy and usability of findings.

Of equal importance is the development of security measures and the creation of backup files. Patient confidentiality is paramount and must be maintained scrupulously, especially when patient names, hospital numbers, or social security numbers are used for longitudinal tracking or matching of data. File access should require the use of a password system. Backup files and code books should be kept in a locked cabinet within a secure office. Additionally, backup files should be appended each time additional data is added to the repository. Backup files can be created, for example, by using diskettes, tape drives, or Zip drives.

Lastly, the results of the outcomes measurement process are reflective of both the rigor of study design and the caliber of the data. Poor data collection and management methods yield results that are likely to be invalid and unreliable. Interdisciplinary health care providers reluctant to change practice because of poor data quality are wise! The bottom line: "Garbage in equals garbage out."

STATISTICAL ANALYSES

Statistical tests are applied to outcomes data to answer the research questions identified by the investigators at the onset of the study. Research questions, then, prescribe the types of statistical analyses that will be used once data has been collected and entered into a computer software program. Because specific statistical tests require certain types of data, the variables collected must be carefully defined to meet the requirements necessary for analysis.

Levels of Data

There are four levels of data. An understanding of data leveling is necessary to correctly identify variables for study and the appropriate statistical analyses that may be used to answer research questions.[15-17] *Nominal data* consists of named categories that lack a defined order.[15-17] Marital status is an example of a nominal variable because the categories of "single," "married," divorced," and "widowed" can be placed in an arbitrary order because no one category is capable of a higher or lower rank. Similarly, racial classification, the presence of a comorbid condition such as diabetes mellitus or atrial fibrillation, or an untoward outcome such as incontinence all represent nominal level variables.

Ordinal data consists of ordered or ranked variables, where differences between categories cannot be considered equal.[16] Many of the variables encountered in health care are ordinal level variables. For example, questionnaires consisting of questions with response choices of "strongly agree," "agree," "disagree," or "strongly disagree" are made up of ordinal variables. Answers may be ranked from best to worst, but there is no mathematically precise measurable difference between each answer. Some ordinal scales may substitute numbers for words, for example, pain may be rated on a scale of 0 (no pain) to 10 (worst possible pain). However, even though numbers are substituted for words, the difference between the values cannot be considered equal.

Interval data consists of variables that have equal distances between values, but the zero point is arbitrary.[15-17] Temperature in degrees Fahrenheit is an example of interval level data. There are equal distances between degrees on the Fahrenheit thermometer, but the zero point has been placed arbitrarily and is not a "true" zero. A *ratio variable* has equal distances between values and has a meaningful zero point. Most laboratory test values are ratio variables, as are height and weight. To illustrate the properties of a ratio level variable, consider that a person weighing 200 pounds is twice as heavy as someone who weighs 100 pounds—even when pounds are converted to kilograms, the ratio stays the same, 2:1.

The level of data determines the statistical methods that may be used for analysis. *Nonparametric tests* are used for the analysis of nominal level data. Nonparametric tests are distribution free; in other words, no assumption is made about the distribution of the variable of interest in the population.[16]

Parametric tests assume that the variable measured in a sample is normally distributed in the population in which findings will be generalized.[16] Originally, fundamentalist statisticians advocated the use of the more powerful and flexible parametric statistical tests on only interval or ratio level data.[18] Today, the use of parametric measures has been extended to ordinal level data, since rarely are relationships between variables distorted by these methods.[16] It is essential, however, to remain alert to the possibility of inaccurate findings when ordinal data are used in parametric analyses.

Descriptive Statistics

Descriptive statistics are used to organize and summarize data. These statistical methods include *measures of central tendency,* which are used to denote a "typical" score for variables within the database, and *dispersion measures,* which describe how scores vary.[15–17] Measures of central tendency include the *mean, median,* and *mode,* each of which describes the middle point among a group of scores.

The mean is simply the mathematical average of a group of scores. Extremes in scores may greatly distort the mean, especially when the sample is small.[16] For example, Table 4–2 presents LOS data for 10 patients admitted to a hospital with a diagnosis of congestive heart failure (CHF). Note the large calculated mean for the sample; the mean inaccurately reflects what most patients experience as a hospital LOS due to the one patient with an extremely long hospitalization. In cases such as this, other measures of central tendency may more accurately reflect reality.

The median is the middle point in a set of ranked scores.[16] To determine the median, scores are listed in order from lowest to highest. The score in the middle represents the median for the group. When an even number of scores is listed, the two middle scores are averaged to determine the median. Table 4–2 also provides the median LOS for the 10 patients with CHF. Note that in this sample, the median is a better indicator of the typical CHF LOS.

The mode is used less often than the mean or median to determine central tendency. However, when nominal level data are used, mode is

TABLE 4–2

Descriptive Length of Stay (LOS) Data

Patient Number	Actual LOS (Hospital Days)	Descriptive Data
1	5	*Sample Mean*
2	4	7 Days
3	4	*Standard Deviation*
4	3	9.56 Days
5	5	*Range*
6	4	2-34 (32 days)
7	6	*Sample Median*
8	34	4 Days
9	3	*Sample Mode*
10	2	4 Days

the only measure that may be applied to determine centrality. The mode is the most common finding among a group, or in the case of numerical data, the most frequently occurring score.[16] See Table 4–2.

Dispersion measures describe how scores within a data set vary.[15–17] *Range* and *standard deviation* are two measures of dispersion that are frequently used to describe data. Range reflects the difference between the highest and lowest scores in the data set. Note the range reported for the CHF LOS data in Table 4–2.

Standard deviation reflects the average variability of scores from the mean score[16] and should always be reported whenever the mean is used as a measure of central tendency. Table 4–3 lists the steps in the calculation of standard deviation from the mean LOS for the sample of 10 patients with CHF. Statistical calculators and software programs are best used to calculate standard deviation, since large samples can make the process labor intensive. Note that the standard deviation from the mean LOS in Table 4–2 is quite large, which is a result of the extreme difference in the one LOS that distorts the mean. By calculating and displaying standard deviation with mean scores, errors in the determination of the typical middle score for a group are easily avoided.

A number of methods may be selected to graphically illustrate descriptive statistics. Figure 4–1 provides an example of a *histogram* used to display the CHF LOS data set from Table 4–2. Histograms, which are commonly used, are bar graphs that display interval or ratio level data.[16] All the bars in a histogram are the same width, denoting equal distance between each variable. A *frequency polygon,* which is created by a line connecting the midpoints of the bars of a histogram, may also be used to present interval or ratio level data[16] (Figure 4–2).

Figure 4–3 illustrates the use of a bar graph to display categorical data. When using a bar graph to display nominal level data, the data

TABLE 4–3

Steps in Calculation of Standard Deviation

LOS (x)	x^2
5	25
4	16
4	16
3	9
5	25
4	16
6	36
34	1156
3	9
2	4
Sum of x = 70	Sum of x^2 = 1312

Step One	Step Two	Step Three	Step Four
$1312 - \dfrac{(70)^2}{n^*}$	$1312 - 490 = 822$	$\dfrac{822}{n-1}$ or $\dfrac{822}{9} = 91.333$	$\sqrt{91.333} = \textbf{9.56}$

Standard Deviation = 9.56

Note: Congestive heart failure length of stay data is taken from Table 4–2.
* n = sample size (i.e., 10)

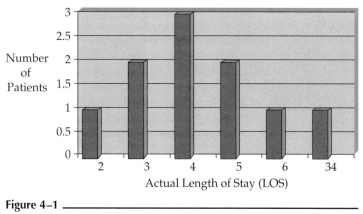

Figure 4–1
Histogram of congestive heart failure length of stay data; $n = 10$.

may be presented in whatever order is deemed reasonable; when bar graphs are used to display ordinal level data, the bars should be arranged from lowest ordinal rank to highest. Bars may be illustrated either vertically or horizontally to display data. *A Pareto chart* is a bar chart that is presented in descending order[15–17] (Figure 4–4).

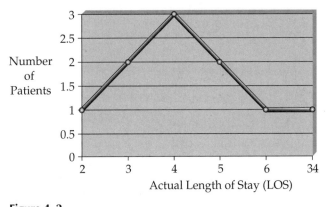

Figure 4–2
Frequency polygon of congestive heart failure length of stay data;
$n = 10$.

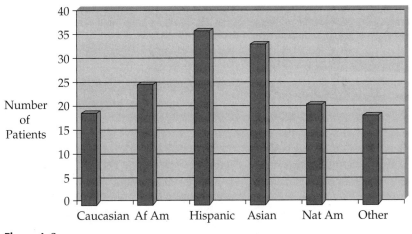

Figure 4–3
Bar graph displaying nominal data; *Af Am* = African American; *Nat Am* = Native American.

Frequency distributions are commonly used to provide a summary of the data set in tabular format.[16] As illustrated in Table 4–4, frequency distributions list all scores for the CHF LOS data from Table 4–2 in ranked order from lowest to highest and present the number of subjects with like scores within the sample.

Correlational tests are used to determine the relationships between variables. Correlation is a measure of the strength of a relationship, but it is important to note that the presence of a relationship does not imply "cause and effect" or "agreement." In other words, a significant relationship between two variables does not guarantee that one variable

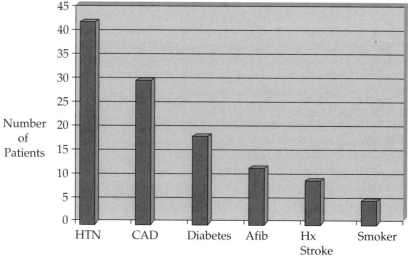

Figure 4–4
Pareto bar graph; *HTN* = Hypertension; *CAD* = Coronary artery disease; *Afib* = Atrial fibrillation; *HX* = History.

TABLE 4–4

Frequency Distribution Table for Congestive Heart Failure Length of Stay (LOS) Data

LOS Score (*n* = 10)	*f*	*Relative f %*	*Cumulative %*
2	1	10	10
3	2	20	30
4	3	30	60
5	2	20	80
6	1	10	90
34	1	10	100
Totals	**10**	**100%**	

Note: *f* = Frequency; *n* = sample size.

caused a change in the other variable, or that the values associated with two variables are identical.[15–17]

The *correlation coefficient 'r'* is used to express the mathematical relationship between variables; *r* may range from −1 to +1, where −1 indicates a perfect negative correlation, 0 represents no correlation, and +1 represents a perfect positive correlation. Rarely are variables perfectly correlated. The direction of a relationship, positive or negative, does not affect the strength of the correlation; a correlation of -0.96 is just as strong as one of $+0.96$.[15-17] Table 4–5 defines the strength of a relationship by *r* value.

In correlation analyses, all variables are assumed to be normally distributed.[16] An example of a correlational test is the Pearson Product Moment Correlation, which requires the use of interval or ratio level data.

Regression analyses are also tests of relationship, but regression tests are used to explain or predict changes in the dependent variable based on findings in one or more predictor or independent variable.[16] *Multiple regression* requires that the dependent variable be continuous, while the independent variables may be continuous or categorical. *Logistic regression* requires a categorical dependent variable, while independent variables may be either continuous or categorical.[15-17]

Inferential Statistics

Inferential statistics are used at higher levels of inquiry to test hypotheses.[16] Hypothesis testing involves the measurement of differences among variables about which the investigator has made an educated guess. Hypotheses are generated when aspects about the phenomenon of interest are known and cited in the literature, forming a theoretic basis for the proposed relationship. Through hypothesis testing, inferential statistical analyses provide a mechanism to generalize or infer findings from a sample to the population.

The term *statistical significance* is used to denote the probability that statistical findings are just a matter of chance.[16] Researchers determine whether results are statistically significant or whether results are from chance alone, using this to determine whether their findings have supported or rejected the hypothesis. Usually the threshold of statistical significance is set at 0.05, which indicates that the probability of results occurring by chance alone is 5 out of 100. Similarly, a threshold of statistical significance of 0.01 indicates that the probability that the results are due to chance is 1 out of 100. The *'p' value* denotes the *probability,* which is used to determine statistical significance.

TABLE 4–5
Degree of Correlation by r *Value*

r Value	Degree of Correlation
0.00-0.25	Very low, if any
0.26-0.49	Low
0.50-0.69	Moderate
0.70-0.89	High
0.90-1.00	Very high

Note: *r* = Statistical value denoting the degree of correlation between variables.

Errors may occur in determining whether a hypothesis has been supported or rejected. The *null hypothesis* proposes that a statistically significant difference or relationship between variables does not exist. A *Type I error* occurs when statistical findings are produced by chance, but the null hypothesis is rejected. In other words, the researchers accept that a statistically significant difference exists between variables, when in reality it does not, and findings were produced by chance. The probability of making a Type I error is termed *alpha (α)*. Type I errors are reduced by lowering the probability level to reduce the risk of findings that are produced by chance.[16]

Type II errors occur when the null hypothesis is accepted, when in reality it should have been rejected. In other words, statistical significance truly exists, but by chance it was not measured in this sample. The risk of making a Type II error may be reduced by increasing the probability level, increasing the sample size, decreasing sources of extraneous variation, and increasing *effect size,* or the amount of effect contributed by the independent variable on the dependent variable.[16]

Power is a term used to describe the likelihood of a test to find a truly significant result, or the opposite of a Type II error.[16] Cohen's (1977) text on power analysis[19] is considered the definitive source for determining sample size. The Cohen approach consists of using effect size, the significance level set by the researcher, and desired power as the three essential elements that should be used to determine sample size. A power of 0.80 is considered "good" and translates to a probability of 0.80 that the null hypothesis will be rejected when it is truly false.[16] Most statistical texts include Cohen's charts, which are highly regarded by scientists for determination of sample size.

Table 4–6 lists criteria for a variety of inferential statistical tests, including the type of analysis provided, type of data required, and assumptions.

THE FINE LINE: "RESEARCH" OR "QUALITY IMPROVEMENT" PROJECT?

Within each health care facility embarking on outcomes measurement, a decision must be made as to whether the project will be classified as "research" or "quality improvement." To assist in making this decision, it is important to relate the aims of the project to the rights and responsibilities of patients and health care facilities.

Patients have the following rights:

- Receipt of information and involvement in health care decision making
- A competent level of care and treatment
- Effectiveness of proposed interventions
- Protection from undue risks

TABLE 4–6

Inferential Statistical Tests

Test	Type of Analysis	Level of Data Required	Assumptions
Chi-Square x^2	Difference Example: *"Is there a difference in the number of children readmitted to the emergency department with exacerbation of asthma from housing complex 'A' vs. housing complex 'B'?"*	Nominal Data are organized into a contingency table; it is determined whether each row variable is independent of or contingent upon the column variables.	1. There is an adequate sample size. 2. Frequency data are available. 3. Measures are independent of each other. 4. There is a theoretic basis supporting the categorization of variables.
Student's *t*-Test	Differences between group means Example: *"Is LOS different for stroke patients with dysphagia, as compared to stroke patients with normal swallow function?"*	Independent variable is nominal; two groups must be available for comparison. Dependent variable is interval or ratio level (ordinal).	1. Dependent measures are interval or ratio level data. 2. Each subject contributes one score to a group's score distribution. 3. The dependent variable is normally distributed. 4. Variances in both groups are similar.
Analysis of Variance (ANOVA) (Multiple Analysis of Variance [MANOVA]—Analysis of more than one dependent variable)	Differences among group means Example (ANOVA): *"Is there a difference in the number of emboli detected by transcranial doppler, by type of cardiopulmonary bypass machine?"*	The independent variable(s) with more than one level are nominal. The dependent variable is interval or ratio level.	Same as those listed for the student's *t*-test.

Note: Commonly used inferential statistical tests.

BOX 4–3   *Guidelines for Differentiating Quality Improvement Efforts from Research*

Classifying the project as "research" should be considered if the answer is "yes" to one or more of the following questions:

- Are subjects placed at any risk for their participation in the project?
- Is the project intended to build scientific knowledge about the phenomena of interest?
- Is a new therapy or practice being compared to an existing standard of care to determine best practice?
- Are the technologies, practices, or interventions planned for implementation different from the currently recognized standard of care for the population of interest?
- Does patient involvement in the project alter care delivery relationships with interdisciplinary providers?

Classifying the project as "quality improvement" should be considered if the answer is "yes" to one or more of the following questions:

- Does the project involve a change in therapy or technology that is considered an extension of the recognized standard of care for the population of interest?
- Is the aim of the project to measure consumer or provider satisfaction in relation to an existing standard of care?
- Does the project involve a data collection instrument that is regularly used in practice for the population(s) of interest?
- Is data collection intended to confirm the use of a specific standard of care already in place for the population of interest?

Modified from: Thurston NE, Watson LA, Reimer MA: Research or quality improvement: making the decision, *JONA* 23(7-8):46-49, 1993.

Today's emphasis on consumer rights in health care has fostered active patient involvement in health care research. Examples include studies of quality of life, consumer satisfaction, and functional status, which are commonly incorporated into care. When asked to participate in research, additional patient rights should include:

- Receipt of information about the purpose of the research and the extent of participation
- Knowledge of potential risks and benefits
- An ability to determine willingness to participate without adversely affecting care delivery

- An ability to withdraw from the project at any time
- A guarantee of confidentiality or anonymity when results are reported

The responsibilities of a health care institution include the provision of safe, effective care by competent providers. Health care institutions must utilize CQI, staff education, and research efforts that aid in the ongoing evaluation of care processes toward the determination of best provider practices. Inclusion of a program of outcomes measurement and management is well suited to support these initiatives.

Box 4–3 provides a set of guidelines to assist providers and health care administrators in differentiating quality improvement efforts from research.[20] Additional considerations for project classification relate to the ability to publish or formally present findings publicly. When presentation or publication of results is desired, a classification as research with approval from an internal review board (IRB) is recommended. Expedited review by an IRB may be negotiated when the project is using accepted national standards of care. Full IRB critique and approval mechanisms should be applied when the standard of care varies from national standards.

| SUMMARY

The measurement of outcomes involves systematic, quantitative observation procedures and should stem from research-based processes. The results generated from outcomes measurement efforts may be used for benchmarking, as measures of CQI initiatives, and as evidence of a program of research generation or utilization.

To be most effective, outcomes measurement and management should be integrated into routine care processes. Redundancy in data generation and collection methods must be prevented; overburdening bedside providers with OM processes reduces their ability to both provide care and manage patient outcomes. Systems should be implemented to support the development and scoring of instruments, data aggregation, and provision of feedback to interdisciplinary grassroots providers in a time-efficient manner.[11] Similarly, interdisciplinary providers should be encouraged to question practice and develop innovative proposals to test new practice methods.

References

1. Kirk R: *Managing outcomes, process and cost in a managed care environment,* 1997, Gaithersburg, Md, 1997, Aspen.
2. Donabedian A: *Explorations in quality assessment and monitoring, Volume I: the definition of quality and approaches to its assessment,* Ann Arbor, Mich, 1980, Health Administration Press.

3. Davies AR et al: Outcomes assessment in clinical settings: a consensus statement on principles and best practices in project management, *Jt Comm J Qual Improv* 20:6-16, 1994.

4. Lohr KN: Outcome measurement: concepts and questions, *Inquiry* 25(1):37, 1988.

5. Hegyvary ST: Outcomes research: integrating nursing practice into the worldview, *NCNR Invitational Conference Proceedings,* Washington, DC, 1992, US Department of Health and Human Services.

6. Greenfield S: Health outcomes research and its interfaces with medical decision making, *Medical Decision Making* 11(4):S19-21, 1991.

7. Lang NM, Marek KD: Outcomes that reflect clinical practice, *Patient outcomes research: examining the effectiveness of nursing practice*, Washington, DC, 1992, US Department of Health and Human Services, NIH Publication No. 93-3411.

8. Ware JE: *SF-36 health survey manual and interpretation guide*, Boston, 1993, New England Medical Center.

9. Deyo RA, Carter WB: Strategies for improving and expanding the application of health status measures in clinical settings: a researcher-developer viewpoint, *Medical Care* 30:MS176-181, 1992.

10. Strickland OL: Measures and instruments, *Patient outcomes research: examining the effectiveness of nursing practice*, Washington, DC, 1992, US Department of Health and Human Services, NIH Publication No. 93-3411.

11. Titler MG, Reiter RC. Outcomes measurement in clinical practice, *MEDSURG Nursing* 3(5):395-420, 1994.

12. DesHarnais S, McMahon Jr. LF, Wroblewski R: Measuring outcomes of hospital care using multiple risk-adjusted indexes, *Health Services Research* 26(4):425-445, 1991.

13. Iezzoni LI et al: The utility of severity of illness information in assessing the quality of hospital care: the role of the clinical trajectory, *Medical Care* 30(5):428-444, 1992.

14. Hopkins DSP, Carroll RJ: Severity adjustment models for CPI. In Hopkins DSP, Carroll RJ, eds: *Clinical practice improvement: a new technology for developing cost-effective quality health care,* New York, 1994, Faulkner & Gray.

15. Norman G, Streiner D: *Biostatistics: the bare essentials*, St Louis, 1994, Mosby.

16. Munro BH, Page EB: *Statistical methods for health care research*, ed 2, Philadelphia, 1993, JB Lippincott.

17. Glaser A: *High-yield biostatistics*, Media, Pa, 1995, Williams & Wilkins.

18. Stevens SS: Mathematics, measurements and psychophysics. In Stevens SS, ed: *Handbook of experimental psychology*, New York, 1951, John Wiley & Sons.

19. Cohen J: *Statistical power analysis for the behavioral sciences*, New York, 1977 (revised edition), Academic Press.

20. Thurston NE, Watson LA, Reimer MA: Research or quality improvement? Making the decision, *JONA* 23(7-8):46-49, July/August 1993.

PART II

Project Implementation

Driving Change to Improve Outcomes

CHAPTER 5

Outcomes Research Methodology

INTRODUCTION

Outcomes research (OR) is a systematic search for knowledge about the end-results of health care processes. OR has its roots in scientific method, the most sophisticated mechanism known to improve knowledge about phenomena of interest. The power of OR lies in the accumulation of scientific evidence, which supports the identification of best provider practices.

OR blends scientific reasoning with evaluative techniques, resulting in a process that, while fallible, generates knowledge more reliably than provider traditions or experience. As demands for provider utilization of best practice increases, health science practitioners will need to embrace scientific method as part of their daily practice routine.

SCIENTIFIC METHOD

Scientific method is a systematic approach to problem solving and knowledge generation that requires the use of disciplined procedures to limit errors and ensure accurate interpretation of findings. Scientists assume that all phenomena have an antecedent, or preceding cause. Scientists, then, are determinists, who seek to achieve an understanding of causality. However, achievement of absolute certainty through the use of scientific method is unfeasible because of the very real possibility of multiple causation. Because of this, the replication of research findings is essential to the generation of scientific knowledge. Replication increases confidence in reported research findings.[1,2]

The goal of scientific research is the achievement of a level of understanding about phenomena of interest that enables the generalization of study findings among other cohorts. Objective, or empirical, evidence is collected through carefully designed methods of observation.[1] Research tools with established validity and reliability or electronic instrumentation are often incorporated into study procedures to enhance the investigator's ability to observe and understand phenomena objectively.

Scientific studies are designed with controls to ensure that researcher biases, as well as effects produced by variables not directly under study, are minimized. In this way, findings that are grounded in reality are more likely to be made evident. However, the complexity of some phenomena may challenge identification and control of all confounding variables. The bottom line is that flaws may be identified in even the best research studies, yet scientific method remains the best procedure available to increase knowledge.

Varying research designs may be selected to outline the strategies that will be used to study phenomena of interest. The selection of a research strategy requires much consideration by the investigator; the research design drives the ability and methods used to measure specific variables of interest, as well as the integrity of study findings. The following questions should be answered by investigators as they contemplate a research design:

- Will an intervention be tested?
- Will a comparison group be used?
- What control measures will be necessary to reduce bias and limit the effects of confounding variables?
- Over what period of time will data be collected?
- What limitations exist within the research setting that may challenge the endeavor?
- What issues surrounding consent are likely to arise?[2–4]

Careful consideration of design selection should be undertaken prior to beginning the research process to improve the power of study findings and their usefulness in practice.

| QUANTITATIVE RESEARCH DESIGNS

Quantitative research methods are concerned with the carefully controlled, systematic collection of numerical data and the statistical analysis of the information collected. Quantitative research emphasizes deductive reasoning, the rules of logic, and measurable attributes of the human experience. Characteristics of quantitative research are listed in Box 5–1. A number of designs fall into the category of quantitative research, namely descriptive, case-control, cohort studies, and experiments.

Descriptive Design
Descriptive design is a research strategy for observing and describing a situation in an undisturbed, naturally occurring setting. The characteristics that define descriptive research include a lack of randomization, usually due to self-selection, and an inability of the investigator to control the independent variable.[3,4] While this research category lacks the rigor of more sophisticated designs, descriptive research often sets the stage for future experimental study by identifying the defining

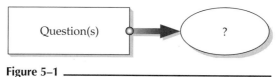

Figure 5–1 ――――――――――――――――――――
Descriptive research design.

characteristics of a cohort, significant relationships between variables of interest, and differences within cohort subgroups. Figure 5–1 illustrates a descriptive research design. An example of descriptive research questions that support construction of a population-specific database is provided in Box 5–2.

The greatest limitation to use of the descriptive research strategy is an inability to infer causal relationships because of loss of manipulative control over the independent variable(s).[3,5] Although it may be determined that a significant relationship exists between two variables of interest, the existence of that relationship does not imply causation, because a number of other uncontrolled variables may have contributed to the significance of the finding.

For example, an investigator might measure a significant relationship between increased length of stay (LOS) and the patient characteristic of insulin-dependent diabetes mellitus (IDDM) in patients undergoing total hip replacement surgery. The investigator cannot assign IDDM to one group of patients and withhold it from another; that is, the manipulation of IDDM variable is not possible. Instead, the two groups were self-selected; patients with IDDM formed one group and those without IDDM formed the other group. This limits the investigator from inferring that having IDDM causes an increase in LOS among patients undergoing total hip replacement. Other factors may have contributed to the

---

Box 5–1   *Characteristics of Quantitative Research*

- The focus is on a limited number of specific concepts.
- The scientist has preconceived assumptions about the interrelatedness of the concepts of interest.
- Structured procedures and formal data collection instruments are used.
- The scientist imposes controls throughout the data collection process.
- Data are collected and analyzed objectively.
- Statistical procedures are used to analyze numeric data.

Adapted from Polit DF, Hungler BP: *Nursing research: principles and methods,* ed 6, Philadelphia, 1999, JB Lippincott.

> ## Box 5–2   *Descriptive Research Questions for the Construction of a Population-Specific Database*
>
> - What is the incidence of "x" within the cohort?
> - Is there a difference in "x" among subgroups of patients within the cohort (e.g., patients with or without specific physiologic, psychosocial, or socioeconomic characteristics)?
> - What are the risk factors for "x" within the cohort?
> - Are there relationships between a finding of characteristic "y" and the occurrence of outcome "x"?
> - What variables predict outcome "x" within the cohort?

increased LOS experienced by the IDDM group, namely, the inefficiency of a specific provider, the occurrence of nosocomial infections, functional limitations, or even social constraints surrounding discharge placement.

The reasons for the selection of a descriptive design usually involve one or more of the following circumstances:

- The inability to manipulate a variable of interest within the cohort due to moral or ethical limitations (e.g., human exposure to second-hand smoke).
- The inability to manipulate a naturally occurring variable of interest (e.g., blindness).
- The inability to randomize patient assignment because of naturally occurring characteristics (i.e., self-selection) that designate group assignment (e.g., diabetics/nondiabetics).
- The inability to randomize patient assignment because of restrictions in the research setting (e.g., using providers A and B, which use different management techniques; limited sample size; provider/patient inconvenience).
- The inability to manipulate a variable of interest because of restrictions in the research setting (e.g., prohibitive cost, provider/patient inconvenience, lack of provider/administrative approval).[4]

The interpretation of descriptive research findings is challenging because of the interrelatedness of a number of complex variables, including physiologic, psychologic, social, and spiritual characteristics. Investigators must use caution in their interpretation of results, placing simply interest, not grandeur, in findings that may—on further study—be found as insignificant contributors to an outcome.

Advantages to the use of descriptive methods include the ease of study execution, the realism of the study setting, the ability to document

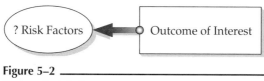

Figure 5–2 _____
Case-control design.

findings that may stimulate further research questions or hypotheses, the relatively low cost involved, and the expedient nature of study completion.[3,4]

Case-Control Design

Case-control designs compare the characteristics and circumstances of similar groups of pair-matched subjects and controls that vary with regard to a specific outcome.[3,4] Case-control studies are designed to identify risk factors for untoward outcomes. A reference group is assembled so that risk factor prevalence can be compared between subjects and controls. By looking backwards, investigators attempt to identify predictive variables that may explain the occurrence of an untoward outcome (Figure 5–2).

A retrospective approach is used in case-control studies. The dependent variable, or outcome of interest, is used to differentiate group assignment of subjects. For example, a case-control design could be used to study the problem of perioperative ischemic stroke in patients that have undergone cardiac surgery. In this case, perioperative ischemic stroke is the dependent variable. Cardiac surgery cases would make up the patient population to be studied. The sample selected would be divided into two groups: *cases*, or patients that developed a perioperative ischemic stroke, and a control group consisting of those patients that did not suffer a stroke perioperatively. The investigator would compare subjects to controls to determine which variables increase the risk or odds for perioperative ischemic stroke in patients undergoing cardiac surgery.

The descriptive information provided by case-control studies is used to define the characteristics of patients that developed an untoward outcome. In case-control designs, investigators estimate the strength of the association between predictor variables and the presence or absence of the untoward outcome. The *odds ratio*, or the approximation of the relative risk for the outcome in relation to the presence of each predictive variable, is used to express this association.[4,5]

Strengths of the case-control design include its ability to provide information about outcomes that are relatively rare events. The case-control design provides an efficient and inexpensive approach to answering questions about problematic outcomes that may otherwise take many years and substantial resources to study.[3,4] The large quantity of predictive variables examined in case-control studies also serves to generate hypotheses about untoward outcomes of interest, stimulating additional research opportunities.

The limitations of the use of a case-control design are a result of the retrospective approach that is used. Since investigators must work backwards, limited information is available to them. Additionally, in a case-control study, only the one outcome for which the reference groups have been formed can be studied. However, the major limitation of case-control studies is an increased susceptibility to bias.[4] In case-control studies, cases are not picked randomly and followed toward development of an outcome of interest. Instead, they are a "known entity," identified through identification of an untoward outcome, and may not be entirely representative of all risk factors under investigation.

Selection of controls must be undertaken cautiously in a case-control design—to limit bias. Matching is often the strategy used by investigators to ensure that cases and controls are comparable. Matching is the investigator's conscious control of subject characteristics to establish equal comparison groups.[4] Matching differs from random assignment in that all possible characteristics cannot be determined. The probability of producing equalized groups by matching techniques is less than with randomization. The use of two or more control groups, each selected by different methods, may also be used to strengthen the study.

The retrospective approach to measurement also contributes to bias in a case-control design.[4,5] Subjects may be asked to recall events or the use of substances. Among case patients, memory of events or substance use may be skewed; that is, case patients may be more likely to recall events or the use of substances than controls because of their knowledge of the untoward outcome. This problem, referred to as *differential recall,* may be overcome by using data recorded prior to the outcome, or by blinding subjects and investigators to both their case/control designation and the risk factors under study.

Cohort Designs

Cohort designs are trended studies that examine outcomes in subpopulations of patients. In cohort designs, a group of subjects are followed over time. Predictor variables are measured at the start of the study, and the subsequent occurrences of the outcome of interest are observed. Cohort studies intend to describe the incidence of specific outcomes over time and analyze the associations between predictor variables and outcome occurrence.[3,4] Two types of cohort designs exist—retrospective and prospective.

Retrospective Cohort Design

The retrospective cohort design uses a previously organized cohort database to answer questions about an unknown outcome.[3,4] All baseline measurements have already been taken and recorded. The investigator identifies a new set of predictor variables from within the database and collects these data for risk factor analysis in relation to the new outcome of interest (Figure 5–3).

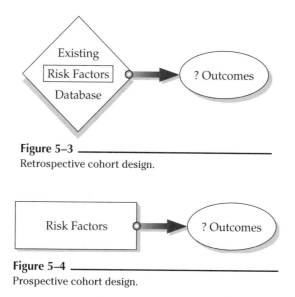

Figure 5–3 —————————————————————
Retrospective cohort design.

Figure 5–4 —————————————————————
Prospective cohort design.

Because the predictor variables are collected before an outcome is known, retrospective cohort studies are able to establish that preexisting conditions preceded the outcome, strengthening causal inference.[3] Investigator bias related to knowledge of the outcome is not a problem in this design, since the outcome is not known at the time of data collection. Retrospective cohort designs are relatively inexpensive and may be conducted in a time-efficient manner because an existing database is used. Bias in the selection of controls and cases is minimized, because all subjects come from the existing database.[3-5]

Weaknesses of the retrospective cohort design derive primarily from the fact that the investigator has no control over the quality of the database because it was assembled in the past.[4] Important data may be missing, limiting the investigator's use of the database.

Prospective Cohort Design

In a prospective cohort design, the investigator selects a group of subjects at the start of a study, prior to the development of a specific outcome of interest. Predictor variables are measured in the subjects at the start of the study. The investigator then follows the subjects over time, periodically evaluating each for the occurrence of a specific outcome[3,4] (Figure 5–4). Comparisons are made between the subjects that developed the outcome and a control group. In the single cohort study, an internal control group consisting of those that did not develop the outcome, is used for comparison. Depending on the investigator's design preferences, an external control group, or second cohort, may be formed for comparison.[3]

Strengths of the prospective cohort design derive from the fact that predictor variables are measured before the occurrence of an outcome.

This sequence strengthens the inference that a specific factor or a combination of factors may have caused the outcome.[4] Because subjects are followed chronologically, each predictor variable may be studied thoroughly and accurately. Problems related to measurement bias are reduced since the outcome is not known in advance.

Major weaknesses of the prospective cohort design are expense and inefficiency. Depending on the availability of subjects, the completion of a prospective cohort study may take many years. This design is best used for studying risk factors for common outcomes.[3,4] Caution must be taken in reviewing results, in that confounding variables associated with both the predictor variable and the outcome may produce misleading findings. By measuring all possible confounding variables and adjusting for their effects, the strength of causal inference is enhanced.

Nested Case-Control Design

A nested case-control design is a study that uses a case-control approach to answer a research question from within a retrospective or prospective cohort study.[3] Following the completion of a cohort study, the investigator reuses the database, organizing it into a case-control format—an outcome of interest is defined, then subjects are divided into cases or controls based on the presence of the outcome. Predictor variables are then measured in both groups, and risk factors in cases and controls are compared (Figure 5–5).

When predictor variables exist that may be expensive to measure using a cohort or experimental approach, the nested case-control design is a useful technique for the investigator to consider. The design is strengthened by all of the benefits of cohort designs. Predictor variables are determined before the outcome occurrence, reducing measurement bias. Sampling bias is also minimized because cases and controls come from within the same database. However, the nested case-control design also shares the same disadvantages of cohort studies.[3] Despite its strengths, the nested case-control design tends to be underutilized by investigators. It should be considered as an effective approach to answering research questions, especially when expensive diagnostic radiology or laboratory data are available from a cohort study.

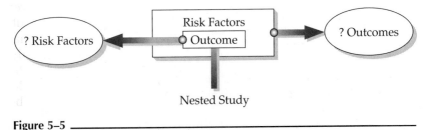

Figure 5–5 ——————————————————————————————————
Nested case-control within a cohort design.

Experimental Design

The true experiment is the most sophisticated research design, requiring the investigator to serve as an active agent in the research process, rather than a passive observer. Experiments are a form of cohort study in which the investigator manipulates an intervention and then observes the effect produced, or outcome[3,4,6] (Figure 5–6). Experimental studies can validate existing clinical practice or indicate the need for a change in practice to improve patient outcomes.

Experiments are well suited for testing cause-and-effect relationships among variables of interest because of the high degree of control, which minimizes the likelihood of alternative explanations. Three criteria must be met to infer causality. First, there must be a relationship between the causal and outcome variables. Second, the causal variable must precede the outcome variable. Third, the relationship between the causal variable and the outcome variable must not be explainable by another variable.[6] The strategies used to set up an experimental design enable a higher degree of confidence in study findings and an ability to generate causal inference better than any other design. While research studies are unable to prove beyond doubt the genuineness of their findings, the true experiment offers the most convincing evidence possible from a research design.

The use of an experimental design is typically reserved for mature research questions, or those that have already been thoroughly studied by the use of observational methods. Experiments are characterized by the following properties: manipulation of the independent variable, control of the experimental situation, and randomization of assignment.

Manipulation

Manipulation implies that the investigator actively treats at least one group of subjects differently from other subjects.[2-4,6] This is accomplished by procedures that prescribe how the independent variable will

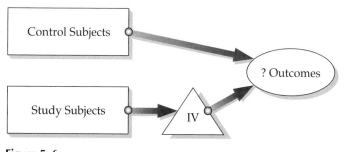

Figure 5–6 _____
Experimental design; *IV* = Independent variable (intervention).

be introduced to study subjects. For example, an investigator interested in the use of guided imagery (independent variable) to reduce patients' perception of the severity of surgical pain (dependent variable) might employ guided imagery in one patient group while withholding it in another. The investigator consciously manipulates the independent variable among different groups of subjects, observing the effect that this produces on the dependent variable of interest.

Control

In an experimental design, the investigator must control the research setting. Several steps are taken to ensure adequate control, including cautious treatment protocol preparation, strategies for manipulation of the protocol, use of a homogeneous sample, random assignment of subjects into study groups, random assignment of study groups to a treatment condition, and the use of a control group.[2,6] Since the control group subjects do not undergo treatment, their outcomes are used as a basis for evaluating the outcomes of the treatment group.

Randomization

Randomization refers to the investigator's selection and assignment strategy for subjects and groups. In an experiment, subjects are randomly assigned to different groups, treatment or control, so that every subject has an equal chance of being assigned to any particular study group.[6] Random assignment controls bias; it equalizes the distribution among groups of extraneous characteristics that may affect study findings. While randomization is designed to create equal study groups, there is no guarantee that the groups that emerge from random assignment are equal. However, randomization remains the best method available to investigators to equalize groups in such a manner.

Randomization often occurs in two phases. First, subjects are randomly assigned to different study groups. Once this has been accomplished, the investigator randomly assigns the groups to a treatment condition. Two common methods used for random assignment are the use of a table of random numbers (Figure 5–7) and the flip of a coin. The numbers represented in Figure 5–7 are randomly ordered. A random sequence of numbers can be selected by movement in any direction, from any point on the table. To illustrate use of the table, the following steps might be used to place a total of 80 subjects into two groups of 40 each:

1. Assign each subject a number from 1 to 80;
2. Pick a point randomly on the table, then move in a specific direction on the table and record each number as it occurs; bypass numbers that have already been written down or those that are higher than the total number of subjects, continuing in the same designated direction. For example, since there are 80 subjects, if the number 93 was encountered on the table, it would be skipped because there is not a subject assigned this number;

							1000 random integers between 0 and 99												
40	23	0	29	10	94	17	58	12	85	13	25	80	84	72	74	54	63	55	31
32	98	49	23	74	97	51	42	21	87	48	64	54	38	84	68	14	17	35	48
84	34	84	14	53	65	67	37	2	45	84	21	71	34	10	80	72	27	11	13
86	37	24	89	23	4	44	40	72	81	44	69	25	44	34	34	34	75	50	50
50	58	85	8	22	24	73	20	63	35	60	87	91	92	96	80	19	22	87	24
1	87	43	82	9	31	40	88	33	28	82	73	18	6	48	64	59	45	34	3
21	19	42	76	84	67	29	68	8	66	93	89	96	28	12	14	38	47	52	65
32	66	33	21	81	97	39	76	67	27	97	22	76	89	41	11	91	29	6	66
16	82	42	75	35	42	92	90	77	24	21	8	36	16	5	54	89	51	57	85
74	32	63	65	93	96	18	36	82	72	39	69	37	97	51	17	36	71	38	30
50	94	4	66	17	37	10	53	8	29	67	74	88	38	11	59	60	91	56	17
71	47	81	18	53	98	7	87	29	37	22	93	13	6	95	7	95	71	14	6
71	93	48	16	33	19	46	21	60	44	52	91	52	58	10	9	41	31	35	18
20	94	13	99	45	6	53	54	1	25	79	28	1	48	36	26	68	37	59	7
75	22	69	56	62	40	64	45	40	99	94	14	98	84	22	38	24	87	43	71
16	87	41	0	88	83	11	37	71	78	22	39	43	37	75	84	84	11	55	58
92	90	80	2	30	37	85	55	56	50	3	71	24	13	62	74	82	44	90	32
96	89	31	32	37	45	70	67	80	55	58	9	55	60	61	55	86	44	27	77
38	29	36	94	65	39	56	29	29	65	88	13	71	38	71	8	81	66	31	44
20	6	61	66	90	13	70	60	92	53	87	49	34	42	14	47	75	33	26	9
63	44	94	21	14	13	41	80	39	72	29	3	25	89	44	88	13	49	18	58
13	32	93	90	31	75	86	95	18	51	61	59	84	95	67	54	40	30	29	63
26	35	48	81	19	24	36	36	76	16	46	5	93	41	97	46	79	54	95	49
89	74	96	95	94	69	31	60	16	69	76	42	28	71	69	34	46	55	20	42
50	39	28	64	20	68	60	33	92	82	61	70	5	68	95	88	12	85	18	94
55	86	5	96	87	69	75	93	54	79	0	57	45	8	86	59	25	21	9	29
75	35	1	2	86	62	70	83	85	13	97	37	13	73	16	38	36	23	54	11
74	50	1	77	87	92	68	87	57	36	17	47	0	97	78	72	72	45	54	51
34	24	35	13	26	42	22	75	47	2	34	87	15	50	65	27	5	72	28	68
73	33	42	65	91	24	44	84	71	55	70	1	27	30	8	61	65	61	18	92
7	55	12	6	61	17	23	95	91	58	60	30	35	61	34	27	75	44	35	64
10	94	18	4	3	19	21	37	28	55	76	25	10	29	80	64	8	81	20	32
20	48	92	87	95	58	57	73	42	1	12	81	94	85	63	97	24	19	93	51
81	10	92	49	70	15	76	4	36	92	62	99	78	32	86	74	43	22	98	46
66	67	82	94	67	75	16	88	84	98	0	52	37	0	43	9	0	51	2	62
64	92	36	11	3	52	44	65	45	67	97	86	92	2	50	5	93	66	73	40
36	29	98	46	88	23	28	44	8	71	69	43	53	16	87	21	56	23	37	24
15	11	82	30	59	94	23	30	40	25	87	26	24	30	44	53	33	65	72	55
89	57	49	79	83	88	42	45	41	93	38	24	15	80	97	18	61	12	13	42
23	36	65	9	64	26	93	37	26	44	42	17	45	68	27	77	74	56	49	34
9	93	90	61	45	40	75	85	64	66	36	89	72	43	99	90	92	10	10	85
53	94	30	31	62	92	82	30	94	56	40	4	50	53	9	74	87	2	36	36
18	69	77	38	89	78	30	68	71	92	22	93	91	74	52	1	97	69	71	42
50	20	76	36	6	20	75	56	36	5	14	70	9	78	23	33	91	33	25	72
30	46	1	10	16	72	69	26	94	39	80	36	36	68	92	74	22	74	41	42
59	47	7	92	77	55	2	12	5	24	0	30	25	62	83	36	92	96	36	75
93	22	3	20	82	44	16	69	98	72	30	57	77	15	90	29	32	38	3	48
9	55	27	41	40	94	77	14	54	10	25	75	1	74	72	15	69	80	33	58
70	8	3	5	46	89	28	86	40	6	25	40	81	26	63	97	87	48	26	41
19	6	89	31	80	60	13	89	17	69	38	93	58	55	54	69	74	33	8	55

Figure 5–7 _____

A table of random numbers. (*From Lo Biondo-Wood, Haber:* Nursing research: methods, critical appraisal, and utilization, *ed 4, St Louis, 1998, Mosby.*)

3. Once enough numbers have been collected to allow for assignment of each subject, break the list into the number of groups to be studied. Since there are two groups of 40 subjects each, the first 40 numbers on the random list could be used to designate group one, while the second 40 numbers could designate group two assignment;

4. Match the assigned subject numbers with their ordered occurrence on the random number list to determine placement of the subjects into groups.

The flip of a coin may also be used to determine subject group assignment. The "heads" and "tails" sides of the coin are used to designate the assignments of group one (e.g., "heads") and group two (e.g., "tails"). A coin flip can also be used to designate which treatment condition the two groups will be assigned to receive. For instance, a flip of "heads" can indicate that group one will be used as the treatment or experimental group, meaning group two will be the control group.

Cluster randomization is a technique that may be used by an investigator to assign groups to different treatment conditions.[3,6] This form of randomization is best employed when subjects enter into a study at varying time frames, in that it prevents the comingling and possible contamination of subjects from different groups.

Blinding is another technique that is used to strengthen experimental designs. With blinding, the investigator and subjects (i.e., in a double-blind study) are prevented from knowing which subjects are in the control group and which subjects are in the study group. Blinding reduces the possibility of an unintended intervention, or a cointervention, being administered to the study group; the investigator is unable to focus any additional attention on the study group because group status is unknown.[6] Unfortunately, blinding may not be possible for all interventions and is best reserved for drug studies, where the experimental drug and placebo may be manufactured to look alike by the sponsoring pharmaceutical company.

There are many different methods by which an experimental design may be executed. Table 5–1 lists a variety of design strategies available to investigators. Experiments typically fall into one of two design categories: between-group designs and within-group designs.[2,3,6] Between-group designs compare the differences in an outcome or dependent variable among two or more groups of subjects that have received different interventions. Within-group designs compare differences in an outcome among the same group of subjects—first, before an intervention, and then again, after the intervention. The between-group design is the most widely used form of clinical research. The randomized controlled trial is a form of between-group design and is held in the highest regard by scientists as the gold standard for clinical research.

Advantages of the use of an experimental design have been highlighted throughout this discussion. The true experiment remains the gold standard for research due to its strength in causal inference. A major disadvantage of the use of an experimental design is the relative artificiality produced by intense control, as compared with "real-world" clinical practice environments. Experiments may also be impractical due to constraints within the work setting, the time frame needed to

TABLE 5–1

Experimental Research Strategies

Strategy	Description
Posttest Only	The period of measurement follows an intervention.
Pretest, Posttest	There are two periods of measurement: Measurements are taken before and after an intervention. This provides data for comparative analysis.
Factorial	Subjects are randomly assigned to specific combinations of treatment conditions. This permits testing of more than one hypothesis in a single experiment. Both the main effects (i.e., those produced by manipulated variables) and interaction effects (i.e., those produced by a combination of treatments) can be measured.
Repeated Measures	Subjects are randomly assigned to receive more than one treatment condition, which are administered in differing orders. This guarantees group equivalency because the same subjects make up both treatment groups. The results may be contaminated by carry over effects; that is, the effects of the first treatment may result in contamination of the effects of the second treatment.

Note: This table is not meant to be all inclusive; commonly used experimental research strategies are represented.

complete the study, and the sample size. The use of an experimental design may also be time consuming and expensive.

Quasiexperimental Design

The term *quasiexperiment* is used to describe an experiment-like design that lacks full experimental control.[6] In the quasiexperiment, the investigator implements an intervention in a similar method to that described in the true experimental design. The difference between the two designs is related primarily to the manner in which subjects are selected and treated in the study. Quasiexperiments often lack randomization of subjects to groups or the random assignment of groups to an intervention. In some cases, quasiexperiments may lack use of a control group altogether (Figure 5–8). Because of these differences, investigator confidence in causal assertion is weakened due to an increased potential for contamination.

An advantage of the use of a quasiexperimental design is practicality in real-world clinical settings. Often, practitioners wish to try new interventions, but meet with resistance from certain factions of the health care team. The use of a quasiexperimental design enables investigators to implement a new intervention among groups of patients where stakeholder buy-in exists. The study can be conducted without use of a control group, or, when possible, patients clinically managed by practitioners uninterested in the new intervention can be used as the control group.

A disadvantage of the use of a quasiexperimental design is the investigator's decreased confidence in causal inference.[6] Caution must be

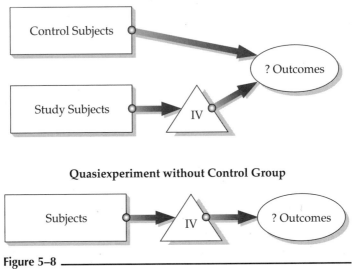

Figure 5–8
Quasiexperimental design; *IV* = Independent variable (intervention).

exercised and all possible alternative explanations for an outcome must be considered. Through the use of well thought-out design methods, controls may be built in to increase investigator confidence; however, replication of findings is paramount.

Evaluation Research

The term *evaluation research* is used to describe an experimental or quasiexperimental approach to studying the end results of program implementation.[2,3,6] Continuous quality improvement (CQI) techniques advocate evaluation research because of the ability to document the effectiveness and efficiency of clinical programs. Evaluation research is typically conducted in either a formative or summative manner. Formative evaluation is concerned with examining the process of program implementation, while summative evaluation deals with the outcomes of a program after completion of the study.

QUALITATIVE RESEARCH METHODS

Human complexity is a challenge to researchers. Human beings are unique individuals with varying degrees of social, economic, and physiologic characteristics. This complexity has moved many scientists away from traditional quantitative research methods toward a model of inquiry within the realm of qualitative research, referred to as *phenomenology*. Phenomenologists seek to understand the human experience as

---

Box 5–3   *Characteristics of Qualitative Research*

1. The scientist attempts to understand the entire scope of a phenomenon.
2. Few preconceived assumptions exist; the subjects' interpretations of events and circumstances are extremely important.
3. Information is collected without formal, structured instruments.
4. Attempts to control the context of the research are avoided to ensure capture of the scope of a phenomenon in its entirety.
5. Subjectivity as a means for understanding and interpreting human experiences is a primary focus.
6. Narrative information is analyzed through organized, intuitive methods.

Adapted from the work of Polit DF, Hungler BP: *Nursing research: principles and methods,* ed 6, Philadelphia, 1999, JB Lippincott.

---

it is lived daily, through the collection and analysis of narrative, subjective materials. Phenomenologists reject the reductionist methods employed by traditional quantitative research methods, suggesting that complex human beings cannot be broken down or reduced to constituent parts to explain a phenomena of interest.[1]

Qualitative research involves the systematic collection and analysis of subjective narrative materials, using procedures in which there is a minimum of researcher-imposed control.[1] Characteristics of qualitative research are listed in Box 5–3. While the primary focus of this book is on the quantitative analysis of health outcomes, a brief discussion of qualitative methods is warranted because of the cumulative way in which scientific knowledge is generated. Qualitative research provides a good foundation for beginning quantitative study of phenomena. Through an understanding of the qualitative experience, variables are identified that may be quantified in subsequent studies as risk factors or outcomes of interest. Similarly, quantitative methods may identify phenomena that are best studied through qualitative methods.[7]

A variety of approaches to qualitative research exist; these methods are often categorized differently by authors of research textbooks. This section explores approaches to qualitative study that may be useful to an outcomes initiative. They are divided into two categories, namely qualitative field studies (supported by phenomenologic methods) and case studies.

Qualitative Field Studies

Field studies are designed to explore and describe phenomena in naturalistic settings, such as patient homes, skilled nursing facilities, hospitals, and rehabilitation centers. Field studies examine practices, attitudes, behaviors, and beliefs of individuals in real-life functional circumstances.[1] The investigator collects narrative materials from observation, review of existing documents, and interviews. The investigator uses subjective judgment to determine the interview schedule, slated questions, and observations to be made. The investigator, then, is the primary instrument of data collection.[1]

Qualitative field studies do not always progress linearly. As the study progresses, new areas for review may be identified, causing the investigator to move in whatever direction is deemed necessary to gather pertinent information. Investigator flexibility is essential to successful construction and subsequent expression of the realities of the subject's experience. Typically, a field study progresses through five stages:

Stage 1: Identify the setting for studying the problem of interest.
Stage 2: Develop strategies for access to the subjects to be studied.
Stage 3: Assume an appropriate role within the setting—this may range from active participation to passive observation.
Stage 4: Collect, record, analyze, and interpret data.
Stage 5: Fulfill commitments that were made to ensure access to the setting and then leave the field.[8]

Phenomenology

Phenomenology is a method of examining the life experiences of a cohort in the field. Phenomenologists are concerned with learning the essence of a phenomenon as experienced by people.[1] An investigator learns about the experience through in-depth interviews or diaries, participation in the experience, direct observation, and introspective reflection.

There are four phases of phenomenologic inquiry. In the first phase, the investigator begins by *bracketing* preconceived beliefs and opinions so that the data may be confronted in a pure state. The second phase, *intuiting*, involves the investigator's ability to stay open to the meanings attributed to the phenomenon by the subjects that have experienced it directly. The third phase involves the *analysis* of narrative materials and categorization of content. Finally, the fourth phase is *description;* the investigator expresses what's been learned and defines the phenomenon.[1]

The strength of qualitative field studies that are supported by phenomenological methods is their realism; studies are conducted in naturalistic settings without imposing structure or controls that may alter findings. These studies provide an understanding of social phenomena related to specific problems of interest.[1] Qualitative researchers advocate the use of this type of study as a form of evaluation research, suggesting that quantitative approaches that have not been supported by qualitative study often miss the identification of the "true" outcomes of interventions.[9] This type of study also assists in the assessment phase of an outcomes initiative by providing program directors with a realistic understanding of the environment, roles, behaviors, beliefs, and attitudes of those to be affected by program change.

The weaknesses of this design are related primarily to the increased potential for bias, because of the depth of the investigator's immersion in the study.[1] These designs are also impossible to replicate, which reduces investigator confidence in study findings.

Case Studies

In-depth investigations of individuals or groups within a particular setting or circumstances of interest are referred to as case studies. Case studies are conducted to explore phenomena that have not been thoroughly investigated, enabling a broader understanding of variables that may contribute to the development of outcomes of interest.[1] Data are often collected over a period of time that allows the investigator to understand how past experiences and the present contribute to the subject's development.

The findings of a case study often stimulate the generation of hypotheses that may be studied through more rigorous research methods. Case studies also benefit the investigator with concept clarification and the uncovering of methods that may be used to study elusive variables.[1] Findings from case studies may be used to support results from quantitative studies, illustrating from a humanistic point of view the power of study conclusions.

The strengths of case studies are related to the depth of the investigation that is made possible through the use of a limited number of subjects. Case studies impart intimate knowledge of subject thoughts, feelings, intentions, conditions, past and present actions, and surrounding environment.[1] The weaknesses of case studies are related to their strengths; that is, the intimacy that develops overtime between the subject and investigator challenges objectivity and increases bias. The greatest disadvantage of case studies is the inability to generalize findings beyond the subject of the study.

| CARRYING OUT AN OUTCOMES STUDY

Getting started in clinical outcomes research may seem a daunting affair to the inexperienced researcher. While an expert research mentor cannot be substituted for, this section offers some guidelines to consider when beginning a research venture. Table 5–2 identifies characteristics that typify sound research methods.

The first and most important step is to define the research problem and develop the research question. The problem must be stated as an answerable question in clear, simple, and—when possible—quantitative terminology. Of equal importance is the need to remain realistic in terms of what the intended research is to accomplish. New researchers often strive for the completion of ambitious projects designed to make important discoveries and contributions to medical science. However, scientific method is complex, requiring cautious and mature skill beyond the grasp of a novice researcher.

TABLE 5–2

Characteristics of Sound Research Methods

Characteristic	Explanation
1. Research question congruent with design	Research problems may be studied with a variety of design strategies; however, many designs may be unsuitable for studying a particular problem. Stating the problem and research question clearly often reveals the best design intuitively.
2. Lack of bias	Bias is an influence that may distort study findings. There is risk for bias that varies with each design strategy, but experimental designs generally limit the amount of bias.
3. Precision	Precision is accomplished through control over extraneous variables; greater control makes a study more precise.
4. Power	Power is the ability of the research design to detect relationships existing among variables. Power is enhanced by increasing sample size, maximizing effect size, and minimizing the threshold of statistical significance.

Once a problem has been identified for study, the investigator should begin the construction of a conceptual model that will be used to guide the outcomes study. The model does not necessarily need to represent a disciplinary-specific theoretic model. Instead, the conceptual model is used to visually map the elements requiring control and the processes that hypothetically are linked to the cause of the outcomes of interest.[10] Figure 5–9 provides a framework for the construction of a conceptual model.

As the conceptual model is constructed, relevant literature should be reviewed thoroughly to bring attention to the body of science currently addressing the problem. It also alerts the investigator to potential confounding variables, which may be measured or controlled, and identifies problems that other researchers have been confronted with while studying similar phenomena.

The third step is the preparation of a study protocol. Study protocols are clearly defined written ideas and procedures that will be used to guide the research process from initiation to completion. The contents of a research protocol typically include the following[1,2]:

1. The research question to be answered and the aims of the study;
2. Discussion of the significance of the study and supportive historical background;
3. The research design, including the number of subjects and selection procedures, data collection and analysis methods, the safeguarding of human subjects, and informed consent;

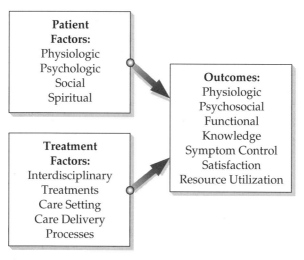

Figure 5–9
Conceptual model construction.

4. The time schedule for completion of the study; and
5. Budget and financial support.

Once the protocol is in writing, it may be evaluated and critiqued by experienced investigators. Consultation regarding study design and protocol often yields the recognition of important problems or limitations. Review by a biostatistician may also prove fruitful in guiding study design and methods for data analysis. The study protocol should then be revised to reflect recommendations and submitted for approval to the appropriate decision-making body.

Pilot testing should be considered before undertaking the study as a whole. Often, problems are identified in this stage that were unforeseen during the construction of the protocol. Pilot testing can save time and resources and promote important protocol revisions that add strength to the study design.

SUMMARY

Health care is becoming more complex than ever before. As providers attempt to uncover best practice, they will become more dependent on scientific methods to support the identification of important health outcomes. While it would be impractical to suggest that expertise in research generation and utilization be attained by all health care providers, clearly future practice paradigms will be developed by those with an ability to put scientific method to work for the benefit of their patients.

References

1. Polit DF, Hungler BP: *Nursing research: principles and methods,* ed 6, Philadelphia, 1999, JB Lippincott.
2. Portney L, Watkins M: *Foundations of clinical research: applications to practice*, Norwalk, Conn, 1993, Appleton & Lange.
3. Hulley SB, Cummings SR: *Designing clinical research: an epidemiologic approach*, Baltimore, 1988, Williams & Wilkins.
4. Friedman GD: *Primer of epidemiology*, ed 4, New York, 1994, McGraw-Hill.
5. Timmreck T: *An introduction to epidemiology*, Boston, 1994, Jones & Bartlett.
6. Grey M: Experimental and quasiexperimental designs. In LoBiondo-Wood G, Haber J (eds): *Nursing research: methods, critical appraisal, and utilization*, ed 4, St Louis, 1998, Mosby.
7. Beck CT: Developing a research program using qualitative and quantitative approaches, *Nursing Outlook* 45(6):265-269, 1997.
8. Wilson HS: *Research in nursing*, ed 2, Menlo Park, Calif, 1989, Addison-Wesley.
9. Swanson JM, Chapman L: Inside the black box: theoretical and methodological issues in conducting evaluation research using a qualitative approach. In Morse JM (ed): *Critical issues in qualitative research methods*, Thousand Oaks, Calif, 1994, Sage Publications.
10. Kane RL: *Understanding health care outcomes research*, Gaithersburg, Md, 1997, Aspen.

CHAPTER 6

Structured Care Methodologies

| INTRODUCTION

Structured care methodologies (SCMs) are tools developed and implemented by health care providers to standardize interdisciplinary care processes for a patient population. A variety of tools may be classified as SCMs, including pathways, algorithms, protocols, standard order sets, and guidelines.[1]

Figure 1–2 identifies Phase II of the outcomes management (OM) model as the phase concerned with the development of SCMs. SCM development should consist of the identification of successful existing practices, review of interdisciplinary literature, and the market analysis of the overall acceptance of proposed practice methods. Practice recommendations should then be presented and negotiated with interdisciplinary team members, with the intended result being the establishment of an agreed upon practice standard.[1]

In keeping with OM process, SCMs should be constructed with a research base that supports the selection of the practice standard that will be prescribed. Where research findings are unclear, measures should be built into the OM process to study the contribution of the SCM toward the defined population outcomes. It is also essential that the problem or population that an SCM has been developed for be clearly delineated. In the case of highly specific SCMs, such as protocols or algorithms, this means the use of an inclusion/exclusion checklist (Box 6–1), which outlines discrete criteria that are used to select or deselect each case for SCM management.

SCMs vary in their ability to control different aspects of care delivery. In Chapter 5, the concept of control in experimental design is discussed in relation to an investigator's ability to infer cause and effect between an intervention and outcome. It is just about impossible to control all aspects of the health care experience; similarly, SCMs that attempt to prescribe care broadly are less likely to achieve any kind of true control, thereby limiting investigators' ability to claim cause and effect between the SCM and outcomes. Conversely, SCMs concerned with control over a narrow aspect of care (e.g., a singular problem or practice occurring within the cohort) are more likely to achieve control,

---

Box 6–1   *rtPA Ischemic Stroke*
Inclusion/Exclusion Criteria

Inclusion Criteria
- Age $\geq$ 18 and functionally independent before current presentation
- Clinical diagnosis of ischemic stroke with measurable neurologic deficit
- Computed tomography (CT) scan negative for intracranial hemorrhage
- Presentation within 180 minutes of symptom onset

Exclusion Criteria
- Rapid improvement in neurologic function before treatment
- CT scan positive for intracranial hemorrhage
- Evolving infarction documented on CT scan with acute hypo-density or mass effect
- Presentation suggests subarachnoid hemorrhage (SAH) in the face of negative CT scan results
- History of seizure prior to or during stroke event
- Extreme moribund presentation
- Inability to maintain systolic blood pressure (BP) < 185 mm Hg or diastolic BP < 110 mm Hg
- Aggressive hypertension requiring sodium nitroprusside
- Serum glucose < 50 mg/dL or > 400 mg/dL
- History of surgery or trauma within the past 14 days
- Arterial puncture at a noncompressible site
- Lumbar puncture within the last 7 days
- History of stroke within the last 3 months
- History of intracranial hemorrhage
- Possible postmyocardial pericarditis
- Lactating or pregnant female

Reprinted with permission from the Health Outcomes Institute, The Woodlands, Texas.

---

thereby enabling inference of a cause-and-effect relationship between the SCM and the outcomes achieved.

This chapter provides an overview of each type of SCM, including recommendations for their construction, organization, and applications in practice. SCMs should be complementary in their design, so that the use of one does not restrict the addition of another. For example, a pathway may be complemented by an algorithm and a protocol, which add further control to the delivery of care processes.

SCMs are dynamic tools that require ongoing revision and refinement. As outcomes are measured in Phase IV of the outcomes manage-

TABLE 6-1

Characteristics of Structured Care Methodologies

Structured Care Methodology (SCM)	Characteristics
Critical Pathway	Represents a sequential, interdisciplinary, minimal practice standard for a specific patient population. Provider is able to alter care to meet individualized patient needs. Abbreviated format; broad perspective. Phase or episode driven. A lack of control prohibits the ability to determine cause-and-effect relationships between the pathway and patient outcomes.
Algorithm	Binary decision trees guide stepwise assessment and intervention. Intense specificity; no provider flexibility. Useful in the management of high-risk subgroups within the cohort. May be "layered" on top of a pathway to control the care practices used to manage a specific problem. May use analytic research methods to measure cause and effect.
Protocol	Prescribes specific therapeutic interventions for a clinical problem unique to a subgroup of patients within the cohort. Multifaceted; may be used to drive practice for more than one discipline. Broader specificity than an algorithm; allows for minimal provider flexibility by way of treatment options. May be "layered" on top of a pathway to control the care practices used to manage a specific problem. May use analytic research methods to measure cause and effect.
Order Set	Preprinted provider orders are used to expedite the order process once a practice standard has been validated through analytic research. Complements and increases compliance with existing practice standards. Can be used to represent an algorithm or protocol in order format.
Guideline	Broad, research-based practice recommendations. May or may not have been tested in clinical practice. Functions as a practice resource that is helpful in the construction of SCMs. No mechanism for assuring practice implementation.

Reprinted with permission from the Health Outcomes Institute, The Woodlands, Texas.

ment model, providers are challenged to return to Phase II to improve upon, or add to, the SCMs in their practice arsenal. Similarly, as science progresses, leading to new practice interventions, technology, and drug therapies, SCMs must be revised to reflect the scientific state of care.

Table 6-1 describes the differences between each type of SCM that is presented in this chapter. The SCM Appendix (see p. 217) provides examples of many different SCMs used to standardize practice for a variety of patient populations. These examples are included to showcase a variety of formats that others have found successful and to stimulate thought related to the construction of SCMs. It is important to emphasize that attempting to use an SCM from one facility in another is challenging. In fact, it is disturbing that SCMs are often sold by their developers, given that their usefulness to the purchaser is generally limited to consideration of a potential format and structural content.

| PATHWAYS

Pathways serve as an abbreviated description of the key events occurring in the care of a specific patient population. The events selected for inclusion in a pathway are thought to be significant contributors toward the achievement of targeted outcomes.

Pathways have their origin in industry, where they have been used to outline specific processes necessary to achieve an outcome. Pathways usually define care delivery patterns according to a series of targeted admission days or by a series of phases in patient populations where length of stay (LOS) may be less predictable. Pathways developed for predictable, simple surgical cases are not only the most simple to construct but also are most likely to reflect accurately the care processes instituted by interdisciplinary providers. When pathways are developed for complex, less predictable populations, they are usually inaccurate in defining with any degree of precision the care delivery requirements on a day-by-day or time-factored basis.

Burns, Daly, and Tice[2] state that the use of a pathway in complex populations is more likely to be marked by variance than by consistency in the use of a prescribed standard of care. The authors note that while this finding is obvious to any practice expert, there is a great deal of pressure placed on bedside providers by noncaregivers to develop pathways for populations in which they will be totally ineffective. They conclude that instead of pathway development, the emphasis should be placed on the selection of true clinical experts to manage the population with state of the science health care practices.[2]

The need to develop a pathway should be evaluated by a collaborative practice team (CPT) brought together to manage the OM process for a population of patients.[1] (Chapter 2 details the CPT development process.) Team members should consider the following when determining if a pathway will meet the needs of the population:

1. Is the population's pathophysiology homogeneous?
2. Is there a consistent degree of disease severity among the population?
3. Is the distribution of comorbidities similar among the population?
4. Is the treatment/management regime consistent within the population?

5. Is the time frame for the execution of therapies consistent among the population?
6. Is the setting in which care is delivered consistent among the population?

An answer of "yes" to all of these questions supports the construction of a pathway outlining the interdisciplinary care regime. An answer of "no" to any of the above questions indicates that pathway management for the population as a whole is most likely contraindicated.

In populations marked by heterogeneity, such as with multiple trauma or aneurysmal subarachnoid hemorrhage, pathway development and use may amount to no more than an exercise in frustration. When this is the case, development of a pathway should not even be considered. Instead, other forms of SCMs should be considered for standardizing practices around more narrow, homogeneous aspects of care.

However, in some cases where heterogeneity is the rule instead of the exception, subgroups may exist within the population that meet the criteria for pathway management. This is a more realistic approach than attempting to fit the care of the whole into a model that is incapable of representing a practice reality. For example, the stroke population is very heterogeneous. Stroke can be broken down into ischemic and hemorrhagic subgroups; clinical management of stroke differs dramatically depending on subgroup classification and the discrete pathophysiologic stroke process involved.

It would not only be unrealistic but also clinically naive to attempt to prescribe the care for all stroke patients on a pathway because of the heterogeneity existing within the population. The ischemic stroke subgroup, however, is more homogenous and thereby may meet criteria for pathway management. Pathway inclusion/exclusion criteria would then be built in to reflect appropriate patient selection.

The severity within a cohort also must be considered. A decision could be made to modify the inclusion/exclusion criteria for selection by pathway management according to specific, objectively measured severity findings. More commonly, however, a decision is made to include patients with a wide variety of disease severity, but to reflect on the pathway only the minimum practice standard; in other words, only the care that is common to all patients regardless of severity is presented on the pathway.

Using the example of ischemic stroke, patients may vary in their presentation from coma with ventilator dependency to minimal neurologic deficit. If a pathway were to reflect all the possible care standards for all levels of stroke severity, it would be too cumbersome a document to be useful to practitioners. When this is the case, the practices represented on a pathway should be limited to those that are common to all patients within the ischemic stroke subgroup; that is, the minimum standard of care for ischemic stroke.

Highly specialized practices, such as the administration of a drug like rtPA, should not be included on pathways. They should be reserved for standardization by protocol for two important reasons. First, not all patients meet candidacy requirements, and second, the strict control necessary to ensure proper procedures can not be presented on a pathway in a practical manner so that it is easy to use. In keeping with the minimum standard criteria, pathways developed for populations that are likely to receive other forms of highly specialized care should prompt providers to review inclusion/exclusion criteria for the addition of specific treatment protocols.

The categories of service and the time frame that will be used to illustrate the care delivery process must also be selected and should be guided by both the literature and expert opinion. The Health Care Financing Administration's recommended LOS data, as well as data from other benchmark sources should be reviewed. Table 6–2 illustrates both the common categories of service and the timing axis, which may be divided into either days or phases of care. The minimum standard of care is then placed within the time frame and service categories.

SCMs should be developed as complementary tools that may be applied as dictated by patient need to tighten control over specific aspects of care. During pathway construction, providers should consider other forms of SCMs that may need to be developed, such as protocols and algorithms. Necessary prompting may then be built into the pathway to direct providers toward the consideration of additional SCMs to tighten control over the delivery of patient care.

By themselves, pathways place limited to no control on practice other than to set a minimum standard of care for a population. Because of this, inference of a cause-and-effect relationship between the use of a pathway and any measurable outcome is not possible. Often the published literature includes papers authored by practitioners attributing reductions in LOS and improved outcomes to pathways. Scientists can easily challenge these claims by not only examining the study design and data collection methods but also the process of pathway use. Pathways lack control and precision; if they were precise instruments and able to execute tight control over care, all patients managed by pathways would be discharged on the targeted LOS, and no additional orders other than those reflected on the pathway would be necessary for patient management.

Instead, when outcome measures change for the better after implementation of a pathway, CPT members should probably give themselves a pat on the back. Measurable improvements in patient care are almost "Hawthornian," in that providers are paying attention to each other's contributions and collaborating, in some cases for the first time, which in and of itself leads to improved outcomes.

Pathways lend themselves to measurement of process variances. As discussed in Chapter 1, variances include alterations in the methods

TABLE 6–2

Example of an Interdisciplinary Pathway Template Showing Common Service Categories and Time Frame

HEALTH OUTCOMES INSTITUTE, INC.

Interdisciplinary Pathway Template
DRG: 00; Population:
Inclusion/Exclusion Criteria:

Addressograph

This pathway is intended to reflect the <u>minimum</u> standard of care for this population and is in no way intended to be all inclusive of the care regime that may be required according to individual patient/family care needs.

DATE	DAY 1 or Phase	DAY 2 or Phase	DAY 3 or Phase	DAY 4 or Phase	DISCHARGE TARGET DAY 5 or Discharge Phase
Consults					
Diagnostics					
Assessments					
Treatments					
Activity					
Nutrition					
Pt/Family Education					
Discharge Planning					

Reprinted with permission from the Health Outcomes Institute, Inc, The Woodlands, Texas.

used to provide care-processes and organizational systems. Because pathways list the minimum standard processes that should occur for patients within a diagnostic category, measurement of variations in process is facilitated by pathway use. It is important to remember that variances in care require definitions to ensure valid and reliable measurement. Secondly, process variances may or may not effect the end results or outcomes achieved by a patient population. For example, a missed laboratory test may not effect an unforeseen development of a complication in some patients, while in others it may significantly affect outcomes.

When CPT members become confident that a pathway's care processes are becoming stable, its content may be modified for use as a consumer education tool. All terminology presented in a consumer pathway must be modified so that medical jargon is replaced with understandable terminology; a sixth grade reading level is desired. While most versions of consumer pathways deal with an illness phase, clearly the growing interest in disease management signals a need to consider pathways as also preventative and wellness-based teaching tools.

| ALGORITHMS

Algorithms are binary decision trees that are used to standardize practice for very specific health care problems. A flowchart format is used to illustrate an algorithm. Step-by-step clinical logic guides practitioners through the clinical management of a specific symptom, laboratory result, or clinical problem.[3]

Because of their narrow focus, algorithms place tight controls on treatment, dictating a stepwise approach to assessment and management of a problem. Algorithms, then, are highly specific and inflexible, making them an ideal choice for use as an SCM designed to manage a high-risk problem associated with a population. In a well-designed outcome study, investigators are able to infer a cause-and-effect relationship between the use of algorithmic management and the occurrence of a specific outcome.

Algorithms, as process flowcharts, may incorporate symbols, which identify the type of specific process occurring each step of the way (Figure 6–1). A sealed, side-lying cylinder is used to represent the starting and ending points of an algorithm. A rectangle represents an action or activity that should occur, and a diamond shape is used to highlight a decision point on the algorithm. Each shape on the algorithm is connected by arrows that point out the next step required according to the clinical logic supporting the tool's construction.[4]

The algorithms that are most well known to health care providers are those associated with the American Heart Association's (AHA) Advanced Cardiac Life Support (ACLS) program. Using these algorithms as an example, a narrow, high-risk problem defines the scope of concern

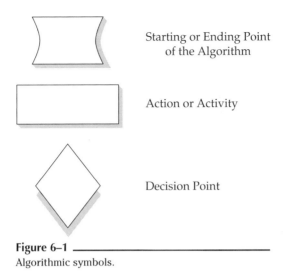

Figure 6–1 ————————————————————
Algorithmic symbols.

for these AHA tools. Separate ACLS algorithms support the care of patients with problems such as ventricular fibrillation, ventricular tachycardia, and asystole, each identifying a stepwise approach to the assessment of and definitive action for solving the problem.

Similarly, algorithms used as SCMs can complement the broad, very general care prescribed by a pathway. For example, a pathway for use in the seizure population could be complemented by an algorithm specifying practice for status epilepticus. The pathway should be designed with prompts to trigger use of the algorithm by providers. These prompts should be based on potential or actual high risk problems that may occur within a population of patients. Figure 6–2 provides an example of an algorithm used as an SCM.

| PROTOCOLS

Similar to algorithms, protocols define the standard of care that is used to manage a high-risk process or specific problem within a population of patients. Most health care providers are well versed in the use of protocols, as they have served as the mechanism for the application of research-based interventions for many years.

Protocols are narrow in their focus, but unlike the algorithm, they may dictate care processes for a number of different disciplines. For example, a protocol for the management of patients with swallowing dysfunction (i.e., dysphagia) might simultaneously direct a registered dietitian, speech and language pathologist, occupational therapist, pharmacist, and registered nurse to provide a very specific standard of care in their management of the patient (Box 6–2).

The use of a protocol in a well-designed outcomes study enables the investigator to infer a cause-and-effect relationship between the

CHF OUTPATIENT MANAGEMENT ALGORITHM

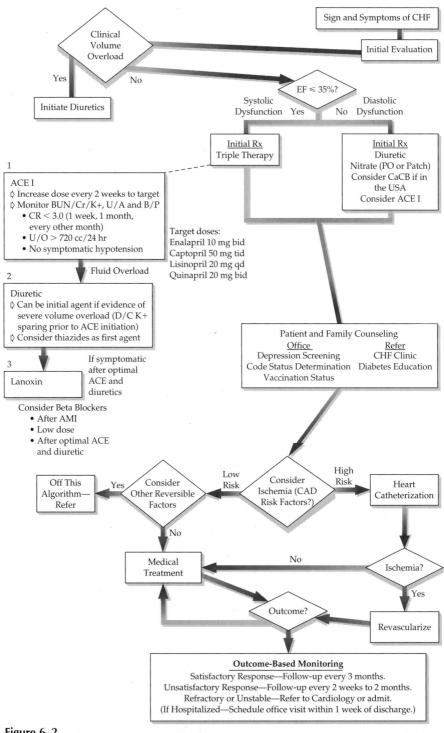

Figure 6–2

Congestive heart failure outpatient management algorithm, used as an SCM, and triple therapy for systolic dysfunction. *(From ACC/AHA Guidelines:* Guidelines for the evaluation and management of heart failure, *Kalamazoo, Mich, November 1995, Burgess Health Alliance.)*

BOX 6–2   *Interdisciplinary Dysphagia Protocol*

Nursing Orders
1. Assess swallowing using Dysphagia Assessment Profile; record findings.
2. Assess potential need for NPO status based on assessment findings or speech and language pathologist's recommendations; notify physician or obtain order.
3. Monitor delivery of all oral substances, noting ability to successfully (without cough) swallow varying consistencies of food substances and liquids; assess for possible aspiration.
4. Maintain head of bed elevated to 30 degrees for a minimum of 30 minutes following delivery of oral intake—or, continually in patients receiving continuous tube feedings.
5. Monitor intake and output every shift; complete calorie counts.
6. Monitor and record patient's weight twice weekly.
7. Assess/document breath sounds every shift and after oral intake; advise physician of findings and potential need for:
    a.   Portable chest x-ray study
    b.   Complete blood count (CBC) with differential
8. Suction apparatus at bedside; suction prn.
9. Provide patient and family education regarding dysphagia.
10. Assess need for pharmacist to review medications for conversion to tube feeding delivery.

Speech-Language Pathologist Orders
1. Determine a suitable route for delivery of enteral nutrition through use of a bedside clinical assessment, review of the Dysphagia Assessment Profile findings, and when indicated, modified barium swallow.
2. Determine treatment category:

Category I—Candidates for Trial Oral Feeding
Description: The patient lacks objective evidence of swallow dysfunction. There is no cough present on intake of water. The patient is alert and able to follow one-step commands. Silent aspiration cannot be ruled out.
• The speech-language pathologist (SLP), in collaboration with the RN, will conduct a trial oral feeding using aspiration precautions. The patient's ability to competently swallow various consistencies of food will be assessed. Findings will be communicated by the SLP both directly and in the patient record on the progress note and will include recommendations for modified oral feedings, tube feedings, or modified barium swallow.

Continued

Box 6–2   *Interdisciplinary Dysphagia Protocol—cont'd*

Category II—Candidates for Modified Barium Swallow (MBS)
Description: The patient tests positive on bedside evaluation for potential swallow dysfunction. This may include coughing on intake of water and successful intake of thicker substances (i.e., no coughing). The patient is alert and able to follow one-step commands.

- The SLP will assess the need for MBS and determine if the patient is an appropriate study candidate. A verbal order for the MBS will be obtained from the attending physician by the SLP. All MBS studies will be conducted and interpreted collaboratively by the SLP and radiologist. Findings will be communicated by the SLP both directly and in the patient record on the progress note and will include recommendations for modified oral feedings or tube feedings.

Category III—Patients Not Eligible for Trial Oral Feeding or MBS
Description: The patient is unable to fully participate in clinical bedside assessment due to alterations in consciousness or cognitive status, gross motor dysfunction, or oral apraxia.

- The SLP in collaboration with the RN and physician will monitor the patient's progress toward potential candidacy for either trial oral feedings or MBS. The patient will receive tube feedings until oral feedings may be safely resumed.

Occupational Therapy Orders
1. Assess trunk, neck, and head positioning to produce an effective swallow; if appropriate, provide adjunctive equipment to ensure proper or modified positioning.
2. Use trial-modified bolus placement techniques for patients cleared for oral intake. Determine effective strategies for feeding.
3. Assess perceptual and cognitive deficits that interfere with feeding; develop a plan for environmental modification to enhance ability to work toward varying levels of independence with oral feeding.
4. Communicate all interventions with patient, family, and interdisciplinary team members, both directly and in the patient record on progress note.

Nutrition Support Dietitian (NSD) Orders
1. Review initial laboratory data including electrolytes, prealbumin, complete blood count (CBC) with differential. Identify additional laboratory data necessary for assessment of nutritional status and communicate with physician or obtain verbal orders.
2. Complete nutritional assessment.

BOX 6–2   *Interdisciplinary Dysphagia Protocol—cont'd*

---

3. Use findings from the nursing and SLP assessments to determine the need for tube feedings. Using the patient's medical history and current assessment, the NSD selects a suitable enteral formula and calculates a tube feeding rate goal to meet 100% of the patient's protein and caloric needs.
4. Inform interdisciplinary team members of assessment findings, plans, and interventions through both direct communication and documentation in the chart progress notes.
5. Use the ongoing assessment made by the SLP to project long-term tube feeding needs and the patient's ability to progress toward oral intake. The NSD's plan should include modification of enteral tube feeding rates in proportion to actual oral intake as the patient progresses.
6. The NSD should include the patient, family, and significant others in the development of a nutrition plan and provide ongoing education regarding all findings and interventions.

Modified from the work of Walton M, Dildy T, Wojner AW: Unpublished practice protocol, 1995.

---

practice delivered and the outcome achieved. Similarly, protocols may be used as an SCM, complementing a pathway. A pathway for ischemic stroke, for instance, may be complemented by a dysphagia protocol when specific clinical signs prompt a high index of suspicion for the presence of swallowing dysfunction.

STANDARD ORDER SETS

Preprinted order sets have been used by clinicians for many years to standardize the clinical approach to common events such as patient admission, routine postoperative care, and transfer from one level of care to another. However, order sets may also be used to enhance compliance with an existing SCM.

Once the care of an SCM has become stable through continuous testing and revision, a decision may be made to display the SCM content on a preprinted order form or computer screen when informatics are used to support the medical record. Displaying SCMs on preprinted forms provides two distinct advantages. First, it lessens the charting and documentation burden on providers. Second, it enhances compliance with the standard of care, in that providers charged with writing orders are not challenged to remember every detail of the protocol for transcription. Box 6–3 provides an example of an rtPA protocol for ischemic stroke that is represented in the form of a standard order set.

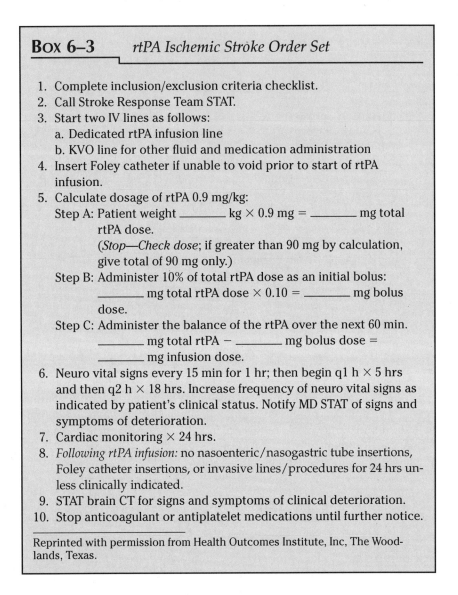

BOX 6–3   *rtPA Ischemic Stroke Order Set*

1. Complete inclusion/exclusion criteria checklist.
2. Call Stroke Response Team STAT.
3. Start two IV lines as follows:
   a. Dedicated rtPA infusion line
   b. KVO line for other fluid and medication administration
4. Insert Foley catheter if unable to void prior to start of rtPA infusion.
5. Calculate dosage of rtPA 0.9 mg/kg:
   Step A: Patient weight _____ kg × 0.9 mg = _____ mg total rtPA dose.
   (*Stop—Check dose*; if greater than 90 mg by calculation, give total of 90 mg only.)
   Step B: Administer 10% of total rtPA dose as an initial bolus:
   _____ mg total rtPA dose × 0.10 = _____ mg bolus dose.
   Step C: Administer the balance of the rtPA over the next 60 min.
   _____ mg total rtPA − _____ mg bolus dose = _____ mg infusion dose.
6. Neuro vital signs every 15 min for 1 hr; then begin q1 h × 5 hrs and then q2 h × 18 hrs. Increase frequency of neuro vital signs as indicated by patient's clinical status. Notify MD STAT of signs and symptoms of deterioration.
7. Cardiac monitoring × 24 hrs.
8. *Following rtPA infusion:* no nasoenteric/nasogastric tube insertions, Foley catheter insertions, or invasive lines/procedures for 24 hrs unless clinically indicated.
9. STAT brain CT for signs and symptoms of clinical deterioration.
10. Stop anticoagulant or antiplatelet medications until further notice.

Reprinted with permission from Health Outcomes Institute, Inc, The Woodlands, Texas.

GUIDELINES

Guidelines are suggestions for practice that may serve as a resource for the development of SCMs. Interdisciplinary providers charged with the development of SCMs are cautioned not to use the terminology "guideline" as the tool's title because if providers consider it to be merely a suggestion, the SCM may not be used.

Published guidelines have been reviewed to determine their method of development, including the scientific base, intended goals, and the degree of precision associated with each tool's recommendations. Unfortunately, findings have revealed that no consistent mechanism exists for the development of guidelines.[3,5] Guidelines abound in the published literature, but the degree of rigor supporting their construction varies from expert opinion to metaanalysis.

When selecting a guideline to provide a framework for the construction of an SCM, providers are encouraged to review the science supporting the practice recommendations carefully. The guidelines produced by the former Agency for Health Care Policy and Research (AHCPR) serve as an excellent model from which to develop and personalize SCMs.

| SCMs—A PERMANENT PART OF THE MEDICAL RECORD?

Rationale supporting the use of SCMs include attempts to decrease practice variation, improve quality of care through practice standardization, and reduce expenses related to poor outcomes and uncontrolled, unnecessary spending.[6] Despite these important goals, the inclusion of SCMs as part of the permanent medical record continues to meet with mixed review.

In many institutions, providers are expected to not only chart in the medical record but also duplicate their documentation on a separate SCM that is not considered part of the chart. This is an unrealistic expectation at a time when resources and personnel are being challenged to provide care efficiently and effectively. In fact, an argument can be made that if SCMs are not intended to be used as a part of the medical record, then why use them at all? Administrators must develop mechanisms to eliminate redundancy in documentation and foster the use of SCMs and data collection methods to support OM.

Friend or Foe in a Court of Law

Defensive medicine is a term that describes medical tests or procedures that are conducted in an attempt to avoid potential liability for medical malpractice. The cost of defensive medicine is substantial in the United States, ranging from an estimated $13.6 to $81 billion dollars annually, or between 1.62% to 11.23% of the aggregate national health expenditure.[6] At present, the effect that SCMs may have on defensive medicine is unclear. However, as research-based SCMs become more commonplace in health care, it is likely that defensive medicine will become a thing of the past.

For a plaintiff to be successful in a medical malpractice case, there must be evidence that the following four conditions have been met in relation to the charge:

1. A duty of care for the patient was owed by the physician;
2. The duty of care was breached by the physician;
3. The physician's breach in duty of care caused the patient's injury;
4. As a result of the injury, the patient suffered damages.[6]

The use of well-constructed SCMs may eliminate the second and third conditions of this argument, in that a physician may be able to clearly demonstrate the medical standard of care that was followed throughout the care regime.

Whether SCMs are included in the medical record or pulled from the final closed version of a chart, they are likely to be discoverable in a court of law because of the following two reasons. First, health care institutions that use SCMs typically have in place policies and procedures that define their purpose and method for use. Since SCMs are by their nature a representation of the standard of care that a patient will receive, a review of the institution's policy and procedure manual will point out to the plaintiff's attorney the importance of their review by an expert witness. Second, even if the SCMs are not mentioned in a policy and procedure manual, attorneys, experts, and plaintiffs have become well aware of SCM use, in particular pathways, to standardize interdisciplinary health care practices. Therefore, it is likely that even if a pathway is pulled from a chart before it is closed, witnesses can be asked in direct testimony whether SCMs were used in the care of the patient.

Often the rationale for not including SCMs as a part of the medical record relates to the fact that variance and untoward outcome data collection may be included as part of the SCM document in some institutions. However, within an OM program, data collection and the use of SCMs should be considered two separate but related processes. The SCM serves as an independent variable in a program of research; data collection mechanisms are carefully designed to maintain the validity and reliability of information. The SCM itself, however, is used solely for the standardization of patient care processes.

Additionally, depending upon how the OM program has been established in an institution, data collection processes may be qualified under quality improvement, thereby making them inaccessible for legal use. However, SCMs used to standardize practice should be retrievable. In fact, when their construction and implementation is supported by sound research findings, SCMs are likely to reduce liability, enhance practice, and improve outcomes. If this is not the case, then they shouldn't be used at all.

Most of the concern about the use of SCMs originated with the development of pathways that were intended to cover 100% of a patient population's care needs. These pathways were so detailed that not only were they confusing to providers who tried to use them but also they prohibited providers from appropriately altering the care regimens to meet the individual needs of patient and families.

As mentioned earlier in this chapter, when pathways are instead used to reflect the minimum standard of practice, interdisciplinary providers are not boxed into a corner. Other interventions may be added as needed to meet individual patient needs without threatening the integrity of the pathway. Pathways should include a statement that demonstrates that they are intended to reflect the minimum interdisciplinary practice standard for the population—that they are not intended to be all inclusive of the total care package that will be provided to meet patient needs.

Medical malpractice may be reduced through the use of SCMs in one of two ways. First, SCMs may reduce the frequency of untoward outcomes. Second, SCMs elucidate the expected standard of care for a patient population. The latter statement makes clear the importance of basing SCMs on research. In fact, without a research base, an SCM found to be associated with an untoward outcome may instead increase the risk of medical malpractice.[6]

When constructing SCMs, interdisciplinary providers must ask themselves, will the content stand up as the standard of care for this population in a court of law under expert testimony? This question basically addresses the importance of research utilization in practice. As the use of SCMs increases in the future, practice that is not research based may place interdisciplinary providers and the institutions in which they practice at substantial risk. Conversely, use of research-based SCMs may reduce the risk of medical malpractice.[6,7]

Lastly, even when the best SCMs have been constructed, they must be used if they are to reduce medical malpractice. At present, physician compliance with the use of SCMs varies. This may be in a large part due to the fact that in some institutions, physicians are not part of the team used to develop SCMs, thereby reducing their acceptance of these tools. Additionally, when SCMs are made to be "comprehensive" and all encompassing, physicians may feel boxed in.

Chapter 3 discusses the importance of interdisciplinary leadership for an OM initiative, including the essential involvement of physicians in the construction of SCMs. Without physician involvement and use of the tools of OM, outcomes are unlikely to be improved and both physician and institutional liability may actually be increased.[6]

| SUMMARY

SCMs, which standardize interdisciplinary practices, come in a variety of formats. SCMs should be considered research-based, dynamic, complementary tools that vary in their ability to control practice delivery. While much remains to be learned about the role that SCMs will play in the legal arena, most believe that well-constructed tools will reduce medical malpractice risk while enhancing patient outcomes.

References

1. Wojner AW: Outcomes management: from theory to practice, *Crit Care Nurs Quart* 19(4):1-15, 1997.
2. Burns SM, Daly B, Tice P: Being led down the critical pathway: a perspective on the importance of care managers vs. critical pathways for patients requiring prolonged mechanical ventilation, *Crit Care Nurse* 17(6):70-75, 1997.

3. Pearson SD et al: The clinical algorithm nosology: a method for comparing algorith-
    mic guidelines, *Medical Decision Making* 12(2):123-131, 1992.
4. Fields WL, Glaser D: Using statistical process control tools in the quality process. In
    Meisenheimer CG (ed): *Improving quality: a guide to effective programs*, ed 2, Gaithers-
    burg, Md, 1997, Aspen.
5. http://www.guidelines.gov
6. West JC: The legal implications of medical practice guidelines: *J Health Hosp Law*
    27(4):97-128, 1994.
7. Lumsdon K: Clinical paths: a good defense in malpractice litigation? *Hospitals and
    Health Networks* 68(13):58, July 5, 1994.

CHAPTER 7

Linking Quality Improvement and Information Technology with an Outcomes Management Initiative

INTRODUCTION

Quality is the degree of excellence possessed by a product, service, process, or workforce. Donabedian (1988) defined quality as the ability to achieve targeted goals using legitimate means.[1] Varying degrees of quality monitoring have always been associated with health care. The very nature of the term care connotes the intent to heal and optimize human health, thereby signaling a need for quality measurement. As a mechanism used to measure and improve practice, outcomes management (OM) provides a research-based framework from which to steer a quality initiative.

The term continuous quality improvement (CQI) emerged in the 1980s and is used to describe activities that incorporate the measurement and management of quality targets to optimize organizational performance.[2] CQI and OM are similar processes in that both use a cycle of measurement and improvement that incorporates process refinement. The rigor associated with the processes used throughout the cycle differentiates the two; OM is wedded to research methodology, while CQI may or may not use a scientific framework. While OM can and should be considered a powerful CQI vehicle, without a research framework, CQI processes alone are not equivalent substitutes for OM.

Measurement capabilities have grown in leaps and bounds over the past two decades and complement an OM-driven quality initiative. Today's information technology systems (ITS) provide a mechanism for rapidly producing and analyzing data from a variety of sources. Improvements in ITS continue to evolve daily, challenging the efficacy and efficiency of systems only a few years old. The growth of ITS has resulted in the development of a variety of quality tracking programs for process measurement and OM. Future advances in ITS will be supported by rigorous scientific framework and will produce powerful outcomes databases to drive pursuit of best practices.

This chapter examines the role played by OM within the context of a quality management program, including the use of ITS to support outcomes measurement and the future implications for strengthening outcomes measurement and management through the improvement of ITS and quality management.

QUALITY: AN OVERVIEW

Patients, payers, and providers are the three primary forces that influence health care systems today. All three groups are placing stringent demands on health care institutions and systems to quantify the quality of their care. A capacity to respond effectively to demands for evidence requires access to integrated quality monitoring and financial systems, as well as collection methods that ensure data integrity. Masters of outcomes-driven CQI are well-positioned to control the health care market.

OM serves as a protector of quality during an era of dramatic cost reduction and should be embraced as a method to document and defend care efficacy and efficiency. Outcome data provide a safety net to ensure quality standards are met, balancing the scales between societal cost and individual health.

Accrediting agencies, such as the Joint Commission on Accreditation of Healthcare Organizations (JCAHO), have made outcomes measurement and management a quality management priority. JCAHO accreditation is focused on organizational performance, shifting the quality movement away from individual performance toward aggregate outcomes assessment. While the JCAHO standards do not mandate the use of a specific outcomes framework, they acknowledge the synergistic effect of an OM initiative on enhancing overall organizational performance.

Accreditation and performance standards, such as those provided by the JCAHO, provide a quantifiable, comparable set of indices that patients, providers, and purchasers of health care can use to identify quality services. Professional specialty organizations are yet another source for performance standards, providing blueprints for constructing and subsequently evaluating provider performance. Employers are major consumers of health care; their collective purchase power has also played a role in promoting construction of health plan standards and measurement of performance. In 1989, a group of employers initiated the development of standardized performance indices, producing a performance measurement system known as the Health Plan Employer Data and Information Set (HEDIS). The intent of HEDIS is to provide evidence of health plan quality through the use of uniform indices.[3]

Methods used to compare quality among health plans, institutions, and providers will continue to evolve. Outcomes measurement and management will ultimately become the backbone of these systems, paving the road for competitive quality contests that will empower the excellent and challenge the existence of substandard performers.

THE STATE OF QUALITY SCIENCE

In 1993, the Health Care Advisory Board (HCAB) predicted that the years 1993 to 1997 would mark the era of reorganization of health care delivery systems and the formation of health networks. While the group anticipated that outcomes measurement would get started and progress through this time period, they also identified that the era of "credible" outcomes tracking would not be recognized until the years 2003 to 2007. The group boldly stated: "The science of tracking is in its infancy; even if quality were all that mattered, no purchaser could confidently use today's data to label one provider's clinical care as superior or inferior [to another's]."[4]

A number of problems with data quality that persist today were identified by the HCAB, including:

- Lack of comparability due to a lack of severity-adjusted data.
- Lack of agreement on study methods and tracking and reporting systems.
- Lack of consensus on which indicators best reflect quality.
- Lack of historical data, which prevents trending of performance over time.
- Poor study controls, which, overall, limits the establishment of cause-and-effect relationships between provider actions and outcomes of interest.
- Difficult data collection methods.
- Bias and vulnerability of data to manipulation.[4]

The HCAB emphasized the importance of severity adjustment of outcomes data and rigorous study design in supporting the usefulness of findings. This visionary group predicted that over time, more—not less —would be expected by consumers and purchasers with regard to health care quality. They also anticipated closure of outlier institutions remaining below the performance mean for quality.[4]

The HCAB recommended that organizations focus on quality indices that accurately measure the variables deemed most important by patients and payers. They emphasized the importance of generating valid and reliable data capable for use as a benchmark with other institutions. They also identified the importance of measurement that is limited to areas within an organization's full control. Lastly, the HCAB predicted that future outcomes measures will shift from measurement by encounter to measurement by disease—and ultimately to measurement of overall population health.[4] Unfortunately, we've yet to move significantly beyond many of the shortcomings noted by the HCAB in 1993; indeed, the period of credible outcomes tracking is yet to come.

| THE STANDARDS CONNECTION

Quality monitoring is divided into three measurement categories: Structure, process, and outcome. The structure category refers to the tools used to bring a process to life, including the equipment, care setting, and budgeted manpower. Processes are the methods and techniques, as well as systems, that are used to deliver care. Lastly, recall that outcomes are end results; Donabedian defined patient outcomes as a change in health status attributed to antecedent health care processes.[5]

Standards provide a framework for judging health care quality structure, process, and outcome. Standards are markers of acceptable performance that should be based on the state of the science, the realistic availability of resources, and unique practice setting conditions.[6] Well-constructed standards should reflect a balance between optimal and acceptable care, while avoiding extremes on either side of the continuum.

Standards are in a constant state of evolution. Modification of standards is dependent on societal values, scientific findings, accrediting bodies, professional organization standards, and the law. Depending on these factors, standards may be quite specific, allowing minimal provider flexibility, or quite broad when less specific findings are available to support strict control of practice.

Because the control of practice is strengthened by the use of standards, practice variability inherently decreases accordingly. Figure 7–1 illustrates this point using the normal curve; as control over practice increases, variability decreases, resulting in a narrow, steeper curve configuration. Strict control, through use of standards that are aligned with best practices, has been shown to not only reduce practice variability but also improve performance outcomes.

Standards should reflect progressively higher levels of acceptable achievement, ensuring continual refinement of care processes. Struc-

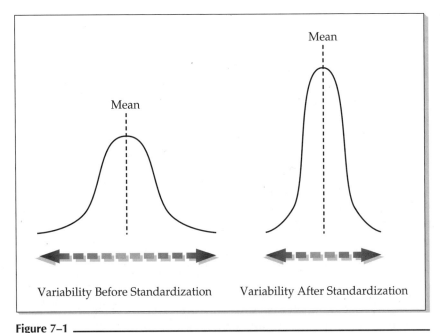

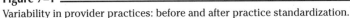

Figure 7–1

Variability in provider practices: before and after practice standardization.

ture, process, and outcome standards should be intertwined logically to produce structured care methodologies (SCMs) such as pathways, algorithms, protocols, and order sets designed to enhance patient outcomes.

ALIGNING QUALITY WITH ORGANIZATIONAL VISION AND MISSION

Quality programs thrive in flexible learning organizations that demonstrate a capacity to assess, design, implement, evaluate, and refine care processes. These organizations actively link their quality efforts to their organizational vision, mission, and strategic plan. An organization's vision describes its preferred future, while its mission is the organization's purpose for existence. The organization's strategic plan is a framework that logically orders strategic initiatives designed to facilitate the accomplishment of the targeted vision.

Health care organizations usually focus their efforts on achieving a vision that is aligned with a specific patient population. Visions are often expressed as goal statements, such as: "To become a regional center of excellence in the provision of acute care services." By logically connecting a quality management program to a strategic plan that targets vision achievement, quality indices serve to measure movement toward or away from the preferred future (Table 7–1).

COMMONLY USED QUALITY MANAGEMENT TOOLS

Organizations committed to learning demonstrate a capacity for accurate self-assessment. These organizations understand their current reality and build their strategic agendas to support service and product excellence for the purpose of maximizing market share and improving

TABLE 7–1

Connecting Organizational Vision, Strategic Planning, and Quality

Vision	Strategic Initiatives	Quality Indices
To be recognized as a regional center of excellence in the provision of acute care services	• Tertiary cardiovascular services • Tertiary high-risk perinatal care services • Tertiary trauma services	Measures associated with each strategic initiative listed (e.g., recidivism, complication rates, functional status measures)

consumer outcomes. Baseline measurement of performance should support identification and implementation of powerful strategic initiatives that will position the organization for future success.

Evaluation of Existing Strategic Initiatives

When the improvement of an existing process is the focus of a strategic initiative, the use of quality tools such as fishbone diagrams and the Serial V may be indicated. Fishbone diagrams, also called Ishikawa diagrams, provide a visual display of potential contributors to an untoward outcome. Well-constructed fishbone diagrams should facilitate the development of hypotheses aimed at understanding the cause and effect relationships among the variables of interest.[7]

The construction of a fishbone diagram consists of drawing a horizontal line with the untoward outcome situated at the "head" of the fish. Contributors associated with the untoward outcome extend from oblique lines, similar to the skeleton of a fish (Figure 7–2). Commonly used categories of contributors to an untoward health outcome include providers, equipment, processes, and patient population—specific variables. The benefit of fishbone diagrams is their ability to present a balanced view of the potential contributors to a problem, as well as the complexity and enormity of the problem solving process.

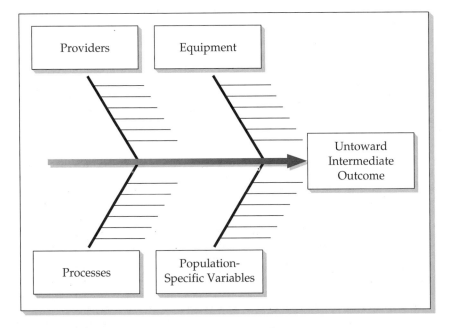

Figure 7–2
Fishbone diagram.

The Serial V concept Fig. 7-3 progressively links measurement, process knowledge, and pilot testing in an improvement cycle. The steps in Serial V are as follows:

- Measure outcomes and identify untoward results.
- Flowchart the basic process.
- Measure the effectiveness and efficiency of the basic process.
- Flowchart high-leverage processes.
- Measure/standardize high-leverage processes.
- Pilot test/implement high-leverage processes.
- Measure the impact on outcomes.[8]

The Serial V Concept is closely aligned with the OM model (Figure 1–2), providing a logical framework for analyzing current processes and organizing new ones aimed at enhancing patient outcomes.

Development of New Strategic Initiatives

The successful implementation of new strategic initiatives should be supported by quality tools that facilitate an understanding of project complexity. Processes and structures that will be necessary to support implementation of each initiative should be carefully identified and mapped out. Flowcharts are quality tools that may assist in the identification of key steps in a process. As discussed in Chapter 6, algorithms

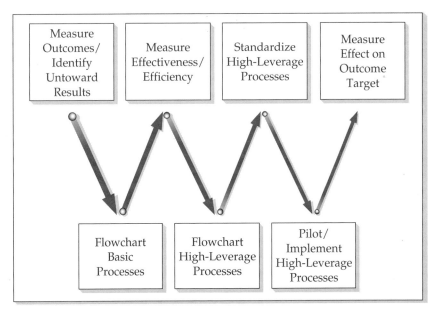

Figure 7–3 ——
The Serial V Concept provides a framework for analyzing processes and implementing new ones to improve outcomes.

are the result of commitment and standardization of a flowchart process, locking providers into the use of a very specific system of care delivery designed to improve outcomes.

Universally accepted symbols are often used to communicate the steps on a flowchart so that narrative language is minimized (Figure 6–3). Flowcharts provide a shared understanding of a process so that it may be critiqued, improved, and easily communicated to stakeholders. Flowchart accuracy is ensured when all disciplines involved with the process take part in their construction and subsequent process refinement.[7]

Statistical Process Control

Quality monitoring of strategic initiatives may call for the assessment of process stability. Stability may be affected by patient heterogeneity and varying degrees of disease severity, provider noncompliance with a practice standard, or fluctuation in structural variables that influence use of the process. Measurement of cause and effect between a process and an outcome is dependent on process stability, or control. To assess stability, control charts may be implemented.

Control charts plot trends in interval or ratio level variables. Control chart construction includes the use of a measure of central tendency (usually the mean) coupled with the upper control limit (UCL) and lower control limit (LCL) values derived through statistical processes. Data variation occurring within the control limits is generally random and is associated with variation that is inherent in the process with 99% confidence. In other words, the data points within the control limits are within statistical control and are associated with only common cause variation. Special circumstances usually are associated with data points outside control limits.[7,9]

It is important to note that statistical control does not denote satisfactory performance. Because a mathematical mean is used to calculate the statistical control limits, statistical control is ultimately influenced by the mean. In other words, if the mean is not satisfactory, then data within statistical control reflect performance that is generally unsatisfactory.

When nonproportional data, such as length of stay (LOS), are to be trended on a control chart, the *individual's control chart* should be used. Box 7–1 illustrates the steps used in preparing an individual's control chart. Of note is the need to consider use of the median when standard deviations are large.[9]

The *p* control chart is used when proportional data, such as infection rates in a surgical population, are to be trended. Box 7–2 illustrates steps for preparing a *p* control chart. The *p* control chart works off of means and standard deviations, instead of medians. When outliers skew data with significant standard deviations from the mean, *p* control charts clearly reflect variability around the upper control and lower control limits.[9]

Control charts stimulate research questions, but they are incapable of providing clear answers to the causes of variation within a process. Instead, control charts readily identify problems that require in-depth

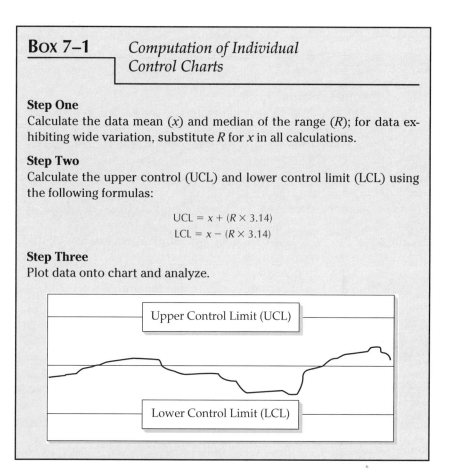

BOX 7–1   *Computation of Individual Control Charts*

Step One
Calculate the data mean (x) and median of the range (R); for data exhibiting wide variation, substitute R for x in all calculations.

Step Two
Calculate the upper control (UCL) and lower control limit (LCL) using the following formulas:

$$UCL = x + (R \times 3.14)$$
$$LCL = x - (R \times 3.14)$$

Step Three
Plot data onto chart and analyze.

Upper Control Limit (UCL)

Lower Control Limit (LCL)

BOX 7–2   *Computation of p Control Chart*

Step One
Calculate the mean (p) and standard deviation of the proportions (SDp).

Step Two
Calculate the upper control limit (UCL) and lower control limit (LCL) using the following formulas:

$$UCL = p + (SDp \times 3)$$
$$LCL = p - (SDp \times 3)$$

Step Three
Plot data onto chart and analyze (plotted similarly to example in Box 7–1).

investigations, as well as draw attention to shifts in process patterns over time. When process changes are made, upper and lower control limits need to recalculated.[7,9]

Measurement Considerations

Thousands of possible quality indicators may be tracked within a health care organization. The temptation to track more than what is absolutely necessary often results in organizations that are data rich but information poor. Organizations bent on improvement should differentiate the "need to knows" from the "nice to knows" to ensure optimal performance and quality program effectiveness.

Each indicator established for monitoring should be supported by criteria that guide study methods. Study design is closely tied to the usefulness of the findings. By wedding a quality initiative with OM, study methods may be strengthened, enhancing the integrity of results and provider incentive to change practice. Establishing an agreement with an institutional review board or committee for the protection of human subjects facilitates research conducted within an OM driven quality program. Mechanisms for expedited review of outcomes studies meeting specific criteria should be established to promote the use of research-based methods.

INTEGRATING ITS WITH QUALITY MANAGEMENT AND OM

In 1993, the HCAB predicted that automated medical record systems would be installed in most institutions by the year 2003. They envisioned an ITS infrastructure that interfaced data from a variety of feeder systems, capable of producing a singular database from which to assess quality;[4] today we call this concept an outcomes data repository (ODR).

Health care ITS integrate patient data, financial data, structure and process information, and outcome indices to facilitate the study of the complex relationships, differences, and end results associated with these variables. From a structural standpoint, ITS should enable accurate determination of cost of care, provide case mix and flexible budgeting processes, and promote environmental utilization trends and clinical and financial forecasting. Within the realm of process measurement, ITS should enable the determination of resource utilization, providing a clear picture of the standard of care and the systems used to achieve outcomes for a given condition. Additionally, ITS should foster utilization review/management and risk management assessment.

From an outcomes perspective, ITS should enable the study of population characteristics, intermediate and untoward intermediate outcomes, process variances, and, within health systems capable of controlling the continuum of care, long-term outcomes. Most importantly, ITS should incorporate methods for adjustment of severity within study populations to enhance the usefulness of findings. These functions are all characteristics of the ODR, a system that enables research-based decision making designed to improve health care for patients and their families.

The prevalence of computers in society has made it imperative for health care providers to integrate their use into the practice arena. Clinicians, educators, researchers, and administrators are all benefiting from computer technology. While computer technology has become an integral part of health care, the field of health care informatics is a relatively new specialty; it is only within the past 10 years that it has been named, defined, and recognized as a specialty. Academic programs to prepare practitioners with expertise in informatics have been established at a number of universities and certification examinations have been developed to credential health care practitioners.[10,11] There is tremendous potential for practitioners within this specialty to have a major effect on the way health care is designed and delivered in the future.

HEALTH CARE INFORMATICS DEFINED

The term informatics was coined from the French word, "informatique." It was first defined by Gorn, as a combination of computer and information science.[12] Informatics is more than just computers; it includes all aspects of technology and science, from the theoretical to the applied. The discovery of new tools, building new computer capabilities, and the study of related ITS, are all important fields of informatics.[10]

The term *health care informatics* refers to that component of informatics designed for, and relevant to, practitioners. Health care informatics integrates interdisciplinary health care science with computer science and information science, enabling identification, collection, processing, and management of data to support practice and business processes, practitioner and patient education, and the growth of evidence-based health care practices.

For more than two decades, practitioners have been working in hospitals and other settings to help with the selection, installation, and evaluation of ITS. This early function continues to be important, but with constant change in health care, the scope of such work has expanded and job opportunities are increasing rapidly. Hersher describes several current and future roles for practitioners in informatics, including:

- Clinical Information Systems Coordinator—A practitioner employed by a health care institution who directs the installation of ITS, including the construction of interfaces with system vendors and users.
- Clinical Information System Installer—A practitioner employed by a vendor who participates in the development and installation of ITS and provides support services for education and troubleshooting.

- Product Manager—A practitioner employed by both vendors and health care institutions who is responsible for constantly updating a current product, keeping abreast of new developments in the field, and interfacing with marketing staff, clients, technical staff, and management.
- Systems Analyst/Programmer—A practitioner employed by the health care institution who assists with the analysis and maintenance of ITS, including programming.[13]

Other roles include the chief information officer, consultant, network administrator, data repository specialist, and clinical information liaison.[13] Settings that incorporate ITS are expanding as continuum-based care delivery evolves into integrated networks and health plans that are responsible for community wellness.

| INFORMATION SYSTEMS IN PRACTICE

ITS are changing the way that health care is delivered, whether in a hospital setting, postacute setting, provider's office, or patient home. With capabilities ranging from advanced instrumentation to high-level decision support, ITS offer clinicians information when and where they need it. Increasingly, ITS facilitate the delivery of patient-centered care and support movement toward the use of electronic medical records (EMR).

In health care settings, definitions of ITS vary significantly. Semancik defined health care ITS as a collection of software programs and associated hardware that supports the entry, retrieval, update, and analysis of patient information and associated clinical information related to patient care delivery processes.[14] Health care ITS may have a patient-focused scope, a departmental scope, or a combination of both.

Automation within the patient-focused domain of an ITS supports patient care processes. Typical applications include order entry, results reporting, clinical documentation, and process accounting. Data entered into the system may be organized into ODRs that can be accessed to assess trends in patient care outcomes. Within the departmental domain of an ITS, programs have evolved to meet the operational needs of specific departments, such as the laboratory, radiology, pharmacy, medical records, and billing departments. Early ITS were typically standalone systems designed for individual departments. A major challenge facing ITS developers is the integration of existing stand-alone systems with all other systems, including those implemented for measurement and support of the patient-focused domain.

Electronic Medical Records
A major component within health care ITS is the EMR. Ideally, the EMR should include womb-to-tomb information reflecting an individual's life-

time health status, the continuum-based health care services that were offered and used, and pertinent health-related environmental and societal factors. The EMR can replace the paper medical record as the primary source of information for health care and must meet clinical, legal, accreditation, and administrative requirements.

EMRs are more than what we know of today's medical record. ITS that interface with EMRs permit input, processing, and integration of greater quantities of data, producing information that is broader than that found within linear paper records. With this in mind, the EMR should not be thought of as a record in the traditional sense; the term "record" connotes a repository with limitations of size, content, and location, the sole purpose of which being the maintenance of health data by event. Although paper records are important resources, EMRs can use individual health data to support the generation and communication of knowledge related to the aggregate health experience among populations of interest. Furthermore, the emphasis today on improving outcomes of care and maintaining health broadens the scope of data maintained within an EMR to reflect not only events related to illness or disease but also wellness.

The womb-to-tomb focus of EMRs should provide a virtual compilation of unique health data (i.e., not redundant) across the lifespan. Health data should include information on allergies; history of illness and injury; functional status information; diagnostic study results; assessments; orders; consultation reports; treatment records; wellness information, such as immunization history, behavioral data, environmental information, demographics, and health insurance; administrative data for care delivery processes; and legal data, such as consents. The "who, what, when, and where" of data capture must also be identified. The structure of the data stored within an EMR should include text, numbers, sounds, images, and full-motion video. These data must be thoroughly integrated, providing an all encompassing picture of individual and aggregate health.

Within an EMR, an individual's health data are maintained and distributed over different systems in different locations, such as a hospital, clinic, physician's office, and pharmacy. Intelligent software agents with appropriate security measures are necessary to access data across these distributed systems. The practitioner retrieving these data must be able to assemble it in such a way as to provide a chronology of health information about the individual, or across a population of patients within a given diagnosis.

EMRs are maintained within systems that capture, process, communicate, secure, and present data about the patient. To increase the capabilities of an EMR, it should be integrated with the health care ITS itself, not maintained as a free-standing computer program. Additional EMR components should include clinical rules, literature for patient education, expert opinions, and payer rules related to reimbursement. When these elements work together in an integrated fashion, the EMR becomes much more than a patient record; it becomes a knowledge tool. The system is able to integrate information from multiple sources and provides decision support for its users.

The Computer-Based Patient Record Institute (CPRI) has identified the following objectives of an EMR[15]:

- Improve individual health and the maintenance of health.
- Facilitate timely, accurate, and comprehensive communication among caregivers.
- Assure confidentiality and integrity of health-related information about individuals.
- Provide ready access to knowledge bases and decision support systems.
- Enhance the productivity and efficiency of the health care delivery system.
- Encourage patient participation in personal health care.
- Support improvement of community health status.
- Encourage and support clinical research and education.
- Support policy and public health responsibilities.[15]

To meet these objectives, the functions of an EMR and its associated ITS must be considered carefully. The CPRI notes that an information infrastructure must be in place to support data input, storage, processing, communication, security, and presentation.[16] The complexity of these issues and the development of systems that are necessary explains why few fully functional EMR systems are in place today.

Components of the Information Infrastructure

Data capture is a term used to describe the collection and entry of data into a computer system. Data may be local or remote, originating from patient-monitoring devices, telemedicine applications, directly from the individual recipient of health care, or from others who have information about the recipient's health or environment, such as relatives, friends, and public health agencies. Data may be captured by multiple means, including key entry, pattern recognition (e.g., voice, handwriting, biological characteristics), and medical device transmission.

All data entered into a computer are not necessarily structured for subsequent processing. Document imaging systems, for example, provide for the creation of electronically stored text but have limitations on the ability to process that text into quantifiable information. Because of this, data capture must include the use of controlled vocabularies (i.e., taxonomies) and code systems to ensure a common meaning for terminology and the ability to process units of information.

A final consideration is the validity and reliability of data. Definitions should support the data targeted for collection to ensure validity of the data entered in the ITS. The number of people charged with entering data must also be carefully thought out; generally, as the number of people entering data increases, the reliability of the data entered decreases.

Measures designed to assess both the intrarater and interrater reliability of data must be implemented on a regularly scheduled basis to ensure data integrity and usefulness over time.

Data storage refers to the physical location of data. In EMRs and integrated ITS, health data are distributed across multiple systems at different sites. For this reason, there needs to be common access protocols, retention schedules, and universal identification mechanisms. Access protocols permit only authorized users to obtain data for legitimate purposes. Additionally, the ITS must have backup and recovery mechanisms established to safeguard the system in the event of computer failure. Retention schedules address the maintenance of the data in both active and inactive forms, as well as the permanence of the storage medium. Lastly, universal identifiers must be established to promote both separation and integration of an individual's health data with a variety of cohorts across multiple systems at a number of sites.

Application functions must also be established to support the ITS and EMR. Data within an ITS are supported by application functions, enabling effective retrieval and processing into useful information. *Application functions* include decision support tools such as alerts and alarms for drug interactions, allergy caution triggers, and abnormal laboratory results highlights. Additionally, reminders can be provided for appointments, necessary pathway or protocol actions, medications to be administered, and other provider or patient activities. Integration of a standard of practice represented on any of the SCM formats may be built into EMR applications and supplemented by the creation of a documentation mechanism.

Information communication refers to the exchange of data across disparate systems and linkages. To integrate health data across multiple systems at different sites, identifier systems (unique numbers or other methodology) for health care recipients, caregivers, providers, payers, and sites are essential. Local, regional, and national health information infrastructures that tie all participants together using standard data communication protocols are key to linkage function. There are hundreds of types of transactions or messages that must be defined and agreed upon by the participating stakeholders. Vocabulary and code systems must permit the exchange and processing of data into meaningful information; additionally, EMR systems must provide access to point of care information databases and knowledge sources, such as pharmaceutical formularies, referral databases, and reference literature.

Security functions ensure the confidentiality of private health information and the integrity of the data. There are three important terms that are used when discussing security: privacy, confidentiality, and security. *Privacy* is the right of an individual to keep information about himself or herself from being disclosed to others, including health care providers, without permission. *Confidentiality* is the act of limiting disclosure of private matters. Once a patient has disclosed private information to a health care provider, that provider has a responsibility to maintain the confidentiality of the information. *Security* is the means of controlling access and protecting information from accidental or intentional disclosure to unauthorized persons, as well as prevention of information alteration, destruction, or loss. When private information is placed in a confidential EMR, the system must have controls in place to maintain security and disallow unauthorized persons access to the data.[15]

EMRs actually provide better protection of confidential health information than paper-based systems, because they support controls that ensure only authorized users with legitimate purposes have access to health information. Security functions must be designed to ensure compliance with applicable laws, regulations, and standards. Security functions also must provide a means to audit for inappropriate access, as well as provide mechanisms for patients to access their records upon request.

Presentation format is another consideration. Given the wealth of information available within EMRs and health care ITS, usable presentation formats are especially important. For example, authorized users may want to view data organized by source, caregiver, encounter, diagnosis, or admission date. Data can be presented in detail or summary format. Tables, graphs, narrative, and other forms of information presentation must be accommodated.

| OUTCOMES DATA REPOSITORIES

Patient outcome capture has been recognized as an essential component of current and future health care systems. Demands for data from policy makers, researchers, administrators, payers, and health care professionals have, historically, outstripped the ability to provide outcomes data. The capabilities of health care ITS and EMRs have made the provision of such data more realistic than it has been in past years.

When designing an ITS for outcomes measurement, common variables of interest, derived from research questions about the target population, should be identified and defined for measurement in all patients within the institution or health care network that meet designated diagnostic classifications. Each variable must be transformed into meaningful data (i.e., nominal, ordinal, interval, or ratio level—see Chapters 4 and 5 for further discussion) that may be aggregated and analyzed using appropriate statistical methods. Variables that support standard quality measures, such as those written by accrediting bodies, should also be identified for inclusion in the ODR, as well as research instruments and severity measures.

Protocols for data collection must be written and implemented. Pilot testing of protocols is recommended—to identify possible problems that may be encountered and that will need to be revised before "going live" with the system. Methods to ensure the validity and reliability of data, as previously discussed, are essential to protocol testing and subsequent implementation.

Next, the schedule for data analysis must be defined. Chapters 4 and 5 provide an overview of methods that may be used to determine sample size, thereby supporting the determination of a data analysis schedule. Since the identification of appropriate statistical analyses should occur with articulation of the research questions and variable definition, data entered into the ODR should be readily available in the formats necessitated for use during analysis. Because the statistical programs contained within most EMR and health care ITS are not capable of supporting sophisticated data analysis to answer each research question of interest, data analysis is best accomplished by shuttling data across infrastructure linkages to statistical software.

Finally, the practice standard that will be tested during the data collection period must be considered. Consistent with Phase II of the OM model, the use of SCMs to standardize and control practice must be defined, agreed upon, taught to those providing direct patient care, and implemented reliably. With this in mind, data analyzed with an ODR reflect outcomes derived from a specific standard of practice, enabling the identification of the state of best practice within an institution or health care network.

When outcomes are not favorable, the standard of practice originally designed in Phase II of the OM model is subject to renovation or the addition of new SCMs. Because each run of the data may reflect differing practice standards, outcome comparisons and intrainstitutional benchmarking should be facilitated by ODRs. Lastly, when new practice standards are implemented, aggregation of data with previous findings must be avoided so that the outcomes achieved reflect only the standard of practice being tested. This speaks to the need for flexibility within the ODR, so that historical outcome data may be saved but not incorporated into a new outcome data file reflecting measurement of outcomes on a new standard of practice.

When designing the EMR component of an ITS, cues must be built into the system to trigger the collection of generic or condition-specific outcome data. Generic outcome data consist of those data that should be collected across all populations of patients (e.g., functional status measures, which are becoming widely accepted among health care professionals as essential to the assessment of end results). Condition-specific outcome data include those data that relate only to certain groups of patients that meet specific operator definitions. For example, measurement of nausea in patients receiving chemotherapy might be selected as a condition-specific outcome.[17]

Variables included within a research instrument may need to be incorporated into the EMR, along with triggers in the system to bring up the instrument at specific points in care for measurement by the bedside provider. Using the example of chemotherapy-induced nausea, an instrument for data collection related to nausea may be triggered by the selection of a chemotherapeutic or antiemetic medication for administration. This example also suggests consideration of the time dimension for measurement of outcomes. Nausea, and similarly pain, are intermediate, proximally-measured outcomes that require triggers to ensure measurement at time intervals that appropriately enable the assessment of treatment effectiveness. Functional status is an outcome that may be measured at both admission and discharge but usually is measured again later in the course of patient treatment and follow-up. Triggers that ensure measurement across time for an outcome such as functional status must also be considered in the design of an EMR.[17]

Outcome data may be generated from multiple sources, including patients, family members, caregivers, health professionals, and medical equipment and instruments. In designing an EMR, the determination of the best sources for outcome data must be considered and built into the system.[17] For example, patients are the likeliest determinants of pain severity; other variables, however, may be tied to laboratory or test values. Similarly, in patients that are unable to participate in data collection due to cognitive impairment, the use of a designated family caregiver for collection of data on functional status after discharge may be required. When a patient or family caregiver records functional status measures directly into a computer at prescribed intervals, the validity and reliability of the data is increased significantly. New technologies that allow the measurement of patient outcomes from home, transferring the data into an EMR at a remote location, are exciting innovations that hold great promise.

The long-term goal of health care ITS is the ability to promote decision support by caregivers. To be effective and useful to stakeholders, these systems must have the ability to aggregate meaningful data that used common definitions, was collected with sound methodology, and was analyzed with appropriate statistical methods. The system must be able to trend data to support decision making yet maintain flexibility, so that variables and different sources of data may be included or excluded as deemed necessary. Ultimately, the system must be capable of spanning the continuum of care, so that patient care, delivered across a variety of locations and providers, is accurately reflected in the system.

Information demands in health care systems are pushing the development of ITS and EMRs. The ongoing development of computer technology—smaller, faster machines with extensive storage capabilities and the ability for cross-platform communication—is making the goal of an integrated health care ITS and EMR a realistic option, not just a dream.

As health care ITS continue to evolve, health care providers will play an important role in their development, implementation, refinement, and evaluation. Knowledge of policies, procedures, and clinical practice is essential as workflow systems are redesigned within an ITS. In particular, those with hands-on interaction with and knowledge of different departmental functions are in the best position to translate important health care functions into electronic systems that provide optimal support to clinical practice.

QUALITY AND OUTCOMES REPORTING

Measuring and reporting results is the foundation of quality improvement. Reports that profile individual provider or provider team performance are a common part of an OM program because of their ability to drive performance improvement. The rapid demand for profiling that occurred in the early 1990s did little to reduce providers' fears of the growing managed care movement in the United States. Instead, reports that profiled provider or team outcomes were viewed as very threatening, often causing providers to disassociate from and distrust the very institutions in which they practiced.

The challenge today is to create strong bonds between providers and health care administrators in the pursuit for optimal performance. At the heart of this challenge is the need to transform thinking regarding quality reporting and profiles, from a punitive philosophy to one that embraces a partnership for the enhancement of practice and system efficiency. Realistically, patient outcomes are derived from such a partnership; whether it is a formal partnership or an informal one that is unrecognized by the parties involved, the products of care are the result of both provider and organizational system contributions. Steps must be taken to formalize and acknowledge the accountabilities of both parties in the reporting process to ensure that providers and system administrators partner for improvement.

BENCHMARK REPORTING

Reporting results and provider profiling are meaningless when unsupported by benchmarks. *Benchmarking* is the continuous process of cross-comparison of products (outcomes), services, and methods (processes) against competitors and industry leaders.[18] The principle driving the benchmark process is a vision of becoming the "best of the best," what the Japanese refer to as *dantotsu*.[19] When optimally conducted, benchmarking produces the tension necessary to support change, moving the workforce from a position of inertia to one of active involvement.[20]

The demand for benchmark reporting in health care has grown significantly in recent years and in all likelihood will continue to increase in sophistication over the next few years. Challenges related to outcomes benchmarking include the following:

- The heterogeneity of patients within discrete diagnostic populations
- The myriad applications of processes, which must be understood to support an understanding of cause and effect
- The dynamic nature of science
- Difficulties with measurement and control across the health care continuum

- Provider resistance to comparison processes and measurement of results

Process benchmarking involves an examination of practices within institutions and is aligned with Phase II of the OM model. Comparative benchmarking is focused on the achievement of targeted outcomes and is therefore an aspect of Phase IV of the OM model. Because the provision of health care comprises the trajectory of a patient from admission to discharge in numerous settings (using a variety of services and personnel), a two-pronged accountability—provider and system—must be acknowledged and quantified. The analysis of profiles must be supported by an understanding of this intricate interplay, which fosters thoughtful dialogue and realistic planning of improvement goals and action strategies.

| SEVERITY ADJUSTMENT

Simply comparing findings from one provider or institution to another does not provide a realistic picture of performance. Instead, differences in patient severity and risk must be addressed and controlled in a manner that fosters comparison of similar groups of patients. Without proper severity adjustment, data are meaningless. There is nothing that will endanger provider-administrative trust more than use of non–severity-adjusted profile data to benchmark performance. Providers are competitive beings by nature and profiles stimulate aggressive competition. Given this, the rules and regulations governing any performance benchmark competition must be fair and square; severity adjustment evens the score.

Severity is a term used to describe a relative loss of function. Functional loss can be described in a number of ways. The most sophisticated severity systems quantify significant physiologic changes associated with a disease state. Other severity measures rely on functional status indices or the ability to perform activities of daily living (ADLs) independently. Risk differs from severity in that it is a term used to describe the predicted potential for poor outcome. Risk-based systems are driven by variables found from analyses of similar series of cases to be predictive of untoward events, such as complications, high resource intensity, and death. Severity measures may be used to establish a baseline for comparison and then reused after the completion of care to assess for differences in functional loss. Pure risk-based systems should be used at the onset of care in an attempt to predict variables that may incur untoward outcomes at some point in the future.

Many commercially available systems overlap severity and risk properties significantly. In fact, the two terms are often used interchangeably in the health care community, as well as within the commercial sector. The growth of industries venturing into the development of risk- and/or severity-based computer systems has been phenomenal in the last 10 years. Many sophisticated, high-cost products are available today on the market, some of which attempt to adjust risk/severity across a wide variety of heterogeneous patient characteristics and diagnoses, the clinical logic of which should be closely scrutinized by the clinician.

Table 7–2 lists some of the more common commercially available severity adjustment systems on the market. A cost/benefit analysis should be conducted to support the decision of purchasing any commercial system. Many fine diagnosis-specific severity measures developed to support clinical trials are available at no cost to the user and should be considered seriously as an alternative to a commercially developed system. The advantage of using clinical trial severity instruments is greater than the cost savings alone. Many demonstrate superior performance in measuring severity in challenging heterogeneous patient populations. Additionally, they are often less time consuming for the provider or data abstractor. Lastly, because of their association with clinical trials, these instruments are often well understood and respected by the very clinicians whose patient outcomes will be measured and benchmarked.

Limitations governing many commercially available systems include the labor intensity associated with data abstraction, product cost, and dependence on a closed medical record's documentation accuracy. Great care should be taken to educate providers in documentation methods that enhance the accuracy of data abstraction. The risk of human error is a limitation that must be addressed in all severity

TABLE 7–2
Commercial Risk/Severity Adjustment Systems

System	Diagnosis Driven	Data Source and Collection Methods
Acute Physiology and Chronic Health Evaluation (APACHE)	No	• Uses clinical data • Focused on the clinically worst values in the first 24 hours of care
All patient-refined–diagnosis-related groups (APR-DRGs)	Yes	• Uses retrospective data collection • Discharge abstract drives the data collection process
Computerized severity index (CSI)	Yes	• Uses clinical data • Based on clinical values collected at different points during hospitalization
Medical Illness Severity Grouping System (MedisGroups)	No	• Uses clinical data • Based on clinical values collected at different points during hospitalization

Note: Not intended to be a comprehensive listing of commercially available systems.

systems through ongoing education and measurement of both inter-rater and intrarater reliability. When choosing a severity adjustment system, the following points should be considered:

- Does science support the variables that are used to adjust for disease severity?
- Is the system logically constructed?
- If a variety of diagnoses are included in the severity model, are they logically comparable for benchmarking?
- Does the system examine the total LOS or a specifically-defined episode within the stay?
- Are data collected retrospectively once the chart has been closed, or are they collected prospectively throughout the stay?
- What is the cost of the system, and are there other clinical tools or research instruments that could be used for severity adjustment at no cost?

| COMMON RISK/SEVERITY ADJUSTMENT TOOLS

One of the earliest attempts to control for patient severity was with the development of the case mix index (CMI). The CMI is used to determine case complexity. The average weight for a hospitalized case is set at 1.0. A CMI of 1.5 would be interpreted as a case that is expected to cost 1.5 times the average treatment cost.[21]

Medicare diagnosis-related groups (DRGs) have been used to severity adjust data, but their ability to effectively level the playing field is limited. Medicare DRGs break out select case mix groups by age, the presence of significant comorbidities or complications (CCs), and discharge disposition. However, the case mix adjustments made because of CCs in Medicare DRGs provide a nonuniform severity adjustment, in that some DRG categories lack the CC classification entirely, others are allotted a CC classification, and a few have a category that allows classification only of major CCs. Severity adjustment by Medicare DRGs disallows adjustment for the presence of multiple significant secondary diagnoses and is limited to patients within the Health Care Finance Administration (HCFA) reimbursement scheme.

3M Health Information Systems (3M HIS) developed all patient-refined–diagnosis-related groups (APR-DRGs) for use in adjusting patient data for severity across a wide variety of diagnoses and in populations beyond those reimbursed by the HCFA. The 3M HIS grouper provides an APR-DRG value and designates both a severity subclass and a risk of mortality subclass for hospitalized inpatients. The APR-DRG system is among the most commonly used systems for severity adjustment within U.S. hospitals.[21]

In Medicare DRGs, the presence of secondary diagnoses drives classification within a CC-designated category. In APR-DRGs, the severity logic adjusts for interactive effects between secondary diagnoses by increasing the overall severity subclassification. The designation of severity of illness and risk of mortality is driven by distinct patient attributes in APR-DRG classification. The extent of physiologic decompensation or organ system loss of function drives the classification of severity of illness, which reflects the total burden of illness for an inpatient stay.

In APR-DRGs, both severity and mortality risk are derived from an evaluation of all secondary diagnoses, which are defined as any diagnoses present on admission (comorbidities) or developed after admission (complications) that affected the treatment received or LOS. Secondary diagnoses are captured using patient discharge abstracts and assigned to one of four complexity levels: no/minor, moderate, major, or extreme. For select principle diagnoses, complexity level assignments for secondary diagnoses may change, in that some secondary diagnoses are logically related to certain principle diagnoses and therefore do not warrant a major increase in classification rank. Lastly, additional adjustments must be made for terminally ill patients designated as "Do Not Resuscitate."

While the APR-DRG score itself may be useful in severity adjusting data, it can also be used to benchmark performance during the course of a hospitalization. For example, one method for benchmarking performance with APR-DRGs is the comparison of a risk of mortality score (based solely on the comorbidities identified at patient admission) with a final risk of mortality score that is based upon all secondary diagnoses at discharge. The initial risk of mortality score reflects the patient risk at the time of admission based on comorbidities alone, before any medical or surgical intervention. This score is compared with the discharge risk score, which reflects both the comorbidities on admission and the complications that occurred over the course of hospitalization. Such a comparison may foster the identification of opportunities for performance improvement.[21]

Severity adjustment methods are likely to evolve over time and look quite different than they do today. With the exception of those methods that involve the use of a clinical research severity tool, there has been limited movement toward establishing methods for severity adjustment of data in the postacute arena. Some changes expected in the future are:

- Inclusion of quality of life and functional status data
- An ability to capture the entire trajectory of an illness across the continuum of care
- Identification of fewer, more specific, and more sensitive data elements for inclusion
- Computer-automated applications that reduce workload
- Mandatory adoption of standardized, uniform severity adjustment methodology that promotes benchmarking

| CONSTRUCTING REPORTS

Report format varies significantly depending on purpose. Considerations for the design of a report should include:

- Target audience(s)
- Ability to visually and narratively describe findings in relation to quality targets aligned with performance improvement
- Regulatory and accreditation requirements/standards
- Methods and mechanisms for benchmarking performance over time
- Potential use for consumer and payer marketing of health services
- The ability to stimulate analysis of future market potential

Two popular formats for reporting overall program quality include the clinical value compass, or instrument panel, and action plans. The traditional compass report format consists of four major categories: clinical outcomes, functional status, patient satisfaction, and cost.[22] The compass report format provides a one-page overview enabling assessment of the balance between cost and quality indices (Figure 7–4).

The action plan is another popular quality reporting format. Table 7–3 illustrates an action plan template used to identify quality targets, goals, findings, significant obstacles, plans, and responsible parties. Action

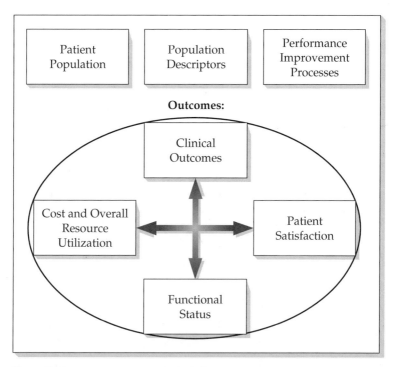

Figure 7–4
Components of the clinical value compass (or instrument panel). Note: Detailed data are written into each section and updated regularly with program refinement.

plan report formats are best complemented by graphic reports, which add a visual dimension to the report's primarily narrative format.

When constructing provider profiles, an additional set of considerations must be made. The provider must be involved in the profile development process; without this key ingredient, the report may not be received in the spirit in which it is offered. Important components of a profile include:

- Mechanisms that ensure privacy for the individual provider and/or team members profiled
- Time allotted for individual consultation regarding findings
- Severity-adjusted benchmarking against peers and/or services providing similar care within the institution—locally, regionally, and nationally
- Examination of practice patterns and processes associated with statistically significant differences in performance
- The use of cost data (charges often have little to no connection to the true cost of services)

TABLE 7–3

Action Plan Format for Reporting Quality

Quality Target	Goals	Findings	Significant Obstacles	Plan	Responsible Parties

As scientists, health care providers are by nature skeptical beings. Expect any report designed to profile and benchmark performance to be closely scrutinized. Report developers should expect that methods will be questioned and critiqued and that replication requests may be issued. Additionally, it is important to acknowledge that, given the forces governing local markets, there may be limited motivation among providers to change high resource practice patterns in settings where *per diem* reimbursement and limited competition exists.

A structured process should be developed to support the manner in which profile information is conveyed. Because the aim of the report is to stimulate performance improvement, the use of descriptors that label providers as "good" or "bad" practitioners must be carefully avoided. The final profile report should include the following elements[21]:

- A description of the methods for data collection and analysis
- A narrative summary of the profiles findings, including sample size, severity, peer and individual percentile rank, contributing provider/system processes, and limitations.
- Graphic display of benchmark data (i.e., outcome and process data)
- Provision of a detailed listing of cases included in the report for provider verification
- An appendix explaining methodology and other pertinent features of the report

Purchasers of care have open access to records of physician and hospital practice patterns and therefore are well positioned to aggregate and benchmark providers and institutions against competitors. Institutions that are successful at using benchmarking as a method to change practice are successful because of a partnership and trust between practitioners and administration, working together to achieve excellence in quality and a competitive market position.

Reports should provide documentation that assures both the general public and regulatory agencies that institutional performance is consistent with community and national standards. Reports should also assist organizations in making informed decisions regarding resource allocation, projected need for services, and opportunities for market expansion. Whatever the format, quality reports must link directly to the vision and mission of an organization. They should develop a plan for improvement, based on objective findings, that is communicated up and down the institution's corporate ladder.

The ultimate goal of quality reporting is public disclosure of health care institution performance.[21] Stakeholders associated with the right to these data include health care providers and administrators, governmental agencies, employers and benefit managers, the media, and the general public. The rationale governing the disclosure of health care performance data relates to the public's right to know the state of both institutional and individual provider quality. The tension developing between the use of reports for the public's information and the use of reports to stimulate quality improvement is rapidly mounting.

Successful release of public data must be supported by a partnership among the stakeholders to ensure consistent, high-quality standards. Significant attention will need to be paid to public education, so that accurate interpretation and use of quality data by lay persons is achieved. Lastly, reports have to assume a standardized format, including severity adjustment measures, to prevent those institutions that care for the sickest patients (e.g., tertiary care centers) from being penalized. While widespread dissemination of findings is central to the mission of research, the exact method and manner of release of quality data to the general public presently evades us.

| SUMMARY

Quality management is a dynamic process based on principles that mandate movement away from simple inspection and reporting to the systematic measurement of outcomes and processes, adoption of methods that reduce variability, and establishment of a provider and administrative partnership for ongoing performance improvement.

Clinical ITS have and will continue to be an important component in the measurement of health care quality. The development of smaller, faster computers with increased storage capabilities is rapidly changing the way patient care information is collected, stored, and retrieved. All institutions, regardless of size or location, are moving toward the implementation of ITS. The EMR is a key element of these systems, which are rapidly developing as knowledge tools for planning and delivering patient care. The linear paper record, as known today, serves mostly to document events and will soon become a remnant of the past.

Changes in the ability to capture, quantify, and report quality carries multiple responsibilities; the security of sensitive, confidential patient data and the assurance of the provider, institution, and public protection are paramount. Stakeholders in health care quality must be aware of these issues and assume leadership for the development of policies and procedures that will enhance overall system improvement and reduce risk for all parties involved.

References

1. Donabedian A: Quality assessment and assurance: unity of purpose, diversity of means, *Inquiry* 25(1):173-192, 1988.
2. Meisenheimer CG: *Improving quality: a guide to effective programs*, ed 2, Gaithersburg, Md, 1997, Aspen.
3. Isaacson SK et al: Health care: employers and individual consumers want additional information on quality, *Journal of Outcomes Management* 3(2):4-9, 1996.
4. Health Care Advisory Board: *Outcomes strategy: measurement of hospital quality under reform*, Washington, DC, 1993, The Advisory Board Company.

5. Donabedian A: *The definition of quality and approaches to its management,* Ann Arbor, Mich, 1980, Health Administration.

6. Larson SA: Standards: the basis of a quality improvement program. In Meisenheimer CG, ed: *Improving quality: a guide to effective programs,* ed 2, Gaithersburg, Md, 1997, Aspen.

7. Fields WL, Siroky KA: Converting data into information, *Journal of Nursing Care Quality* 8(3):1-11, 1994.

8. Batalden PB, Nelson EC, Roberts JS: Linking outcomes measurement to continual improvement: the Serial "V" way of thinking about improving clinical care, *Journal on Quality Improvement* 20(4):167-180, 1994.

9. Wheeler DJ: *Advanced topics in statistical process control,* Knoxville, Tenn, 1995, SPC Press.

10. Ball MJ, Douglas JV, Newbold SK: Integrating nursing and informatics. In Ball MJ et al, eds: *Nursing informatics: where caring and technology meet,* ed 2, New York, 1995, Springer-Verlag.

11. Gassert CA: Academic preparation in nursing informatics. In Ball MJ et al, eds: *Nursing informatics: where caring and technology meet,* ed 2, New York, 1995, Springer-Verlag.

12. Gorn S: Informatics (computer and information science): its ideology, methodology, and sociology. In Machlup F, Mansfield U, eds: *The study of information: interdisciplinary messages,* New York, 1983, John Wiley & Sons.

13. Hersher BS: Careers for nurses in health care information systems. In Ball MJ et al, eds: *Nursing informatics: where caring and technology meet,* ed 2, New York, 1995, Springer-Verlag.

14. Semancik M: The history of clinical information systems: legacy systems, computer-based patient record and point of care. In Semancik M, ed: *Clinical information systems,* Seattle, 1997, Scapulas Medical.

15. Computer-Based Patient Record Institute: *Work Group on Confidentiality, Privacy, and Security: guidelines for establishing information security policies at organizations using computer-based patient records,* Schaumburg, Ill, 1995, The Association.

16. Computer-Based Patient Record Institute: *Framework for the definition and modeling of the computer-based patient record environment.* Schaumburg, Ill, 1997, The Association.

17. Zielstorff RD: Capturing and using clinical outcome data: implications for information systems design. In Saba VK, Pocklington DB, Miller KP, eds: *Nursing and computers: an anthology, 1987-1996,* New York, 1998, Springer.

18. Camp RC: *Benchmarking: the search for industry best practices that lead to superior performance,* Milwaukee, Wis, 1989, Quality Press.

19. Camp RC, Tweet AG: Benchmarking applied to health care, *Journal on Quality Improvement* 20(5):229-238, 1994.

20. Mohr JJ et al: Clinical benchmarking for best patient care, *Journal on Quality of Improvement* 22(9):599-616, 1996.

21. Goldfield N, Boland P: *Physician profiling and risk adjustment,* Gaithersburg, Md, 1996, Aspen.

22. Nelson BC et al: Report card or instrument panels: who needs what? *Journal of Quality Improvement* 21:155-166, 1995.

CHAPTER 8

Effect of Technology on Costs and Outcomes in Critical Care

INTRODUCTION

Major efforts have been made in the past decade to reduce the costs associated with acute and critical care. These efforts grew in earnest at a time when health care reform was in its earliest stages. One of the major goals that has driven the reform movement is a reduction in the cost of U.S. health care. In comparison to other countries, the United States spends far more of its gross national product (GNP) on health care (Figure 8–1). Many ideas have been put forth on how to control costs. One area that frequently comes under the attention of cost control is technology utilization. Is this attention on technology utilization justified? The answer to this seemingly simple yet complex question is "yes."

When examining the costs in acute and critical care, technology utilization certainly plays a measurable role. The moment a patient enters an acute care area, technology is immediately put into action (Figure 8–2). This action can range from the use of electrocardiograph (ECG) monitoring, pulse oximetry, and intravenous pumps to venous and arterial access devices. In addition, less visible technology, such as the suction and oxygen systems built into the walls of most hospital rooms, are widely available. All this technology costs the hospital and patient money. Is the technology used in day-to-day practice worth the money invested in its application?

The value of technology has rarely been assessed. However, the effect of technology is probably best reflected by the following statement: "Technology is only as good as the skills and knowledge of the clinicians using it." The effect of technology varies between hospitals as a result of the different methods used to prepare and teach the clinicians to use it.

An example of this is demonstrated by the current debate over the value of the pulmonary artery catheter (PAC).[1] PAC usage can illustrate potential problems with technology. The appropriate use of PACs is driven by knowledge and skill, yet standardized educational methods, teaching strategies, and accreditation of clinicians have not been adopted across all practice sites that use this technology. In addition, though the use of PACs is higher in the United States than anywhere else in the world (Figure 8–3), well-designed outcomes studies that are able to link the use of PACs to optimal patient results have not been

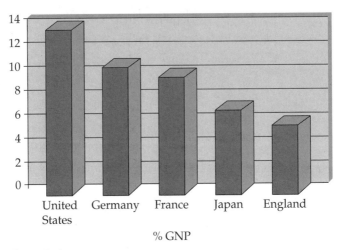

Figure 8–1 ——————————————————————————
Gross national product of the United States in comparison to other countries.

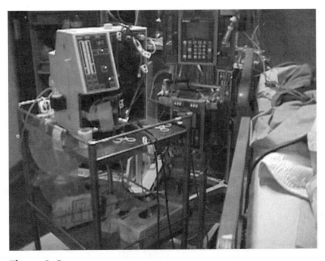

Figure 8–2 ——————————————————————————
Technology and critical care frequently intertwined.

executed. If problems with PACs do exist, they most likely stem from clinicians' skills in working with catheters rather than a problem with the technology itself.[2–4]

This chapter analyzes the actual and potential effects of technology and evaluates key steps to employing technology, which are applied in case study examples. The focus of this analysis is to help clinicians identify what is necessary to use technology appropriately. The appropriate use of technology clearly results in cost reduction without harming the quality of care provided. As this analysis unfolds, the use of

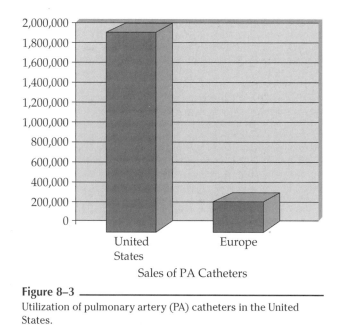

Figure 8–3
Utilization of pulmonary artery (PA) catheters in the United States.

technology in the "average" patient as well as the "outlier" will be clarified. For technology to be used appropriately, prioritizing technology utilization for optimum results must be done at each hospital. This chapter presents the foundation for developing this prioritization schema.

| DEFINITION OF TECHNOLOGY

Technology is a term that can be used to describe many of the techniques used to evaluate and treat acutely ill patients. For the purpose of this chapter, the focus of technology will be on patient monitoring technologies.

| ROLE OF TECHNOLOGY IN COSTS

Who Should Receive Technology?

The determination of who should receive technologies is a critically important point for patients, clinicians, and hospitals. One key point should guide the application of technology: the technology should have some direct effect on the patient being monitored. It is important to have clear expectations of technology and avoid using technology just because it is available. To illustrate this point, consider the widespread use of pulse oximetry. In many intensive care units (ICUs) and intermediate care units, pulse oximetry is performed on virtually every patient

(Figure 8–4), regardless of admitting problem or symptom. For example, patients with a gastrointestinal (GI) bleed or uncomplicated myocardial infarction (MI) are likely to have a pulse oximeter in place. Because pulse oximeters are primarily a technology that monitors lung function (or the effects of other organs on lung function), the use of this technology will not have much value in the assessment of the patients described above. The same can be said of routine ECG monitoring and many other technologies.

Critical thinking should support the selection of technologies employed in patient care. Patients should be evaluated at admission to determine the types of technology that will best suit their monitoring needs. If a patient is at risk for pulmonary dysfunction, then pulse oximetry monitoring is appropriate. However, if lung function is unlikely to be a factor in the patient's condition, then pulse oximetry use is unnecessary. Such an approach is not the standard in many clinical settings. Some technologies are applied more often than necessary due to a lack of critical thinking.

One of the most important responsibilities facing a clinician is determining when technology is no longer beneficial. Removal of technology that is no longer beneficial is important for several reasons. If the patient has technology that is generating information, clinicians will be prone to treat changes detected by the technology. Treatment of this nature is fine as long as it benefits the patient's outcome. However, technologies have the tendency to encourage over-treatment by simply providing information that, although available, is not necessarily important. Keep in mind the following concept: "The ultimate goal of any treatment should be improvement of the patient's prognosis, comfort,

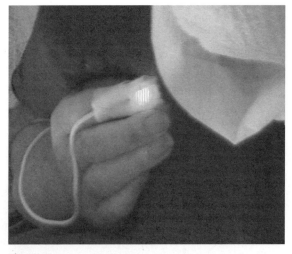

Figure 8–4 _____
Pulse oximetry application is often overused.

well being, or general state of health. Not every measurable physiologic effect is beneficial if it fails to meet this goal."[5]

Identifying when a technology will no longer benefit a patient is a key step in cost control. Patients with life-threatening conditions that are so severe that survival is unlikely no longer benefit from the technology that is used to monitor their physiologic status. However, clinicians tend to be hesitant about removing technologies once they are put in place.

The PAC is once again a good example of this problem. When the flow-directed PAC was developed by Dr. Swan and Dr. Ganz, the goal was to use the technology for short periods of time (i.e., to identify rapidly which therapies work) and then remove the catheter. An examination of current practice reveals that PACs are left in place for days instead of hours. This practice is driven by the ability to obtain data that is unavailable after the catheter has been removed.

EFFECT OF TECHNOLOGY ON "AVERAGE" PATIENTS

The effect of technology on the "average" patient varies. Keep in mind that the majority of patients have short stays in the hospital or ICU. Technology can only modestly affect the length of stay (LOS) on a patient that is only in the ICU for a few days. The manner in which technology can affect patient and cost outcomes is illustrated below in three case studies that highlight technologic effect.

CASE STUDY I   *Guiding Therapies to Allow for Rapid Titration of Drugs*[6]

A 72-year-old man is admitted to the unit with the diagnosis of acute exacerbation of congestive heart failure (CHF). Initial therapy with diuretics does not relieve his shortness of breath. A flow-directed PAC is inserted to help improve evaluation of the condition. Dobutamine therapy is started at 3 µg/kg/min. After 15 minutes, hemodynamic parameters are repeated. No physical changes have occurred except the patient feels "a little better." The following changes in the patient are measured:

Parameter	Before dobutamine	After dobutamine
SvO_2 (mixed venous oxyhemoglobin)	0.48	0.68
Stroke index	22	31
Cardiac index	2.2	2.5

Note that the SvO$_2$, stroke index, and cardiac index have all returned to normal. The therapy has been successful and can stop at this point. Keep in mind that none of these parameters are available by physical assessment. The data obtained from the PAC technology has allowed immediate assessment of the therapy plus identified that therapy does not need further adjustment. Without this information, further titration of the drug may have occurred since no measurable physical changes took place.

CASE STUDY II   *Providing Information that Accelerates Diagnosis and Early Intervention*[7]

A 43-year-old man underwent coronary angioplasty 8 hours ago and is doing well. His femoral sheath is removed by the physician, during which time the patient complains of nausea. He states he is "squeamish when he sees blood." Within an hour of the sheath removal, the patient's nausea increases. He is very anxious and afraid that something is wrong. The physician has left instructions for the patient to call him and the cardiac catheterization personnel immediately if he shows evidence of occlusion at the angioplasty site. The evidence available to the nurse is the data provided by ST segment monitoring technology. Evaluating the ST segment program indicates that the patient's ST segments are unchanged.

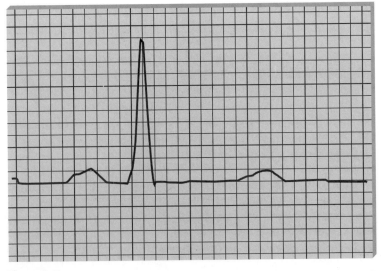

Figure 8–5
ST segments are unchanged indicating noncardiac origin of chest discomfort.

This information allows the nurse to focus on relieving noncardiac-induced nausea and monitor the patient continuously via the ST segment program for further changes. The patient recovers uneventfully and is discharged a few hours later. Without the ST segment information, the physician would have been more inclined to treat this as a cardiac event. Now the nurse and physician can feel comfortable that there is a noncardiac source for this patient's nausea.

CASE STUDY III	*Detecting Events that are Undetectable, yet Clinically Important, by Physical Assessment*

A 27-year-old man with a history of asthma and anxiety becomes short of breath. The clinician must differentiate an anxiety episode from physiologic origin; is the problem anxiety-based or physiologic in nature?

Parameter monitored	Value
Ve (i.e., minute ventilation—amount of air inspired or expired in one minute)	13.5 L/min
$PaCO_2$ (i.e., arterial carbon dioxide level)	37 mm Hg
RR (respiratory rate)	34 bpm

Note the $PaCO_2$ level, obtained from an arterial blood gas measurement, is normal despite an elevated minute ventilation. Keep in mind that neither $PaCO_2$ levels or minute ventilation (i.e., respiratory rate multiplied by tidal volume) are detectable by physical examination alone. Normally, in the case of an anxiety attack, $PaCO_2$ levels fall while minute ventilation increases. Noting that this has not occurred, anxiety is determined to be an unlikely source for the patient's problem, which is probably related to an increase in physiologic deadspace, thereby producing shortness of breath. The use of technology to measure minute ventilation (e.g., flow meters, spirometers) and arterial carbon dioxide levels (e.g., arterial blood gas measurements) facilitates this interpretation. Without this information, clinicians may select incorrect therapies, such as anxiolytic agents, which would not only fail to relieve the problem but also likely increase the hospital LOS and costs.

EFFECT OF TECHNOLOGY ON "OUTLIERS" OR "ATYPICAL PATIENTS"

Technology utilization in a hospital is markedly affected by a group of patients called "outliers." *Outliers* are patients who consume disproportionate amounts of technology, resources, and costs in comparison to other patients; a typical definition is a patient who is more than two standard deviations off the mean in terms of cost per case.

Outliers are atypical representatives of the average patient within a given diagnostic category. They are not rapidly discharged from the ICU or the hospital and they do not recover or die quickly. Their clinical course is marked by deviations from "normal." Outlier care cannot be mapped out on a pathway, as their course is marked with complications. Their mortality and morbidity rates are much higher than the average patient and outlier cost per case is markedly higher than that of more typical patients (Figure 8–6). Outlier patients often suffer prolonged and complex clinical courses that are marked by lack of achievement of desired patient, family, or clinician outcomes. This group's management commonly evokes ethical dilemmas and eventually placement problems within both the acute care system and postacute settings.

Outlier data distorts the assessment of the appropriate use of technology. This group consumes resources so significantly that their presence in data representing technology utilization may result in misleading values compared to typical patients with similar primary diagnoses (Figure 8–7). Consider the experience of one hospital during an attempt

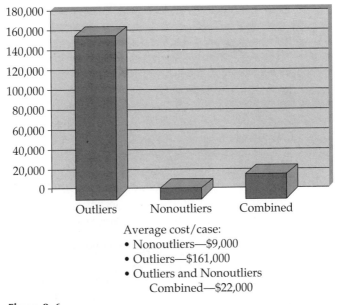

Average cost/case:
- Nonoutliers—$9,000
- Outliers—$161,000
- Outliers and Nonoutliers
  Combined—$22,000

Figure 8–6
Cost per case for outliers is much higher than for average patients.

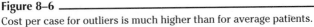

to reduce the number of arterial blood gas measurements taken in the medical ICU. The hospital administrative staff identified that the medical ICU used 5709 blood gases in a year, or an average of 4.5 per patient. The goal was to eliminate 1000 blood gases (saving about $5000 in costs and $65,000 in charges) and reduce the average blood gas volume to about 3.5 per patient. Had outliers been considered in the initial assessment, the strategies proposed for this situation would have been completely different.

The outliers in the ICU (62 patients) had an average blood gas usage of 43 tests per patient, while the nonoutlier patients (1202) averaged three tests per patient. Outliers were responsible for almost 50% of the blood gases ordered for this patient group, while average patients had already reached the desired threshold per patient. The use of three blood gases per patient reflected appropriate care needed to safely monitor average cases. However, in the outlier group, poor outcomes resulted regardless of the number of blood gases ordered. This example illustrates the importance of accurately assessing data to determine opportunities for cost control. Efforts at blood gas reduction across all patients may have placed over 90% of patients at risk for a reduction in the quality of care, while not truly identifying the source of the problem.

IDENTIFYING WHERE TO ACHIEVE "BIGGEST BANG"— PRIORITIZING EFFORTS

Prioritizing efforts for appropriate utilization of technology will vary between hospitals. However, many hospitals have a major problem in terms of outlier management. In most cases, controlling outlier management has a major effect on the reduction of costs associated with technology. For example, reducing unnecessary use of technology in the

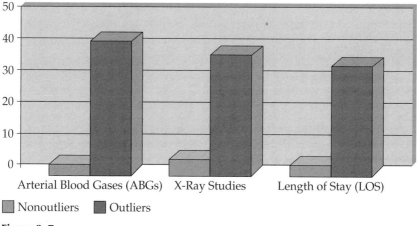

Figure 8–7
Outliers distort use of resources on an "average" patient.

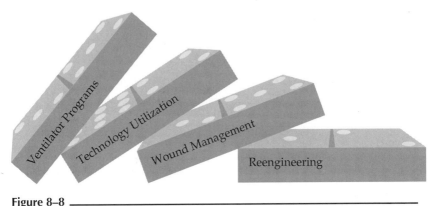

Figure 8–8 _____
Domino effort of controiling outliers.

outlier group by 10% will have a major effect on cost. In the blood gas example given above, 270 arterial blood gases would have been avoided with a 10% reduction in outlier use. However, the "domino effect" may also occur—a reduction in the use of routine ECG monitoring, fewer pulse oximetry probes, a decrease in central venous access devices, fewer specialty beds, and fewer IV pumps (Figure 8–8).

The effect of reducing technology utilization in the outlier group by 10% is equivalent to implementing a series of programs that affect a much larger patient population. Reducing technology utilization in the outlier group by 10% might involve addressing a handful of patients. However, to obtain an equivalent cost effect by working solely with changes in practice for average patients, the volume of patients affected would need to increase significantly, as well as the control measures put in place to enforce the appropriate use of technology. The bottom line is that addressing outliers requires far less effort for changing a hospital's infrastructure and the behavior of clinicians than does a program that must address larger numbers of patients.

Outlier management should be planned carefully (Table 8–1). Identifying current practice (e.g., occupancy patterns), outlier effects, key clinicians and administrators, and potential barriers to change are all key steps in the development of a process to effectively manage outliers. The effects of outlier technology utilization is a critical aspect of cost control that cannot be ignored.

COSTS ASSOCIATED WITH TECHNOLOGY ACQUISITION

Costs associated with technology can be divided into several segments. These include the following:

- The cost of purchasing the technology
- The cost of educating staff to use the technology

TABLE 8–1

Outlier Program Occurs in Planned Stages

Temporal Order of Stages	Person Responsible
Developing awareness of outlier problem • Evaluation of current effect of outliers • Identification of survival characteristics in ICUs (as program develops, expand to other units)	Champion of the program (e.g., advanced practice nurse [APN], physician, manager)
Developing sense of urgency to address the problem • Presentation to key clinical and administrative personnel • Explanation of effects, if addressed	Champion
Developing solution • Presentation of current science (best practices) • Adaptation of current science to individual hospital • Identification of barriers to success • Development of incentives for key personnel • Development of a continuous quality improvement (CQI) program to assess the need for changes in a program as it is implemented	All team members
Implementing solution • Pilot phase • Adaptation of original program to address problems found in pilot phase • Implementation of adapted program • Adjustments as necessary based on CQI program	All team members
Measuring effects	The champion, information systems, statistician
Interpretation of results	All team members—emphasis is on the champion
Presentation of results • To internal customers • Publication in scientific journals	Champion

• Maintenance costs
• Adverse events from using the technology

The use of ST segment monitoring serves as an example for the costs associated with the use of technology (Table 8–2). The cost of ST segment monitoring is about $2000 per bed. If an ICU with 12 beds incorporates ST segment monitoring into all of its beds, the cost to the hospital will be $24,000. However, factoring in costs related to staff

TABLE 8–2

Costs Associated with ST Segment Monitoring

Cost Concepts	Cost Factors
Cost of the technology (assume 12 monitors purchased)	$24,000
Maintenance costs ($500/monitor)	$ 6,000
Education costs	$ 2,400
Assumptions:	
• 4 hours per clinician	
• Average salary $20/hour	
• Number of clinicians = 30	
Adverse event costs	None expected
Total costs	$32,400
Life span of monitor	10 years
Number of patients used on in 10 years	1000
Assumptions:	
• Average LOS = 3 days	
• Occupancy = 80%	
Average Patient Cost	$32.40

education and maintenance adds approximately $8400 to total costs. Often the "soft" costs associated with technology, namely staff education and maintenance, are not considered when determining overall costs of technology.

| EFFECT OF TECHNOLOGY ON OUTCOMES

The primary mechanism through which technology reduces cost is through improved patient outcomes. Does technology such as ECG or ST segment monitoring, pulse oximetry, or PACs improve patient outcomes? Research evidence is lacking in this regard. Studies that have assessed the accuracy of technologies (e.g., pulse oximetry) in detecting clinical problems are available in the literature, but the ability of technology to actually cause improvement in patient outcomes is unclear.[8] Positive effect on patient care is cited in association with almost every form of technology documented in medical literature,[9–15] but the studies making these claims tend to have small numbers of patients enrolled and are nonrandomized or prospective in design, limiting the ability to generalize findings.

It seems unlikely that thoughtfully applied technologies would fail to have an effect on patient outcome. All technologies have the potential to improve patient outcomes. For example, capnography can reduce the number of deaths and brain injuries occurring from inadvertent esophageal (as opposed to tracheal) intubation. However, the incidence of such a problem may be too infrequent to make this effect obvious. Nonetheless, for each esophageal intubation that is avoided, costs are reduced and patient outcomes are improved.

| ROLE OF EDUCATION

Improving patient outcomes is related to the application of technology in situations where it will have greatest benefit. A combination of education and changes in practice behaviors support this goal. Education of clinicians in the appropriate and safe use of technology is paramount, making it surprising that so little attention and support is given to this in the clinical arena. Education of clinicians is usually performed initially by representatives of the manufacturer and is often supplemented thereafter by hospital personnel. The quality and quantity of these programs vary significantly and are usually not supported by standards to guide practice implementation or outcomes assessment. Instead, most technology educational programs tend to focus primarily on operational issues. This focus is important during initial learning phases, but the focus should shift to optimal clinical application once operational mastery has been achieved. In most settings, the educational process supporting appropriate technology utilization and management is in need of significant improvement.

Clinicians rapidly learn the basics of how a technology is used. While the basics are important, the full effect of technology cannot be assured if basics remain the only foundation for use in clinical practice.[16] Education must increase to ensure that technology in complex clinical areas, such as the critical care unit, is used to its fullest potential. When education time is cut in an attempt to control costs and time is not allocated for supplemental education, the benefits of technology may not be realized.

This is illustrated by the following example involving the use of capnography. Capnography is the measurement of exhaled carbon dioxide. It is an essential technology for the assessment of tracheal intubation and is a good indicator of the adequacy of resuscitation and survival during resuscitation. Appropriate use of capnography can reduce the number of necessary arterial blood gas measurements and other assessments of intubated patients. However, the introduction of capnography in critical care areas failed to fully develop the primary application (intubation) and incompletely addresses other applications. The result of this oversight is an inability of this technology to consistently reach its full effect. Avoiding improper placement of an endotracheal tube once in 10 years can save the hospital hundreds of thousands of dollars in clinical and legal costs. The education associated with the use of this technology is well worth the added time in paying clinicians to attend educational sessions aimed at optimizing the use of this technology in clinical practice.

INFRASTRUCTURE REQUIREMENTS (COMMITMENT TO USE)

The commitment to use technology optimally is a major one, requiring cooperation between management and key clinicians. Managers must be willing to invest in the technology as well as provide the resources necessary to educate clinicians optimally. Clinicians must have a clear understanding of what the technology can do and then use it in such a way that patient management is improved.

For example, if SvO_2 monitoring is acquired by the hospital, clinicians must agree as to how this technology will change and improve practice. In the past, assessments might have relied more on blood pressures and cardiac output values. But if SvO_2 technology is available, this should dramatically effect the level of significance that was previously placed on parameters such as arterial blood pressure and cardiac output values, altering practice patterns for the better.

Appropriate utilization of technology requires interdisciplinary commitment. Key clinicians, such as nurses and physicians, must come to agreement on essential concepts. These concepts include such things as agreeing upon which aspects of a technologically-derived parameter are to be treated, which require notification, and which can safely be ignored. In addition, it must be made clear how technologically-derived information will be utilized in practice. Will basics be the goal or will advanced application occur? This agreement is the cornerstone of effective utilization of information derived from technology.

The manner in which the technology is to be implemented needs to be addressed as well. Two examples will help illustrate this point. First, if outliers or challenging populations are to be addressed, the use of a collaborative practice team (CPT) charged with protocol development may be appropriate. Teams work well when a complex, focused topic is to be addressed (i.e., the management of outlier cases, challenges associated with weaning from mechanical ventilation).

Protocols work well when the parameter to be monitored is easily defined. Use of pulse oximetry to titrate oxygen concentrations is a good example of an area where protocol management would be successful in supporting the appropriate utilization of technology. For example, a recommendation to reduce oxygen content until the SpO_2 is 0.93 could be written into protocol format. This supports easily manageable and measurable processes, minimizing deviations from the standard. In addition to identifying how technology should be implemented, it should be clear as to when the technology should be removed. Excessive and unnecessary use of technology leads to both increased costs and patient risk. Protocols also support termination of technology in a manner that reduces unnecessary risk related to cost.

Once a method for implementing the technology has been agreed upon, a timeline for implementation is necessary. In addition, it is essential that specific responsibilities and expectations be clearly woven into the timeline. As part of the timeline, incentives for achieving success, such as an employee recognition program, may help ensure participation and achievement of appropriate technology utilization.

Barriers to technology implementation can be structural in nature (e.g., unavailable supplies) or related to personnel (e.g., individual knowledge levels, failure to participate). How well barriers are surmounted dictates how much success will be achieved in the utilization of any technology.[17]

| QUALITY MONITORING

When any technology is introduced, efforts to ensure that the technology is positively affecting patient care must be taken. To ensure the effective utilization of technology, a quality monitoring program should be developed and implemented. Recommendations for the development of a quality monitoring program for measuring the effects of technology on patient outcomes are as follows:

1. Measure baseline practice outcomes prior to the implementation of new technology and other process or system changes that will occur.
2. Identify the outcome variables that will be effected by the new technology.
3. Acquire the technology and develop clinicians in its use.
4. Implement the new technology and associated practice changes.
5. Measure the effects of the technology and new practices on the outcome variables.
6. Evaluate the cost/benefit of the new technology based on accumulated outcomes data.

| COMMUNICATION BETWEEN CLINICIANS, PATIENTS, AND FAMILIES

Ensuring that patients and families understand the technology used to manage care is an essential responsibility of clinicians. Learning needs should be assessed and the presentation of unnecessary or unwanted technical information should be omitted or delayed until the timing is right for receipt of more in-depth information.[18] Written materials may enhance understanding and allow meaningful dialogue with patients and families.

Clinicians should reflect on methods to improve their ability to communicate effectively with patients and families. Overly technical discussions should be avoided and clinicians should encourage patients and family to ask questions and seek clarification as needed. In the case of outlier management, which may involve removal of technologies, clear, two-way communication regarding achievable outcomes and appropriate management strategies should be sought. Because removal of technology may be an early step in allowing a patient to die, patients (when able to communicate) and their family should clearly understand the differences between supportive care and curative management strategies.

Rarely do patients and families make decisions regarding the type of technology that will be used in their care. Instead, patients articulate outcomes of the care process that they hope to achieve. It is the clinician's responsibility to make decisions that are guided by a patient or family's articulated, desired outcomes regarding the optimal use of technologies. Providing patients and families with clear treatment recommendations and a basic understanding of the technologies that will be used to deliver care is an important step in partnering with consumers of health services in the decision-making process.

| SUMMARY

Technology utilization reduces costs and improves practice quality. Appropriate utilization of technology is facilitated by optimal development of key clinicians and administrators. In addition, clinicians and administrators must focus efforts where they will have the greatest potential for effect. The management of outliers, for example, can have a major effect on technology utilization, improving patient management and overall institutional costs. Specific technologies may be optimally utilized in practice when supported by protocols or clinical team management, reducing the need to disrupt the overall patient management infrastructure.

References

1. Connors AF et al: The effectiveness of right heart catheterization in the initial care of critically ill patients, *JAMA* 276:889-97,1996.
2. Vincent JL et al: Is the pulmonary artery catheter misused? A European view, *Criwt Care Med:* 26:1283-87, 1998.
3. Ahrens TS: Is nursing education adequate for pulmonary artery catheter utilization? *New Horiz* 5:281-85, 1997.
4. Papadakos PJ, Vendor JS: Training requirements for pulmonary artery catheter utilization in adult patients, *New Horiz* 5:287-91, 1997.
5. Weber LJ, Campbell ML: Medical futility and life-sustaining treatment decisions, *J Neurosci Nurs* 28:56-60, 1996.
6. Powers C, Ahrens TS: The use of SvO_2 monitoring in assessing cardiac drug therapy, *Transport* 3:1-5, 1992.
7. Ahrens TS: Changing perspectives in the assessment of oxygenation, *Crit Care Nurse,* 13:78-83, 1993.
8. Severinghaus JW, Kelleher JF: Recent developments in pulse oximetry, *Anesth* 76:1018-38, 1992.
9. Patel DJ et al: Long-term prognosis in unstable angina: the importance of early risk stratification using continuous ST segment monitoring, *Eur Heart J* 19:240-9, 1998.

10. Langer A: Prognostic significance of ST segment shift early after resolution of ST elevation in patients with myocardial infarction treated with thrombolytic therapy: the GUSTO-I ST Segment Monitoring Substudy, *J Am Coll Cardiol* 3:783-9, 1998.

11. Kremzar B et al: Normal values of SvO_2 as therapeutic goal in patients with multiple injuries, *Intensive Care Med* 23:65-70, 1997.

12. Hassan E, Roffman DS, Applefeld MM: The value of mixed venous oxygen saturation as a therapeutic indicator in the treatment of advanced congestive heart failure, *Am Heart J* 11:743-9, 1987.

13. Williamson JA et al: The Australian Incident Monitoring Study. The capnography: applications and limitations—an analysis of 2000 incident reports, *Anesth Intensive Care* 21:551-7, 1993.

14. Holland R, Webb RK, Ruchman WB: The Australian Incident Monitoring Study. Esophageal intubation: an analysis of 2000 incident reports, *Anesth Intensive Care* 21:608-10, 1993.

15. Levine RL, Wayne MA, Miller CC: End tidal carbon dioxide and outcome of out-of-hospital cardiac arrest, *N Engl J Med* 337:301-6, 1997.

16. Ahrens TS: Technology utilization in the cardiac surgical patient: SvO_2 and capnography monitoring, *Crit Care Nurs Quart* 21:24-40, 1998.

17. Ahrens TS: Impact of technology on costs and patient outcome, *Crit Care Nurs Clin* 10:117-125, 1998.

18. Gilligan T, Raffin TA: Physician virtues and communicating with patients, *New Horiz* 5:6-14, 1997.

CHAPTER 9

Building Support for Outcomes Management Implementation

INTRODUCTION

The development and implementation of an outcomes management (OM) program must be supported by institution-wide commitment. Numerous employees, at varying levels within an institution, must be educated regarding the overall structure of the program, the organization's philosophy of OM, and their individual roles and responsibilities in an OM initiative. A sense of employee ownership of the OM process must be developed to drive individual commitment in the continuous improvement of practice.

This chapter focuses on building support for an OM initiative, including measures that facilitate staff involvement like development of objective performance criteria and employee educational strategies.

EMPLOYEE PERFORMANCE CRITERIA SUPPORTING OUTCOMES MANAGEMENT

Health care institutions employ a variety of interdisciplinary direct care providers and ancillary service personnel. While OM leadership is essential, program success is often determined by the level of commitment among direct care providers. Direct care providers make up the bulk of any health care institution's work force; without their support and involvement in OM, the program is likely to fail regardless of its sophistication and good intent.

Direct caregiver support for OM is driven by two essential components: employee ownership and employee accountability. A sense of employee ownership is built through a shared leadership philosophy.[1] Leaders behind the organization of OM must collaborate with interdisciplinary staff to create an atmosphere that invites involvement and team ownership of both the process and the outcomes achieved. A member of each group of interdisciplinary providers directly involved in the care of an OM patient population should be identified for membership on a collaborative practice team (CPT).[1,2] The responsibilities of staff CPT members are identified in Box 9–1.

> **Box 9–1**   *Responsibilities of an Interdisciplinary Staff Collaborative Practice Team Member*
>
> - Serves as the voice for the discipline represented.
> - Demonstrates a collaborative practice, shared leadership philosophy.
> - Maintains current knowledge of research and practice literature affecting the discipline's delivery of care to the assigned population.
> - Collaborates on the development of new practice interventions designed to enhance patient outcomes.
> - Presents and negotiates use of evidence-based practices to replace methods of care that are not scientifically sound.
> - Assists with the development of strategies to enhance acceptance of practice changes.
> - Writes definitions for study variables to enhance validity and reliability.
> - Constructs and revises structured care methodologies (SCMs).
> - Assists with data collection as needed.
> - Participates in the design of research methods and the critique of study findings.
> - Disseminates study findings to members of the discipline represented, administrators, and other interdisciplinary staff.
> - Participates in the presentation of study findings through professional lectures or publication.
>
> Reprinted with permission from the Health Outcomes Institute, Inc, The Woodlands, Texas.

Staff should be encouraged to contribute research questions for study and participate in the planning, development, implementation, evaluation, and revision of OM strategies. A top-heavy, administratively controlled program is less likely to be successful and will be incapable of fully understanding clinical problems, their contributors, and possible solutions from a relevant caregiver viewpoint.[1] Instead of decisions being made at the point furthest away from the patient, the leadership pyramid must be turned upside down, enabling those closest to the patient to redefine their care practices and environments (Figure 9–1).

Performance expectations should support direct caregiver and ancillary staff involvement in OM. Specific criteria should define the accountabilities of staff in a variety of positions. Staff should participate in the development of their position's performance criteria and share in the accountability associated with attainment or lack of success in managing targeted population outcomes.[1]

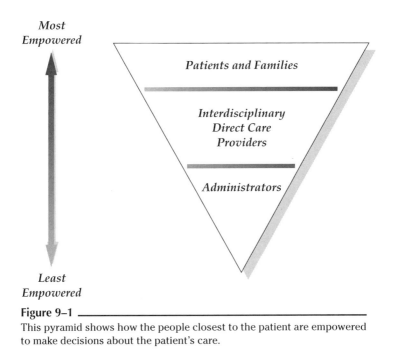

*Most
Empowered*

*Least
Empowered*

Figure 9–1 _____
This pyramid shows how the people closest to the patient are empowered
to make decisions about the patient's care.

Interdisciplinary Direct Caregivers

The role of the interdisciplinary staff should include participation in the development and organization of an outcomes data repository, consistent with Phase I of the OM model (see Figure 1–2). Direct caregivers are also key to the development, implementation, and revision of structured care methodologies (SCMs) in Phase II. They must achieve mastery of new procedures implemented in Phase III and provide feedback in Phase IV regarding needed improvement strategies to further enhance care delivery.

When documentation processes have been altered to include specific SCMs, direct caregivers should be consulted to advise the development of methods that do not add to the documentation burden, but rather reduce or streamline charting processes. They must then support the use of new documentation tools and become proficient in their use to further support the initiative.

Data collection is often identified as a responsibility of direct caregivers. However, OM leaders are cautioned to limit the number of data collectors because of problems that may emerge related to the reliability and validity of data. Caregivers that may qualify for participation in data collection include those who repeatedly provide highly competent or expert-level practice, exercise a sound understanding of the pathophysiology managed, and demonstrate an interest in clinical research and continuous quality improvement (CQI).

Caregivers involved with data collection should only be required to capture data related to their specific area of practice. For example, an untoward intermediate outcome (UIO) related to the development of malnutrition should be defined, measured, and collected by a registered dietitian; similarly, activity intolerance interfering with participation in physical therapy is best defined, measured, and collected by a physical therapist. Administrators should consider the development of clinical ladder criteria to support identification of caregivers that may be empowered to assist with this important aspect of OM programs. Caregivers participating in data collection should be credentialed and measurement of interrater reliability should be conducted regularly.

As data are processed and findings are revealed, direct caregivers should receive timely feedback related to patient outcome attainment. Sharing data with staff on a regular basis enhances program ownership, participation, and pride; it also enhances appreciation for the research process, stimulating staff development of pertinent clinical questions or research utilization strategies.[1,3]

Interdisciplinary direct caregivers should be evaluated throughout the year and annually on their contribution to the OM process. Box 9–2 identifies performance criteria that may be incorporated in a position description to enhance accountability for direct caregivers aligned with an OM initiative.

The Nurse Manager

Nursing staff make up the largest volume of employees within most health care institutions. Because of this, nursing staff and managerial contributions supporting OM are paramount to program success. The nurse manager role has changed dramatically over the past several years. Whereas once a nurse manager had authority for one patient care unit, today these individuals act as executives, managing a number of units supporting a clinical service. Because of this, nurse manager oversight may be delegated to unit-based nursing positions, which should also be aligned with the roles and accountabilities associated with OM.[1]

Chapter 3 discusses the accountabilities of the primary leaders for an OM initiative, namely the outcomes manager, physician, and service line manager. It is essential to note that the relationship between these OM leaders and the nurse manager is vital to the success of the program.

On an organizational ladder, the nurse manager usually is positioned laterally to the outcomes manager. As the peer of the outcomes manager, the nurse manager position should be considered instrumental in fostering active nursing staff participation and support for OM. Whereas the outcomes manager focuses on clinical CQI, the nurse manager's emphasis is on clinical operations. The outcomes manager and nurse manager should share a collegial and collaborative relationship, supported by common clinical service and population-specific goals.[1] Table 9–1

BOX 9–2   *Outcomes Management Performance Criteria for a Direct Caregiver*

- Assesses, provides care, and documents patient progress using select structured care methodologies (SCMs) for targeted patient population(s).
- Notifies appropriate interdisciplinary team members of patient needs; obtains necessary orders and consultations as specified by SCMs.
- Consults with the outcomes manager regarding the management of complex, high-risk patients.
- Informs the case manager of issues related to resource utilization, discharge planning, and systems or provider variances.
- Stays informed regarding outcomes research findings and implications for practice.
- Contributes to the development of research questions within the study population.
- Actively pursues continuous quality improvement (CQI) of clinical practice as demonstrated by mastery of new clinical practice standards for study population.
- Participates in data collection to support research initiatives as requested by collaborative practice teams (CPTs).
- Participates as a member of the CPT as requested by the manager or CPT leadership.

Note: Direct caregivers include all licensed clinical positions involved in providing health care services to the target population (e.g., physicians, nurses, respiratory therapists, pharmacists, physical therapists, occupational therapists, speech and language pathologists, social workers, and registered dietitians). Reprinted with permission from the Health Outcomes Institute, Inc, The Woodlands, Texas.

---

identifies the complementary processes used by nurse managers and outcomes managers to support an OM initiative.

Outcomes managers should serve as clinical experts, while nurse managers must operate as expert administrative leaders for their specific clinical service area. Nurse managers successfully supporting an OM initiative demonstrate effective interpersonal communication, mentoring, and negotiating skills; business expertise; objectivity; patient/family and staff advocacy; and systems thinking.[1]

Nurse managers should serve as essential "reality checkpoints," validating performance expectations that can be accomplished realistically and identifying the best strategies for enhancing staff ownership of the OM program. By working collaboratively with the outcomes manager,

TABLE 9–1

Complementary Processes of the Nurse Manager and Outcomes Manager

Nurse Manager	Outcomes Manager
• Is accountable for clinical management and operations.	• Is accountable for collaborative practice team (CPT) performance and clinical outcomes.
• Undertakes role modeling and staff development related to leadership, collaboration, and professionalism.	• Undertakes role modeling of expert clinical practice, research utilization, collaboration, and professionalism.
• Facilitates the development and implementation of unit-based outcomes management (OM) programs; ensures staff participation and ownership.	• Leads CPT development of interdisciplinary interventions for testing within a service-wide OM program.
• Creates a unit-based shared leadership council structure to implement clinical continuous quality improvement (CQI) programs driven by outcomes research findings.	• Presents research findings related to study populations in a manner that promotes research utilization and facilitates the generation of research questions or hypotheses for testing.
• Evaluates staff nurse participation in the service-wide OM program.	• Provides opportunity for staff ownership of the OM program.
• Budgets and engineers service-wide structural changes driven by outcomes findings, including position allocation, supplies, and capital equipment.	• Collaborates with members of the CPT to plan new programs for patient populations.

Reprinted with permission from the Health Outcomes Institute, Inc, The Woodlands, Texas.

nurse managers set the tone for administrative expectations and define performance success for their staff. A self-directed, goal-oriented nurse manager can lead the nursing staff and those from other support areas toward a commitment to teamwork and enhanced patient outcomes.[1]

The nurse manager's business expertise should be used by the service line manager in the development of service-wide goals and budgeting.[1] The collaborative efforts of the nurse manager and CPT leaders culminates in the development of a strategic plan that will carry the service into the future, addressing both clinical and business organizational priorities.

The Case Manager

In Chapter 1, the differences of outcomes and case management are discussed. Chapter 3 focuses on leaders of an OM program, including the role of the outcomes manager. Case management, or the process of overseeing individual patient care coordination, provides an ability to apply research-based OM strategies on a case-by-case basis.[3]

Functions of a case manager include utilization review, facilitation of patient movement through the health care system, collaboration with patients and other interdisciplinary health care providers to organize a discharge plan that meets the approval of designated payers, and the recording of system or provider variances that prevent timely movement of the patient through the health care system.[1,3]

Often when case manager positions are conceived, utilization review/utilization management (UR/UM) becomes the primary position responsibility, and the traditional case management functions involving discharge planning and care coordination are dropped from the role. However, separation of UR/UM functions from these other key responsibilities translates into a position that serves solely as the bearer of payer coverage information, which is often perceived as unwelcome news.[1]

To increase case manager effectiveness, the three functions—UR/UM, discharge planning, and care coordination—should be combined, placing these essential individuals in the position to not only obtain information but also take action, as necessary, to facilitate patient movement through the system. Additionally, the combination of these important functions heightens the awareness of glitches in the system or inappropriate provider responses that interfere with patient progress, placing these key individuals in the best position to document provider and system variances. Lastly, combining the UR/UM role with other traditional case management functions is cost effective at a time when health care institutions are challenged to control operating expenses.[1,3]

Performance criteria for the case manager role are listed in Box 9–3. Qualifications for case managers should include a baccalaureate nursing degree, direct care experience in clinical management of the targeted patient population, a collaborative practice philosophy, excellent communication skills, and experience with quality improvement and data management.[1]

It is important to distinguish the role of the case manager from that of the outcomes manager. The outcomes manager is an expert clinician and researcher with a masters or doctoral degree that functions as an attending nurse for a population of patients. Case managers, on the other hand, apply the strategies developed in response to a program of outcomes research on an individual case-by-base basis, as well as troubleshoot individual payer and discharge issues that may arise during the course of care. The use of a nurse with a masters or doctoral degree in the role of case manager is a waste of expertise and limits program success; that is, the nurse with graduate education is an expensive full-time equivalent (FTE) allocated to UM/UR and discharge planning instead of building a program of research and ensuring excellence in clinical practice.[1]

There is clearly a synergistic relationship that exists between case managers and outcomes managers. The two roles should work closely together with patients, families, and clinical staff to optimize care delivery. Additionally, combining the case manager's variance data with outcomes data often reveals important opportunities for CQI.[1,3]

Box 9–3   *Case Manager Performance Criteria in Outcomes Management*

- Conducts utilization review on assigned caseload of patients.
- Consults with interdisciplinary providers regarding resource utilization and discharge planning for assigned caseload.
- Seeks expertise of outcomes manager with regard to clinical care, interpretation and utilization of research findings, and change management.
- Works with collaborative practice team (CPT) to write valid and reliable definitions supporting systems and provider variances; collects variance information on assigned caseload of patients.
- Identifies trends in variance information and consults with interdisciplinary team members to determine potential solutions.
- Consults with payers to obtain preapproval for admissions, transfers, and procedures.
- Actively participates as a member of the CPT for the assigned patient population.

Note: Variances are defined as alterations in systems and processes from an established standard of care.
Reprinted with permission from the Health Outcomes Institute, Inc, The Woodlands, Texas.

The Social Worker

Social workers are credited with the historical development and implementation of case management. Traditionally, these key individuals established significant rapport with patients and families, enabling them to develop discharge plans that were meaningful, therapeutic, and well coordinated. As case management functions have grown in their sophistication, and UR has become commonplace, social workers have struggled to find a place within the system that enables position effectiveness and security.

The use of the case manager position for UR/UM, discharge planning, and variance data collection does not in anyway threaten the position of the social worker. Instead, it allows the social worker increased time for assessment, counseling, and the building of an effective therapeutic relationship, something that patients and families often feel deprived of in today's rapid-transit health care system. Additionally, it enables time for collaboration with other interdisciplinary team members and the organization of patient/family conferences that promote improved care coordination. It also eliminates from the role the burden of spending numerous hours on the phone with payers. This promotes more effective use of social workers, especially those with masters degrees that have expertise in therapeutic counseling.

INSTRUCTIONAL METHODS

Once an administrative decision has been made to initiate OM, program leaders must be selected and oriented to their roles and responsibilities. Chapters 2 and 3 describe this process and orient the reader to the organization and functions of the CPT.

However, for OM to be successful, all employees must be educated regarding program goals for related populations and necessary changes in individual performance accountabilities to support the initiative. While the depth of education required varies according to employee position, a variety of teaching/learning strategies should be considered to bolster both employee knowledge and employee ownership in the OM process.

A number of theories of learning have evolved that may be used as a framework to guide educational methods.[4] Methods of instruction are largely based on what is believed about human behavior and learning capacity. Box 9–4 identifies major themes that have emerged from learning theories that should be considered when developing an educational program. Teachers have little control over the learning process; they should not attempt to manipulate the learner, but must instead assist and guide learning in an environment that promotes exploration and facilitates active discovery.

Educational psychologists have categorized human behaviors according to cognitive, affective, and psychomotor domains of learning. The *cognitive domain* of learning focuses on intellectual behaviors, including knowledge, comprehension, application, analysis, synthesis,

---

BOX 9–4   *Common Themes from Learning Theories*

- Learning requires application and practice to ensure mastery.
- Application and practice that produce satisfying effects result in retention of learned behaviors; similarly, frustration results in rejection of the concepts assigned for learning.
- Praise, reward, and a feeling of inclusiveness related to learned behaviors promotes retention of new concepts.
- Learning requires reinforcement on the part of the teacher.
- Drive and motivation are secondary responses to learning that will only be evident when lower-level needs, such as position security, have been attained.
- Learning is driven by a need to attain a goal; the significance of the goal to the individual drives the rate and the quality of learning exhibited.
- The intellectual, physical, social, and emotional involvement of the learner increases the likelihood that learning will take place.

and evaluation. At the lower end of the cognitive continuum, knowledge is the simple remembering of previously learned information; evaluation, which sits at the upper end of the continuum, reflects an ability for systems thinking and value judgment.[4]

Within the *affective domain*, learned responses include attitudes, opinions, beliefs, values, and feelings. Affective learned responses are mastered early in life and are reflected in overt actions and behaviors.[4] Often, success in the learning process is stifled because of conflict with the affective domain. Internal values and attitudes can be challenging to overcome; when learners are presented with circumstances that threaten the integrity of their personal beliefs, the learning process may be slowed or abruptly halted.

The *psychomotor domain* focuses on motor skill attainment. Psychomotor skill is the result of reception and analysis of new information, decision making, and output responses.[4] It links together underlying chained behaviors that must occur in proper order and time sequence. Learning is the result of both practice and positive reinforcement.

There is overlap and interplay between the three learning domains that must be acknowledged when instructional methods are selected for teaching the OM process. Additionally, individual learning differences and styles must be supported to promote effective mastery of new information and skills. Principles of adult learning should be used to support the instructional style and environment (Box 9–5). Clinical CPT leaders and members must serve as teachers and mentors to interdisciplinary staff to enhance learning and overall program effectiveness.

The teaching/learning process must be driven by objectives that identify the learning outcomes as evident once the program of instruction has been completed. Learner objectives should reflect the performance criteria supporting each position within an OM program. In

---

Box 9–5   *Adult Learning Principles*

- Past experience, knowledge, skills, motivation, interests, and competencies shape adult learning and behavior.
- Adults learn best through methods that foster the application of new concepts and social interaction.
- Adults commit to learning when targeted goals are perceived as useful, realistic, and relevant to personal and professional objectives.
- Ownership and involvement in the teaching-learning process enhances adult learning.
- Individualized and personalized teaching methods enhance adult learning.

this way, staff are informed of their performance expectations at the start of the educational program.

A number of teaching strategies may be used to impart learning. The method of teaching should be aligned with the characteristics of the target audience, the defined learner outcomes or staff performance criteria, available resources, and the intended subject content. The use of a variety of teaching methods has been found to enhance adult learning. In fact, when information is transmitted by two separate sensory channels (e.g., auditory and visual, auditory and tactile), perceptual capacity and rate of learning have been found to increase.[4]

Retention of new information is enhanced when active learning strategies are used by the teacher to directly involve the learner.[4] Despite this, lecture continues to be the most widely used instructional method, primarily because of its efficiency. Self-instructional methods have also grown in popularity because of their cost-effectiveness and efficiency and the ability to progress at an individually determined pace.

Lecture and Discussion

The lecture is the most common form of educational instruction. Lecture methods consist of the provision of one-way communication to impart new information. The greatest limitation to the use of the lecture as an instructional method is its one-sidedness.[4] In other words, the lecturer must assume that what is communicated is learned.

Because of this limitation, it is recommended that lecture content be divided into sound-bites of no more than 20 minutes.[4] After each 20-minute session, learners should be engaged in discussion to keep them involved and focused. Discussion allows for personalization of content, direct learner participation, and clarification of information. The use of audiovisual aids and handouts to support the lecture content is also recommended. Box 9–6 provides an example of content that might be included in an introductory OM workshop for licensed interdisciplinary, direct care providers.

Self-Instructional Media

Self-instructional media (SIM) are gaining in popularity as instructional methods that allow individuals to progress at their own pace through an educational program. SIM may take a variety of forms, including paper, video, or computer-based methods. The uses of video and computer-based simulation, including virtual reality, have also gained popularity among educators as tools capable of building both knowledge and psychomotor skill.[4] Given the cost of professional video development, few are likely to select this method of course development. However, the explosion in computer technology and internet-based instruction will likely lead to an increased use of this medium for the development of educational programs.

SIM development should follow a logical course, beginning with the identification of the target audience and development of module objec-

---

Box 9–6 *Sample Content Outline for an Introductory Program on Outcomes Management*

I. Why Outcomes Management (OM)
   A. Evolving health care system
   B. The relationship of research to practice improvement
II. OM Defined
   A. Ellwood's definition
   B. OM quality model
   C. Institutional OM philosophy
   D. Effect of OM on current practice roles and accountabilities
      1. Performance criteria
      2. Outcomes defined
      3. Building the data repository
      4. Structured care methodologies (SCMs) and related documentation systems
      5. Use of research findings to change practice
      6. Connection with the continuous quality improvement (CQI) program

Note: Target audience includes licensed, interdisciplinary, and direct caregivers.

---

tives that are suitable to audience level. Objectives are then used to drive development of the module's content. Because SIMs are intended to educate, an evaluation of learning should also accompany each module. Evaluation may take the form of a pretest/posttest or simply provide posttest evidence of learning.[4] Continuing education units or credit hours should whenever possible be attached to each SIM developed. An example of a SIM developed as an introduction to the process of OM for licensed interdisciplinary, direct care providers is provided in Appendix A.

Advantages to the use of SIM include reduced employee training hours and instructional efficiency. Disadvantages to the use of SIM include the inability of a student to ask questions or verbally interact with an instructor and other participants, module development time, participant inexperience with technology (for computer-based systems), learner procrastination, and, in some cases, development and implementation costs.[4]

Grand Rounds Presentations

Once an OM program has been up and running for a period of time, CPT leaders should involve their members and other staff in the development and delivery of an educational program for grand rounds. Grand rounds presentations may take a variety of formats, but usually are organized using a lecture/discussion strategy, supported by audiovisual aids and a case study presentation.

Interdisciplinary grand rounds presentations showcase OM program achievements, highlighting staff contributions that have resulted in improved patient outcomes. Grand rounds presentations foster *ésprit de corps* among direct caregivers, as well as a sense of accomplishment and pride. Lastly, grand rounds serve as an effective means of communicating important CQI findings throughout a health care institution.

Evaluating Learning

Because of the dynamic nature of OM, processes and procedures for the delivery of patient care are always changing. This implies that lifelong learning must be a commitment made by staff engaged in an OM program.

The evaluation of learning may take several forms. Learning may be evaluated by assessing staff reliability in the conduction of a psychomotor procedure such as the use of a new protocol for promoting urinary continence. Similarly, satisfaction with a new procedure, a documentation tool, or role accountabilities may be used to evaluate the affective domain. Lastly, evaluation of learning also includes the level of staff performance attained at year end on a performance appraisal.

Both the learner and the teacher hold responsibility for learning. Interpretation of evaluation results must take into consideration the effectiveness of teaching strategies, the perceived value held by the learner for the new concepts, and the environmental culture affecting the learning process.

| SUMMARY

Successful implementation of an OM program is largely dependent on staff involvement and support. Administrators and CPT leaders are challenged to foster a sense of ownership of the OM program among direct caregivers. Clear, objective performance criteria must be developed for each interdisciplinary position involved with the production of patient outcomes. Staff education regarding new roles, accountabilities, and performance expectations should then be provided to enhance participation, involvement, and ongoing development of the OM initiative.

References

1. Wojner AW, Rauch P, Mokracek M: Collaborative ventures in outcomes management: roles and responsibilities in a service line model, *Crit Care Nurs Quart* 19(4):25-41, 1997.
2. Grady GF, Wojner AW: Collaborative practice teams: the infrastructure of outcomes management, *AACN Clinical Issues* 7:153-158, 1996.
3. Wojner AW: Widening the scope: From case management to outcomes management, *The Case Manager* 8(2):77-82, 1997.
4. Van Hoozer HL et al: *The teaching process*, Norwalk, Conn, 1987, Appleton-Century-Crofts.

PART III

Looking Ahead:
Complementary
Next Steps

CHAPTER 10

Long-Term Outcomes Measurement and Management

INTRODUCTION

Long-term outcomes measurement requires an ability to conduct research across the health care continuum successfully. To facilitate meaningful longitudinal study, the uniqueness of each care setting must be acknowledged using a systematic approach to clinical inquiry and practice standardization. Within each level of care, mastery of intermediate-level outcomes measurement and management should precede attempts to study long-term outcomes. Longitudinal study that is attempted before maximizing control across care settings is likely to provide investigators with meaningless and confusing findings that may prove challenging to manage.

This chapter focuses on methods that may be used to measure and manage long-term outcomes. The unique characteristics of the post-acute continuum are presented and strategies for longitudinal study are discussed.

LONGITUDINAL OUTCOMES MEASUREMENT AND MANAGEMENT

Chapter 4 outlines the process of outcomes measurement as the collecting and analyzing of data for the purpose of identifying the results of interdisciplinary health care interventions. Measurement may be confined to a phase of care to study intermediate outcomes or it may be carried out longitudinally across the health care continuum to study long-term outcomes.[1]

Long-term outcomes are considered the "end results" of health care interventions. Box 10–1 lists a variety of long-term outcomes that are commonly of interest to health care providers. Because long-term outcomes are measured over a prolonged period of time, the sample studied is likely to be subjected to a number of conditions that may challenge the validity of study findings.[1,2]

Movement across the health care continuum exposes study subjects to care that is provided by a number of different interdisciplinary providers whose skill level, education, and licensure vary significantly.

Box 10–1   *Commonly Studied Long-Term Outcomes*

- Functional Status
- Quality of Life
- Caregiver Burden
- Severity of Illness
- Resource Utilization
- Depression

- Social Reintegration
- Pain Control
- Return to Employment
- Mortality
- Satisfaction with Health Care Services

Reprinted with permission from the Health Outcomes Institute, Inc, The Woodlands, Texas.

Staffing patterns within different care settings also vary dramatically. For example, consider the differences in registered nurse staffing between intensive care units (ICUs), general care units, inpatient rehabilitation centers, skilled nursing facilities (SNFs), and in-home care settings.[2]

The measurement and analysis of long-term outcomes is further complicated by the lack of practice standardization that exists across the health care continuum. For example, within an acute care setting, patients at risk for a particular complication may be managed using a standard of care that differs from that used within a subacute facility; still another practice standard may be used to prevent the same complication should the same patients be moved to a SNF.[2]

The sociocultural characteristics of the cohort adds yet another challenging dimension to meaningful study of long-term outcomes. Subjects with extensive financial or personal resources may exhibit different patterns of health maintenance than those with limited resources, such as improved follow through with provider recommendations for clinic visits and use of prescribed medications. Precise measurement of a cause-and-effect relationship between a specific standardized practice that *may* be inconsistently used by subjects, and an outcome of interest would be challenging in these circumstances.[2]

Controls may be applied to some of these variables, but others may be near impossible to manage. Because of the challenges to the validity of long-term outcomes, a systematic approach to longitudinal study should be undertaken, acknowledging the unique attributes of patients, providers, and systems that characterize the many phases of care along the health care continuum.[2]

Getting Started

Long-term outcomes measurement undertaken without some degree of control yields useless information. However, many providers eager to begin measuring outcomes often begin by launching programs of long-term outcomes measurement that are not supported by sound research methods. Unfortunately, measurement without structure and clear purpose produces results that are anything but clear. Untoward outcomes are likely to be identified, originating from unknown sources, thereby frustrating and limiting practitioners' abilities to develop and implement meaningful interventions.[2] While measurement of long-term results is appealing, a systematic approach to the continuum of care must be used so that study findings take on greater significance and usefulness.

Outcomes management (OM) is the process of actively changing health care practices based on findings obtained through measurement procedures. As illustrated in Figure 1–2, OM is a continuous four-phase process that begins with the development of a database system or outcomes data repository (ODR) in Phase I. Phases II through IV involve the development and implementation of practice standards, which are tested through the achievement of outcome targets. Practice standardization is usually accomplished through the use of structured care methodologies (SCMs). When Phase IV findings fall short of expectations, revisions or additions of SCMs occur through a return to Phase II. The OM process then begins a new cycle of implementation and measurement of outcomes attainment. Regardless of the care setting along the continuum, the process of OM remains unchanged.[1,2]

Within each care setting identified for participation in the study protocol, initiation of Phase I database development should occur. Once Phase I has been completed, each study site should have developed complementary data repositories to assist with identification and management of untoward results for the cohort of interest.

Descriptive research methods are first used to enable understanding of the characteristics that make up the cohort, including significant relationships and differences among subgroups and untoward intermediate outcomes (UIOs) occurring within each care setting. Descriptive findings are then used to drive the development of SCMs for the enhancement of cohort outcomes. As SCMs are implemented, experimental designs may be used to test their effectiveness on the targeted outcomes of interest. Continuous improvement of SCMs and the addition of new practice standards occurs within each setting until cohort outcomes are optimized.[2]

Because the selection of care settings is typically driven by disease severity, the characteristics and UIOs associated with a population in one care setting are likely to differ from those that define the same population in a different level of care. Similarly, practice strategies associated with improved outcomes in one setting may be unsuccessful or impractical because of the staffing mix or the geographic layout in a different care setting.[2]

Because of the complexity of the continuum and the number of variables that can affect findings, practice within each level of care should be optimized before attempting to find meaning in long-term results. An ability to merge databases between different care settings signals a significant accomplishment in practice standardization and an ability to begin well-controlled, longitudinal measurement.[2]

TABLE 10–1

Services Provided along the Postacute Care Continuum

Services	Home	Nursing Facilities	
	Home Health Care	Skilled Nursing Facility (SNF)	General Subacute Care
Patient/Resident Services	24-hr home support	Daily skilled nursing and rehabilitation	Daily skilled nursing and rehabilitation
Physician Visits	N/A	Monthly to every 60 days	Recommended weekly to 3 times/wk
Direct Nursing Care Hours	3-5 visits/wk	2.5-3.0 hrs	3.5-5.0 hrs
Respiratory Therapy Services	N/A	Rarely available	24-hr contract availability
Rehabilitation Services	3 visits/wk	3-5 times/wk	Daily for 6 days/wk; PT, OT, and ST
Pharmacy, Lab Services	N/A	Contract staff only	Contract staff only
ALOS	3-4 wks	60-90 days	10-40 days
Discharge Target Site	Home or outpatient clinic	LTC or home	LTC or home

Adapted from the work of Mark A MacCutcheon; reprinted with permission from the Health Outcomes Institute, Inc, The Woodlands, Texas.

A number of instruments may be used to measure long-term outcomes. Disease-specific severity measures should be used whenever possible to enable measurement of the effect of interventions on disease severity and to facilitate understanding of the relationship between disease severity and important outcomes such as those listed in Box 10–1.

Measurement Considerations within the Postacute Continuum

The post-acute continuum consists of a variety of care settings, including inpatient rehabilitation centers, subacute care, long-term care (LTC), and home care. Admission criteria for inpatient rehabilitation require medical prescription of a variety of therapies, including but not limited to physical, occupational, and speech therapy, as well as the patient's ability to tolerate 3 or more hours of continuous therapy.[2]

In the United States each state defines what services and care are classified as LTC, but in most cases, LTC is synonymous with skilled nursing care. LTC is usually provided in facilities that are licensed by their state. Staff mix for LTC facilities consists of a minimal number of registered nurses and a majority of certified nurse assistants that serve as primary caregivers. The patients that typify LTC facilities are quite debilitated, requiring assistance with activities of daily living (ADLs).[2]

	Hospital-Based Facilities	
Acute Rehabilitation	Transitional Subacute Care	Acute Care
Intensive rehabilitation nursing; 3 hrs/day PT, OT, and ST	Daily skilled nursing and rehabilitation	Medically unstable; invasive procedures; most complex level of care
Daily	Daily	Daily
5.5-7.0 hrs	5.0-6.0 hrs	6.5 or more hrs
24-hr on-site availability	24-hr on-site availability	24-hr on-site availability
High intensity, multi-disciplinary; 3 hrs/day	Daily; PT, OT, and ST	Daily; PT, OT, and ST
24-hr on-site availability	24-hr on-site availability	24-hr on-site availability
14-21 days	<20 days	4-6 days
Home, subacute, or outpatient	Home (LTC rare)	Home, transitional subacute, rehab, or SNF

Subacute care is a level of care that blends both acute and long-term care philosophies and skills. The vast majority of subacute care is provided in SNF beds, which may be located in a hospital or in a freestanding nursing facility. In the United States subacute care is not currently recognized as a specific reimbursement category, nor is it governed by regulatory or designated licensure requirements in most states. However, this is in the process of changing.[2]

Patients managed in subacute units and LTC settings carry a combination of medical, nursing, and rehabilitation care needs. Length of stay (LOS) in subacute care and LTC varies according to the type of care provided. The average LOS for subacute units within hospital settings is approximately 12 days, while the average LOS in subacute units in freestanding nursing facilities or specialty hospitals is 25 days. In contrast, LTC residents may be admitted for a year or more.[2]

Home health care services were designed to provide varying levels of care based on both patient and caregiver needs. Table 10–1 highlights the differences in patient/resident services among home health care, SNFs, inpatient rehabilitation centers, and subacute and acute care settings.

The measurement of outcomes and the utilization of findings to improve care is mandated for postacute providers by the Joint Commission on Accreditation of Healthcare Organizations (JCAHO), the Health

Care Finance Administration (HCFA), and the Commission on Accreditation of Rehabilitation Facilities (CARF). Each organization must develop an outcomes-based performance improvement program as part of the regulatory requirements of these agencies.[2]

The CARF requires use of the Functional Independence Measure for Adults (Adult FIM) and the Functional Independence Measure for Children (WeeFIM) to measure outcomes within rehabilitation settings. At present, the Functional Independence Measure (FIM) is considered to be the most widely used system in the world for documenting the severity of patient disability and the outcomes of medical rehabilitation. FIM's comparative database is reported to be based on over 800,000 cases. FIM uses an ordinal scale with seven levels, ranging from least independent to most independent, and is used to measure self-care, sphincter control, mobility, communication, psychosocial adjustment, and cognitive function. The administration and scoring of FIM is conducted by the facility's interdisciplinary care team on admission, at least once more prior to discharge, and as a follow-up measure 60 to 90 days after discharge.[2]

Federal standards, implemented as part of the Omnibus Budget Reconciliation Act of 1987 (OBRA-1987) regulated by the HCFA, mandate the use of the Resident Assessment System (RAS) as an outcome and performance improvement measure within LTC facilities and subacute units. The RAS is a standardized system of measurement that uses a core set of elements known as the Minimum Data Set (MDS). The MDS is combined with Resident Assessment Protocols (RAPs), which are triggered by specific assessment findings. Proper use of the MDS and RAPs produces comprehensive, standardized, comparable, and reproducible assessments of the functional capabilities of LTC residents.[2,3]

A four-level ordinal scale is incorporated into the MDS for rating physical functioning, cognitive patterns, communication/hearing patterns, ADLs, self-performance items, continence, weight variances, types and stages of pressure ulcers, and chemical or physical restraint utilization.[2] MDS findings may be tracked and benchmarked regularly as quality indicators and outcomes measures. Federal regulations mandate MDS completion under the following circumstances[2]:

- Resident admission to LTC
- At a minimum, every 12 months unless otherwise indicated
- When there has been significant clinical change in a resident's status
- When a resident returns to a facility following hospitalization for a significant clinical change

The MDS currently includes more than 300 items that assess functional status, comorbid health findings, and care services provided to residents. Reliability of the MDS has been found to be excellent in the categories of cognition, ADLs, nutritional status, hearing and vision patterns, medication use, and disease diagnoses.[4,5] However, estimates of the reliability of the MDS have been low in the capture of important elements such as pain, mood distress, and delirium.[4] Additionally, the

MDS fails to detect psychiatric symptoms including delusions, halluci-nations, mania, paranoia, and social withdrawal.[6]

A number of factors have contributed to the slow development and implementation of outcomes measurement and management within the postacute aspects of the health care continuum. First, the small number of registered nursing staff used in postacute settings reduces available expertise in assessment beyond that mandated by regulatory agencies. Limited availability of advanced practice nurses (APNs) with research experience is quite typical in postacute practice settings. When present, APNs may function as nurse practitioners, performing clinical services with limited time for research.[2]

Stringent documentation guidelines mandated by accrediting agencies also contribute to the limited development of outcomes programs in postacute settings; coupled with the decreased number of available registered nurses in LTC, the documentation burden limits time to use additional documentation measures such as critical pathways. Pathways and other SCMs have the ability to decrease documentation through the elimination of nursing care plans (NCPs), but LTC accreditors have not universally accepted their use as a substitute for the NCP, often necessitating double documentation by the registered nurse.[2]

The relative absence of automated clinical documentation systems and computerized technology is but another contributor to the slow emergence of OM systems across the postacute continuum. Presently, most outcomes data must be manually tracked, reducing process efficiency. Patients/residents in postacute settings may also be unable to

---

Box 10–2   *Intermediate Outcome Measures of Interest within Long-Term Care Settings*

- Health status (e.g., physical, psychologic, social)
- Functional status
- Untoward intermediate outcomes (UIOs) (e.g., complications)
- Length of stay (LOS)
- Emergency Department or Urgicare visits
- Rehospitalization
- Discharge disposition
- Total cost of stay
- Resource utilization
- Cost per patient day
- Facility-acquired infection rates
- Falls, with and without serious injury
- Resident nutritional status
- Facility-acquired pressure ulcer rates

Adapted from the work of Mark A MacCutcheon; reprinted with permission from the Health Outcomes Institute, Inc, The Woodlands, Texas.

participate in completion of commonly used instruments, such as the Medical Outcomes Study Short Form–36, due to debilitation, problems with cognition or level of consciousness, and difficulty in identifying family or caregivers who could participate in data collection.[2]

On a positive note, researchers interested in setting up outcomes studies in postacute settings are often welcomed by program administrators, as long as additional burdens are not placed on staff. Postacute care administrators have learned to value the measurement of outcomes that demonstrate improved quality of life and functional status for patients/residents at lower costs than those incurred by acute care providers.[2]

Box 10–2 lists intermediate outcomes of interest within LTC and subacute settings. Significant LTC process measures include the number of residents requiring restraint (physical or medicinal) and the use of any of the following medications: antidepressants, anxiolytics/hypnotics, and psychotropics.[2]

| SUMMARY

Long-term outcomes measurement involves the collection of data across a continuum of care services in a patient cohort. To provide meaningful findings, measurement and management of intermediate outcomes within the varied acute and postacute care settings should precede measurement of long-term outcomes. Once connected across a continuum of services, measurement of long-term outcomes produces powerful findings that may be used to optimize the health care experience for patients and their families. The postacute continuum is ripe with opportunities to conduct research, which should be pursued with vigor by investigators interested in understanding the contributions of this segment of the continuum to the production of patient outcomes.

References

1. Wojner AW: Outcomes management: from theory to practice, *Crit Care Nurs Quart* 19(4):1-15, 1997.
2. Wojner AW, MacCutcheon MA: Longitudinal outcomes measurement and management: standardizing practices across the continuum of care, *Crit Care Nurs Clin N Am* 10(1):33-40, 1998.
3. UB Foundation: *Getting started with the Uniform Data System for Medical Rehabilitation*, Buffalo, NY, 1994, Uniform Data System.
4. Hawes C et al: Reliability estimates for the Minimum Data Set for nursing home resident assessment and care screening, *Gerontologist* 35:172-178, 1995.
5. Haratmaier SL et al: The MDS cognition scale: a valid instrument for identifying and staging nursing home residents with dementia using the Minimum Data Set, *J Am Geriatr Soc* 42:1173-1179, 1994.
6. Frederiksen K, Tariot P, DeJonghe E: Minimum Data Set Plus (MDS+) scores compared with scores from five rating scales, *J Am Geriatr Soc* 44:305-309, 1996.

CHAPTER 11

Disease Management: Outcomes-Driven Continuum-Based Care

INTRODUCTION

The concept of disease management (DM) takes its origins from the pharmaceutical industry, which sought to partner with managed care organizations in the early 1990s for the development of comprehensive health strategies for a variety of diseases.[1] While DM has become a commonly used term to describe the delivery of comprehensive integrated health care services, the ability to successfully manage diseases across a continuum of care is anything but a simple process. At the core of DM is a need to continuously measure and manage outcomes; without this, practitioners could never know with any degree of certainty the effect of their interventions on a target population. In other words, claims to truly manage a disease are dependent on the measurement of outcomes.

This chapter defines DM and relates the development of a DM program to both outcomes and case management systems. The goals, as well as the power, of a well-orchestrated DM program are explored, including the ability to effect reform of health care legislation.

DISEASE MANAGEMENT DEFINED

Meanings associated with DM vary according to the source (Table 11–1). However, the theme most commonly associated with DM suggests that it provides a comprehensive approach to health care and reimbursement—based on the natural course of a disease—within service settings designed to maximize treatment effectiveness and efficiency.[2] A DM program unites the concepts of outcomes research and management with the continuous quality improvement (CQI) of continuum-based health care services toward the discovery of methods that reduce the incidence and severity of common chronic diseases and enhance quality of life.[3,4]

Figure 11–1 identifies the relationships between DM, outcomes, and case management strategies. To be effective, DM must be viewed as a continuous process that unites services within both the acute and postacute continua to provide comprehensive, interdisciplinary

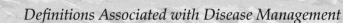

TABLE 11–1

Definitions Associated with Disease Management

Source	Definition of Disease Management (DM)
Managed Care Organizations	A method of standardizing practice and medical management for specific patient populations with measures that foster good clinical outcomes at acceptable cost levels.
Manufacturers	The selection and application of appropriate medications or medical devices in specific disease states, which acts to optimize both patient outcomes and resource consumption.
Providers	A process of preventing, predicting, and managing disease states to ensure optimal quality of life for patients and their families.
Payers	A systematic method of providing rational medical care in an efficient and cost-effective manner.

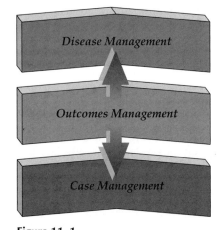

Figure 11–1

The relationship between disease, case, and outcomes management. Note that outcomes management (OM) drives development of both disease management (DM) and case management programs.

management of a disease. Assumptions supporting the development and implementation of a DM initiative include the following:

- When the natural course of a disease is known, standardized health care processes may be constructed that provide maximum benefit to stakeholders.
- Cost and quality are market driven; the quality of a DM program reflects the value propositions of its stakeholders.

- Accurate reflection of stakeholder values fosters support for costs associated with DM program development, implementation, and ongoing refinement.
- Health care delivery is driven by the disease process, not by reimbursement.
- Outcomes measurement and management guides ongoing DM process improvement.
- Consumer education improves appropriate usage of health care services.
- Partnerships with pharmaceutical and medical device manufacturers strengthens DM.

In its purest form, DM rivals traditional health care models that value the impact of services on individuals. The focus of DM is on maximizing the health of populations.[4] This "greatest good for the greatest group" philosophy may challenge the traditional health care consumer's value system.

A health care system built on a pure DM model eliminates the consumer's right to select medical services independently without the consumer's regard for the potential benefit of the service. DM models assume consumer acceptance that outcomes measurement will direct the delivery of care that has been found to be most effective—to those with the greatest potential for benefit. Such a philosophy supports achieving a balance between cost and quality and removes the possibility of delivering futile care to patients unlikely to achieve beneficial outcomes. In a society that has grown accustomed to the belief that death can be warded off at all costs, this marks a significant change in thinking.

Programmatic Steps of Disease Management

The process of organizing a DM program can be divided into five developmental steps (Figure 11–2). In Step I, an emphasis is placed on public health education with a focus on preventative services, early screening, diagnosis, and treatment. Step II consists of the development and implementation of processes that support ongoing symptom management for chronic illnesses, as well as the prevention and early detection of associated complications. Step II programs should include a variety of services, such as patient education, diet and exercise programs, psychosocial counseling services (including behavioral modification), and close monitoring and management of the medication regimen. During Step II, patients and interdisciplinary teams of providers should work toward the development of a close working relationship to foster ongoing trust and communication over time.

In Step III, the emphasis is shifted toward patient transition to maintenance management, incorporating measures that prevent complications and disease exacerbation. Step IV focuses on the development of patient ownership for health maintenance, including long-term health planning,

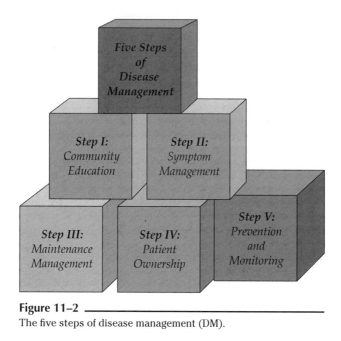

Figure 11–2 _____

The five steps of disease management (DM).

end-of-life decision making, and resource support. Lastly, Step V of DM focuses on preventative therapies and ongoing patient monitoring.

| GETTING STARTED

Because high volume, common chronic diseases such as asthma, diabetes, stroke, and congestive heart failure generate most of the health care system's business, most DM programs identify chronic diseases as program targets. Of special interest are those populations with a high incidence of inappropriate or avoidable emergency department use related to disease exacerbation, which may be prevented through education and other measures. However, getting the system's "hands" around a chronic disease process is a monumental task.

Chronic diseases are complex to manage; they challenge the traditional focus of health care on a single, simple disease model with a single, proximate cause. Instead, chronic illness models are complex, continuous, chaotic, and irregular processes, with multiple risk factors and biopsychosocial origins.[5] It would be illogical to assume that one size/treatment standard would fit all patients within the same chronic disease category. To best meet the needs of these patients, the cycle of chronic illness must be understood in such a way that specific outcomes may be predicted based on sets of patient and environmental characteristics. At present, few if any providers have this capability.

The costs associated with chronic diseases are highly visible and are driven by many factors, including[2]:

- Patient inability to access/use necessary health services
- Lack of preventative services and early screening/diagnosis
- Exacerbation cycles associated with the disease process

Combined, these factors promote recidivism within high-cost, acute care settings. Disease progression and exacerbation cause health care system reentry in extreme states via highly accessible high-cost routes, such as the emergency department. At the heart of the problem are rudimentary reimbursement systems that overlook the complexity of chronic illness, as well as the need for ongoing treatment and access to services to prevent high-cost, intensive health utilization.

Most of today's DM programs have focused on provision of Step I and Step II services. By opening access to services such as regular clinic and home care visits, they aim to lower the rate of recidivism and improve overall functional status. These programs have boldly made the decision to spend money in the postacute continuum to save money in acute care costs and many are meeting with success by doing just that.[6] However, the ability to manage completely the natural course of a disease starts well before diagnosis and, logically, continues after diagnosis toward the prevention of associated disease states; it is on this side of the DM service continuum that much work has yet to be done.

Disease modeling should support the construction of services and the identification of care delivery points for each disease selected for management. Disease modeling is the ability to map out the precursors of a disease, factors that precipitate onset, factors effecting early identification/diagnosis, potential complications, and the potential for resolution (Figure 11–3). Disease modeling promotes the pinpointing of essential services that, if delivered at critical periods, may reduce the incidence of unfavorable outcomes and enhance quality of life.

Building an Integrated System

Management of a disease implies an ability to move across the health care continuum into a number of different care delivery settings. Because of this, integrated health care systems are well situated to move toward delivery models based on the principles of DM. Formation of integrated health care systems, or strategic alliances for the management of diseases, enables health care organizations and providers to reach across the health care continuum.

The formation of alliances has been described in terms of a marital relationship; potential partners progress through attraction, dating, engagement, and ultimately marriage, which is often accompanied by a prenuptial agreement in case of divorce.[1] Although continuum-based alliances are necessary to support DM, the competitive nature of health care providers and organizations often makes the process of uniting

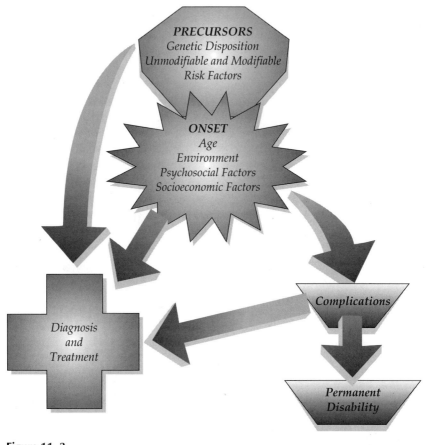

Figure 11–3 _____
Disease modeling.

services a painful one. In addition, once alliances have been formed, development and implementation of complementary processes within each sector of the continuum requires strong leadership and direction to realize. Simply "collecting" services across the continuum does not amount to integration; careful planning and coordination coupled with an intense commitment to collaboration are necessary to truly integrate.

To be successful at DM, health care administrators and providers across all sectors of the continuum must use a systematic process of program development supported by ongoing measurement and management of patient outcomes. Controls should be implemented to allow for effective and equitable program administration; these include:

- The use of scientifically sound, standardized practices and structured care methodologies (SCMs)
- Drug and device formularies
- Authorization programs
- Patient education protocols and compliance monitoring

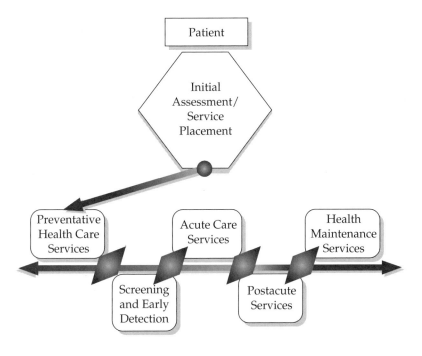

 = Control points in progression through disease-managed services;
ensures appropriate level of care is provided to optimize health
and wellness

Figure 11–4 _____
Program development and control mechanisms.

- Expert business management and coordination of continuum-based practice sites
- Programs in health promotion and disease prevention
- Linked multisite information systems

Figure 11–4 highlights DM program development based on targeted population outcomes. Processes and controls that promote the attainment of population outcomes are built into the program to ensure the effectiveness and efficiency of services.

Business processes should also be closely tied to a DM program to facilitate identification of necessary resources, appropriation of funding, monitoring of service reimbursement, marketing, and trend analysis and benchmarking. Figure 11–5 identifies the inputs and outputs associated with DM. Population outcomes serve as the major input to a DM program; program outputs reflect the business and health care processes designed to improve the health of the population. Outcomes measurement and management serve as the backbone of DM program development; the processes illustrated in the OM model (see Figure 1–2) direct development and ongoing refinement of a DM program.

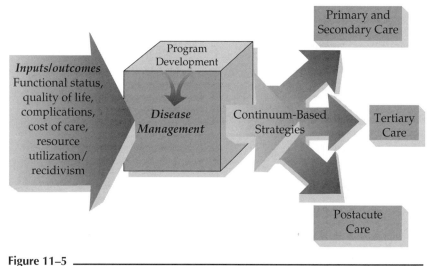

Figure 11–5

Disease management (DM): inputs and outputs.

| BUILDING VALUE

A DM program should reflect the values of its stakeholders. An overall definition of *value*, in relation to DM, is the provision of optimal care delivery services (e.g., systems, methods, providers) for the least amount of resources (Box 11–1).

Stakeholders supporting a DM program have been defined according to the seven "Ps," namely **p**atients, **p**ractitioners, **p**urchasers, **p**roduct producers, **p**rovider programs, **p**ayers, and **p**olicy makers.[1] The value propositions differ for each of these DM stakeholders and must be reflected in the quality of the program to ensure relevance, buy-in, and ultimately success. Providers of a DM program must also stay alert to signs of value migration, identifying necessary service adaptations to meet stakeholder needs.

Box 11–2 identifies specific value propositions for each of the seven groups of stakeholders. Up front, DM program administrators must recognize that health care consumers will determine the success of their program. For patients, quality of life, functional status, ability to return to work (productivity), timeliness of care delivery, service accessibility, and quality of the patient-practitioner relationship are among the values used to judge a DM program. Coupled with the growing accessibility of consumer health care information, future patients will be well positioned to judge DM quality through an improved understanding of disease conditions, risk factors, available state-of-the-science treatment options, and reported practitioner competency ratings.

Business consumers will judge DM program value through another set of criteria. Corporate business leaders acknowledge the benefits

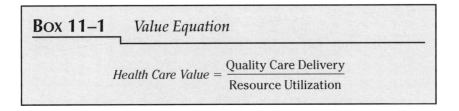

BOX 11–1   *Value Equation*

$$\text{Health Care Value} = \frac{\text{Quality Care Delivery}}{\text{Resource Utilization}}$$

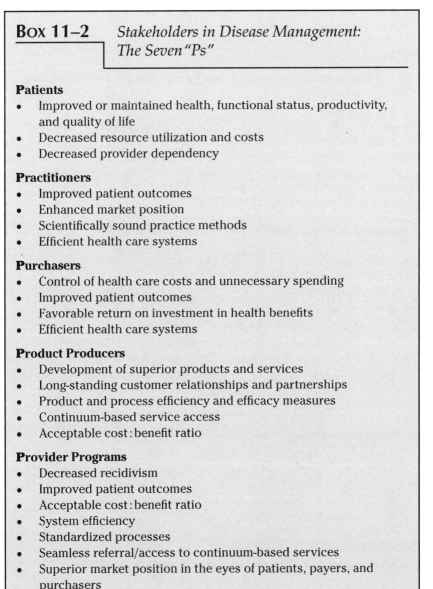

BOX 11–2   *Stakeholders in Disease Management: The Seven "Ps"*

Patients
- Improved or maintained health, functional status, productivity, and quality of life
- Decreased resource utilization and costs
- Decreased provider dependency

Practitioners
- Improved patient outcomes
- Enhanced market position
- Scientifically sound practice methods
- Efficient health care systems

Purchasers
- Control of health care costs and unnecessary spending
- Improved patient outcomes
- Favorable return on investment in health benefits
- Efficient health care systems

Product Producers
- Development of superior products and services
- Long-standing customer relationships and partnerships
- Product and process efficiency and efficacy measures
- Continuum-based service access
- Acceptable cost : benefit ratio

Provider Programs
- Decreased recidivism
- Improved patient outcomes
- Acceptable cost : benefit ratio
- System efficiency
- Standardized processes
- Seamless referral/access to continuum-based services
- Superior market position in the eyes of patients, payers, and purchasers

Continued

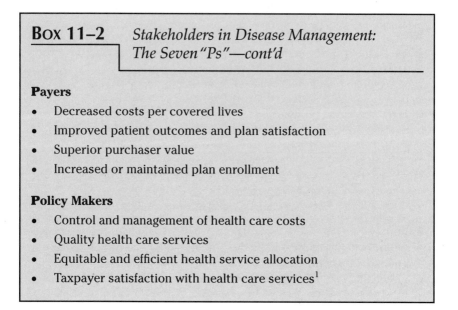

BOX 11–2 *Stakeholders in Disease Management: The Seven "Ps"—cont'd*

Payers
- Decreased costs per covered lives
- Improved patient outcomes and plan satisfaction
- Superior purchaser value
- Increased or maintained plan enrollment

Policy Makers
- Control and management of health care costs
- Quality health care services
- Equitable and efficient health service allocation
- Taxpayer satisfaction with health care services[1]

associated with maintaining and improving the health of both their employees and their employees' families. Optimal health drives increased worker productivity and lowers overhead related to absenteeism and disability costs. The association between healthy workers/families and improved work output is so strong that many businesses are beginning to partner with health plans in the development of outcomes-based DM initiatives, which will generate quality data to drive continuous improvement of both business and health care processes.

Health care systems that achieve success with DM recognize it as a philosophy that drives ongoing transformation of business programs, provider practices, care delivery strategies, and systems. Couch states that "DM provides a new way of aligning the inputs and outputs of customers and suppliers, up and down the value chain, that ultimately results in demonstrably better value care to patients and those who subsidize overall costs of care."[1] A sound DM initiative should create a culture that is determined to know the needs of its stakeholders and willing to build strategies to meet those needs. It requires a fluid, dynamic, and critical work ethic that moves continuously towards bettering itself in the eyes of its consumers.

The concept of total health management (THM) may become the end product of DM. Management of total health stretches across the health care continuum and the life cycle, providing womb-to-tomb public health services that encompass all the major elements of DM, including prevention, screening, early diagnosis, treatment, and ongoing monitoring/management. What THM will add to DM is a focus on wellness care.

Stakeholders for THM will resemble those identified for DM, with the addition of healthy populations. To be successful, THM will require significant stakeholder partnership to manage a wide variety of hetero-geneous populations, both well and ill, with varying degrees of disease severity, and differing health, personal, and socioeconomic characteristics. A THM program will require significant financial commitment to support human resources, information technology, and alliance management systems.

CHALLENGES TO SUCCESSFUL PROGRAM DEVELOPMENT AND IMPLEMENTATION

There are several reasons why achieving success with DM program development and implementation remains a challenge. Provision of health care practices based on tradition is by far the most common hurdle that must be overcome. In some institutions, movement into DM may mean sacrificing a variety of "sacred cows," which carries significant risk and political implications. However, movement away from provincial care delivery, based on institution/provider history or habit, is paramount to achieving success with DM.[3]

Secondly, a lack of standardized medical information technology systems (ITS) capable of crossing the care continuum challenges integration and analysis of meaningful outcomes data. While ITS have matured greatly in the acute care arena, their presence within the postacute continuum remains relatively invisible.[3]

The need for standardized methods to quantify and adjust disease severity across a variety of medical diagnoses also challenges development and implementation of DM programs. This is coupled with the need for standardized medical diagnosis-based data sets, associated taxonomy, and rigorous measurement techniques to enhance the quality and usability of findings in the development of a DM program.[3]

Reimbursement systems currently challenge DM as a financially viable model of care delivery in that they are often lacking incentives for health care providers to build health maintenance and prevention services. Additionally, pharmaceutical and medical device manufacturers are not always willing partners with health care providers in efforts to lower costs and share financial risk.[3]

Lastly, a number of patient-related factors challenge the ability to manage diseases effectively. Within a DM health care model, patients must accept accountability for the unhealthy behaviors that have contributed to their health care status. In other words, patients must accept accountability for the health and lifestyle decisions they have made that improve or promote a decline in their health status. Without patient acceptance of accountability, the burden is placed solely on the health care provider to work toward attainment of what may be unrealistic health goals. The paternalism that has dominated medical care delivery throughout its history must give way to patient-practitioner partnerships that acknowledge and accept patient/family health-related decisions as the final word.[3]

NEXT STEPS: PATIENTS, PROVIDERS, AND PUBLIC POLICY

As the health care system continues to change, market position among competitors will be determined by an ability to identify and respond rapidly to market trends. A noteworthy trend is the growing hostility among both consumers and interdisciplinary providers with the health care system at large.

As the U.S. "baby boomer" generation ages, expectations related to the role of providers, payers, and health care institutions are changing markedly. The patient "passivity" and acceptance of paternalistic provider-directed health care that typified previous generations is likely to come to an end. This heralds the emergence of a new health care culture in which both providers and institutions must respond to demands for patient-driven services.

What do patients want from health care providers and institutions? The simplistic answer to this question is quality health care services. Health care quality can be divided into two spheres: technical quality (e.g., provider skill and competence, effectiveness and efficiency of processes and systems) and subjective quality (e.g., patient perceptions of personal well-being and the nature of the care experience).[7]

Research conducted by the Picker/Commonwealth Program for Patient-Centered Care sought to define the subjective quality experience. Published in a book titled *Through the Patient's Eyes*, their findings identify seven critical dimensions of patient care that serve to measure the subjective quality of a patient's health care experience.[7] The seven dimensions are as follows:

- *Respect for patient values, preferences, and expressed needs*— Consists of the health care team's concern for patient individuality, acceptance of the patient's/family's definition of quality of life, patient involvement in treatment decisions, maintenance of personal dignity, and understanding the patient's needs, expectations, and desire for autonomy.
- *Coordination and integration of care*—Consists of the ability of the health care team to work together in an integrated, organized, and cohesive manner so that the patient perceives seamless care delivery.
- *Information, communication, and education*—Consists of both the provision of information and care choices, as well as the subjective quality of the communication, including an ability for effective patient/family teaching, honesty, and delivery of information in a caring manner.
- *Physical comfort*—Consists of comprehensive pain management, which includes traditional and alternative therapies, assistance with activities of daily living (ADLs), and enhanced physical surroundings to promote healing and maintain privacy.

- *Emotional support and alleviation of fear and anxiety*—Consists of recognition by the health care team of the significant emotional effects of disease on the patient and family, as well as the provision of supportive measures such as referrals, support groups, patient/family teaching, and the use of caring therapeutic conversations.
- *Involvement of family and friends*—Consists of accommodation of family and friends by the health care team to enhance the use of existing support systems, involvement in care decisions and care delivery, recognition of unique family needs, and support for family caregivers.
- *Transition and continuity of care*—Consists of provision of information related to the ongoing delivery of health care as the patient moves across the care continuum, coordinated planning, and the establishment of support systems to troubleshoot problems.[7]

By looking at the care experience through the patient's eyes, it becomes clear that downsizing highly educated, bedside caregivers in an attempt to reduce health care costs will dramatically affect the perceived subjective quality of the health care experience. In fact, as health care systems move closer toward patient-driven care in a DM model, the need for bedside caregivers may increase dramatically.

The chaos in the current health care system has caused many interdisciplinary health care workers to perceive, whether accurately or inaccurately, that they have been disenfranchised by the institutions in which they practice. Clearly, institutional administrators are under extreme pressure today to keep afloat in a system that demands high quality as well as significant cost control and cost reduction. However, often the measures used to manage costs have had dramatic effects on both technical and subjective quality.

The business of health care is primarily conducted through clinical operations. Reduction of clinical staff, coupled with an expectation that the remaining staff should "do more with less," translates into provision of poor clinical services. When clinical staff are downsized, provision of care that meets the humanistic needs of patients and families (i.e., subjective quality) must be traded off in an attempt to maintain the highest possible technical quality. Interestingly, the natural history of institutions that have downsized nursing staff aggressively reveals that within a 2 to 3 year period, aggressive rehiring strategies are employed due to a measurable decline in quality.

Given the heightened value of the patient-practitioner relationship identified by health care consumers and the increased demand among health care workers for highly satisfying practice environments, changes in the way health care institutions operate are inevitable. It is likely that health care workers will reexamine and strive to redefine their relationships with patients. Powerful patient-practitioner alliances that will foster redesign of health care services are a likely outcome.[8,9]

Within the practice setting, increased work demands associated with clinical staff downsizing have forged unheralded collaborative relations among interdisciplinary health care workers. As teamwork continues to evolve among the disciplines, it is promoting the organization of specialty-based, interdisciplinary group practices. The implications of this movement may be quite significant, in that the bulk of health care workers presently employed by institutions may shift into the private practice sector. Contracted interdisciplinary care provision may be the end result. Evidence of this cultural shift is mounting; interdisciplinary provider groups continue to form and separate themselves from hospital control.

Effects of Disease Management on Public Policy

The effects of DM on community health and the cost of health-related services will be monitored with growing interest by legislators. As health care consumers become more savvy and vocal, legislative mandates for system redesign will arise. Bedside practitioners, in partnership with patients, will be in a strong position to participate in the creation of a new health care system driven by the needs of patients.

Political action is defined as the process of influencing the allocation of scarce resources. Resource consumption in health care is driven by a number of variables. Some of the more visible contributors to resource consumption include:

- Technologic and pharmaceutical advances
- The need for highly educated, competent interdisciplinary staff
- Disease severity and the aging population
- Inaccessibility of services promoting early screening, preventative care, and health maintenance
- Inefficiency of health care services and fragmentation
- Provision of futile care
- Lost productivity on the part of the patient and/or caregiver

The need for control of health resource consumption has fueled much of the work to date on development and implementation of disease, case, and outcomes management programs. As DM, in particular, continues to evolve, highly successful models for predicting and controlling resource consumption are likely to be identified. Improved community health status is the inevitable result of widespread DM, but only if program results are made visible to those writing health legislation.

A number of interest groups are likely to be involved in the construction of health system legislation and the political goals attached by these groups to the distribution of resources are likely to differ significantly. Health care workers have traditionally represented a variety of separatist, fragmented interest groups, commonly targeting goals that directly challenge the interests of one another.

Health care consumers will become increasingly active in establishing mechanisms for health care reform.[8,9] However, their ability to create a system that uses all health care practitioners to their fullest potential, for the benefit of the patient, is limited without the collaborative involvement of interdisciplinary caregivers. The health professions must learn to work in unity toward the construction of future health care systems or their roles will be handed to them by outsiders.

In the United States the federal government's role in public health is derived from broad phrases in the Preamble to the U.S. Constitution, which outline the intent of government to "promote the general welfare" of the nation. The authority of the federal government is so broad that, if deemed necessary, the U.S. Congress could pass legislation affecting almost every aspect of national health care delivery.[10] In reality, however, the federal government has limited their role to actions in response to problems of nationwide concern. The Social Security Act of 1935, for example, was enacted in the aftermath of the Great Depression of the 1930s. Subsequent amendments to the act included Medicare and Medicaid legislation in 1965, which opened the door for direct federal reimbursement of health care services meeting specific quality criteria.[10]

DM offers a mechanism to explore the ability of a variety of interdisciplinary models and practice settings to effect improved population outcomes. The results of DM-based care systems must be made highly visible to attract legislator attention to the power of patient-practitioner partnerships. Special interest groups promoting collaborative partnerships between patients and practitioners should lobby actively for specific changes in health care system legislation as concrete methods for improved community health emerge.

Outside the realm of federal government lobbying, a number of actions should be considered to improve the visibility of DM-based initiatives. Simple measures that market the value of collaborative interdisciplinary care delivered in partnership with patients and families should be considered within the community setting.[11] Networks that unite stakeholders to build strategic alliances to effect a change in health policy should be established. Professional associations that promote stakeholder groups should be approached for the purpose of developing position statements and resources that enhance DM initiatives. Lastly, demonstration projects promoting the utilization of DM should be implemented and made highly visible through publications and community and professional presentations.

SUMMARY

DM is the product of outcomes measurement and management across the health care continuum. The ability to positively affect community health is greatly improved through DM programs, which are driven by ongoing outcomes assessment and strive for continuous improvement of health care services. A number of challenges must be overcome to ensure the widespread implementation of DM. Through patient and provider partnership, health care reform based on the principles of DM may be accomplished.

References

1. Couch JB: *The physician's guide to disease management*, Gaithersburg, Md, 1997, Aspen.
2. The Zitter Group: *Disease management: in principle, in practice, in partnership*, San Francisco, 1995, The Zitter Group.
3. Wojner AW: Outcomes management: from theory to practice, *Crit Care Nurs Quart* 19(4):1-15, 1997.
4. Kozma CM, Kaa KA, Reeder CE: A model for comprehensive disease state management, *J Outcomes Management* 4(1):4-8, 1997.
5. Pawlson LG: Chronic illness: implications of a new paradigm for health care, *J Quality Improvement* 20(1):33-39, 1994.
6. Heimoff S: A promising beginning: an uncertain future, *Healthcare Forum J* 41(5):23-26, 1998.
7. Gerteis M et al: *Through the patient's eyes*, San Francisco, 1993, Jossey-Bass.
8. Rodwin MA: Patient accountability and quality of care: lessons from medical consumerism and the patients' rights, women's health, and disability rights movements, *Am J Law Med* 20(1-2):147-167, 1994.
9. Rodwin MA: Consumer protection and managed care: the need for organized consumers, *Health Affairs* 15(3):110-123, 1996.
10. Stephenson DG et al: *American government*, New York, 1988, Harper & Row.
11. Goldwater M, Zusy MJL: *Effective political action*, St Louis, 1990, Mosby.

CHAPTER 12

Creating an Outcomes-Oriented Culture: Leading Behind the Lines

| INTRODUCTION

Leadership is the critical element that generates and focuses the human energy needed to design, manage, and continuously improve a patient-driven health services model. Successful outcomes management (OM) requires collaborative leadership from nurses, physicians, administrators, and other interdisciplinary caregivers to create and sustain a practice environment committed to and competent in outcomes research, interdisciplinary teamwork, practice redesign, and the continuous pursuit of best practice. In the quest to meet patient needs, leadership is a high leverage factor.

The importance of the leadership challenge should not be underestimated. Without a critical mass of effective leaders in key areas in an organization, it is not realistic for a health care institution to expect success from OM, continuous quality improvement (CQI), team-based strategy, reengineering, or other initiatives designed to improve results. Without clinical and administrative leaders who are able to communicate a clear vision, build a team, generate commitment, and manage change effectively, health care institutions will find it very difficult to develop patient-driven health services within the constraints of a payer-driven environment.

Because OM is an interdisciplinary initiative, it requires a fundamental shift in thinking about leadership. The traditional top-down, hierarchical style of leadership will not be effective. OM needs collaborative leadership that supports interdisciplinary ownership of the process (see Chapter 3). The objective is for clinical and business leaders to empower collaborative practice teams (CPTs) to work together to manage specific patient populations, continuously improve the quality of care, and pursue best practice. The OM process breaks down when decision-making authority is removed from the CPT and resides primarily at the top of a hierarchical structure.

The importance of empowering CPTs in OM is amplified by the fact that they are the primary point of contact between the health care institution and specific patient populations. A health care institution cannot be truly responsive to the needs of the patients it is designed to serve unless front-line professionals are given the authority and support to make decisions that affect patient outcomes. This is the reason that the traditional top-down, hierarchical style of leadership is not effective. Top-down leaders, if they withhold power from clinical professionals on the front line, restrict the ability of those professionals to use the expertise and data vested in them to respond directly to the needs of patients and families.

To be successful, OM requires the support and collaborative leadership of nurses, physicians, and service line managers. However, many health care institutions have had so many "flavor-of-the-month" improvement initiatives from management that new programs are quickly dismissed. This kind of cynicism may generate compliance, but it will never create commitment. If OM is to be successful, it must be viewed as more than "just another program." Commitment is necessary, not just compliance.

| PRIORITIES FOR EFFECTIVE LEADERSHIP

To drive effective change and move successfully toward a patient-driven health services model, an effective leader focuses on seven priorities.

Priority One: Becoming an Architect of Change

Leadership is about being a pioneer—discovering, exploring, and paving new pathways. Leadership is about working with people—motivating a team or an organization to move from where they are to where they need to be. Leadership is about being an architect of change—challenging the status quo and developing new and better ways of doing things.

Leaders in health care recognize that the past is an increasingly inadequate guide to the future. American humorist Will Rogers put it succinctly when he said, "The future just isn't what it used to be." Consequently, leaders in health care are not preoccupied with protecting the status quo. Rather, they are on a continuous search for more effective ways to produce improved outcomes and they are willing to pursue the changes necessary to produce those outcomes.

Health care leaders realize that change is not easy. There will be obstacles. Effective leaders, therefore, work diligently to identify and overcome obstacles such as resistance to change, structural impediments, organizational politics, resource limitations, and discouragement. Indeed, leadership is very much about enabling individuals and empowering an organization to manage the gap between the current state of health care delivery and the future vision.

Managing the Gap: The Heart of Leadership

At the personal level, the principle of "managing the gap" teaches that personal and professional growth require a certain degree of tension; that is, the tension between our current state (where we are today) and our future state (where we want to be). As Figure 12–1 illustrates, some people manage the gap by reacting to tension with negative emotion. These people become preoccupied with negative feelings, which does nothing to effect productive change. Other people manage the gap by responding to the tension with creative action. These people are leaders, and they focus on what needs to be done.

At the organizational level, growth and change also require a certain degree of tension; that is, the tension between an institution's current state (where it is today) and its future state (where it wants to be or needs to be). As illustrated in Figure 12–2, successful leaders are those who do specific things to enable an organization and empower people to manage the gap successfully.

OM requires leaders who are able to manage the gap between the current and future states of health care delivery. OM requires leaders who have the ability to create a compelling, interdisciplinary vision for continuously improving health care services across the continuum of

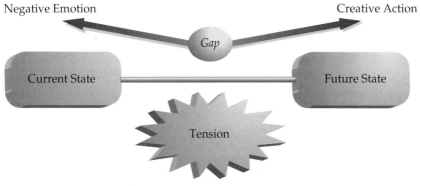

Figure 12–1

Responses to tension. *(Reprinted with permission from the Management Resource Group, Fallbrook, Calif.)*

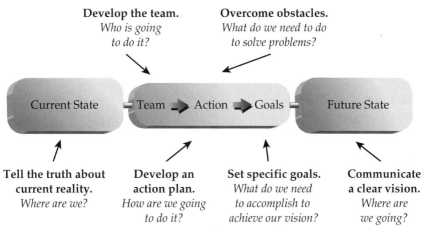

Figure 12–2

Managing the gap: the current and future state of health care. *(Reprinted with permission from the Management Resource Group, Fallbrook, Calif.)*

care, and who also have the ability to build and manage a team that will translate the vision into sustained action.

Priority Two: Earning Trust Through Character and Competence

Leadership is a relationship between leaders and the people they aspire to lead. Trust is the essential element in that relationship. Without trust, people will not commit to the vision that a leader communicates; nor will they embrace the change for which a leader asks. People need to know that a leader is worth following; they simply will not follow leaders they do not trust. Leadership is not power derived from status or position. Leadership is influence built on character and competence.

Trust is not based on technique. It is based on character and competence. Character is an issue of integrity, as in the consistency of what a leader says and what a leader does. Trust is built when people see that a leader is a person of integrity whose words and deeds are consistent. Competence is an issue of ability, as in the practical evidence of a leader's expertise. Trust is built when people see that a leader is a person of ability who can get things done. Character and competence together establish a leader's credibility and trustworthiness. When people see and experience a leader's integrity and ability, a foundation of trust is built. A foundation of trust then gives a leader the credibility to challenge the status quo, communicate the vision, build a team, and manage the change process. Figure 12–3 illustrates how the absence or presence of trust determines the effects of leadership on an organization and its people.

When Trust is Not Present	When Trust is Present
• Effective communication and cooperation are nearly impossible.	• Communication and cooperation levels are high.
• Information is withheld and distorted.	• Information is shared quickly and easily.
• People are cynical and suspicious.	• People are enthusiastic and candid.
• Motivation is undermined.	• Motivation is high.
• Negative things are amplified and positive things are diminished.	• Positive things dominate and negative things are openly discussed and resolved.
• People hesitate to share new ideas or challenge the status quo.	• People are encouraged to share new ideas and challenge the status quo.

Figure 12–3

Effects of the absence or presence of trust. *(Reprinted with permission from the Management Resource Group, Fallbrook, Calif.)*

The interdisciplinary nature of OM requires high levels of trust in those leading the initiative. Leadership for OM must be collaborative and must come from clinical professionals and administrative staff who have established their credibility within the institution and thus earned the confidence of the people and disciplines who will participate in the project. This trust is not static—it must be earned and reinforced continuously as the initiative moves forward.

It is important to note that in any change initiative, there will be crisis points. It is too late for a leader to establish credibility and trust at the moment of crisis. Trust cannot be called upon at the moment of need if it has not been earned in the time leading up to the crisis. Building trust is not an event; it is a process.

Priority Three: Developing the Team

Leadership is not a solo act. Leaders understand that people produce results. Leaders recognize that teams outperform individuals. No matter how talented, gifted, or committed an individual may be, no one person or mere group of people can achieve what an effective team can accomplish. The performance potential of a team of people, fully committed to their goal and to each other, is nearly unlimited.

Clearly OM is a team-based strategy for health care delivery. The activities that drive OM cannot be accomplished by one person or by a single discipline. The success of OM is largely dependent on the ability of multiple disciplines to coordinate their efforts to optimize patient care delivery.

Therefore, the leadership challenge is to develop an effective team that fully supports the OM model. The most successful leaders work hard to build teams with the following attributes.

Commitment

Everyone is committed to the purpose of the team, the performance of the team, and the people on the team. The team purpose is paramount; personal agendas are not. Note also that the best leaders are careful about who gets on the team. Every person on the team is important to the team's performance. Every person contributes to shaping team dynamics and outcomes. No leader can compensate for people who are not committed to the team's purpose or who lack the competence to perform.

Competence

A successful team requires specific skills and competencies to accomplish its mission. The competencies required by a team fall into three basic categories:

1. Technical—A team must have the specific technical knowledge and skills required by its mission.
2. Interpersonal—Because teamwork is highly relational, interpersonal skills are a necessity.

3. Problem solving—A team must have the ability to solve problems and overcome obstacles.

Communication

Successful teams are effective at team-based communication, which includes: listening (i.e., they hear what is being said), sending (i.e., they say what will be heard), debating (i.e., they avoid group thinking and engage in healthy debate), and deciding (i.e., they work together to make decisions).

Cooperation and Coordination

Successful teams coordinate their efforts to accomplish the mission. This means that politics and personal agendas are subordinated to the team's purpose; all members contribute to the development of a working plan; and the roles, relationships, and responsibilities of team members are clarified. Team members understand and are committed to their particular roles, relationships, and responsibilities within the team. They know where they fit in and what is expected of them.

Conflict Resolution

All teams have conflict. This is because teams are made up of people with different backgrounds, personalities, experiences, and paradigms. Effective teams learn to resolve conflict.

Priority Four: Building Culture

"Culture" refers to the dominant concepts that shape and direct the attitudes and actions of people in an organization. Culture is the combination of what an organization says about its mission and core values, what people believe about the organization, and how people actually behave. Leaders pay very careful attention to building and sustaining a strong culture. Indeed, the most successful leaders are conceptual leaders. They understand that the direction and performance of an organization must first be created and shaped conceptually, so that it can be acted upon operationally. The bottom line is that people will not work with enthusiasm and commitment in a direction in which they don't genuinely believe.

The Law of Roots and Fruit

An organization's "root system" ultimately shapes and determines the performance of its "fruit system." The root system is the cultural foundation that supports and feeds everything an organization does. It is a law of organizational life that what people believe shapes how people behave, that the collective attitudes of people in an organization direct institutional action, that the level of commitment people have to an organization's purpose and principles has a direct effect on how people and the organization perform, and that corporate character determines corporate conduct.

If a health care organization desires an effective and efficient health care delivery system, then its leaders must cultivate and manage an organizational root system that directly supports its delivery system. A health care organization must be well managed "below ground" if it is to function effectively "above ground." Patient-driven OM at the operational level begins with and is sustained by a commitment to patient-driven health services at the conceptual and cultural level.

Unfortunately, many executives and managers tend to manage almost exclusively "above ground" and thus fail to cultivate a strong and effective root system in their organizations. As a result, "above ground" managers fail to capture and harness the full intellectual and emotional energy of people and neither the people nor the organization reach their full potential.

Mission and core values are the heart of an organization's cultural foundation. When people in an organization or on a team are driven by different missions and values, they pursue different and often conflicting agendas. Under such conditions, teamwork and communication are disrupted, politics and personal agendas tend to dominate, and there is very little alignment or empowerment. This is illustrated in Figure 12–4 by the large arrow on top, where the people (the small arrows) are directed by different core concepts and are thus working in different directions.

But when people in an organization or on a team are driven by commitment to shared mission and values, the indispensable human capital and energy of the organization are focused in the same direction and a major precondition for success has been achieved. In Figure 12–4, this

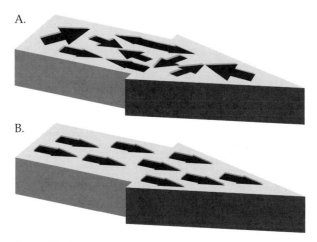

Figure 12–4 _____
A, Organization driven by different missions and values.
B, Organization driven by commitment to shared missions and values. *(Reprinted with permission from the Management Resource Group, Fallbrook, Calif.)*

is illustrated by the large arrow on the bottom, where the people are directed by the same mission and values and are thus working in the same direction. Shared mission and values produce alignment, which is the necessary foundation for effective communication, teamwork, and empowerment—all essential ingredients for success in today's competitive health care environment.

OM requires culture that places a high value on patient-driven care, interdisciplinary teamwork, communication, innovation, and research-based CQI. It is important not to underestimate how much time and energy are necessary to build and sustain this culture. The leadership challenge is to communicate the mission and core values of OM clearly, consistently, and creatively.

Priority Five: Telling the Truth About Current Reality

An effective leader tells the truth about current reality. Indeed, true leadership is reality-based. It doesn't obscure, manipulate, or distort the facts. Leaders understand that the more accurately they see reality, the more effectively they can respond to it. Leaders recognize that people want and need to know (1) where they are, and (2) how they are doing. People want and deserve an honest and accurate assessment of the current state of the organization or department in which they work.

Successful leaders want people to know the truth about current reality. If results are good, leaders want people to know so they will feel good about their accomplishments and keep up the good work. If results are poor, leaders want people to know this so they will be challenged to seek solutions for improvement. Leaders who hide or distort the truth about current reality create an atmosphere of uncertainty, resentment, discouragement, and distrust. The irony is that, sooner or later, people discover most of the truth anyway—and when they do, they don't feel very good about their leaders.

The concept of "vision" is as much about seeing current reality as it is about seeing the future. It is very difficult to inspire commitment to a shared vision of the future without communicating a clear vision of the present. It is very difficult to become the organization you want to be if you do not see and take responsibility for the organization you are.

An effective system for measuring performance is an important element in telling the truth about current reality. Successful leaders track key performance indicators and key performance drivers to evaluate performance. They see the critical connection between these two kinds of measures. *Key performance drivers* are the actions taken and activities engaged in to produce end results. *Key performance indicators* are the end-results (the outcomes) of the actions.

Leaders recognize that to change outcomes it is necessary to change actions. Leaders therefore use performance indicators to focus on, manage, and improve performance drivers. Leaders are always cognizant of the performance management axiom, "If you always do what you always did, you will always get what you always got." This same performance principle has been expressed by defining insanity as "doing the same thing over and over again and expecting different results." Telling the truth about current reality thus means measuring outcomes to manage and improve the actions that produce the outcomes.

In many ways, OM is the ongoing process of telling the truth about current reality. Indeed, OM is driven by research that measures the outcomes of care by continuously comparing actual findings against desired results (see Chapter 1). Success in OM thus requires clinical and business leaders who have the courage and commitment to utilize outcomes data to identify opportunities to continuously improve health services, improve resource allocation decisions, and even enable patients to choose among treatment options.

Priority Six: Communicating the Vision

A distinctive attribute of effective leadership is the willingness and ability to create and consistently communicate a clear and compelling vision of the desired future state of the organization. An empowering vision is a powerful mechanism that stimulates effort and commitment. Most organizations have some kind of "vision" that they espouse, but very few are able to communicate the vision effectively. Leaders provide a vision that is clear and compelling, that serves as a unifying point of focus and effort, and that creates immense team spirit.

A classic example of such a compelling vision in our generation is the commitment to put a man on the moon. U.S. President John F. Kennedy declared on May 25, 1961, that "this nation should commit itself to achieving the goal, before this decade is out, of landing a man on the moon and returning him safely to Earth." This vision captured the attention of the American people and focused the efforts and resources of the U.S. space program. Such was the collective commitment of the nation that, indeed, the United States landed a man on the moon within the same decade.

Stretch Goals

Goals are specific results the team must achieve *en route* to achieving the vision. Goals are critical because they are the stepping stones to achieving the vision. Goals translate the vision into specific, concrete objectives. Effective leaders establish stretch goals that require high commitment from the team.

An effective stretch goal is clear and compelling and requires little or no explanation:

- It is a goal that the team will actively pursue—like climbing a mountain or going to the moon. It is not merely a statement.
- It is a goal that can not be accomplished by one person or a few people; it requires the commitment and active participation of the whole team.
- It is a goal that is often outside the team's comfort zone.

- It is a goal that is consistent with the organization's mission and core values.

Strategy and Action Plan

Strategy is the action plan a team uses to accomplish its goals and achieve its vision. Leaders work with the team to develop and continuously adjust a strategy for producing results. Leaders understand that strategy development and implementation is not an event—it is an ongoing process. Very few strategies work exactly the way they were designed to work. The best strategies evolve over time as the team and its leadership discover what works best in the real world.

Strategy focuses on productive action. It is not merely theoretical. It is practical. Strategy continuously asks of its users, "What do we need to do to accomplish our goals and achieve our vision?" The best leaders help people see the linkage between strategy and vision. Leaders don't want people to take action simply out of a sense of obligation or compliance. Rather, leaders want people to see the vision, understand the strategy, and take action out of a sense of commitment to and passion for the mission of the organization.

Priority Seven: Creating a Learning Organization

Continuous improvement never happens without continuous learning. Leaders therefore focus on individual and organizational learning as key factors in determining how well a health care institution will respond to the needs of the community and to the realities of the health care market. Successful leaders pay as much attention to developing and managing an approach to learning as they do to building culture, developing strategy, or measuring results.

Leaders create an environment of continuous learning. They create a learning organization. A learning organization, as illustrated in Figure 12–5, takes advantage of a health care institution's clinical experience

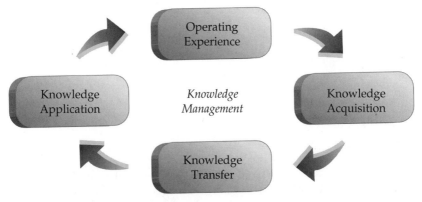

Figure 12–5

The knowledge management process. *(Reprinted with permission from the Management Resource Group, Fallbrook, Calif.)*

to accelerate learning and manage the acquisition, transfer, and application of knowledge.

This process is called *knowledge management* and is essential to everything a health care organization does—care for patients, build and manage culture, measure and manage outcomes, and continuously improve health services. It captures and utilizes a health care organization's most valuable asset—the intellectual capital of its practitioners.

Leaders drive knowledge management. Knowledge management enables a health care organization to capture its many learning experiences for use in future problem-solving and improvement initiatives anywhere in the organization. Knowledge management allows an organization to "recycle" its learning so that it may use it again to solve similar problems and respond to similar improvement opportunities it may face. This is an important competency, because knowledge management is faster, more effective, and much less expensive than knowledge creation.

Competitive Advantage Through Learning

A health care organization is a reservoir of experiences. Every day the organization comes into contact with new patients and new people, learns more about clinical and organizational processes, thinks up new ways to solve problems, and explores practice strategies. The leadership challenge is to learn from these experiences. What differentiates health care institutions is not so much the relative quality or depth of their experiences but the institution's relative capacity to learn from each experience. Some organizations are capable of extracting significant learning from their experiences. Some institutions are simply more effective at learning and knowledge management. The capacity to acquire ideas for improvement and innovation from each and every incremental experience is a critical component of resource leverage.

OM is a strategy of knowledge management. It is a strategy of continuous improvement through continuous learning. OM thus requires leaders who drive a process of systematic clinical learning where interventions are developed, implemented, and tested toward outcomes achievement. As the process moves through successive stages, it is the CPT's ability to learn that determines the scope, scale, and speed of improvements. The capture of untoward intermediate outcomes (UIOs) data and system/provider variances are key learning elements; they provide valuable data for practitioners by identifying untoward occurrences that may be resolved through new interventions (see Chapter 1).

The capacity to learn from experience depends on many factors:

LEADERS WHO UNDERSTAND AND CHAMPION THE LEARNING PROCESS. Leaders must understand that learning is not simply taking in more information. Learning is the process of developing knowledge and skills in order to take more effective action.

HAVING A FORUM WHERE PEOPLE CAN IDENTIFY COMMON PROBLEMS AND SEARCH TOGETHER FOR HIGHER-ORDER SOLUTIONS. Effective learning requires focus, teamwork, and time to think about and discuss critical issues.

THE WILLINGNESS TO "UNLEARN." Unlearning must often take place before learning can begin. An organization cannot be overly committed to protecting the past. The potential for leveraging the experiences of every person in the quest for competitive advantage exists only when leadership declares open season on precedent and orthodoxy. Each new experience and each success or failure must be seen as an opportunity to learn.

BEING WILLING TO FIX THINGS BEFORE THEY'RE BROKEN. The most effective organizations are proactive in their learning. They don't wait for something to go wrong before they seek improvement. Learning is driven by the pursuit of superior outcomes and not simply by problems.

CONTINUOUS BENCHMARKING AGAINST BEST PRACTICES. Learning from best practices is a proven method of accelerated learning and continuous improvement. Best practices provide objective standards against which to measure performance, practical ideas about how to improve, and real-world evidence that best practice is attainable.

The bottom line is that successful leaders focus on learning as a key driver of continuous improvement. They create an organizational environment where learning and knowledge management are an integral part of the way the organization operates.

| SUMMARY

Successful OM requires clinical and service line leaders who have the credibility and capability to create a compelling, interdisciplinary vision for continuously improving health care services across the continuum of care. It also requires leaders who have the ability to build and manage a team that will translate the vision into sustained action. Leaders must build a culture that supports OM and must develop the ability of the organization to systematically improve through effective learning.

Self-Instructional Module: Introduction to Outcomes Management

Reprinted with permission from the Health Outcomes Institute, Inc, The Woodlands, Texas.

CONTENT DESCRIPTION

This module is designed to assist the learner in understanding the principles and methods used to develop and implement an outcomes management (OM) program. The learner is introduced to the concept of OM, the differences between OM and case management, and a framework to support an OM initiative. This module is suitable for learners from a variety of disciplines and roles.

Learning Outcomes
1. Discuss the concept of OM, identifying differences between OM and case management.
2. List the four phases of OM, defining the steps taken in each phase to move toward achievement of best practice.
3. Identify the role of the administrator, advanced practice nurse (APN), physician, and case manager within an OM initiative.
4. Discuss the principles supporting collaborative practice team (CPT)–managed OM programs.
5. Identify differences between structured care methodologies (SCMs), as wells as how these tools can be used to standardize practice for a patient population.

SECTION ONE: INTRODUCTION

The cost of health care has prompted mandates by payers and consumers to reform the delivery system. Payers have made themselves the gatekeepers of consumer access to health care services and are closely scrutinizing consumer needs and provider services. In response, nursing case management (NCM) was promoted in the early 1980s as "second generation primary nursing,"[1] advocating the addition of financial advocacy to the existing primary nursing principles of authority, accountability, and autonomy.[2] Early NCM programs limited their study to rudimentary outcomes, namely length of stay (LOS), cost of care, and patient satisfaction with health care services. The use of severity-adjusted data and significant clinical indices was often lacking, prohibiting meaningful interpretation of data. While NCM programs met with some successes, they were primarily viewed as grassroots, nursing strategies to facilitate care coordination.[3]

OM was first theorized in the literature in 1988, by Dr. Paul Ellwood. Ellwood's theory for OM differed significantly from NCM, advocating a research-based model for practice assessment and ongoing enhancement. Ellwood defined OM as a "technology of patient experience, designed to help patients, payers, and providers make rational, medical care–related choices based on better insight into the effect of these choices on the patient's life."[4] Four principles for inclusion in an OM program were sighted by Ellwood:

1. An emphasis on standards that physicians can use to select appropriate interventions.
2. The measurement of patient functioning and well-being with disease-specific clinical outcomes.
3. A pooling of clinical and outcomes data on a massive scale.
4. The analysis and dissemination of the database to appropriate decision makers.[4]

The process of OM can be summarized as the enhancement of physiologic and psychosocial patient outcomes through the development and implementation of exemplary health practices and services, all driven by outcomes assessment.[3] Outcomes are produced by processes or interventions. Favorable outcomes are achieved when specific population goals have been attained.[5] The process of OM provides a mechanism for identifying differences among subgroups of patients within a population that may benefit from a specialized care regimen. It also enables measurement of relationships between patient conditions and specific interdisciplinary interventions, fostering continuous quality improvement (CQI) of care delivery toward the achievement of best practice.[6]

Collectively, OM and NCM produce a powerful mechanism for movement toward patient-driven health care. OM produces findings that may be shared with patients and families to enhance decision making regarding health care options. It enables the prediction of necessary resources for specific patient populations. Through OM, nurse case managers and other grassroots providers are able to bring best practice to life by providing care that has been validated through research. Finally, when optimal patient outcomes are produced, health care costs drop dramatically. Complications, recidivism, altered functional status, and consumer dissatisfaction drive health care costs. When these untoward outcomes are resolved, cost decreases dramatically, thereby reducing financial risk and optimizing institutional marketability within the managed health care arena.[7]

| SECTION ONE: CONTENT REVIEW

Select the best answer to the following questions on Section One:

1. Nursing case management (NCM) is best defined as:
   a. A process of sophisticated outcomes management and measurement.
   b. Interdisciplinary primary nursing care.
   c. A technology of patient experience designed to help patients, payers, and providers make rational care-related choices.
   d. A nursing process supported by the principles of autonomy, accountability, authority, and financial advocacy.
2. Outcomes management (OM) is:
   a. Synonymous with NCM.
   b. A research-based process that complements and drives a grass-roots case management initiative.
   c. A mechanism to support payer-driven health care systems.
   d. Second-generation primary nursing.
3. A benefit of an OM initiative is:
   a. Informed patient and family decision making related to treatment options.
   b. Reduced patient and family accountability for health status.
   c. The rightful restoration of power to health care providers.
   d. Enhanced payer control over health care access and service delivery.
4. Outcomes are best defined as:
   a. Processes used to provide care.
   b. The result of interventions.
   c. System and provider efficiencies.
   d. Variances.
5. Favorable outcomes are best defined as:
   a. Efficient systems and processes.
   b. Provision of expert, interdisciplinary care to a specific patient population.
   c. Attainment of defined patient population goals.
   d. Best practice.

| SECTION ONE: KEY

Check your answers against the following key for Section One; repeat the section if further clarification is necessary.

1. d
2. b
3. a
4. b
5. c

| SECTION TWO: THE PROCESS OF OM

Patient populations are selected at the beginning of the process of OM. Usually these populations represent either high volume or high financial loss cases within a health care institution. Once a population has been selected, the next step involves the formation of an interdisciplinary CPT. The disciplines represented within a CPT should reflect all of those involved in providing care to the specified patient population.[8,9]

An APN with expertise in the care of the selected population should be identified to serve as an outcomes manager. Outcomes managers act as attending nurses for their assigned patient populations, overseeing the provision of interdisciplinary care and serving as expert clinicians and researchers for team members.[3,7,10] Physician leadership should also be identified for the CPT. The physician selected may be the chief of service or a powerful advocate or champion for the process. A case manager for the population should also be identified to provide utilization review and discharge planning services, as well as to assist with the capture of system and provider-specific inefficiencies that influence outcome attainment.[7,8] Table A–1 provides an example of CPT membership for a neurosurgical patient population.

It is essential that administrators set the tone for OM within their institutions at the start of the project. First, outcomes measurement must be sanctioned and made policy as part of the quality review process;

TABLE A–1

Neurosurgical Collaborative Practice Team Membership

Regular Membership	Ad Hoc Members
Neuroscience outcomes manager (advanced practice nurse)	Laboratory representative
Neuroscience case manager	Radiology representative
Neuroscience nurse manager	Radiation oncologist
Neuroscience staff nurses (one per unit)	Medical physicist
Neuroscience Operating Room staff nurse	Medical oncologist
Neurosurgeons	Neurologist
Occupational therapist	Emergency Department physician and nurse representatives
Physical therapist	Emergency Medical Services representative
Speech-language pathologist (SLP)	
Registered dietitian	
Licensed medical social worker	
Pharmacist	
Rehabilitation Unit nurse manager	
Rehabilitation Unit staff nurse	
Physiatrist	
Home care nurse	

that is, whether or not interdisciplinary providers elect to participate in the use of new practices developed by the CPT, their patients' outcomes will be measured. This facilitates the ability to examine differences in patient outcomes between the users (study group) and nonusers (control group) of CPT processes. Secondly, administrators must delegate total authority to the CPT membership for determining the strategies that will be used to improve practice. Administrators may measure the success of an OM program by the population outcomes produced, which reflect the commitment and ability of CPT members. Thirdly, administrators must eliminate departmental territoriality, encouraging cooperation and collaboration between interdisciplinary stakeholders.[8]

A shared leadership philosophy must be valued by CPT members ensuring individual as well as team ownership and accountability for program outcomes. Successful OM initiatives are guided by the following fundamental principles:

- Team commitment to the pursuit of patient-driven health care
- Identification of a variety of heath outcomes for measurement
- Standardization of interdisciplinary practices for the purpose of health outcomes measurement
- Prudent and effective use of human and material resources
- Commitment of interdisciplinary providers to collaborative practice
- Commitment to pursue best practice through CQI of standardized practices, driven by outcomes assessment[11]

The process of OM follows an orderly sequence of steps from which to study a patient population, create new health care interventions for testing, and continuously improve interdisciplinary practice. An outcomes management quality model can be used to frame the OM process (Figure A–1).

Phase I

The CPT begins the OM process in Phase I, where population-specific outcomes are defined. There are two main outcomes categories: long-term outcomes, or those achieved at some point beyond the completion of all levels of care (e.g., 3, 6, 12, or 24 months); and intermediate outcomes, or those *proximal* outcomes that can be measured at the point of completion of a phase of care (e.g., at hospital discharge, prior to transfer to rehabilitation services).

Long-term outcomes usually measure functional status (e.g., the ability to participate in activities of daily living [ADLs]), quality of life, consumer satisfaction with health care services, consumer resource utilization, and changes in physiologic measures over time. A variety of instruments exist for the measurement of long-term outcomes.

Intermediate outcomes measure the achievement of defined physiologic and psychosocial goals. They are often best measured by the study of untoward intermediate outcomes (UIOs). UIOs represent all

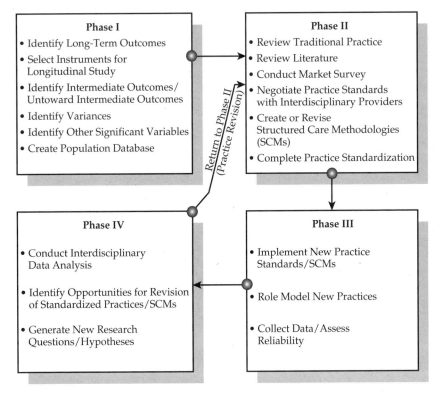

Figure A–1

likely occurrences (specific complications and psychosocial problems) that prohibit the attainment of intermediate outcomes. By measuring the occurrences of UIOs, attainment of desired intermediate outcomes can be determined in a "documentation by exception" format, providing rich information that reveals specific problems within high-risk subgroups of patients. Definitions must accompany each UIO. For example, the use of "pulmonary complications" as a UIO is inadequate, because sensitivity is lost. It would be impossible to interpret how many cases of pulmonary embolism, pneumonia, respiratory arrest, and inability to wean from mechanical ventilation occurred within the cohort. Instead, the CPT might define specific problems such as "radiographically diagnosed pneumonia, not present at the time of admission" as a pulmonary UIO.

Variances are also defined for measurement during Phase I. Variances are provider and system inefficiencies that prohibit timely movement of the patient cohort through the health care institution. Similar to UIOs, variances need definitions that support their objective retrieval and aggregation. Generally, the best source for defining variances is the staff nurse provider, who can quickly identify provider and system problems that stifle patient management.

Variables that represent outcomes measures and variances are then used to create a population database that will enable study of the cohort's health care experience. Other essential physiologic, psychosocial, and demographic variables are also identified at this time for inclusion in the database. For example, within a cardiac surgery population, left ventricular ejection fraction and pump time are two examples of variables that should be targeted for inclusion. Within the stroke population, locations of any brain infarction and the presence of a tube feeding-dependent dysphagia would be important. The list of possible significant variables is endless. When a fully automated informatics system is in place, a long list of variables is usually not problematic, but in semiautomated institutions a limit may need to be placed on the number of variables that can be realistically retrieved through data collection.

Ongoing descriptive study of the population is conducted to identify targets for the development and implementation of new interdisciplinary practice interventions. The findings of these studies are used to drive the analytical research methods used throughout Phases II, III, and IV.

Phase II

In Phase II, descriptive findings are used to support the need for practice standardization through the use of SCMs. SCMs include a variety of tools such as pathways, protocols, algorithms, and order sets that vary in their degree of provider flexibility and practice specificity (Table A–2). SCMs are best used when they are designed in a layered fashion that allows practitioners to begin with basic minimal interdisciplinary practice standardization (e.g., a pathway) and add layers of more specific care as needed by a subgroup of patients within the cohort (e.g., algorithms, protocols, and order sets). For example, within the myocardial infarction population, a pathway can be developed to support care for all patients. However, a protocol that strictly controls the administration of rtPA can be layered on top of the pathway when thrombolytic therapy is indicated. Similarly, a generic pathway for seizure patients may be complemented by a status epilepticus algorithm to strictly control the management of this life threatening disorder, should it occur.

An orderly process is used to design SCMs, as illustrated in the quality model. Phase II ends when a new interdisciplinary practice standard has been negotiated and locked into place.

Phase III

In Phase III, the new practice standard developed in Phase II is implemented. CPT members are involved with educating their peers within each discipline, role modeling the new practice, and ensuring the validity and reliability of data collected for OM.

TABLE A–2

Characteristics of Structured Care Methodologies (SCMs)

SCM	Characteristics
Critical Pathway	• Represents a sequential, interdisciplinary, minimal practice standard for a specific patient population • Provider flexibility to alter care to meet individualized patient needs • Abbreviated format, broad perspective • Phase or episode-driven • Lack of control prohibits the ability to measure cause-and-effect relationship between pathway and patient outcomes; changes in patient outcome are directly attributable to the efforts of the collaborative practice team (CPT)
Algorithm	• Binary decision tree that guides stepwise assessment and intervention • Intense specificity; no provider flexibility • Useful in the management of high-risk subgroups within the cohort • May be "layered" on top of a pathway to strictly control care practices used to manage a specific problem • May use analytical research methods to measure cause and effect
Protocol	• Prescribes specific therapeutic interventions for a clinical problem unique to a subgroup of patients within the cohort • Multifaceted; may be used to drive practice for more than one discipline • Broader specificity than an algorithm; allows for minimal provider flexibility by way of treatment options • May be "layered" on top of a pathway to control care practices used to manage a specific problem • May use analytical research methods to measure cause and effect
Order Set	• Preprinted provider orders used to expedite the order process once a practice standard has been validated through analytical research • Complements and increases compliance with existing practice standards • Can be used to represent the algorithm or protocol in order format
Guideline	• Broad, research-based practice recommendations • May or may not have been tested in clinical practice • Practice resources that are helpful in the construction of SCMs • No mechanism for assuring practice implementation

Reprinted with permission from Health Outcomes Institute, Inc, The Woodlands, Texas.

Phase IV

Phase IV involves the analysis and interpretation of data collected from the cohort, facilitating completion of the analytical research cycle. Results of the data analysis should be reviewed by the interdisciplinary team; expertise and ability to identify clinically significant findings may vary among provider disciplines. During Phase IV, CPT members validate whether they have attained best practice through the use of the SCMs implemented, but more often than not, they identify further room for improvement in clinical services, as well as new research questions. This sends the CPT back to Phase II, where new interventions are created and older ones are fine-tuned, reflecting the endless cycle of CQI supported by OM.

| SECTION TWO: CONTENT REVIEW

Match the following phases of OM with the defining characteristics. Each phase may be used more than once.

a. Phase I
b. Phase II
c. Phase III
d. Phase IV

1. Completion of analytical research
2. Development of pathways for patient management   _____
3. Development of a population database   _____
4. Role modeling of new practices   _____
5. Identification of outcome measures   _____
6. Completion of market surveys and literature review _____
7. Generation of new research questions   _____
8. Monitoring of the validity and reliability of data _____

                                                    _____

Please select the best response to the questions below.

9. An example of a SCM that strictly controls practice, prohibiting practice variation and provider flexibility is:
   a. Pathway
   b. Algorithm
   c. Protocol
   d. Order set
   e. Guideline

10. A _____ is best described as a broad, minimal, interdisciplinary practice standard for a patient population.
   a. Pathway
   b. Algorithm
   c. Protocol
   d. Order set
   e. Guideline

11. A _____ serves as a resource for developing standardized practices, but by itself, carries no guarantee that its practice recommendations will be used.
   a. Pathway
   b. Algorithm

    c. Protocol
    d. Order set
    e. Guideline

12. Effective CPTs:
    a. Embody a shared leadership philosophy.
    b. Ensure territorial control over practice revisions.
    c. Acknowledge the value of maintaining practice traditions.
    d. Are always chaired by the medical chief of service.

13. The CPT's attending nurse or outcomes manager:
    a. Chairs the CPT meetings.
    b. Acts as clinical expert and researcher for the CPT.
    c. Functions as a case manager for the CPT.
    d. Carries sole responsibility for the effectiveness of an OM initiative.

14. Variances:
    a. Are synonymous with untoward intermediate outcomes (UIOs).
    b. Are physiologic complications that affect patient outcome.
    c. Represent patient psychosocial untoward occurrences.
    d. Reflect system and provider inefficiencies in patient management.

15. To ensure success of an OM initiative, administrators should:
    a. Limit outcomes measurement to only those providers using CPT interventions.
    b. Govern the CPT's processes and run its meetings.
    c. Limit risk taking to avoid errors that may jeopardize the process.
    d. Delegate all authority for development of the OM program to the CPT.

| SECTION TWO: KEY

Check your answers against the following key for Section Two; repeat the section if further clarification is necessary.

1. d
2. b
3. a
4. c
5. a
6. b
7. d
8. c
9. b
10. a
11. e
12. a
13. b
14. d
15. d

References

1. Zander K: Second-generation primary nursing, *J Nurs Admin* 15:18-24, 1985.
2. Marram G, Barrett MW, Bevis EO: *Primary nursing: a model for individualized care*, St Louis, 1979, CV Mosby.
3. Wojner AW: Outcomes management: an interdisciplinary search for best practice, *AACN Clinical Issues* 7:133-145, 1996.
4. Ellwood PM: Outcomes management: a technology of patient experience, *New Engl J Med* 318:1549-1556, 1988.
5. Davies AR et al: Outcomes assessment in clinical settings: a consensus statement on principles and best practices in project management, *Journal of Quality Improvement* 20:6-16, 1994.
6. Wojner AW: Outcomes management: from theory to practice, *Crit Care Nurs Quart* 19(4):1-15, 1997.
7. Wojner AW: From case management to outcomes management, *The Case Manager* 8(2):77-82, 1997.
8. Wojner AW, Rauch P, Mokracek M: Collaborative ventures in outcomes management: roles and responsibilities in a service line model, *Crit Care Nurs Quart* 19(4):25-41, 1997.
9. Grady GF, Wojner AW: Collaborative practice teams: the infrastructure of outcomes management, *AACN Clinical Issues* 7(1):153-158, 1996.
10. Wojner AW, Kite-Powell D: Outcomes manager: a role for the advanced practice nurse, *Crit Care Nurs Quart* 19(4):16-24, 1997.
11. Hedberg A-M, Wojner AW: *Integrating nutrition into critical pathways for improved outcomes*, Columbus, Ohio, 1994, Ross Products Division: Abbott Laboratories.

Structured Care Methodologies

This section contains examples of different types of structured care methodologies (SCMs) submitted by various health care organizations and individuals. Their inclusion does not imply acknowledgment of best practice but rather is intended to stimulate thought and generate ideas about formats for presenting standardized interdisciplinary practices.

Contents

Congestive Heart Failure (Uncomplicated) Clinical Pathway

Jewish Hospital
217 E. Chestnut Street
Louisville, Kentucky 40202

This pathway is initiated in the Emergency Department. All disciplines identifying the patient's appropriateness for inclusion are responsible for initiating the pathway. Nurses review the pathway, verify completion of patient goals, use appropriate follow-up measures, and document variances. Variances are summarized, analyzed, and shared with the collaborative practice team (CPT).

Modified from Jewish Hospital, Louisville, Kentucky. Used with permission.

Jewish Hospital
Clinical Pathway—DRG 127
Congestive Heart Failure (Uncomplicated) Clinical Pathway
Target LOS 3 Days

(Addressograph)

	Day 1/ER Date_____	Day 2 Date_____	Day 3 Date_____
Patient Goals and Clinical Outcomes	Patient diuresing. Y___ N___ Patient weighed. Y___ N___ Pt/SO explained signs and symptoms of disease and teaching plan initiated? Y___ N___ Is patient diabetic? Y___ N___	Are breath sounds clear? Y___ N___ Is patient's weight down? Y___ N___ Activity and rest periods allow for independent ADLs w/ SaO$_2$ at 92% and HR <30 beats over resting rate? Y___ N___ Is O$_2$ weaned per Protocol? Y___ N___ If no, QRM for Home O$_2$	Pt/SO verbalizes understanding of medications; diet and signs and symptoms instructed to daily weights. Y___ N___ Pt/SO verbalizes MD follow-up visit. Y___ N___ Was an ECHO, Nuclear Study, or Cardiac Cath ordered this admission? Y___ N___
Consults	Cardiology? Pharmacy screening Dietitian		Verbalizes understanding of follow-up MD visit. Y___ N___
Tests	CXR ECG REP CBC SaO$_2$		
Assessments and Treatments	Monitored bed, if indicated. Daily weights Strict I&O V/S q4h O$_2$ per protocol Saline lock	Off monitor, if indicated. Daily weights Strict I&O V/S q4h O$_2$ per protocol Saline lock	Verbalizes understanding of home daily weights. Y___ N___
Medications	Diuretic IV/PO K$^+$ supplement Cardiac medications IV/PO Ace inhibitors Nitrates Digoxin	Evaluate and change medications to PO. •	Verbalizes understanding of home medications. Y___ N___
Nutrition	Healthy Heart diet. Fluid restriction, if needed.	Additional diet instruction needed?	Verbalizes understanding of discharge diet. Y___ N___
Activity	Assess activity level. Independent as possible with ADLs.	Ambulate 3+ minutes four times daily, as tolerated. Assess SaO$_2$ status. HR not > than 20-30 beats over resting rate.	Verbalizes understanding of periods of rest and activity. ADLs with minimal SOA.
Education and Discharge Planning	CHF teaching plan QRM for D/C needs Assess for home health follow-up for reinforcement and compliance	CHF teaching plan Reinforce education for S/S diet, instruction; daily weights QRM for D/C needs Assess for home health follow-up	Has written discharge information.
		Signatures	
	_____	_____	_____

This Clinical Path has been developed as a guideline for management of patients hospitalized for this diagnosis or procedure. Care may be revised to meet the individual patient's needs.

Coronary Intervention Documentation Standards and Clinical Pathway

Dartmouth-Hitchcock Medical Center
1 Medical Center Drive
Lebanon, New Hampshire 03756

Documentation standards are guidelines for care practitioners for the use of the related clinical pathway. The coronary intervention clinical pathway is an interdisciplinary plan used to guide the care of the various practitioners with patients undergoing coronary angioplasty, coronary atherectomy, or coronary stent placement. Note that discharge outcomes are stated along with interventions and patient data.

Coronary Intervention Clinical Pathway Documentation Standards

Dartmouth-Hitchcock Medical Center

POLICY STATEMENT

1. The Coronary Intervention Clinical Pathway is initiated by an RN during the preprocedure visit or once it's recognized that an inpatient will have this procedure.
2. The pathway is a permanent part of the patient's medical record. It is kept at the inpatient's bedside to facilitate ongoing intershift report, physician rounds, and discharge planning. At discharge, the pathway is filed at the front of the progress note section of the medical record.
3. The pathway will replace, for documentation purposes, the following forms:
   - Standard Nursing Care Plan
   - Follow-up Care Instructions
   - Post-Catheterization Contact Form
   - MHMH Outpatient Cardiac Catheterization/Coronary Angioplasty Flow Sheet
   - SDP Outpatient Cardiac Catheterization/Coronary Angioplasty Preprocedure Assessment Data Form
   - SDP Health Survey Assessment Form
4. All health care team members will use the pathway as a plan to manage care for the PTCA/PDCA/stent patient throughout the patient's contact with us for this procedure. This will usually include the following care arenas: Same Day Program, ICCU, CCU, Cardiac Catheterization Lab, ASCU, and Cardiology Clinic.
5. For patients who do not achieve the established outcomes or require significant changes in their plan of care, the pathway will be discontinued and a new plan of care will be developed by the health care team (e.g., the patient who needs CABG surgery after PTCA). When a patient is removed from the pathway, the reason for discontinuing the pathway will be documented in the Progress Notes.
6. The "Referral for Continuing Health Care at Home" portion of the pathway document is used for the transmission of orders and information to the VNA.
7. Variances are noted at the top of the pathway. Interventions for continuous quality improvement will be implemented and evaluated by trending patient outcomes and variance patterns. The clinical pathway is reviewed and revised annually and as needed.

PROCEDURE

1. The RN in Cardiology Clinic, Same Day Program, CCU, or ICCU will initiate the Coronary Intervention Clinical Path, ensuring that it is addressographed and dated and that appropriate patient data on page 2 is completed. Clinical pathway forms are available in appropriate care arenas.

2. The pathway is kept at the patient's bedside in SDP, ICCU, CCU, and ASCU.

3. New medical orders are compared to the pathway. Process of care steps that are not ordered for this patient are to be crossed off the plan. Additional orders unique to the patient are to be transcribed onto the pathway when appropriate. The clinical pathway does not replace the need for the Physician Order Sheet.

4. Members of the health care team will review the plan and expected patient discharge criteria as they pertain to the patient for additions or deletions, individualizing the plan. For example, a patient with history of back pain may have measures to reduce back discomfort added to the pathway.

5. The abbreviation "N/A" may be used for events or discharge criteria that are not applicable or not achievable by the patient.

6. Any member of the health care team who notes a variance will state the variance on the day it occurs. Patient-related variances are to be documented in the variance section at the top of the pathway. Further descriptive information about the variance and the revised plan of care must be written in the progress notes. When documenting a variance on the pathway, include the name of the person identifying the variance, date, and time.

7. All members of the health care team should complete data on the pathway as it pertains to their care. The person completing an activity in the process of care initials the appropriate box (e.g., "☐ Remove dressing, cleanse site, and apply bandage"). Descriptive information is entered in the designated space (e.g., lung sounds, color of limb). Assessment orders are not included on the pathway, in general, because it is assumed that each caregiver will perform those assessments necessary for his/her practice.

8. The RN or tech accountable for the care of the patient during the time period will sign one's initials at the top of the column along with the shift. This signifies that the patient's care has been implemented according to the plan below and that variances have been documented.

9. Upon completion of the procedure, the Cath Lab RN/technician completes the "Status at Transfer from Cath Lab" section. This can be used to facilitate telephone reporting to the ASCU or CCU RN.

10. Discharge criteria on the pathway are initialed as they are met. The discharging RN is accountable for all criteria being met or stated as N/A. If a discharge criterion is not met, a progress note is

written to explain the reason. The discharging RN also completes any of the requested descriptive information (e.g., TPR and peripheral pulses in the involved leg) and signs at the bottom right of page 2 along with the date.

11. If a patient stays for additional days after the sheaths are out, the several dates are written at the top of the "Sheaths Out" column.

12. The discharging physician adds all discharge medications to the pathway form and signs the bottom right of page 2.

13. If a referral is made for continuing care, the RN and physician complete the needed information on the far right of page 2.

14. The patient signs the bottom of the page 2 of the pathway form prior to discharge. The patient does not receive a copy of the pathway but receives a copy of the discharge instructions.

15. At discharge, the two sections to the right on page 2 of the pathway are torn off and faxed to Referral Services, the appropriate clinic, and to the home health agency if used.

16. During the follow-up telephone call, the Cardiology nurse/technician writes his or her findings onto a progress note.

Dartmouth-Hitchcock Medical Center
Coronary Intervention Clinical Pathway (Page 1)

	VARIANCES

CATEGORY	DATE:		
	PREPROCEDURE VISIT/UPON ADMISSION		
	RN INITIALS:　SHIFT:	RN INITIALS:　SHIFT:	RN INITIALS:　SHIFT:
EDUCATION/PSYCHOLOGIC SUPPORT	☐ Review revascularization strategies ☐ Obtain informed consent ☐ Assess patient expectations and document ☐ Review with patient/family preop orders and activities ☐ Show patient/family PTCA videotape ☐ Give patient/family PTCA pamphlet ☐ Give patient/family Heartlines packet ☐ Give patient/family "Back Pain" handout Encourage patients/family to ask questions and express concerns about procedure ⎯⎯ Teach patient stress reduction techniques as needed		
CONTINUING CARE	☐ CRC referral PRN re: discharge, financial, or psychosocial needs Identify discharge needs of patient/family and how needs are to be met Initiate appropriate support service referrals		
CARDIAC STATUS	Vital signs Obtain preop assessment of angina Describe: Assess for risk factors: ☐ Current smoker　　　　☐ Lipid disorders ☐ High stress　　　　　　☐ Hypertension ☐ Diabetes　　　　　　　☐ Family history		
ACTIVITY/FUNCTIONAL STATUS	Assess home activity Perform usual home activity ☐ Complete patient admission survey		
PAIN MANAGEMENT (back, groin)	Discuss back discomfort and management strategies		
NUTRITION/ELIMINATION	NAS, low cholesterol diet Other: Assess for history of difficulty voiding: ☐ No　☐ Yes - Check with physician for catheterization order Describe:		
VASCULAR STATUS	Assess for presence of PVD and previous vascular surgery ☐ No　☐ Yes Describe:		
MEDICATIONS	Evaluate need for H_2 blocker　　　　　　　　　Check for history of problems Start antiplatelet regimen 24 hrs before procedure　with previous diagnostic procedures Ca^+ channel blocker　　　　　　　　　　　　☐ No　☐ Yes　　Describe: Usual cardiac medications Sleeping medication　　　　　　　　　　　　　Bleeding precautions Antianxiety medication prn RBOs		
FLUID STATUS	Admission weight: Admission height: Lung sounds:		
DIAGNOSTIC PROCEDURES	Type and screen Ensure Blood Lok tag is in place ECG CBC, electrolytes, BUN, and creatinine within 30 days CXR done within 6 mo and on file		

VARIANCES	
DATE:	**ARRIVAL TIME IN CATH LAB:**
SDP ARRIVAL TIME: **TO CATH LAB TIME:**	**PROCEDURE:**
IMMEDIATE PREPROCEDURE	**RN/TECH INITIALS:** **SHIFT:**
RN/TECH INITIALS: **SHIFT:**	

	Provide simple introduction to: • Lab • Equipment • Personnel • Sensations and sounds to expect • Symptoms to report Review results of procedure with patient
Outline plan of the day with patient Instruct patient to: ☐ Keep eye glasses, dentures, and hearing aid in place ☐ Not wear snap gown ☐ Instruct family where to wait and how they will be contacted ⟶	⟶
Vital signs **"Same Day Only"** Recent change in frequency and severity of "angina" symptoms? ☐ No ☐ Yes Recent SOB, cough, ankle swelling, or weight gain of more than three pounds? ☐ No ☐ Yes Recent signs of infection or fever? ☐ No ☐ Yes Recent bleeding? ☐ No ☐ Yes Recent vomiting or diarrhea? ☐ No ☐ Yes Recent change in medication use? ☐ No ☐ Yes If on warfarin, has it been stopped? ☐ No ☐ Yes	☐ Complete NNE data form Monitor ECG, BP, SpO$_2$, and chest pain status continuously Continuous arterial pressure monitoring per standard of care O$_2$ prn at 2L/min NP
Bedrest after preop sedation	
Assess back discomfort	Assess back discomfort q1h Administer pain medication and assess response Reposition patient as allowed Back rub prn
NPO after midnight Void on call to Cath Lab	

☐ Mark pedal pulses bilaterally			☐ Clipper prep and surgical scrub to groins
			prn evaluation of peripheral circulation

Leg	R	L
Color		
Temperature		
Sensation		
Movement		
Dorsalis pedis pulse		
Posterior tibial pulse		

☐ Apply sterile dressing to groin and cap ports of sheath at end of procedure

Preop sedation Continue to take cardiac medications—hold diuretic if ordered Adjust insulin dose if diabetic **"Same Day Only"** Medications AM of procedure:	Analgesia prn Antacid prn IV NTG Sedation prn Heparin IV Antiplatelet medication Reevaluate and reorder routine medications Follow DHMC IV Conscious Sedation Guidelines
Insert two 18 g IV catheters in left arm and cap with SafSite T connector D$_5$NS at 100/hr with macrodrip, extension tubing, and regular bore SafSite T connector 2 hrs before procedure Daily weight: Lung sounds:	
Fasting glucose via fingerstick if diabetic Protime/PTT STAT if ordered **"Same Day Only"** ☐ History and physical ☐ ECG ☐ Labs ☐ CXR ☐ Type and screen	ACT after heparin q1h; maintain level > 300 seconds ⟶

(continued)

Dartmouth-Hitchcock Medical Center
Coronary Intervention Clinical Pathway (Page 1)—cont'd

VARIANCES		ADDRESSOGRAPH			
		ARRIVAL TIME IN RECOVERY UNIT:			
	STATUS AT TRANSFER FROM CATH LAB	SHEATHS IN			
	TRANSFER RN/TECH:	RN INITIALS:	SHIFT:	RN INITIALS:	SHIFT:
EDUCATION/ PSYCHOLOGIC SUPPORT		Review results of procedures with patient and family			
		☐ Teach patient/family symptoms to report, activity restrictions			
		Encourage patient and family to ask questions and express concerns about recovery			
CONTINUING CARE		☐ Review results with referring MD			
CARDIAC STATUS	Vital signs: Rhythm: Angina during procedure:	Check BP, pulse q15″ × 4, q30″ × 4, q1h × 4, then q2h; assess resp q2h Titrate oxygen to keep SpO$_2$ > 90% Check SpO$_2$ on admission, q8h, and prn Continuous bedside ECG monitoring in lead showing ischemia Defibrillation for VT and VF, cardiovert, and external pacing per standing order Monitor for chest pain and initiate protocol Check cuff BP on admission and q8h Continuous arterial pressure monitoring, level to femoral artery catheter, zero balance, and dynamic response; continuous flush			
ACTIVITY/FUNCTIONAL STATUS		Bedrest with HOB no greater than 30° Immobilize extremity with sheet tuck Instruct patient to avoid activities that put pressure on groin			
PAIN MANAGEMENT (back, groin)	Pain during procedure (back, groin): Status of pain:	Assess back discomfort q1h Administer pain medication and assess response Reposition patient prn Back rub prn			
NUTRITION/ ELIMINATION	Voided:	Stent: Liquids first meal Reorder diet if necessary (finger food)—NAS, low cholesterol diet Other: If sheaths out same day, do not feed until 2 hrs later If sheaths out in AM, NPO after 0300 and until 20 hrs after sheaths out ☐ Diet consult for discharge diet information if necessary Insert foley catheter if difficulty voiding			
VASCULAR STATUS	Groin accessed: Groin assessment:	Assess for bleeding Dressing to groin; change prn Check groin and distal pulses; assess temperature, sensation and movement q15″ × 4, q30″ × 4, then q1h while sheaths in Temp on admission and q8h Utilize sheath removal protocol: ☐ Early ☐ AM Clamping procedure per protocol If fever, look under dressing			
MEDICATIONS	Medications given during procedure: Medications currently being infused and rates: Discharge criteria for IV conscious sedation met: ☐ Yes ☐ No ☐ N/A	K$^+$ supplement per protocol Sleeping medication prn Administer and wean NTG per protocol Antianxiety medication prn Adjust and wean heparin per protocol Analgesia prn Premedicate for sheath removal Antiplatelet drug as ordered Lidocaine and atropine per standing orders Mylanta II 10-15 ml PO prn RBOs Follow DHMC IV Conscious Sedation Guidelines			
FLUID STATUS	IV fluids infusing and rates:	1 liter of PO fluids for the remainder of the day if ordered IV maintenance fluid as ordered Move maintenance IV from peripheral to venous access. Note: Leave heparin and NTG in peripheral sites I&O q2h Hang 500 cc NS at KVO prior to sheath removal			
DIAGNOSTIC PROCEDURES	Last ACT:	CBC electrolytes, BUN, creatinine in AM ☐ Blood cultures and fever work-up if temp > 38.5°C ABG if respiratory or circulatory condition changes ☐ EKG on arrival and in AM ☐ STAT K$^+$ if diuresis > 500 cc over 2 hr and 1 hr after K$^+$ therapy completion ☐ CPK and LDH on arrival and in AM ☐ PTT and ACT per Sheath Removal Protocol and Heparin Protocol Avoid renipuncture; draw blood through venous sheath if present; reinfuse discard volume Test urine, stool, and emesis for blood qd If patient receiving abciximab, platelets at 2 hrs and 24 hrs after bolus			

Dartmouth-Hitchcock Medical Center
Coronary Intervention Clinical Pathway (Page 2)

DATE: _____ | DATE: _____

ADDRESSOGRAPH

	DATE:	TIME SHEATHS OUT:	DATE:	TIME AMBULATORY:

	SHEATHS OUT: BEDREST			SHEATHS OUT: AMBULATORY		
CATEGORY	RN INITIALS: SHIFT:	RN INITIALS: SHIFT:	RN INITIALS: SHIFT:	RN INITIALS: SHIFT:	RN INITIALS: SHIFT:	RN INITIALS: SHIFT:
EDUCATION/ PSYCHOLOGIC SUPPORT	Review the plan of the day—emphasize activity restrictions ☐ Teach patient/family information to meet discharge outcomes			Review the plan of the day ☐ Teach patient/family information to meet discharge outcomes ☐ Assemble appropriate material into Heartlines packet Encourage patient and family to ask questions and express concerns about discharge		
CONTINUING CARE				☐ Inform patient of follow-up appointments with MD and/or procedures		
CARDIAC STATUS	Check pulse, BP q5" while clamp occlusive, then q15" × 4, q1h × 4, q4h × 24 hrs Resp q4h for 24 hrs Defib for VT and VF, cardiovert, and external pacing per standing order Monitor for chest pain and initiate protocol Continuous ECG monitoring for 24 hrs after PICA			Check pulse, BP, resp q4h × 24 hrs, then q8h ⟶ ⟶ ⟶		
ACTIVITY/ FUNCTIONAL STATUS	☐ Cardiac Rehab consult Bedrest with HOB no greater than 30° for ____hrs Immobilize extremity for 6 hrs			Up to BR with assistance, then advance activity as tolerated ☐ CRP walks patient 5 minutes and up and down stairs prior to discharge ☐ Early ☐ Delayed activity protocol		
PAIN MANAGEMENT (back, groin)	Assess back discomfort q1h Administer pain medication prn and assess response Reposition patient prn Back rub prn			⟶		
NUTRITION/ ELIMINATION	NAS, low cholesterol diet (finger food) 2 hrs after sheaths out Other: Insert foley catheter if difficulty voiding			⟶		
VASCULAR STATUS	Clamping procedure per protocol Assess for bleeding ☐ Sandbag or sheet tuck × 6 hrs Check groin and distal pulses q5" while clamp occlusive, then q15" × 4, q30" × 4, q1h × 4 DSD to site after clamp removed ☐ Remove dressing, cleanse site, and apply bandage once sandbag removed Temp q8h ☐ Transfer from ASCU when criteria met Check for bruit prior to ambulation ☐ + ☐ −			Check groin and distal pulses q1h × 1, q4h × 2, then q8h for 24 h and at discharge Temp q8h until discahrge		
MEDICATIONS	Atropine and lidocaine per standing orders Sleeping med prn Analgesia prn Antianxiety medication prn RBOs Mylanta II 10-15 ml PO prn ☐ Low ☐ High anticoagulation protocol Follow DHMC IV Conscious Sedation Guidelines Bleeding precautions			☐ Write prescriptions ⟶ ⟶ ⟶ ⟶ ⟶ ⟶		
FLUID STATUS	Cap peripheral IVs when VS stable after sheath removal I&O q2h while in ASCU/CCU; then discontinue when patient voiding without difficulty 1 liter of PO fluids day of procedure if ordered			Capped peripheral IV(one if low intensity anticoagulation; two if high intensity) Daily weights		
DIAGNOSTIC PROCEDURES	Hgb and Hct if hematoma or blood loss ☐ CBC, electrolytes, BUN, creatinine, CPK, LDH in AM POD 1 ☐ ECG in AM POD 1 Test urine, stool, and emesis qd for blood High intensity anticoagulation protocol: PIT per Heparin Protocol CBC qa or qod while on heparin PT qd if on warfarin If patient receiving abciximab, platelets at 24 hrs after bolus			☐ CBC, electrolytes, BUN, creatinnine, CPK, LDH in AM POD 1 ☐ ECG in AM POD 1 ⟶		

(continued)

Dartmouth-Hitchcock Medical Center
Coronary Intervention Clinical Pathway (Page 2)—cont'd

DISCHARGE DATE:	DISCHARGE TIME:

THE PATIENT MAY BE DISCHARGED WHEN

EDUCATION/ PSYCHOLOGIC SUPPORT	☐ Strategies for future reviewed by MD

Patient or family member describe care at home R/T:
☐ Site care ☐ Activity ☐ Has a phone number to call with questions or problems
☐ Risk factor modification ☐ Medications ☐ Is eager to leave
☐ Follow-up ☐ Bleeding precautions ☐ All questions have been addressed
☐ S/S of complications and appropriate actions ☐ Has received medication materials
    ● Infection ● Altered circulation in extremity ☐ Has received pamphlet about intervention performed
    ● Bleeding ● Angina

CONTINUING CARE	☐ Physician follow-up has been identified Name: _____ in _____ weeks	Date:	Fax to: ☐ Referral Services ☐ DHMC Clinic

☐ MD discharge summary is dictated
☐ A person to drive the patient home is identified
☐ VNA ☐ NA
☐ Fax received

CARDIAC STATUS	☐ No angina postprocedure ☐ ECG rhythm at baseline ☐ BP and pulse are reviewed and acceptable Vital signs at discharge: T: P: R: BP: Rhythm:

ACTIVITY/ FUNCTIONAL STATUS	☐ At least at preprocedure activity level or ☐ Walked 5 minutes continuously and up and down 26 stairs without symptoms Activity level at discharge:

PAIN MANAGEMENT (back, groin)	☐ Has nothing more than minimal discomfort at operative site

NUTRITION/ ELIMINATION	☐ Diet information given in low cholesterol, low saturated fat, moderate salt diet Comprehension: ☐ Excellent ☐ Very good ☐ Good ☐ Fair ☐ Poor ☐ Denies need ☐ No difficulty voiding Last BM _____

VASCULAR STATUS	☐ No signs of fresh bleeding from any insertion site for 12 hrs after sheath removal ☐ If hematoma, no signs of progression ☐ If hematoma, not pulsatile ☐ No impairment in peripheral circulation from baseline ☐ Temperature <38.5°C

Leg	R	L
Color		
Temperature		
Sensation		
Movement		
Dorsalis pedis pulse		
Posterior tibial pulse		

MEDICATIONS	☐ No longer receiving IV cardiac medications ☐ Has receive prescriptions ☐ Has received prescription for SL NTG prn ☐ Has plan to obtain medications

FLUID STATUS	☐ Capped IV catheter, D/C'd Discharge weight: Lung sounds:

DIAGNOSTIC PROCEDURES	☐ No acute ECG changes indicative of significant cardiac damage ☐ Hgb and Hct > 10 g/dl and 35% or at preop level ☐ Enzymes are reviewed and are not greater than upper level of normal ☐ BUN and creatinine stable ☐ K⁺ > 3.5 mEq ☐ If on warfarin, INR 2-2.5	Latest INR Date

Admit Date:	ADDRESSOGRAPH
Allergies:	

Medical history:	Address:
	Telephone:

Functional deficits/limitations

Psycho/social history:

Admission medications:

Cath data:

Admission: wt: _____ ht: _____ TPR: _____ B.P.: _____

Procedure:

Interventionalist:	Date of intervention:
Cardiologist:	Primary care provider:

REFERRAL FOR CONTINUING HEALTH CARE AT HOME   NA ☐

Home health orders:

PT/INR follow-up:

HOME HEALTH AGENCY/FACILITY

Name:

Telephone:	FAX:

Insurance:

Clinical Resource Coordinator: Beeper:

Transferred to home health agency ☐   Patient is homebound ☐

Routine discharge instructions provided ☐   4-week F/U appt. with _____ to be mailed to patient ☐

MEDICATIONS

I understand and have been given a copy of discharge instructions.
I authorize DHMC to make a home health referral for continued care, if necessary, as ordered above.

Patient/agent:

Discharging nurse:	Discharge date:

Physician:

Cardiac Surgery Documentation Standards and Clinical Pathway

Dartmouth-Hitchcock Medical Center
1 Medical Center Drive
Lebanon, New Hampshire 03756

Documentation standards are guidelines for care practitioners for the use of the related clinical pathway. The cardiac surgery clinical pathway is used to guide the care of various practitioners with cardiac surgery patients regardless of the procedure. Note that outcomes are stated for the intensive care period and for discharge, as well as daily for the Intermediate Cardiac Care Unit. The form is also used to convey information to the home health nurse, the follow-up clinic, and the referring physician at discharge.

| Cardiac Surgery Clinical Pathway Documentation Standards

Dartmouth-Hitchcock Medical Center Cardiothoracic Surgery Service

1. Cardiac Surgery Clinical Pathway forms are available on the following units: CT ICU, ICCU, CCU, Preadmission Testing, and Same Day Program.
2. The Cardiac Surgery Clinical Pathway is initiated upon determination of the patient's need for cardiac surgery, either as an inpatient or in Preadmission Testing. The nurse initiating the clinical path ensures that it is addressographed, dated, and completed with appropriate baseline patient data.
3. An exclusion criterion for the initiation of the Cardiac Surgery Clinical Pathway is any preexisting preoperative diagnosis that requires extended postoperative evaluation and treatment.
4. The clinical pathway replaces the Standard Nursing Care Plan and the Interdisciplinary Patient Discharge Instruction Sheet for documentation purposes. The clinical pathway does not replace the need for the Physician Order Sheet.
5. The pathway is kept on the patient clipboard in the CT ICU/CCU and in the patient's bedside notebook on the ICCU to facilitate ongoing intershift/daily report, physician rounds, and discharge planning. The pathway is a permanent part of the patient care record.
6. All health care team members use the clinical pathway to manage care for cardiac surgery patients throughout their hospitalization. It is also used to track a patient's progress toward daily outcomes, as well as those at the time of transfer from CT ICU/CCU and discharge from ICCU.
7. The RN responsible for care of the patient places a check mark in the boxes on the pathway as interventions are completed and fills in any objective data requested (e.g., preop SpO_2). All others who complete interventions are to sign their initials in the respective box. Since interventions are checked on the pathway no duplicate documentation of this needs to occur on the Flow Sheet. Most of the objective physiologic data should continue to be written though on the Flow Sheet or Clinical Record. Expected patient assessments are not included on this pathway, since it is assumed that all health care team members will perform timely assessments of patients appropriate for their discipline.
8. Documentation of signatures representing initials on the clinical pathway can be found on the Signature Sheet for staff RNs. All other caregivers who initial the pathway should write their signature at the bottom of page 3 or 5.

9. The interventions on the pathway should be individualized for each patient based on physician's orders. The responsible RN reviews the plan and makes changes as needed based on the patient's individual needs, variances, and complications. These changes may be documented by category or in the "Change of Plan" space.

10. To document that daily outcomes (shaded areas) have been met, the RN responsible for care of the patient places a check mark in the related boxes within the categories. If the patient is in Preadmission Testing, this is completed during that visit. If the patient is an inpatient, this is completed by the night RN as it relates to the status of the patient at midnight. If all daily outcomes have been met the responsible RN checks the respective box at the top of the column. If one or more daily outcomes have not been met, the box "Not met" is to be checked instead.

11. At any time, if it is recognized that outcomes are not being met or variances are occurring, the accountable practitioner should determine what assessments and interventions need to take place and document them in the "Change of Plan" section, a progress note, or the Flow Sheet.

12. At the end of each shift, the responsible RN is to sign his or her initials and shift worked, signifying that the plan of care is individualized and up to date. Initials by the night RN also indicate that daily outcomes have been evaluated.

13. The abbreviation "N/A" may be used for interventions or outcomes that are not applicable to the patient.

14. Upon transfer from the CT ICU, the RN assigned to the patient completes the section "Pertinent CT ICU History and Patient Status at Transfer," checking off the individual outcomes that have been achieved (shaded area), checking off the summary box concerning all outcomes, and completing the patient assessment data. The complete signature of the RN should be written.

15. When a patient follows the pathway but exceeds the expected length of stay, the extra columns on pages 3 through 6 should be used to plan and document the patient's care.

16. For patients who do not achieve the established outcomes or require significant changes in their plan of care, the pathway will be discontinued and a new plan of care will be developed by the health care team in accordance with institutional policy. When a patient is removed from the clinical pathway, the reason for discontinuing the pathway will be documented in the "Progress Notes" section by the responsible physician. A patient requiring readmission to the CT ICU is automatically removed from the clinical pathway and resumed on the pathway as soon as the clinical condition warrants.

17. The Clinical Resource Coordinator (CRC) is responsible for reviewing the clinical pathway, facilitating the completion of assessments and interventions with the aim of achieving identified outcomes, and recording and tracking variance data.

18. Discharge outcomes are initialed as they are met. The discharging RN is accountable for all baseline data being entered on page 1. Also, he or she ensures/documents that discharge outcomes have been met, enters the requested discharge data and writes his or her signature on the pathway at the bottom of page 2. If discharge outcomes have not been met, rationale for discharge and any follow-up should be documented in the progress notes.

19. The "Referral for Continuing Health Care at Home" portion of the path is completed by the discharging MD, responsible RN, and CRC. It is used for transmission of orders and information to the VNA.

20. The discharging physician adds all discharge medications to the clinical pathway and writes his or her signature on the bottom of page 1 even if the patient does not have a referral for continuing care. Medications do not need to be written elsewhere.

21. The patient must sign the bottom of the first page of the pathway prior to discharge. The patient does not receive a copy of the pathway but will receive a copy of the "Discharge Instructions for the Cardiac Surgical Patient."

22. At discharge, pages 1 and 2 of the pathway are faxed to Referral Services, the appropriate Hitchcock Clinic, and VNA if a referral is initiated. Then the complete pathway is filed in front of the "Physicians' Order" section of the medical record.

23. Variances from the clinical pathway are reviewed. Interventions for continuous quality improvements (CQI) are implemented and evaluated by trending patient outcomes and variance patterns. The clinical pathway is reviewed and revised annually and as needed.

Dartmouth-Hitchcock Medical Center
Cardiac Services
Clinical Pathway: Cardiac Surgery
Page 1

Admit Date:	Addressograph
Allergies/ADRs:	Address:
Age:	
Past Medical History: Diabetes ☐ Type 1 ☐ Type 2 ☐ None	Telephone:
	Name of Home Caregiver:

♡ Risk Factors:

Functional Deficits/Limitations:

Psycho/Social History:

Admission Medications:

Cath Data:	LV EF: %

Admission/
Preop: Wt: _____   Ht: _____   TPR: _____   BP: _____

Intervention:	Date:	Interventionalist:
Surgical Procedure:		Date of Surgery:
Surgeon: Phone: 603-650-7390		Primary Care Provider:
Clinical Resource Coordinator:	Phone: 603-650-5789 Beeper #:	

REFERRAL FOR CONTINUING HEALTH CARE AT HOME   N/A   ☐

Home health orders: ☐   2x/wk x 2 wk and prn   ☐   Other   Additional referrals:

Check incisions, cardiopulmonary status, vital signs, effectiveness of medications, and rehabilitation progress.

PT/INR follow-up:

Other:

HOME HEALTH AGENCY/FACILITY

Name:

Telephone:	FAX:

Insurance:

Transferred to home health agency: ☐   Pt. is homebound: ☐   Routine discharge instructions provided: ☐

4 week F/U appt. with _____ to be mailed to pt. ☐   Other appointments:

DURABLE MEDICAL EQUIPMENT

Vendor:

Telephone:

Equipment:

MEDICATIONS

I understand and have been given a copy of discharge instructions. I authorize DHMC
to make a home health referral for continued care, if necessary, as ordered above.

Patient/Agent:	
Discharging Nurse:	Disc. Date:
Physician:	Disc. Time:

At discharge, fax to Referral Services, DHMC clinic, and VNA if ordered. Original at front of progress notes in medical record.

	The Patient May Be Discharged When:	Discharge Data
Cardiac Status	Cardiac status is stable. Stability is defined for the patient by: ☐ Resting heart rate >60 and <100 bpm for 24 hrs ☐ NSR for 24 hr., determined by ECG or telemetry ☐ Angina-free condition ☐ Systolic BP >90 but <160 mm Hg ☐ Temperature is <38° for 24 hrs	Pulse:_____ BP: _____ Rhythm:_____
Respiratory Status		Respiratory rate: _____ Lung sounds at discharge: _____
Nutrition/ Elimination	☐ Resumed eating usual diet Diet comprehension: ☐ Excellent ☐ Very Good ☐ Good ☐ Fair ☐ Poor ☐ Denies Need	Diet: _____ _____ Last BM: _____
Wound/ Sternum	☐ There are no signs/symptoms of wound infection ☐ The sternum is stable	Describe incisions: _____ _____ Temperature: _____
Pain Mgmt.	☐ Pain controlled to permit activity progression, pulmonary hygiene, and sleep	Usual pain 0-10:
Fluid Status	☐ No gross pitting edema ☐ Weight decreasing toward baseline	Weight: _____
Functional Status	☐ Can walk unassisted and continuously for 5 min ☐ Can walk up and down one flight of stairs These activities are accomplished: ☐ Without pulse increasing more than 25 bpm above resting level ☐ With pulse returning to resting level in 3 min ☐ With O$_2$ sat. ≥90% breathing room air ☐ With no dizziness or lightheadedness ☐ With no angina ADLs are evaluated	Admit Disc Feeding _____ _____ Bathing _____ _____ Toileting _____ _____ Dressing _____ _____ Key 0 Independent 1 Uses equipment or devices 2 Needs assistance or supervision 3 Needs assistance and special equipment 4 Dependent; does not participate
Medications	☐ The medications have been reviewed by the intern or NP to determine necessity and accessibility ☐ The prescriptions have been written and discussed with patient	
Diagnostic Tests	The following tests are performed and reviewed: ☐ Chest x-ray study—one PA and lateral must be done, reviewed by a physician or NP, and judged to be satisfactory within 4 days of discharge ☐ WBC <15,000 and falling within 4 days of discharge ☐ K+ ≥4.0 mmol/L within 4 days of discharge ☐ ECG performed during post-op period ☐ Hgb ≥8 g/dl within 4 days of discharge	Last INR: _____ Date: _____
Education	Can demonstrate knowledge of the following: ☐ Wound care, sternal healing ☐ Activities/rest ☐ Exercise plan ☐ Medication regimen ☐ Pain management ☐ Follow-up care/ appointments ☐ Warning signs and actions to take ☐ Risk factor modification ☐ Psychologic adaptations ☐ DHMC person or local physician to call with problems ☐ Care of leg edema ☐ Patient able to massage scar ☐ Patient able to count pulse with exercise ☐ Patient has received medication pamphlets, Med Card, Med Schedule ☐ Patient/family have watched homegoing video	
Continuing Care	☐ Patient and family feel patient is ready ☐ There is a specific person(s) identified who will assist with meals, transportation, personal care, and home maintenance ☐ Adequate shelter is assured	

At discharge, fax to Referral Services, DHMC clinic, and VNA if ordered.

(continued)

	Date:_____ Preadm/Preop	Date:_____ CT ICU: Day of Surgery/ POD 1	Pertinent CT ICU History and Status at Transfer
Category Signatures	RN: _____ Shift:____ RN: _____ Shift:____ RN: _____ Shift:____ ☐ All outcomes met ☐ Not met	RN: _____ Shift:____ RN: _____ Shift:____ RN: _____ Shift:____	RN: _____ Shift:____ RN: _____ Shift:____ RN: _____ Shift:____ ☐ All intermediate outcomes met ☐ Not met
Cardiac Status			☐ Cardiac index >2L/min/m^2 ☐ Resting heart rate >60 bpm and <120 bpm ☐ No life threatening arrhythmias ☐ Systolic BP >90 but <160 mm Hg ☐ No central monitoring lines
	Admission vital signs	Continuous ECG and hemo-dynamic monitoring VS q1/2h x 4 then q1h x 12 and prn, then q2h and prn Rewarm using lights, Bair Hugger, warm fluids ☐ Discontinue PA catheter after extubation if CI >2.2 and off all inotropic support for >4 hrs	Vital signs: Rhythm: ☐ Preop LV EF:_____%
Respiratory Status	☐ Describes need for and demonstrates (when possible) incentive spirometry and C&DB exercises		☐ Resting SpO$_2$ ≥90% on NP O$_2$ ☐ SpO$_2$ ≥85% on O$_2$ with activity ☐ Effective cough and airway clearance
	☐ Preop SpO$_2$ on room air: _____ ☐ O$_2$ on way to OR (inpatients only) ☐ Anesthesia consult	ET suction prn Initiate weaning protocol Extubate within 6 hrs ☐ or 12 hrs ☐ of CT ICU admission O$_2$ to maintain SpO$_2$ ≥90% Continuous SpO$_2$ monitoring CDB, incentive spirometry q1-2h WA Chest physiotherapy if significant atelectasis or consolidation	O$_2$ requirement: Lung sounds: SpO$_2$ on room air:
Nutrition/ Elimination			
	☐ Instruct in supplemental nutrition as needed; give booklet "Tips to Better Food Intake" Usual home diet NPO per anesthesia guidelines	NG/OG tube while intubated Advance diet as tolerated	Diet: Bowel sounds:
Wound/ Sternum			
	☐ Hibiclens shower/bath	Chest tubes to 10cm H$_2$O pressure ☐ Remove chest tubes (if no air leak and CT drainage <30 cc/hr × 4hrs) Dry sterile dressings to incisions × 24 hrs Betadine to incisions bid after 24 hrs ☐ ☐ Ace wrap in figure 8 to vein harvest leg(s)	Incisions:
Pain Management	☐ Identifies pain management concerns r/t chronic and current health conditions ☐ Describes understanding of pain scale		☐ Pain controlled to permit activity progression, pulmonary hygiene, and sleep Usual pain 0-10:_____ Pain control:
		IV/PO pain medication per order	Last pain med:
Fluid Status			☐ Urine output >30 cc/hr
	☐ Weight morning of surgery ☐ Height	Hourly I&O IV fluids per MD orders Foley to CD	DTV: Edema: Weight:

KEY: SHADED areas indicate intermediate outcomes to be met.

Signatures of other than staff RNs:	Init.:	Signature:	Init.:	Signature:	Init.:

CT ICU Date:_____	CT ICU Date:_____	Date:_____ ICCU: Day of Transfer	Date:_____ ICCU: Day 2
RN: _____ Shift:___ RN: _____ Shift:___ RN: _____ Shift:___	RN: _____ Shift:___ RN: _____ Shift:___ RN: _____ Shift:___	RN: _____ Shift:___ RN: _____ Shift:___ RN: _____ Shift:___ ☐ All outcomes met 2400 ☐ Not met	RN: _____ Shift:___ RN: _____ Shift:___ RN: _____ Shift:___ ☐ All outcomes met 2400 ☐ Not met
		☐ Resting heart rate >60 bpm and <120 bpm ☐ No life threatening arrhythmias ☐ Systolic BP >90 but <160 mm Hg	☐ ———————➤ ☐ ———————➤ ☐ ———————➤
		☐ ☐ Epicardial pacing wire care bid Check P, R, and BP q4h for 24 hrs ECG monitoring	☐ ☐ Epicardial pacing wire care bid Check P, R, and BP q4h for 24 hrs and then every shift ☐ Discontinue ECG monitoring (48 hrs postop if rhythm stable, mediastinal tubes out, and EF >30%)
		☐ Resting SpO$_2$ >90% on NP O$_2$ ☐ SpO$_2$ >85% on O$_2$ with activity ☐ Effective cough and airway clearance	☐ ———————➤ ☐ ———————➤ ☐ ———————➤
		O$_2$ via NP; wean as long as O$_2$ sat. ≥90% ☐ SpO$_2$ qd at rest CDB, incentive spirometer q1-2h WA Chest physiotherapy if significant atelectasis or consolidation	O$_2$ via NP; wean as long as O$_2$ sat. ≥90% ☐ SpO$_2$ qd at rest CDB, incentive spirometer q1-2h WA
		Able to tolerate full liquids	☐ Able to tolerate regular/NCS diet
		Clear liquids when bowel sounds present Diet consultation for supplements and discharge diet information Dietary supplements if needed: ☐ Consult completed ☐ Supplements added RBOs	☐ Progress to regular diet as tolerated; no concentrated sweets for diabetics ☐ MOM 15 ml PO if no BM
		☐ Free of signs/symptoms of infection	☐ ———————➤
		☐ ☐ Betadine to incisions bid ☐ Remove chest tubes ☐ Take sternal and leg dressings off (at 24 hours) Check temperature q4h; if >38.5° call HO ☐ ☐ Ace wraps in figure 8 to legs if leg incision; rewrap q12h	☐ ☐ Betadine to incisions bid ☐ Remove chest tube dressings (24 hrs after chest tubes out) Check temperature q4h for 24 hrs, then every shift; if >38.5° call HO ☐ ☐ Ace wraps in figure 8 to legs if leg incisions; rewrap q12h
		☐ Pain controlled to permit activity progression, pulmonary hygiene, and sleep	☐ ———————➤
		PO analgesic q3-4h prn	PO analgesic q3-4h prn
		☐ Weight is decreasing	☐ ———————➤
		Weigh qd Foley to constant drainage Capped IV	Weigh qd ☐ Remove foley catheter (POD2 in AM) Capped IV
Signature:	Init.: Signature:	Init.: Signature:	Init.: Signature:

(continued)

	Date:_____ Preadm/Preop	Date:_____ CT ICU: Day of Surgery/ POD 1	Pertinent CT ICU History and Status at Transfer
Functional Status			☐ Up in chair for 1 hr

	Activity as tolerated	While intubated:
		  HOB 30°
		  Turn q2-4h prn
		When extubated:
		  Dangle at bedside ☐
		  Up in chair tid ☐ ☐ ☐
		  March in place ☐
			Activity:

Medications			☐ Antibiotics complete
	Medications on call to OR as ordered PO H$_2$ blocker if ordered hs sedation Consider usual medications	Medications as ordered by physician/NP Vasoactive IV medications per order and protocol If diabetic with glucose >200mg/dl, initiate insulin protocol If diabetic, consider sliding scale insulin at transfer	If diabetic, medications:
Diagnostics Tests	ECG (within past 6 months) PA and LAT chest x-ray study (within past 1 year) Blood tests per anesthesia guidelines (within past 45 days)/MD orders ☐ If diabetic, fingerstick BG morning of surgery	☐ Check x-ray study postop ☐ ECG postop ☐ Chest x-ray study after chest tube removal ☐ Postop labs; ABG with bicarb, Hct/Hgb, K+, glucose ☐ Hct/Hgb 4 hrs postop	Last K+: If diabetic, last fingerstick:
Education	☐ Describes basic understanding of surgical procedure/purpose and expected recovery process and information resources ☐ Identifies expected discharge time frame and potential resources needed at discharge Share plan of care ☐ Provide patient/family with preop video ☐ Provide patient/family with preop booklet ☐ Discuss with patient/family: Preop orders Postop: Pain management/activity regimen Sensory/perceptual changes Weight gain and anasarca ☐ Provide incentive spirometer and instruct in use	Share plan of care	Other:
Continuing Care	Disposition identified ☐ Home ☐ Rehab ☐ ECF ☐ CRC (Office of Care Management) referral prn regarding disc., financial, or psychosocial concerns Chaplain referral prn		☐ CT ICU data completed on NNECVDSG Data Collection Form _____ _____
Change in Plan	_____ _____ _____ _____	_____ _____ _____ _____	_____ _____ _____ _____

Addressograph

CT ICU Date:_____	CT ICU Date:_____	Date:_____ ICCU: Day of Transfer	Date:_____ ICCU: Day 2
		☐ Cardiac Surgery Exercise Class if appropriate ☐ ☐ ☐ Up in chair tid, with legs elevated if leg incision ☐ Walk 1-2 min assisted; monitor SpO$_2$ ☐ Flexibility exercises with PT	☐ Cardiac Surgery Exercise Class When in chair legs elevated if leg incision ☐ ☐ ☐ Walk tid, increase 1-3 min/day; monitor SpO$_2$ Encourage patient to walk ad lib when able ☐ ☐ Flexibility exercises bid
		☐ ASA 81 mg PO qd, except with mechanical valve and normal coronary arteries ☐ With mechanical valve, consider anticoagulation Consider diuretic until preop weight Antibiotic IV to complete series ☐ Evaluate to restart preop medications H$_2$ blocker PO If diabetic, restart oral agent or insulin	Continue meds as ordered
		☐ AP portable chest x-ray study after chest tube removal	☐ Potassium while diuresing
		Explain usual care activities to patient Share plan of care	☐ Give postop Heartlines packet and review With valve include as appropriate: ☐ Bacterial Endocarditis prophylaxis ☐ Medic Alert ☐ Warfarin ☐ Have patient/family watch homegoing videotape prior to discharge Explain usual care activities to patient Teach patient daily to meet discharge outcomes Share plan of care
		Cardiac Rehab consultation If diabetic, consult Diabetes CNS as needed	
_____ _____ _____ _____ _____	_____ _____ _____ _____ _____	_____ _____ _____ _____ _____	_____ _____ _____ _____ _____

(continued)

CLINICAL PATHWAY: Cardiac Surgery—cont'd   Page 5

	Date:_____ ICCU: Day 3	Date:_____ ICCU: Day 4	Date:_____ ICCU: Day 5
Category Signatures	RN: _____ Shift:_____ RN: _____ Shift:_____ RN: _____ Shift:_____ ☐ All outcomes met at 2400 ☐ Not met	RN: _____ Shift:_____ RN: _____ Shift:_____ RN: _____ Shift:_____ ☐ All outcomes met at 2400 ☐ Not met	RN: _____ Shift:_____ RN: _____ Shift:_____ RN: _____ Shift:_____ ☐ All outcomes met at 2400 ☐ Not met
Cardiac Status	☐ Resting heart rate >60 bpm and <120 bpm ☐ No life threatening arrhythmias ☐ Systolic BP >90 but <160 mm Hg Check P, R, and BP every shift ☐ Remove pacing wires (if off telemetry 24 hrs) or ☐ clip (if on warfarin)	☐ ──────► ☐ ──────► ☐ ──────► Check P, R, and BP every shift	☐ ──────► ☐ ──────► ☐ ──────► Check P, R, and BP every shift
Respiratory Status	☐ SpO2 ≥90% on room air at rest and with activity ☐ Effective cough and airway clearance ☐ SpO2 qd at rest ☐ Discontinue oxygen CDB, incentive spirometer q1-2h WA	☐ ──────► ☐ ──────► CDB, incentive spirometer q1-2h WA	☐ ──────► ☐ ──────► CDB, incentive spirometer q1-2h WA
Nutrition/ Elimination	☐ Able to tolerate regular/NCS diet Progress to regular diet as tolerated; no concentrated sweets for diabetics ☐ Dulcolax suppository if no BM	☐ Had BM Regular diet; no concentrated sweets for diabetics ☐ Diet information given on low cholesterol, low saturated fat, and moderation in salt diet ☐ Enema if no BM	Regular diet; no concentrated sweets for diabetics
Wound/ Sternum	☐ Temperature is less than 38°C ☐ Free of signs/symptoms of infection ☐ ☐ Betadine to incisions bid Check temperature every shift; if T >38.5°C call HO ☐ ☐ Ace wraps in figure 8 to legs if leg incision; rewrap q12h	☐ ──────► ☐ ──────► ☐ ☐ Betadine to incisions bid Check temperature every shift; if T >38.5°C call HO ☐ ☐ Ace wraps in figure 8 to legs if leg incision; rewrap q12h ☐ Remove chest tube sutures	☐ ──────► ☐ ──────► Check temperature every shift; if T >38.5°C call HO ☐ ☐ Ace wraps in figure 8 to legs if leg incision; rewrap q12h
Pain Management	☐ Pain controlled to permit activity progression, pulmonary hygiene, and sleep PO analgesic q3-4h prn	☐ ──────► PO analgesic q3-4h prn	☐ ──────► PO analgesic q3-4h prn
Fluid Status	☐ Weight is decreasing Weigh qd ☐ Discontinue capped IV if off telemetry >24 hrs	☐ ──────► Weigh qd	☐ ──────► Weigh qd
Signatures of other than staff RNs:	Init.:	Signature:	Init.:	Signature:	Init.:

Addressograph

Date: _____ ICCU: Day _____	Date: _____ ICCU: Day _____	Date: _____ ICCU: Day _____

RN: _____ Shift:_____
RN: _____ Shift:_____
RN: _____ Shift:_____
☐ All outcomes met at 2400
    ☐ Not met
	RN: _____ Shift:_____
	RN: _____ Shift:_____
	RN: _____ Shift:_____
	☐ All outcomes met at 2400
	    ☐ Not met
		RN: _____ Shift:_____
		RN: _____ Shift:_____
		RN: _____ Shift:_____
		☐ All outcomes met at 2400
		    ☐ Not met

☐ ————————▶ ☐ ————————▶ ☐ ————————▶ Check P, R, and BP every shift	☐ ————————▶ ☐ ————————▶ ☐ ————————▶ Check P, R, and BP every shift	☐ ————————▶ ☐ ————————▶ ☐ ————————▶ Check P, R, and BP every shift

☐ ————————▶
 	
☐ ————————▶
 	
CDB, incentive spirometer q1-2h
  WA
	☐ ————————▶
	
	☐ ————————▶
	
	CDB, incentive spirometer q1-2h
	  WA
		☐ ————————▶
		
		☐ ————————▶
		
		CDB, incentive spirometer q1-2h
		  WA

Regular diet; no concentrated
  sweets for diabetics
	Regular diet; no concentrated
	  sweets for diabetics
		Regular diet; no concentrated
		  sweets for diabetics

☐ ————————▶
☐ ————————▶
 	
Check temperature every shift;
  if T >38.5°C call HO
☐ ☐ Ace wraps in figure 8 to
legs if leg incision; rewrap
q12h
	☐ ————————▶
	☐ ————————▶
	
	Check temperature every shift;
	  if T >38.5°C call HO
	☐ ☐ Ace wraps in figure 8 to
	legs if leg incision; rewrap
	q12h
		☐ ————————▶
		☐ ————————▶
		
		Check temperature every shift;
		  if T >38.5°C call HO
		☐ ☐ Ace wraps in figure 8 to
		legs if leg incision; rewrap
		q12h

☐ ————————▶ PO analgesic q3-4h prn	☐ ————————▶ PO analgesic q3-4h prn	☐ ————————▶ PO analgesic q3-4h prn
☐ ————————▶ Weigh qd	☐ ————————▶ Weigh qd	☐ ————————▶ Weigh qd
Signature: Init.:	Signature: Init.:	Signature:

(continued)

CLINICAL PATHWAY: Cardiac Surgery—cont'd   Page 6

	Date: _____ ICCU: Day 3	Date: _____ ICCU: Day 4	Date: _____ ICCU: Day 5
Functional Status		☐ Walked 5 minutes continuously ☐ Gone ↑ and ↓ stairs	☐ ———————→ ☐ ———————→
	☐ Cardiac Surgery Exercise Class When in chair, legs elevated if leg incision ☐ ☐ ☐ Walk tid, increase 1-3 min/day; monitor SpO_2 until ≥90% off O_2 Encourage patient to walk ad lib when able ☐ ☐ Flexibility exercises bid	☐ Cardiac Surgery Exercise Class When in chair, legs elevated if leg incision ☐ ☐ ☐ Walk tid, increase 1-3 min/day ☐ Once walking 5 min and off O_2, go up and down stairs Encourage patient to walk ad lib when able Shower after pacing wires out ☐ ☐ Flexibility exercises bid	☐ Cardiac Surgery Exercise Class When in chair, legs elevated if leg incision ☐ ☐ ☐ Walk tid, increase 1-3 min/day ☐ Once walking 5 min and off O_2, go up and down stairs Encourage patient to walk ad lib when able Shower after pacing wires out ☐ ☐ Flexibility exercises bid
Medications	☐ Pre-op medications have been restarted Continue medications as ordered	Continue medications as ordered	Continue medications as ordered Write prescriptions
Diagnostics Tests	☐ Potassium while diuresing qd If diabetic, fingerstick ac and hs	☐ Potassium while diuresing qd ☐ CBC, lytes, BUN, creatinine ☐ ECG ☐ PA and LAT chest x-ray study ☐ Review POD 4 tests	☐ Potassium while diuresing qd
Education	☐ Have patient/family watch nutrition videos Teach patient daily to meet discharge outcomes Share plan of care ☐ Have patient/family watch homegoing video prior to discharge	☐ ———————→ Teach patient daily in order to meet discharge outcomes Share plan of care ☐ ———————→	☐ ———————→ ☐ Discuss bacterial endocarditis prophylaxis with appropriate patients ☐ Discuss anticoagulation, precautions, and follow-up plan with appropriate patients ☐ ———————→ Teach patient daily in order to meet discharge outcomes Share plan of care
Continuing Care	Disposition confirmed ☐ Home ☐ Rehab ☐ ECF ☐ Referral to outpatient cardiac rehabilitation program ☐ Cardiac risk factor counseling		Date: Fax to: _____ ☐ Referral Services _____ ☐ DHMC Clinic _____ ☐ VNA ☐ NA _____ ☐ Fax received ☐ If anticoagulated, arrange PT follow-up with referring MD
Change in Plan	_____ _____ _____ _____	_____ _____ _____ _____	_____ _____ _____ _____

Addressograph

Date:_____ ICCU: Day_____	Date:_____ ICCU: Day_____	Date:_____ ICCU: Day_____
☐ ——————→ ☐ ——————→	☐ ——————→ ☐ ——————→	☐ ——————→ ☐ ——————→
☐ Cardiac Surgery Exercise Class When in chair, legs elevated if leg incision ☐ ☐ ☐ Walk tid, increase 1-3 min/day ☐ Once walking 5 min and off O_2, go up and down stairs Encourage patient to walk ad lib when able Shower after pacing wires out ☐ ☐ Flexibility exercises bid	☐ Cardiac Surgery Exercise Class When in chair, legs elevated if leg incision ☐ ☐ ☐ Walk tid, increase 1-3 min/day ☐ Once walking 5 min and off O_2, go up and down stairs Encourage patient to walk ad lib when able Shower after pacing wires out ☐ ☐ Flexibility exercises bid	☐ Cardiac Surgery Exercise Class When in chair, legs elevated if leg incision ☐ ☐ ☐ Walk tid, increase 1-3 min/day ☐ Once walking 5 min and off O_2, go up and down stairs Encourage patient to walk ad lib when able Shower after pacing wires out ☐ ☐ Flexibility exercises bid
Continue medications as ordered	Continue medications as ordered	Continue medications as ordered
☐ Potassium while diuresing qd	☐ Potassium while diuresing qd	☐ Potassium while diuresing qd
Teach patient daily to meet discharge outcomes Share plan of care	Teach patient daily to meet discharge outcomes Share plan of care	Teach patient daily to meet discharge outcomes Share plan of care
_____ _____ _____ _____ _____	_____ _____ _____ _____ _____	_____ _____ _____ _____ _____

| Acute Ischemic Stroke Clinical Pathway

Jewish Hospital
217 E. Chestnut Street
Louisville, Kentucky 40202

This pathway is initiated in the Emergency Department. All disciplines identifying the patient's appropriateness are responsible for initiating the pathway. Nurses review the pathway to verify completion of patient goals, take appropriate follow-up measures, and document variances. Variances are summarized, analyzed, and shared with the collaborative practice team (CPT).

Jewish Hospital
Clinical Pathway—DRG 14A
Acute Ischemic Stroke Clinical Pathway
Target LOS 6 Days   (Addressograph)

	DAY 1/ED Date_____	DAY 2 Date_____	DAY 3 Date_____	DAY 4 Date_____	DAY 5 Date_____	DAY 6 Essential D/C Outcomes Date_____
Patient Goals and Clinical Outcomes		Breath sounds clear. BP within 90-180 and diastolic B.P. within 50-100. If on heparin, PTT therapeutic. Pt teaching plan initiated and documented in computer (Education Record).	BM within last 72 hrs. Activity progressing as planned. Pt/family makes decision regarding D/C plan.	Eating at least 2/3 of meals without choking or coughing. If pt to be D/C'd home, pt/family demonstrates ability to care for pt at home. If not met, reevaluate D/C plan.		INR 2-3 without bleeding. Y___ N___
Consults	Neurologist Speech/PT D/C planner Primary Care if none on case	Physiatrist Dietitian				Verbalizes need for follow-up with MD. Y___ N___
Tests	SpO₂/Accucheck CT (unenhanced) GBC, SMA-18, PT, PTT ECG Stroke Profile CXR	Carotid US MRI/MRA PT/PTT Carotid US 12/24 Holter 2D Echo/TEE Hgb-A1C if BG elevated	Lipid Profile Video Swallow, if indicated EEG PT/PTT Arch/arteriogram	PT/INR F/U CT, if indicated	PT/INR	See "Medications" and "Consults"
Assessments and Treatments	Accuchecks every shift if BG > 120 × 24 hrs DVT precautions/TEDs Cardiac Monitor × 24 hr Saline Lock I&O NIHSS within 72 hrs VS/NC q4h and prn Weight Skin assessment q8h	DVT precautions/TEDs I&O D/C cardiac monitor if no arrhythmia Saline lock Skin assessment q8h	DVT precautions/TEDs I&O Saline lock Skin assessment q8h	DVT precautions/TEDs I&O Saline lock Skin assessment q8h	DVT precautions, D/C when ambulatory I&O Saline lock Skin assessment q8h	Demonstrates ability to perform ADLs with minimum assistance. Y___ N___ If no, D/C plan appropriate. Y___ N___ Skin intact without decubitus. Y___ N___
Medications	Antiplatelet/anti-coagulant therapy as indicated Home medications Antihypertensives as indicated Consider tPA if acute onset <3 hrs Consider for clinical trial	Antiplatelet/anti-coagulant Home medications Stool softener DVT prophylaxis if nonambulatory	Antiplatelet/anti-coagulant Home medications IV medications to PO Stool softener DVT prophylaxis if nonambulatory	Antiplatelet/anti-coagulant PO Stool softener DVT prophylaxis if nonambulatory	Antiplatelet/anti-coagulant PO D/C heparin if NR >2 PT therapeutic Stool softener DVT prophylaxis if nonambulatory	Pt verbalizes understanding of D/C medications; given written info if D/C'd on antiplatelet/anticoagu-lant. Y___ N___
Nutrition	NPO until RN observes swallow with medications; call MD if demonstrates risk of aspiration If swallow okay; Healthy Heart diet as tolerated Add NCS diet if diabetic Prealbumin if nutrition score ≥9	Healthy Heart diet as tolerated Speech tx for bedside evaluation IF PO intake <50%, oral supplement ordered (dietitian or RN)	Healthy Heart diet as tolerated If Video Swallow (+) place DHT and use Dysphagia Addendum	Healthy Heart diet as tolerated	Healthy Heart diet, as tolerated	Meets dietary goals Y___ N___ Pt/family verbalize understanding of D/C diet. Y___ N___ Adequate hydration and route for medication administration. Y___ N___

(continued)

Acute Ischemic Stroke Clinical Pathway—cont'd

	DAY 1/ED Date_____	DAY 2 Date_____	DAY 3 Date_____	DAY 4 Date_____	DAY 5 Date_____	DAY 6 Essential D/C Outcomes Date_____
Activity	Bedrest Assess ADL level	Evaluate pt at B/S Chair for 15 min Assists with ADL (RN/OT) BRP with assistance only	Obtain assistive devices prn Ambulate with assistance BRP; increase activity as tolerated	ADLs with assistance Chair bid Ambulate with assistance as tolerated	ADLs with minimum assistance Ambulate with assistance as tolerated	See "Assessments and Treatments"
Education and Discharge Planning	Discuss diagnosis and plan of care. Discuss safety measures. Orient pt/family to JH Stroke Center. Discuss purpose and use of medications.	Reinforce diagnostic information. Discuss clinical path and plan of care. View stroke film, WYNK Ch. 14, 3:30 PM. Assess home/self-care abilities; note NIHSS. Verify payor source/benefits.	Discuss risk factor teaching. Educate on assistive devices. Reevaluate D/C plan.	Reinforce teaching as needed.	Reinforce teaching as needed.	D/C to appropriate facility: Home ___ Home with OP or Home Health ___ IP Rehab ___ Subacute Rehat ___ SNF ___ Has written information regarding D/C Plan, when/how to contact MD. Y___ N___ Verbalizes S&S of stroke. Y___ N___ Verbalizes own risk factors. Y___ N___ All valuables with pt. Y___ N___
Signatures						

This Clinical Path has been developed as a guideline for management of patients hospitalized for this diagnosis or procedure.
Care may be revised to meet the individual patient's needs.

Elective Infrarenal Abdominal Aortic Aneurysm Repair Clinical Pathway

Dartmouth-Hitchcock Medical Center
1 Medical Center Drive
Lebanon, New Hampshire 03756

The development of the Elective Infrarenal Abdominal Aortic Aneurysm Repair Clinical Pathway was an interdisciplinary effort led by the chief of Vascular Surgery. The pathway is designed to commence the same day of surgery, when the patient enters the hospital, and concludes on the day of discharge. It is presented in a traditional format, with time expressed on the x-axis and body systems on the y-axis, creating a grid through which patient progress is documented. Unique features include display of the desired outcomes in shaded format at the top of each box. This pathway is accompanied by standing physician orders (see p. 314), as well as a unique "front page," which highlights outcomes and allows the user to see, at a glance, the patient's progress or lack of progress through the pathway. The goal of this pathway is to standardize the approach to care and guide nursing and physician interventions to achieve expected outcomes.

CLINICAL PATHWAY: Abdominal Aortic Aneurysm Repair

Baseline Data	Date: _____

BP _____   RA SpO$_2$ _____
HR _____   RR _____
Hb _____

Pulses (0-2):　Fem　　DP　　PT

Left　　_____　_____　_____　Diet _____
Right　　_____　_____　_____　Living situation _____

(ICU Admission)　　Date: _____

Circulatory	D/T: _____ [12°] I: _____ No vasoactive infusion × 6 hrs	D/T: _____ [+12°] I: _____ No vasoactive infusion × 6° Extubated Spontaneous UO > 30 cc/hr × 6° No active myocardial ischemia
Respiratory	D/T: _____ [6°] I: _____ Extubation criteria met FiO$_2$ = .40 PEEP ≤5 cm H$_2$O IMV ≤4 breaths/min. PSV ≤5 cm H$_2$O RR ≤25 breaths/min SpO$_2$ ≥90%	D/T: _____ [+1°] I: _____ Extubated
Fluid/ Electrolyte/ Kidney	D/T: _____ [24°] I: _____ Urine >30 ml/hr × 6 hrs	
Gastrointestinal	D/T: _____ [48°] I: _____ NG output <350 cc/12° No abdominal distention	D/T: _____ [+2°] I: _____ NG tube removed
Skin Integrity/ Wound Healing		D/T: _____ [48°] I: _____ Abdominal incision dry
Neuro/Psych	D/T: _____ [2°] I: _____ Follows commands	D/T: _____ [+4°] I: _____ Oriented × 3
Functional Ability	D/T: _____ [12°] I: _____ Up to chair	D/T: _____ [+12°] I: _____ Ambulate with assistance
Pain Management	D/T: _____ [4°] I: _____ Adequate analgesia ☐ Epidural ☐ Parenteral	
Patient Education/ Continuing Care		

KEY:　　Shade in box when intermediate outcome met.　　Number in box indicates target for achieving outcome.
　　　　Green = Outcome met within target time　　　*Red* = Target time exceeded
Pain Scale (0-10):　0 = No pain　　10 = Worst imaginable pain
Activity Scale:　0 = Independent　　　　　　　　　1 = Uses equipment or devices
　　　　　　　　2 = Needs assist. or supervision　3 = Needs assistance and special equipment
　　　　　　　　4 = Dependent, does not participate
Neuro Scale:　1 = Alert and oriented　2 = Intermittantly confused　3 = Confused　4 = Disoriented
Pulses:　　　0 = Absent　　1 = Diminished　　2 = Normal

Weight	_____	Activity (0-4):	
Neuro (0-4)	_____	Walking	_____
Pain (0-10)	_____	Feeding	_____
		Bathing	_____
		Toilet	_____
		Dressing	_____
		Stairs	_____

Time:_____			Total Time
D/T: _____ I: _____ [+1°] PA catheter removed	D/T: _____ I: _____ [+12°] VS ± 20% baseline × 4 hrs	D/T: _____ I: _____ [+36°] VS ± 20% BL × 24 hrs (no IV medications)	Day 3
D/T: _____ I: _____ [+30°] SpO2 >90% on FiO2 ≤0.50	D/T: _____ I: _____ [+36°] Room air SpO2 >90% or baseline	D/T: _____ I: _____ [+48°] No SOB during baseline ADL	Day 5
D/T: _____ I: _____ [+72°] Foley removed	D/T: _____ I: _____ [+6°] Voids OK	D/T: _____ I: _____ [+48°] Weight ± 5% baseline	Day 5
D/T: _____ I: _____ [+24°] Tolerates liquid diet	D/T: _____ I: _____ [+24°] Tolerates baseline diet	D/T: _____ I: _____ [+24°] Bowel movement	Day 4
	D/T: _____ I: _____ [+24°] Groin incision dry		Day 3
D/T: _____ I: _____ [+42°] Baseline function			Day 2
	D/T: _____ I: _____ [+72°] Baseline mobility	D/T: _____ I: _____ [+24°] Baseline ADL met	Day 4
D/T: _____ I: _____ [+70°] Epidural removed PCA or D/C'd	D/T: _____ I: _____ [+0°] Adequate PO analgesia		Day 3
	D/T: _____ I: _____ [+72°] D/C disposition confirmed	D/T: _____ I: _____ [+48°] D/C teaching; IDF completed	Day 5
		Discharge	Day 6

(continued)

CLINICAL PATHWAY: Abdominal Aortic Aneurysm Repair—cont'd

| Baseline Data | Date/Time: _____ | RA SpO₂: _____ | Wt: _____ | Neuro (0-4): _____ | Hb: _____ |

Pain (0-10) _____

BP: _____   Fem   DP   PT

HR: _____   Pulses (0-2): LEFT: _____ _____ _____

RR: _____   RIGHT: _____ _____ _____

Other Medical Issues: _____

ICU Admission Date/Time: _____   ☐ Pathway implemented   ☐ Pathway continued

Cagetory	0-12 Hrs Postop Date: _____	12-24 Hrs Postop Date: _____	POD #2 Date: _____	POD #3 Date: _____
Circulatory Outcomes	Time: _____ Init: _____ No vasoactive infusion × 6 hrs	Time: _____ Init: _____ PA catheter and A-line removed when extubated, UO >30 cc/hr × 6 hrs and no active myocardial ischemia	Time: _____ Init: _____ VS ± 20% baseline × 4 hrs	Time: _____ Init: _____ VS ± 20% baseline × 24 hrs without need for IV antihypertensives
Assessments	VS q15" × 4; q30" × 4; q1h × 4; q1-2h A-line, CVP, PA, SpO₂ and cardiac monitoring with continuous ST segment monitoring LE motor and sensory exam Postop assessment per ICU standard Admission: Doppler ankle pressure _____ ECG _____	VS q2h A-line, CVP, PA (until lines removed), SpO₂, and cardiac monitoring Continuous ST segment monitoring LE motor and sensory exam Doppler ankle pressure with morning assessment = _____ ECG in morning prior to transfer, if ordered _____	VS q4h • DP/PT _____ • CSM _____ SCDs while in bed or chair > 2 hrs _____	VS q12h • DP/PT _____ • CSM _____ SCDs while in bed or chair > 2 hrs _____
Interventions	SCDs _____ Call CCS HO if BP >180 mm Hg or <100 mm Hg; HR >100 bpm or <50 bpm; T >38.5°C; ST up or down ≥2mm; cardiac index, 2.0 Call Vascular HO for change in LE motor, sensory, or doppler exam	Call CCS HO if BP >180 mm Hg or <100 mm Hg; HR >100 bpm or <50 bpm; T >38.5°C; ST up or down ≥2mm; cardiac index, 2.0 Call Vascular HO for change in LE motor, sensory, or doppler exam		
Respiratory Outcomes	Time: _____ Init: _____ Extubation criteria met per weaning protocol Time: _____ Init: _____ Extubated	Time: _____ Init: _____ SpO₂ ≥ 90% on FiO₂ ≥0.50 Maintains patent airway		Time: _____ Init: _____ Room air SpO₂ ≥90% or baseline
Assessments	Admission ABG: _____ Admission CXR: _____	CXR in morning prior to transfer: _____	q4h SpO₂ and lung sounds	q12h SpO₂ and lung sounds
Interventions	Vent wean protocol if intubated: standard _____, rapid _____, or N/A _____ Secretion management Initial vent settings per CCS When extubated, O₂ per facemask _____, NC _____ to maintain SpO₂ ≥90% Bronchodilators as ordered IS turn, cough, deep breathe q1h WA Call CCS HO if RR >30 breaths/min or <12 breaths/min; SpO₂ <90%	Secretion management When extubated, O₂ per facemask _____, NC _____ to maintain SpO₂ ≥90% Bronchodilators as ordered IS turn, cough, deep breathe q1h WA Call CCS HO if RR >30 breaths/min or <12 breaths/min; SpO₂ <90%	Titrate O₂ to maintain SpO₂ ≥90% Pulmonary toilet prn Bronchodilators as ordered	Titrate O₂ to maintain SpO₂ ≥90% Pulmonary toilet prn Bronchodilators as ordered

Activity Scale: 0-4	
	Admit
0 = Independent	Toilet _____
1 = Uses equipment or devices	Feeding _____
2 = Needs assistance/supervision	Bathing _____
3 = Needs assistance & special equipment	Dressing _____
4 = Dependent, does not participate	Walking _____
	Stairs _____

POD #4 Date: _____	POD #5 Date: _____	POD #6 Date: _____	POD #7 Date: _____
VS q12h • DP/PT _____ • CSM _____	VS q12h • DP/PT _____ • CSM _____	VS q12h • DP/PT _____ • CSM _____	
SCDs while in bed or chair > 2 hrs _____	SCDs while in bed or chair > 2 hrs _____	SCDs while in bed or chair > 2 hrs _____	
	Time: _____ Init: _____ No SOB during baseline ADL		
q12h SpO$_2$ and lung sounds Titrate O$_2$ to maintain SpO$_2$ ≥90% Pulmonary toilet prn Bronchodilators as ordered	q12h SpO$_2$ and lung sounds Titrate O$_2$ to maintain SpO$_2$ ≥90% Pulmonary toilet prn Bronchodilators as ordered	q12h SpO$_2$ and lung sounds Titrate O$_2$ to maintain SpO$_2$ ≥90% Pulmonary toilet prn Bronchodilators as ordered	

(continued)

CLINICAL PATHWAY: Abdominal Aortic Aneurysm Repair—cont'd

Cagetory	0-12 Hrs Postop Date: _____	12-24 Hrs Postop Date: _____	POD #2 Date: _____	POD #3 Date: _____
Electrolyte/ Kidney Outcomes		Time: _____ Init: _____ Urine >30 cc/hr × 6 hrs		
Assessments	Admission labs: lytes, glucose, BUN/Cr, CBC, PT/PTT, Mg++, Ca++ _____ I&O per ICU standard	AM labs prior to transfer: CBC, lytes, BUN/Cr I&O q2h Morning wt _____	Wt: _____ I&O q4h 24-hr I: _____ O: _____	Wt: _____ I&O q12h 24-hr I: _____ O: _____
Interventions	IV fluids as ordered Postop weight _____ Call CCS HO if urine output < 60 cc/2 hrs Foley care per standard _____	IV fluids as ordered Foley care per standard _____	IV fluid as ordered Foley care per standard _____	IV fluid as ordered Hep cap IV when tolerating liquids _____ Foley care per standard _____
Gastroin- testinal Outcomes			Time: _____ Init: _____ NG output <350 cc/12 hrs No abdominal distension NG tube removed	Time: _____ Init: _____ Tolerates liquid diet
Assessments	Bowel sounds q4h Check NG output q2h Heme check all stools	Bowel sounds q4h Check NG output q2h Heme check all stools	Bowel sounds, flatus, NG output q4h	Bowel sounds, flatus, NG output q12h
Interventions	NGT to LCS, flush 20cc NS q4h and check pH For NG pH <6: Antacid as ordered H2 blocker as ordered NPO except ice chips Call Vascular HO if Heme + stool	NGT to LCS, flush 20cc NS q4h and check pH For NG pH <6: Antacid as ordered H2 blocker as ordered NPO except ice chips Call Vascular HO if Heme + stool	NGT to LCS Obtain order; D/C NGT when output <350 cc/12 hrs; advance to sips—self-limiting diet; 1/2 portions	Advance diet as tolerated Consider dietary consult if not advancing _____ Routine bowel orders
Skin Integrity/ Wound Healing Outcomes			Time: _____ Init: _____ Abdominal incision dry	Time: _____ Init: _____ Groin incision dry
Assessments	Check dressings with VS assessments Braden score: _____	Check dressings with VS assessments	Check skin q8h: IV site, wounds, pressure points Braden score: _____ (follow protocol)	Check skin q12h: IV site, wounds, pressure points
Interventions	Notify Vascular HO of bloody dressings	Notify Vascular HO of bloody dressings	Remove dressing if incision dry _____ DSD for incisional drainage	Remove dressing if incision dry _____ DSD for incisional drainage
Neuro/Psych Outcomes	Time: _____ Init: _____ Follows commands Oriented x3		Time: _____ Init: _____ Baseline neurologic function = _____	
Assessments	Mental status assessment ____	Mental status assessment ____	Mental status assessment q4h	Mental status assessment q12h
Interventions	Reorient prn	Reorient prn		

POD #4	POD #5	POD #6	POD #7
Date: _____	Date: _____	Date: _____	Date: _____
Time: _____ Init: _____ Foley removed, voids O.K.		Time: _____ Init: _____ Weight ± 5% baseline	

Wt: _____
I&O q12h
24-hr I: _____
      O: _____
	Wt: _____
	I&O q12h
	24-hr I: _____
	      O: _____
		Wt: _____
		I&O q12h
		24-hr I: _____
		      O: _____	

Obtain order to D/C foley: If no void within 6 hrs, straight cath and notify Vascular HO Foley D/C'd _____	Obtain order to D/C hep cap Hep cap; D/C'd _____		
Time: _____ Init: _____ Tolerates baseline diet	Time: _____ Init: _____ Bowel movement		
Bowel sounds, flatus q12h			
Advance diet as tolerated _____ Consider dietary consult if not advancing _____ Routine bowel orders	Advance diet as tolerated _____ Consider dietary consult if not advancing _____ Routine bowel orders	Advance diet as tolerated _____ Consider dietary consult if not advancing _____ Routine bowel orders	
	Time: _____ Init: _____ Wound edges approximated; no drainage, erythema, edema		
Check skin q12h: IV site, wounds, pressure points			Staples out: _____
Remove dressing if incision dry _____ DSD for incisional drainage			
Mental status assessment q12h _____ _____	Mental status assessment q12h _____ _____	Mental status assessment q12h _____ _____	

(continued)

CLINICAL PATHWAY: Abdominal Aortic Aneurysm Repair—cont'd

Cagetory	0-12 Hrs Postop Date: _____	12-24 Hrs Postop Date: _____	POD #2 Date: _____	POD #3 Date: _____
Functional Ability Outcomes	Time: _____ Init: _____ Bedrest maintained	Time: _____ Init: _____ Ambulate with assistance		Time: _____ Init: _____ Bathes and dresses self with minimal assistance
Assessments	Assess pain management prior to mobilization	Assess pain management prior to mobilization	Sensory/motor assessment	
Interventions	Bedrest overnight; HOB 30° Turn q2h Upper and lower extremity ROM	Turn q2h Upper and lower extremity ROM Up to chair in morning Stand, pivot to chair bid	Turn/reposition q4h _____ Up to chair with assistance _____ Ambulate at least bid _____	Ambulate 4 times a day with assistance _____ Advance distance as tolerated _____ Assist with ADLs/shower prn _____ Consider PT consult if pt. not progressing _____
Pain Management Outcomes		Time: _____ Init: _____ Adequate analgesia (0-3/10 at rest) _____ Epidural _____ Parenteral	Time: _____ Init: _____ Epidural removed or PCA D/C'd Adequate po analgesia	
Assessments	Pain assessment (0-10): _____	Pain assessment (0-10): _____	Pain assessment (0-10): _____	Pain assessment (0-10): _____
Interventions	Thoracic epidural per APS: _____ PCA: _____ Notify APS for uncontrolled pain _____ Splint/position for comfort	Thoracic epidural per APS: _____ PCA: _____ Notify APS for uncontrolled pain _____ Splint/position for comfort	Thoracic epidural per APS: _____ PCA: _____ Position for comfort Teach splinting/relaxation Obtain order to D/C epidural or PCA _____ Notify APS for uncontrolled pain _____	Obtain order to D/C epidural or PCA _____ Advance to po analgesia as ordered
Patient Ed/ Cont. Care Outcomes		Time: _____ Init: _____ Pt. demonstrates use of IS, C&DB Pt. verbalizes understanding of activity/rest expectations Pt./family questions/concerns addressed		
Assessments	Evaluate pt./family level of understanding regarding plan of care _____	Evaluate pt./family level of understanding regarding plan of care _____	Assess continuing care needs	
Interventions	Orient pt./family to ICU environment _____ Review IS, C&DB technique _____ Review activity progression _____ Involve pt./family when applicable	Review IS, C&DB technique _____ Review activity progression _____ Involve pt./family when applicable	Initiate D/C teaching _____ Med Review _____ Activity _____ Diet _____	Continue D/C teaching _____ Establish D/C disposition _____ _____ _____
Change in Plan	_____ _____ _____ _____	_____ _____ _____ _____	_____ _____ _____ _____	_____ _____ _____ _____
RN Signature:	07-19 _____ 19-07 _____	07-19 _____ 19-07 _____	07-19 _____ 19-07 _____	07-19 _____ 19-07 _____
KEY: Neuro Scale:	1 = Alert and oriented	2 = Intermittently confused	3 = Confused	4 = Disoriented
Pulses:	0 = Absent	1 = Diminished	2 = Normal	

Addressograph

POD #4	POD #5	POD #6	POD #7
Date: _____	Date: _____	Date: _____	Date: _____
Time: _____ Init: _____ Baseline mobility	Time: _____ Init: _____ Baseline ADL = _____		D/C Activity (0-4) Walking _____ Toilet _____ Feeding _____ Dressing_____ Bathing _____ Stairs _____

Ambulate 4 times a day with
  assistance _____
Advance distance as
  tolerated _____
Assist with ADLs/shower
  prn _____
Consider PT consult if pt. not
  progressing _____
	Ambulate 4 times a day with
	  assistance _____
	Advance distance as
	  tolerated _____
	Assist with ADLs/shower
	  prn _____
	Consider PT consult if pt. not
	  progressing _____
		Ambulate 4 times a day with
		  assistance _____
		Advance distance as
		  tolerated _____
		Assist with ADLs/shower
		  prn _____
		Consider PT consult if pt. not
		  progressing _____	

Pain assessment (0-10): _____
 	
Advance to PO analgesia as
  ordered
	Pain assessment (0-10): _____
	
	PO analgesia as ordered
		Pain assessment (0-10): _____
		
		PO analgesia as ordered
		Pt. education on post-D/C
		  pain medications (e.g.,
		  Percocet, Tylenol, Advil)
			Pain assessment on D/C with
			  PO analgesia (0-10): _____

		Time: _____
		Init: _____
		Interdisciplinary discharge
		  completed
		D/C disposition established
		Pt./family verbalize
		  understanding of D/C plan
			Pt./family verbalize
			  understanding of D/C plan
			  _____
			
			F/U return visit: _____
			
			VNA _____

Continue D/C teaching _____	Continue D/C teaching _____		
_____ _____ _____ _____	_____ _____ _____ _____	_____ _____ _____ _____	_____ _____ _____ _____
07-19 _____ 19-07 _____	07-19 _____ 19-07 _____	07-19 _____ 19-07 _____	07-19 _____ 19-07 _____

At discharge, photocopy clinical pathway and mail to Office of Care Management   Original to Medical Records

| Stroke Management Clinical Pathway

Ruttonjee and Tang Shiu Kin Hospitals
266 Queen's Road East
Wanchai, Hong Kong

The Stroke Management Clinical Pathway was initiated by the Department of Geriatrics to provide quality care for the third greatest cause of death in Hong Kong. The acute phase has been managed by the Acute Integrated Medical Services of the Department of Medicine while the rehabilitation phase is under the care of the Geriatrics wards or the Geriatric Day Hospital.

The clinical pathway is a standardized spectrum of care provided through a multidisciplinary approach. The Bladder Training Protocol is a list of procedures for nurses to optimize patients' bladder function once they enter the rehabilitation phase (see p. 298). The Swallowing Screening Algorithm commences as soon as possible after admission by nurses and is followed by a speech therapist's assessment (see p. 290). The Order Set is provided to doctors to facilitate immediate and effective interventions as soon as the patient is admitted.

RUTTONJEE HOSPITAL—Stroke Management Clinical Pathway

	Acute Phase (max 7 days—Week 1)				Rehab Phase (max 4 weeks)		
Admission Date	Day 1	Days 2-3	Days 4-5	Days 6-7	Week 2 Days 8-14	Weeks 3-4 Days 15-28	Week 5 Days 29-35
Consults	♦ Admit under Neurology bed ♦ Consider **neurosurgical opinion** ♦ **PT and OT, MSW**	♦ Consider **speech therapist** for swallowing or speech problems			♦ **Consult** all rehab team members ♦ Consider: - **Continence nurse** - **Dietitian** - **Psychiatrist** - **Pastoral care** - **Podiatrist**		♦ Consider: - **CNS** - **CGAT**
Diagnostic	♦ **Blood Tests:** CBP, ESR RFT, LFT, Ca, Sugar PT/APTT/INR Lipids, cholesterol Consider T$_4$ ♦ ECG, CXR ♦ CT scan brain (plain) Urinalysis	♦ Consider **investigations:** Echocardiogram Carotid doppler MRI			♦ PT/APTT/INR if on warfarin	♦ PT/APTT/INR if on warfarin	
Assessment	**Clerking Proforma and Functional Assessment Forms** ♦ **Neuro-obs q1-4h** ♦ **Swallowing Screening Test** ♦ **Bladder, bowel** > ♦ **Skin, body weight** > ♦ **Relatives' concern and needs** >		♦ **Consider Predischarge functional assessment by team**	>	♦ **Functional assessment by team** ♦ **Weigh patient**		♦ Predischarge functional assessment by team ♦ **Weigh patient**
	♦ Continue **nutritional, swallowing, skin, emotional, bowel, and bladder assessment** ♦ Weekly or biweekly case conference (Ward round and discuss discharge plan if necessary — Acute Phase)						
Treatment & Activity	♦ **Consider Surgery** if necessary ♦ Consider **Aspirin** or **LMWH** in suitable cases Administer **mannitol** for 2-4 days (in the first and second day) in indicated cases. ♦ **Foley catheter** if ROU ♦ **Risk factor** modification ♦ Avoid **overtreatment of initial hypertension** ♦ Maintenance **PT and OT** ♦ Consider **bed rest** ♦ **Safety precautions**	♦ Consider **swallowing training** if necessary ♦ Consider **bed sore prevention program** ♦ PT and OT as tolerated ♦ Activity as tolerated	♦ Consider **off foley** ♦ Consider **off IVF** ♦ Consider **NGT** if dysphagia persists > > > >	♦ If pending discharge: ♦ Consider **prescribing aides** ♦ Consider **home visit** > > > >	♦ Consider **warfarin** for secondary prevention in suitable cases ♦ Consider: **Pressure sore prevention** program if necessary **Bowel and bladder training** if necessary **Swallowing and speech training** if necessary **Communication with relatives** **Psychosocial support** **Ward rehabilitation activities** ♦ **Bed mobility** → Transfer → Sitting balance → Standing balance → Level ground walking → Stairs/slopes/outdoor (i.e., PT) ♦ **Bed mobility** → Bedside self-care → Basic self-care → IADL if tolerated (i.e., OT) ♦ Consider **Fine hand function** training ♦ Consider **aides/home visit** if discharged		

(continued)

RUTTONJEE HOSPITAL—Stroke Management Clinical Pathway—cont'd

	Acute Phase (max 7 days—Week 1)				Rehab Phase (max 4 weeks)		
Admission Date	**Day 1**	**Days 2-3**	**Days 4-5**	**Days 6-7**	**Week 2 Days 8-14**	**Weeks 3-4 Days 15-28**	**Week 5 Days 29-35**
Nutrition	◆ DAT if no swallowing problem ◆ NPO and IVF, as well as Ryles tube feeding if swallowing test failed	>	>	◆ NGT if dysphagia persists		◆ Discuss PEG feeding if failed swallowing training	
Education (Patient and Relatives)	◆ Ward orientation ◆ Stroke pamphlet	◆ For cases with swallowing and speech problems	◆ Risk factor modification ◆ Discharge instructions and FU arrangements	> >	◆ Orientation of Rehab Ward	◆ Self-care/ADL, home exercise aids usage ◆ Self-help group ◆ Sharing Section	◆ Discharge instructions and FU arrangements
Discharge Planning	◆ Notify MSW for problem cases	>	◆ Pre-discharge checklist	◆ If for discharge, FU/refer to: **Geriatric Stroke Rehab Program**		◆ Pre-discharge checklist ◆ Consider CNS	◆ Discharge instructions and FU arrangements ◆ Hotline service
GOAL	Stabilization of medical condition and prevention of complications				Rehabilitation for full integration to the community		
Data Collection	◆ Hong Kong Island Stroke Data Bank ◆ PRG						

<u>Remarks:</u> The average length of stay of the acute phase is around 4 days, after which patients are transferred to the Geriatric Stroke Rehab Team.

KEY:
LMWH	:	Low–molecular weight heparin
ROU	:	Retention of urine
PRG	:	Patient-related group (similar to a DRG)
NGT	:	Nasal-gastric tube
PEG	:	Percutaneous entero-gastrostomy
IADL	:	Instrumental activity of daily living
FU	:	Follow-up
PT	:	Physiotherapy
OT	:	Occupational therapy
>	:	Item has been carried forward from previous day

| Renal Transplant Clinical Pathway

Dartmouth-Hitchcock Medical Center
1 Medical Center Drive
Lebanon, New Hampshire 03756

The Renal Transplant Clinical Pathway (RTCP) is used for those individuals with chronic renal failure who meet the criteria to have renal transplantation. The pathway covers both living related or cadaveric kidney donation. The pathway is also used for patients with or without diabetes.

The pathway is individualized for each patient. This specific clinical pathway states the outcomes, assessments, and intervention for this population and is used for documentation of the care planning process for the patient's entire length of stay. The pathway includes a Fluid/Electrolytes/Kidney Function Algorithm to deal with symptoms of oliguria, anuria, or rising/unchanged creatine (see p. 276). Adjunctive forms include preprinted preoperative and immediate postoperative standing orders (see p. 300).

Renal Transplant Clinical Pathway Instructions For Use

Clinical pathways are tools to guide quality care. Accepted care practices may vary with each individual patient, including a variety of responses that are not reflected by the pathway. Individualizing the clinical pathway may consist of one or more of the following: adding or deleting treatments, tests, supplies, or medications; or other orders based upon specific patient problems that are not reflected in the pathway. Decision-making authority regarding additions or deletions to the clinical pathway rests with the physicians accountable for the care of the patient.

1. The Renal Transplant Clinical Pathway (RTCP) is individualized for each patient based upon a physician's order.
2. The RTCP is used for documentation of the care planning process for the patient's entire length of stay. Adjunct forms that are used in conjunction with the pathway include: (1) Preprinted Preoperative and Immediate Postoperative Standing Orders, (2) Acute Care Flow Sheet, (3) Medication Administration Records, and (4) Renal Transplant Teaching Tool.
3. The RTCP and corresponding orders are initiated by the Transplant Coordinator in either the Same Day Program or PACU dependent upon where the patient enters the system.
4. The RTCP is a permanent part of the patient's medical record and should be documented in ink. It is kept in the patient's blue notebook on 4 West. At discharge, a photocopy of the pathway should be sent to the Transplant Office. The original should be filed in front of the "Progress Notes" section of the chart.
5. All pathway content, including algorithms, must be guided by appropriate physician orders.
6. The "Baseline Data" section, located at the top of the RTCP, is completed by the Transplant Coordinator on admission.
7. All staff involved in the care of a patient on the RTCP should time and initial on the blank lines as appropriate, indicating that the outcome(s) occurred. Specific data points to be documented on the pathway include: (1) Daily weight, (2) BUN/Cr, and (3) the frequency of VS and I&O. These data points do not need to be documented doubly on the flow sheet. The abbreviation "N/A" (not applicable) may be used to indicate that a particular assessment, intervention, or outcome does not apply to the patient.
8. Patient rounds are formatted according to the system categories on the pathway. Each column (POD) is reviewed during rounds. Orders are written daily, depending upon the patient's status and identified plan of care. The shaded areas indicate outcomes to be met. Documentation of outcomes met within the target time are indicated by a black check mark in the left box. If the outcome was not met within the target time, a red "X" should be marked in the right box with the actual time frame identified.

9. If an identified outcome has not occurred within the prescribed time frame, the accountable practitioner should evaluate why the event has not occurred and plans should be executed and documented at the bottom of the appropriate pathway column to facilitate completion of the assessments and interventions that need to take place. If the stated outcomes do not occur, a revised plan of care should be documented in the 'Changes in Plan' section at the bottom of the appropriate day.

10. For symptoms of oliguria, anuria, or rising/unchanged creatinine, the "Fluid/Electrolytes, Kidney Function Algorithm" should be followed. Consideration for this algorithm is denoted by a delta symbol to the left of the hour boxes on the pathway. The algorithm is a guide for the medical team and should be physician driven to differentiate potential patient problems. This should assist the care team to revise the plan of care as appropriate to maintain the patient on the pathway.

11. The Registered Nurse assigned to the patient is responsible for assuring the completion and individualization of the clinical pathway activities, documentation, and daily outcome achievement.

12. The CRC is responsible for reviewing the clinical pathway, facilitating the completion of assessments and interventions and recording and tracking variance data.

13. If a patient follows the pathway but exceeds the five day length of stay, documentation of the plan of care should continue on the "Extended Stay" form and should be consistent with the format on the preprinted pathway.

14. Removal of the patient from the RTCP can be determined by the physician, RN, Transplant Coordinator, or CRC in the event of any of the following:

- The patient develops complications or diagnoses unrelated to the renal transplant (e.g. renal artery thrombosis causing the patient to require a nephrectomy).
- The plan of care deviates from the original clinical pathway, so that the path is no longer representative of the actual care the patient is receiving.

If a patient is removed from a clinical pathway, a plan of care must be developed in accordance with institutional policy.

Dartmouth-Hitchcock Medical Center

CLINICAL PATH: Renal Transplant

Baseline Data	Date: _____		BP: _____ HR: _____
	Weight (dry): _____		Allergies/ADR: _____
			Dialysis access: _____
BUN/CR: _____			Surgical procedure: _____
Diabetes: ☐ IDDM ☐ NIDDM ☐ Non-DM			Other medical issues: _____
			CMV Rx: _____

	Date: _____ PACU Criteria 0-6 hrs	Date: _____ PACU Criteria 0-6 hrs	Date: _____ POD #2
Circulatory	T: _____ [+] [-] I: _____ BP & HR within ± 20% of baseline Normothermic	T: _____ [+] [-] △* I: _____ BP <200/100 mm Hg or within circulatory ± 20% baseline Anti-HTN regimen initiated	T: _____ [+] [-] I: _____ BP <200/110 mm Hg or within ± 20% baseline Afebrile
		VS q2° or q4° Pedal pulses on arrival to unit DP: R: _____ L: _____ PT: R: _____ L: _____ ☐ Note no BP or blood draw __ arm Call HO if BP <110/60 mm Hg or <10% of baseline or >190/100 mm Hg, p ≥120	VS q4° or q8° or q12° Max BP: _____ Max T°: _____
Respiratory	T: _____ [+] [-] I: _____ Awake, able to protect airway and follow commands Pulse Ox ≥90% on FIO_2 ≤40% RR within ± 20% of baseline		T: _____ [+] [-] I: _____ Pulse Ox >90% No SOB at rest
		Assess lung sounds/RR _____ Pulmonary toilet as needed Titrate 0_2 for SpO_2 >90%	Assess lung sounds/RR _____ Pulmonary toilet as needed Titrate 0_2 for SpO_2 >90%
Fluid/Electrolyte	T: _____ [+] [-] △* I: _____ Electrolytes WNL or treatment plan	T: _____ [+] [-] △* I: _____ Electrolytes WNL or treatment plan	T: _____ [+] [-] △* I: _____ Tolerating PO, liquids

		I&O: q2° or q4° 24° Total I____
		                                    O____
		Weight: _____
		Replace/maintain IV fluids as
		ordered
			I&O: q4° or q8° 24° Total I____
			                                    O____
			Weight: _____
			Hep cap IV when tolerating liquids

GU Liche procedure U-P Anastomosis (U-P)	T: _____ [+] [-] I: _____ Foley patent JP drainage ≤300 cc/2 hrs	T: _____ [+] [-] I: _____ U-P: Foley D/C'd Liche: Foley patent	T: _____ [+] [-] I: _____ U-P: Voiding independently JP drainage D/C'd if <100 cc/24 hrs
	Assess JP drainage _____	Assess foley patency. If foley D/C'd, assess voiding pattern Of output <100 cc/hr, irrigate foley with physician present If JP drainage >150 cc/hr initiate wall suction. Assess drainage _____	Assess foley patency/voiding patterns Assess JP drainage D _____ N _____

KEY: SHADED areas indicate outcomes to be met.   ☑ in left box if outcome met within target time.

T: Time outcome met

At discharge, photocopy clinical pathway and mail to Transplant Office. Original in medical record.

RR: _____ Pulse Ox: _____

Urine output pretransplant: _____

_____

_____

_____

Activity Scale: 0-4
0 = Independent
1 = Uses equipment or devices
2 = Needs assistance/supervision
3 = Needs assistance & special equipment
4 = Dependent, does not participate
_____ Ambulation _____ Feeding _____ Stairs
_____ Dressing _____ Bathing _____ Toileting

Date: _____ POD #3	Date: _____ POD #4	Date: _____ POD #5
T: _____ [+] [-] I: _____ BP <200/110 or within + 20% baseline Afebrile VS q4° or q8° or q12° Max BP:_____ Max T°:_____	T: _____ [+] [-] I: _____ BP <200/110 mm Hg or within ± 20% baseline Afebrile VS q8° or q12° Max BP:_____ Max T°:_____	T: _____ [+] [-] I: _____ Anti-HTN regimen in place BP <200/110. VS q12° Max BP:_____ Max T°:_____
	T: _____ [+] [-] I: _____ No SOB on exertion	T: _____ [+] [-] I: _____ Lung CTA or at baseline No SOB on exertion
Assess lung sounds/RR _____ Pulmonary toilet as needed Titrate O_2 for SpO_2 >90%	Assess lung sounds/RR _____ Pulmonary toilet as needed Titrate O_2 for SpO_2 >90%	
		T: _____ [+] [-] I: _____ Electrolytes WNL or receiving replacement therapy CVP line D/C'd
I&O: q8° or q12° 24° Total I___ O___ Weight: _____	I&O: q8° or q12° 24° Total I___ O___ Weight: _____	Discharge wt:___
T: _____ [+] [-] I: _____ Liche: Foley patent	T: _____ [+] [-] I: _____ Liche: Foley D/C'd	T: _____ [+] [-] I: _____ Liche: Voiding independently JP D/C'd if <100 cc/24 hrs or outpt. plan
Assess foley patency/voiding patterns Assess JP drainage D _____ N _____	Assess voiding patterns Assess JP drainage D _____ N _____	Assess voiding patterns Assess JP drainage D _____ N _____

[X] in right box if outcome not met in target time.
I: Initials of person documenting the information

△ * See Fluid/Electrolytes/Kidney Function Algorithm on p. 000

(continued)

Dartmouth-Hitchcock Medical Center

	Date: _____ PACU Criteria 0-6 hrs	Date: _____ POD #1 6-24 hrs	Date: _____ POD #2

Kidney Function	T: _____
	I: _____ [+] [-] △*
	
	U/O ≥100cc/hr.
		T: _____
		I: _____ [+] [-] △*
		
		U/O ≥100cc/hr.
		
		CVP reading if U/O <100 cc/hr
		BUN/Cr _____
		Medication doses based on Cr/Cl
		Review circulation, GU, and fluid
		  status assessments
		Refer to fluid management
		  algorithm if appropriate
			T: _____
			I: _____ [+] [-] △*
			
			U/O >1.5 liters/day
			Renal ultrasound +/normal
			
			BUN/Cr _____
			Medication doses based on Cr/Cl
			Encourage PO fluids
			Review circulation, GU, and fluid
			  status assessments
			Refer to fluid management
			  algorithm if appropriate

GI	T: _____
	I: _____ [+] [-]
	
	Sips of clear liquids
	Free of nausea and vomiting
		T: _____
		I: _____ [+] [-]
		
		Tolerating clear liquids
		⊕ BS
		
		Assess bowel sounds, flatus,
		  distention
		_____
		N/V (+/-) _____
		Toleration of PO fluids _____
		Clear liquid diet _____
		Dulcolax tabs as ordered
			T: _____
			I: _____ [+] [-]
			
			Tolerating regular food
			⊕ flatus
			
			Assess bowel sounds, distention,
			  flatus, bowel movement activity
			_____
			N/V (+/-) _____
			Advance diet as tolerated _____

**Skin Integrity/
Wound Care**
	T: _____
	I: _____ [+] [-]
	
	Minimal drainage from incision
		Assess CVP site, JP site, surgical site,
		  and Braden score/protocol _____
		If applicable, peritoneal catheter
		  exit site
		CVP dressing M-W-F _____
		JP site care and DSD _____
		DSD to incision _____
			Assess CVP site, JP site, surgical site
			_____
			If applicable, peritoneal catheter
			  exit site
			CVP dressing M-W-F _____
			JP site care and DSD _____

Endocrine	T: _____
	I: _____ [+] [-]
	
	Blood glucose stabilizing
		T: _____
		I: _____ [+] [-]
		
		Blood glucose managed by insulin
		  SQ or oral agent
		
		If insulin qtt or sliding scale, FS as
		  ordered
		Glucose level or range: = _____
		Adjust insulin as ordered
			Glucose level or range = _____
			Transition to standard insulin dosing
			Establish glucose monitoring
			  schedule and target range for
			  blood glucose _____
			Consult Diabetes CNS if necessary
			_____

Functional Ability		T: _____ I: _____ [+] [-] Up to chair Sensory/motor assessment _____	T: _____ I: _____ [+] [-] Ambulate with assistance ADLs with minimal assistance _____

Date: _____	Date: _____	Date: _____
POD #3	**POD #4**	**POD #5**
T: _____ I: _____ [+] [-] △*	T: _____ I: _____ [+] [-] △*	T: _____ I: _____ [+] [-] △*
U/O >1.5 liters/day	U/O >1.5 liters/day	U/O >1.5 liters/day
BUN/Cr _____ Medication doses based on Cr/Cl Encourage PO fluids Review circulation, GU, and fluid status assessments Refer to fluid management algorithm if appropriate	BUN/Cr _____ Medication doses based on Cr/Cl Encourage PO fluids Review circulation, GU, and fluid status assessments Refer to fluid management algorithm if appropriate	BUN/Cr _____ Medication doses based on Cr/Cl Encourage PO fluids Review circulation, GU, and fluid status assessments Refer to fluid management algorithm if appropriate
	T: _____ I: _____ [+] [-] Tolerating regular diet, including 2 liters/day; BM prior to D/C Dietary instructions given	T: _____ I: _____ [+] [-]
Assess bowel sounds, distention, flatus, BM activity _____ N/V (+/-) _____ Advance diet as tolerated _____ Renal dietary consultation _____	Assess bowel sounds, distention, flatus, BM activity _____ N/V (+/-) _____	Assess bowel sounds, distention, flatus, BM activity _____ Renal dietary discharge plan
T: _____ I: _____ [+] [-] Incision clean and dry, no signs of lymphocele		T: _____ I: _____ [+] [-] Incision clean and dry Afebrile
Assess CVP site, JP site, surgical site _____ If applicable, peritoneal catheter exit site CVP dressing M-W-F _____ JP site care and DSD _____	Assess CVP site, JP site, surgical site _____ If applicable, peritoneal catheter exit site CVP dressing M-W-F _____ JP site care and DSD _____	Assess CVP site, JP site, surgical site _____ If applicable, peritoneal catheter exit site CVP dressing M-W-F _____ JP site care and DSD _____
T: _____ I: _____ [+] [-] Blood glucose within patient target range		T: _____ I: _____ [+] [-] Blood glucose stable with appropriate diabetes management
Glucose level or range = _____ Consult Diabetes CNS if necessary	Glucose level or range = _____ Consult Diabetes CNS if necessary	Glucose level or range = _____
T: _____ I: _____ [+] [-] Baseline mobility achieved	T: _____ I: _____ [+] [-] Baseline independence with ADLs achieved	
ADLs with minimal assistance _____	ADLs achieved _____	

(continued)

Dartmouth-Hitchcock Medical Center
CLINICAL PATH: Renal Transplant—cont'd

	Date: _____ PACU Criteria 0-6 hrs	Date: _____ POD #1 6-24 hrs	Date: _____ POD #2
Pain Management	T: _____ [+ | -] I: _____ Patient reports <4/10 or acceptable level of pain	Pain assessment (0-10): D _____ N _____ MS04 PCA Position to comfort Teach splinting/relaxation	T: _____ [+ | -] I: _____ Patient reports <4/10 or acceptable level on PO analgesia Pain assessment (0-10): D _____ N _____ D/C PCA _____ Advance to PO analgesia
Patient Education	T: _____ [+ | -] I: _____ Able to use PCA appropriately Able to demonstrate TC and DB PCA and TC and DB teaching	Reinforce postop care Begin med teaching	T: _____ [+ | -] I: _____ Patient recording I&O and begins identification of medications Give patient record book to review Teaching tool—medication focus
Continuity of Care		T: _____ [+ | -] I: _____ Discharge plan initiated Discharge assessment by CRC in collaboration with transplant coordinator Outpatient medication plan (order/ identification of meds)	Social worker update on identifying resources to obtain and pay for medications Identify need for lodging or transportation
Immuno-suppression Treatment	T: _____ [+ | -] I: _____ (please circle) CyA, Imuran, Solumedrol Cellcept Antibody R$_x$ (OKT3, ATG)	T: _____ [+ | -] I: _____ Check CBC _____ Taper/protocol dose _____ Check WBC per protocol _____ Per protocol	T: _____ [+ | -] I: _____ Check CBC _____ Taper/protocol dose _____ Check WBC per protocol _____ Nurse to administer medication - Dose 3
Change in Plan	_____ _____ _____ _____ _____ _____	_____ _____ _____ _____ _____ _____	_____ _____ _____ _____ _____ _____
Category Signatures: MD:I/Signature/ Time:	07-19 RN: _____ 19-07 RN: _____	07-19 RN: _____ 19-07 RN: _____	07-19 RN: _____ 19-07 RN: _____

Date: _____ POD #3	Date: _____ POD #4	Date: _____ POD #5
T: _____ [+] [-] I: _____ Patient reports <4/10 or acceptable level on PO analgesia Pain assessment (0-10): D _____ N _____		
	Pain assessment (0-10): D _____ N _____	Pain assessment (0-10): D _____ N _____
T: _____ [+] [-] I: _____ Identifies and administers medications State symptoms of rejection/infection Independantly recording I&O Teaching tool; medications Symptoms of rejection/infection	T: _____ [+] [-] I: _____ Identifies and administers medications Daily monitoring, independently or SO (e.g., BP, temp, Wt., I&O, and palpate kidney) Dietary teaching Teaching tool	T: _____ [+] [-] I: _____ Passed discharge exam Able to state/identify medications and state symptoms of rejection/ infection and contact numbers Teaching tool completed Pharmacist review of medications
Outpatient medication availability	T: _____ [+] [-] I: _____ Discharge disposition confirmed and in place; if patient receiving OKT3 plan outpatient treatment	Supply of medications and cards are reviewed Written discharge instructions with appropriate follow-up appointment(s) and lab slips; in collaboration with transplant coordinator Community referral as needed
T: _____ [+] [-] I: _____ Check CBC _____ Taper/protocol dose _____ √ LFT's _____ Check WBC per protocol _____ Address CyA use	T: _____ [+] [-] I: _____ Check CBC _____ Taper/protocol dose _____ Check WBC per protocol _____ Per protocol	T: _____ [+] [-] I: _____ Check CyA level _____ Check CBC _____ Change to oral _____ Check WBC per protocol _____ Per protocol
_____ _____ _____ _____ _____ _____ _____ _____	_____ _____ _____ _____ _____ _____ _____ _____	_____ _____ _____ _____ _____ _____ _____ _____
07-19 RN: _____ 19-07 RN: _____	07-19 RN: _____ 19-07 RN: _____	07-19 RN: _____ 19-07 RN: _____

Acute Myocardial Infarction Care Track

Ruttonjee and Tang Shiu Kin Hospitals
266 Queen's Road East
Wanchai, Hong Kong

The Acute Myocardial Infarction Care Track was developed by the Department of Medicine as a standardized measure to provide efficient and effective care to patients affected by the second greatest cause of death in Hong Kong. The care track maps outs the standardized spectrum of care provided through a multidisciplinary approach to patients with acute myocardial infarction. The protocol on thrombolytic therapy (see p. 296) is observed by doctors and nurses to intervene effectively at the CCU and the Acute Integrated Medical wards. The algorithm for postthrombolytic assessment (see p. 278) is activated once patients are put on thrombolytic agents in the CCU and Acute Integrated Medical wards.

Modified from Ruttonjee and Tang Shiu Kin Hospitals, Wanchai, Hong Kong. Used with permission.

	RUTTONJEE HOSPITAL Department of Medicine Acute Myocardial Infarction Care Track		
DATE	DAY 1: _____ CCU/General Ward	DAY 2: _____ CCU/General Ward	DAY 3 to Discharge : _____ General Ward
CONSULTS	Cardiac Team	Physiotherapist; dietitian prn	MSW prn; occupational therapist prn
DIAGNOSTICS	ECG within 1 hr of admission and q8h pre- and postthrombolytic recurrent chest pain CPK with MB q8h × 3 times Urgent electrolytes, glucose, ABG (prn) CBP/LFT/RFT PT/APTT/INR (baseline and q6h after heparinization until stable) CXR Echocardiogram prn Cardiac catheterization prn	ECG qd and prn CPK qd Fasting lipids profile, glucose CBP, RFT PT/APTT/INR qd and q6h CXR prn	ECG qd (D3-D4); prn and before discharge CPK qd (D3-D4) and prn RFT; Hb; glucose; APTT prn CXR prn Predischarge echocardiogram Predischarge stress ECG or echocardiogram Arrange cardiac catheterization prn
ASSESSMENTS	Visual analog (0-10) chest pain assessment Hemodynamic assessment q1h I&O Cardiac monitoring SaO$_2$, CVP, PAWP prn	Visual analog (0 -10) chest pain assessment Hemodynamic assessment Cardiac monitoring	Visual analog (0-10) chest pain assessment Hemodynamic assessment q4h-qid Cardiac monitoring/telemetry prn
TREATMENTS	Aspirin (chewed) and PO qd Consider thrombolytic protocol (SK/rtPA) Medications - consider: B-Blocker. ACEI, heparin, nitrate, diuretics, morphine, antiarrhythmics, inotropes, magnesium, Ca antagonists Oxygen prn	Medications: also consider lipid lowering agents	Cardiac Rehabilitation Phase I
ACTIVITY	Bed rest	Early mobilization, sit out	Low-intensity exercise program
NUTRITION	NPO / Diet as tolerated / Therapeutic diet	Diet as tolerated / Therapeutic diet	Diet as tolerated / Therapeutic diet
PATIENT/ FAMILY EDUCATION	What is AMI? Characteristics of chest pain Management and prognosis of AMI Effects and side effects of thrombolytics and treatments	Management plan explanation Risk factor identification	Risk factor modification for secondary prevention; Hyperlipidemia, HTN, and DM control; smoking cessation; diet advice; stress management; return to work; exercise; sexual activities; advice on medications; and symptoms of ischemia.
DISCHARGE PLANNING	Discuss long-term management plan	Reinforce disease knowledge and control of risk factors	Consider referring to Cardiac Rehab.

Hemorrhagic Stroke (Nonsurgical) Clinical Pathway

Jewish Hospital
217 E. Chestnut Street
Louisville, Kentucky 40202

This pathway is initiated in the Emergency Department. All disciplines identifying the patient's appropriateness are responsible for initiating the pathway. Nurses review the pathway, verify completion of patient goals, take appropriate follow-up measures, and document variances. Variances are summarized, analyzed, and shared with the collaborative practice team (CPT).

Jewish Hospital
Clinical Pathway—DRG 14B
Hemorrhagic Stroke (Nonsurgical) Clinical Pathway
Target LOS 6 Days   (Addressograph)

	DAY 1/ED Date_____	DAY 2 Date_____	DAY 3 Date_____	DAY 4 Date_____	DAY 5 Date_____	DAY 6 Essential D/C Outcomes Date_____
Patient Goals and Clinical Outcomes		Pt teaching plan initiated and documented in computer (Education Record).	Activity progressing as planned. Pt/family makes decision regarding D/C plan.	Eating at least 2/3 of meals without choking or coughing. If pt to be D/C'd home, pt/family demonstrate ability to care for pt at home. If not met, reevaluate D/C plan.		D/C'd to home or appropriate facility.
Consults	Neurosurgeon Neurologist Speech/PT D/C planner Primary Care if none on case	Dietician Physiatrist				Verbalizes need for follow-up with MD Y___ N___
Tests	SpO₂/Accucheck CT (unenhanced) CBC, SMA-18, PT, PTT bleeding time ECG Stroke profile CXR	If on mannitol, serum osmolarity 1 hr prior to dose; hold if >350 Angiogram, if indicated* MRI, if indicated 2D Echo, if indicated *If angiogram demonstrates need for surgical intervention, see alternate clinical pathway.	Lipid profile Video Swallow if indicated Dilantin level	Repeat noncontrast CT		See "Medications" and "Consults"
Assessments and Treatments	DVT precautions/TEDs Cardiac monitor × 24 hrs Saline lock I&O NIHSS within 72 hrs VS/NC q2h and prn Weight Skin assessment q8h	DVT precautions/TEDs I&O D/C cardiac monitor if no arrhythmia Saline lock Skin assessment q8h Breath sounds clear VS/NC q4h and prn if stable	DVT precautions/TEDs I&O Saline lock Skin assessment q8h BM within last 72 hrs	DVT precautions/TEDs I&O Saline lock Skin assessment q8h Reassess limited fluid intake	DVT precautions, D/C when ambulatory I&O Saline lock Skin assessment q8h	Demonstrates ability to perform ADLs with minimal assistance. Y___ N___ If no, D/C plan appropriate. Y___ N___ Skin intact without decubitus. Y___ N___
Medications	H₂ blockers (PO or IV) Home medications Antihypertensives as indicated Treat if systolic BP > 170 mm Hg or diastolic BP > 110 mm Hg Consider for clinical trial Phenytoin/ dexamethasone Mannitol	Home medications Stool softener	Home medications IV medications to PO Stool softener Wean dexametha-sone? Wean mannitol?	Stool softener	Stool softener	Pt verbalizes understanding of D/C medications given written info if D/C'd on phenytoin. Y___ N___

(continued)

Jewish Hospital
Clinical Pathway—DRG 14B
Hemorrhagic Stroke (Nonsurgical) Clinical Pathway – cont'd
Target LOS 6 Days

	DAY 1/ED Date_____	DAY 2 Date_____	DAY 3 Date_____	DAY 4 Date_____	DAY 5 Date_____	DAY 6 Essential D/C Outcomes Date_____
Nutrition	NPO Add NCS diet if diabetic Prealbumin if nutrition score ≥9	NPO until RN observes swallow with medications; call MD if demonstrates risk of aspiration If swallow okay; Healthy Heart diet as tolerated Add NCS diet if diabetic If PO intake <50%, oral supplement ordered Speech treatment for bedside evaluation	Healthy Heart diet as tolerated If Video Swallow (+) place DHT and use Dysphagia Addendum	Healthy Heart diet as tolerated	Healthy Heart diet as tolerated	Meets dietary goals. Y___ N___ Pt/family verbalize understanding of discharge diet. Y___ N___ Adequate hydration and route for medication administration. Y___ N___
Activity	Bedrest Assess ADL level	Pt evaluated at B/S Chair for 15 min. Assists with ADL (RN/OT). BRP with assist only.	Obtain assistive devices pm Ambulate with assistance BRP; increase activity as tolerated	ADLs with assistance. Chair bid Ambulate with assistance as tolerated	ADLs with minimum assistance Ambulate with assistance as tolerated	See "Assessments and Treatments"
Education and Discharge Planning	Discuss diagnosis and plan of care. Discuss safety measures. Orient pt/family to JH Stroke Center. Discuss purpose and use of medications.	Reinforce diagnostic information. Discuss clinical pathway and plan of care. View Stroke film, WYNK Ch. 14, 3:30 PM. Assess home/self-care abilities; note NIHSS. Verify payor source/benefits.	Discuss risk factor teaching. Educate on assistive devices. Reevaluate D/C plan.	Reinforce teaching as needed.	Reinforce teaching as needed.	D/C to appropriate facility: Home Home with OP or Home Health Inpatient Rehab Subacute Rehab SNF Has written information regarding D/C plan, when/how to contract MD. Y___ N___ Verbalizes S&S of stroke. Y___ N___
	Signatures					
	_____	_____	_____	_____	_____	_____
	_____	_____	_____	_____	_____	_____

This clinical pathway has been developed as a guideline for management of patients hospitalized for this diagnosis or procedure. Care may be revised to meet the individual patient's needs.

| Total Knee Replacement Clinical Pathway

Jewish Hospital
217 E. Chestnut Street
Louisville, Kentucky 40202

This pathway is initiated in the Emergency Department. All disciplines identifying the patient's appropriateness are responsible for initiating the pathway. Nurses review the pathway, verify completion of patient goals, take appropriate follow-up measures, and document variances. Variances are summarized, analyzed, and shared with the collaborative practice team (CPT).

Jewish Hospital
Total Knee Replacement Clinical Pathway—DRG 209
Target LOS 3 Days Postop

(Addressograph)

	Preadmission Day Date _____	SHA/OR/PACU Day of Operation Date _____	Ortho Unit Day of Operation Date _____	Postop: Day 1 (Ortho Unit) Date _____	Postop: Day 2 (Ortho Unit) Date _____	Postop: Day 3 (Ortho Unit) Date _____	Postop: Day 4 (Ortho Unit–Home) Date _____
Patient Goals and Clinical Outcomes	Pt teaching completed. Y___ N___ Preop tests/labs completed. Y___ N___ Consent form signed. Y___ N___	**SHA** Pt to SHA on time—1 1/2 hrs prior to scheduled OR start time. Y___ N___ **PACU** Pt tolerates operation without complications. Y___ N___ Breath sounds clear. Y___ N___ VSS Y___ N___ Pain level controlled <3. Y___ N___ NV status 5 preop. Y___ N___ Abx. initiated as ordered postop. Y___ N___ Knee immobilizer as indicated. Y___ N___ Plexipulse/SCD/ TED as indicated. Y___ N___	VSS Y___ N___ Pain level controlled <3. Y___ N___ Tolerates diet without N/V. Y___ N___ NV status 5 preop. Y___ N___ Breath sounds clear. Y___ N___ Abx. initiated as ordered. Y___ N___ Knee immobilizer as indicated. Y___ N___ Plexipulse/SCD/ TED as indicated. Y___ N___	Tolerates diet without N/V. Y___ N___ Exercise program begun. Y___ N___ Pain level controlled <2. Y___ N___ Breath sounds clear. Y___ N___ Activity is initiated. Y___ N___	Comfortable with PO pain medications (pain level <2). Y___ N___ Uses BSC. Y___ N___ Breath sounds clear. Y___ N___ Activity is progressing. Y___ N___	Demonstrates adaptive equipment (if needed). Y___ N___ Breath sounds clear. Y___ N___ Activity is progressing. Y___ N___	Pt and caregiver independent with transfers if going home after D/C. Y___ N___ D/C teaching completed. Y___ N___ Follow-up appointment scheduled if going home. Y___ N___ Verbal understanding of D/C medications and instructions. Y___ N___ Given written information if on anticoagulant. Y___ N___ Breath sounds clear. Y___ N___
Consults	Anesthesiologist Case Manager Physical Therapy Dietitian Nursing Social Work as indicated RT Assessment as indicated	**SHA—Anesthesia** Check if epidural will be placed	Acute Pain Service (if pt has epidural catheter) RT assessment as indicated	Acute Pain Service (if pt has epidural catheter) RT assessment as indicated	Acute Pain Service (if pt has epidural catheter)	RT assessment as indicated	Move patient to rehab pathway if moving to rehab.
Tests	H&P ECG with chart copy if indicated. X-ray studies—LL films; Chest PA/Lat; 2-view knee AP/Lat wt. bearing, on 7317 films w/ knee centered, if indicated. Lab: CP18, CBC, PT PTT, UA, TSH 2 U.	**OR** X-ray studies intraop (prn). **PACU** H&H (optional)		H&H	RT assessment as indicated H&H (optional) PT if on warfarin	H&H (optional) PT if on warfarin	PT if on warfarin
Medications	Review home medications Preop medications per anesthesia	**SHA** IV fluids Preop per anesthesia: ANcef 1 gm IV (to OR with pt). **OR** Anesthesia drugs after induction **PACU** IV fluids Antibiotic IV Pain medication IV DVT prophylaxis as indicated	IV Fluids Antibiotic IV Pain medication IV DVT prophylaxis as indicated Home medications as indicated	Antibiotics IV IV fluids Pain medication DVT prophylaxis Home medication as indicated	Pain medication (PO) ABX IV as indicated DVT prophylaxis Home medications as indicated	Pain medication (PO) DVT prophylaxis Home medications as indicated	Pain medication (PO) DC IV Heplock DVT prophylaxis Home medications indicated

Jewish Hospital
Total Knee Replacement Clinical Pathway—DRG 209
Target LOS 3 Days Postop

(Addressograph)

	Preadmission Day Date _____	SHA/OR/PACU Day of Operation Date _____	Ortho Unit Day of Operation Date _____	Postop: Day 1 (Ortho Unit) Date _____	Postop: Day 2 (Ortho Unit) Date _____	Postop: Day 3 (Ortho Unit) Date _____	Postop: Day 4 (Ortho Unit-Home) Date _____
Assessments & Treatments	Autologous Blood Donation: 2 Units for TKR. 3 Units for Revision TKR.	**SHA** IV Access. Shave Prep **OR** Knee immobilizer Plexipulse/ SCD/TED, as indicated. **PACU** Standard PACU setup & care. Ortho Evac per protocol, as indicated. NV checks, as indicated. Wound Drain, as indicated. NPO	CDB q2h WA Standard PACU setup and care Ortho Evac per protocol as indicated. VS q15" until stable, then q1h VS q2 × 2, then q4 NV checks as indicated NV checks q4 × 24 hrs Wound drain as indicated Skin assessment q8h Plexipulse/SCD/ TED as indicated PCA/EPI pump	Wound drain as indicated VS and NV checks q4h WA CDB q2h WA Skin assessment q8h Plexipulse/ SCD/TED as indicated PCA/EPI pump	CDB q4h WA D/C wound drain as indicated VS and NV checks every shift. Skin assessment q8h Heplock IV Plexipulse/SCD/ TED as indicated D/C PCA/EPI pump	Heplock IV CDB q4h WA VS and NV checks every shift Skin assessment q8h Plexipulse/SCD/ TED as indicated	CDB pm VS and NV checks every shift Skin assessment q8h Plexipulse/SCD/ TED as in-dicated
Nutrition	NPO at midnight before surgery.		Diet as indicated	Diet as indicated	Diet as indicated	Diet as indicated	Diet as indicated
Activity	AAT	Bedrest	Bedrest	Isometrics q2h WA OOB to chair with appropriate weight bearing restrictions bid Immobilizer at night and with ambulation as indicated Pt Acute Care Assessment Initial ambulation	Isometrics q2h WA OOB to chair with appropriate weight bearing restrictions bid Immobilizer at night and with ambulation as indicated CPM initiated to pt tolerance as indicated Progressed ambulation	Isometrics q2h WA OOB to chair with appropriate weight bearing restrictions at least bid OOB for meals as tolerated Immobilizer at night and with ambulation as indicated When able to SLR, may be OOB without immobilizer Therapeutic exer-cise program CPM increased 10 degrees per day, minimum AAROM knees and SLR bid Progressed ambulation	Isometrics q2h WA OOB to chair with appropriate weight bearing restrictions at least bid OOB for meals as tolerated Immobilizer at night and with ambulation, as indicated Therapeutic exercise program Stair climbing CPM increased 10 degrees per day, minimum AAROM knees and SLR bid Progressed ambulation
Education	Total joint class Preop instruc-tions video JH orientation	Reinforce preop education Instruct family of waiting area.	Isometrics Reinforce pain control and CDB Instructions.	Reinforce isometrics. Reinforce pain control and CDB instructions.	Reinforce isometrics. Reinforce pain control and CDB instructions.	Home care instructions	Patient handouts D/C instructions
Discharge Planning	Home Care Evaluation Rehab pre/screen as appropriate Home Health prescreen as appropriate		Review D/C plan.	Review D/C plan and discuss with patient and family. Rehab evaluation as appropriate.	Review D/C Plan and discuss with patient and family. Rehab evaluation as appropriate. Initiate transfer forms if moving to rehab unit.	Review D/C Plan and discuss with patient and family. Implement "DME Protocol" if patient to go home and needs equipment.	Notify HHA at D/C if appropriate. Signatures

Signatures

_____ _____ _____ _____ _____ _____ _____

_____ _____ _____ _____ _____ _____ _____

This clinical pathway has been developed as a guideline for management of patients hospitalized for this diagnosis or procedure. Care may be re-vised to meet the individual patient's needs.

Fluid/Electrolytes, Kidney Function Algorithm

Dartmouth-Hitchcock Medical Center
1 Medical Center Drive
Lebanon, New Hampshire 03756

The Fluid/Electrolytes, Kidney Function Algorithm deals with symptoms of oliguria, anuria, or rising/unchanged creatine. It is used in conjunction with the Renal Transplant Clinical Pathway (see p. 259).

Fluid/Electrolytes, Kidney Function Algorithm

Symptoms: Oliguria, Anuria, Rising/Unchanged Creatinine

I.   Early Phase
PACU ---> POD #1 (first 18 hrs)
Differential: Mechanical obstruction
                                 Incomplete resuscitation
                                 ATN
                                 Thrombosis/rejection (both extremely rare)

Assessment/Criteria: CVP >10   ☐ Yes   ☐ No
                           BP >110/60   ☐ Yes   ☐ No
                           Foley in place?   ☐ Yes   ☐ No
                           Foley irrigated - clot? ☐ Yes ☐ No

Algorithm:
☐ If CVP <10, BP <110/60   • Complete resuscitation
☐ If foley obstructed   • May need replacement with larger foley
                                  • Irrigation regimen
☐ Suspected ATN
      Suggested order changes:
      • Restrict fluids to 1500 cc/day
      • K+, PO4 restriction
      • Renal duplex ultrasound—R/O thrombosis, R/O hydronephrosis (NOTE: if R/I—emergency OR)
      • Assess need for dialysis, notify Nephrology
      • Alternagel PO 30 cc qid
      • Review medications for renal dosing
      • Consider change in immunosuppression treatment   (if R/O—follow the other orders)

II.   Late Phase
POD #2 ---> Discharge (>24 hrs)
Differential Diagnosis: Rejection
                           Thrombosis
                           Nephrotoxicity (CyA)
                           Ureteral obstruction/hydronephrosis
                           Bladder dysfunction
                           Infection

Assessment: Circulation
              Respiratory
              Foley functional/postvoid residuals
              Temperature, wound
              Medication review for renal dosing with transplant pharmacist

Algorithm:
Orders: 1.   Urgent renal duplex—R/O thrombosis, R/O hydronephrosis
              2.   Laboratory tests: U/A, Amylase, Lipase, LFTs, CyA level

☐ If nephrotoxicity   • Adjust medication dosage
                                   • Repeat laboratory tests
                                   • R/O HUS (hemolytic uremic syndrome)

☐ If bladder dysfunction   • Straight catheter regimen

☐ If infection   • Culture and work up
                                   • Initiate appropriate therapy

☐ If hydronephrosis/ureteral obstruction   • Surgical revision
                                             • Percutaneous stent
☐ If thrombosis   • Emergent OR

☐ If rejection   Order Solu-Medrol IVP 500mg
                      _____ Consider renal biopsy
                      _____ Consider Antibody Rx and patient assessment for initiation of therapy
                      • Dialysis assessment
                      • Consider CellCept therapy

| Postthrombolytic Therapy Assessment Algorithm

Ruttonjee and Tang Shiu Kin Hospitals
266 Queen's Road East
Wanchai, Hong Kong

This algorithm was developed to guide the assessment of patients that have received thrombolytic therapy for acute myocardial infarction. It is used in conjunction with the myocardial infarction pathway (see p. 268).

Postthrombolytic Therapy Assessment Algorithm

Assessment of the Effectiveness of Thrombolytic Therapy

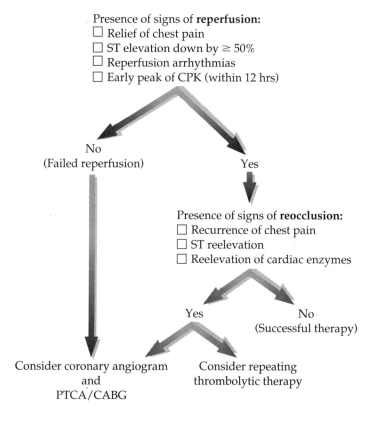

Presence of signs of **reperfusion:**
☐ Relief of chest pain
☐ ST elevation down by ≥ 50%
☐ Reperfusion arrhythmias
☐ Early peak of CPK (within 12 hrs)

No
(Failed reperfusion)

Yes

Presence of signs of **reocclusion:**
☐ Recurrence of chest pain
☐ ST reelevation
☐ Reelevation of cardiac enzymes

Yes

No
(Successful therapy)

Consider coronary angiogram
and
PTCA/CABG

Consider repeating
thrombolytic therapy

Convulsive Status Epilepticus Treatment Algorithm

Dartmouth-Hitchcock Medical Center
1 Medical Center Drive
Lebanon, New Hampshire 03756

This protocol is used to guide quick intervention to prevent status epilepticus (SE) and the potentially serious complications of prolonged or repetitive convulsive seizures. When patients are admitted for video/EEG monitoring, antiepileptic medications are routinely reduced or discontinued to promote seizure activity, therefore increasing the risk of developing SE. The protocol is initiated for patients at risk.

The nursing staff are educated to identify the various presentations of SE. SE is diagnosed and treated within 3 minutes or it is treated after three seizures without mental clearing between. After this initial intervention, the nurse contacts the attending physician for further recommendations.

Modified from Dartmouth-Hitchcock Medical Center, Lebanon, New Hampshire. Used with permission.

Convulsive Status Epilepticus Treatment Algorithm

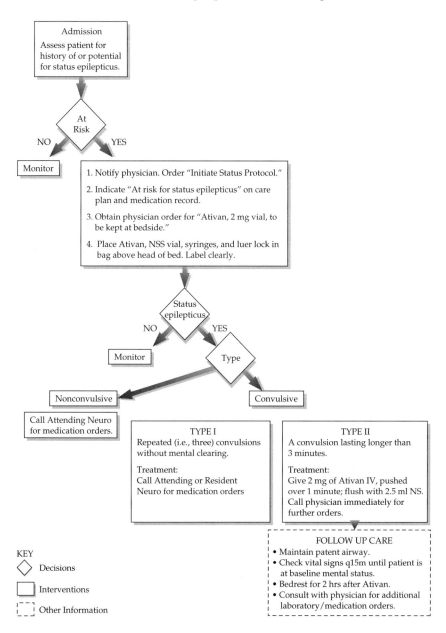

| Seclusion/Restraint/Protective Intervention Algorithm

University of Michigan Health Systems
1500 Medical Center Dr.
D4206 Medical Profession Building
Ann Arbor, Michigan 48109-0718

Patients can be a challenge when they present with behaviors that require seclusion, restraint, or protective intervention to ensure their own or others' safety or to maintain therapies. This algorithm assists the nurse in making decisions and implementing specific policies, procedures, and guidelines to meet that challenge.

Seclusion/Restraint/Protective Intervention Algorithm

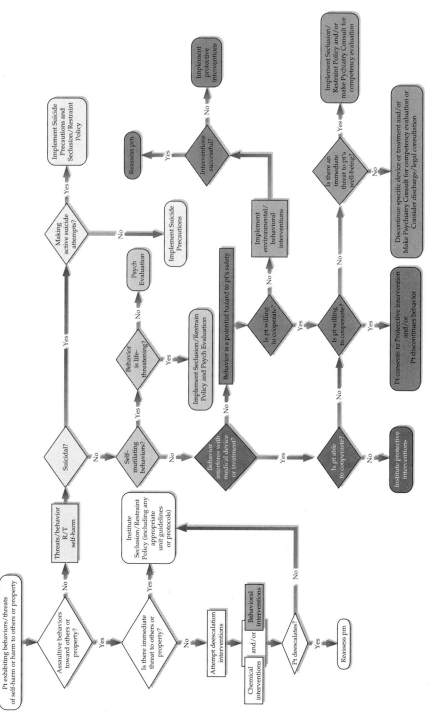

Process for Obtaining Equipment and Preparing Patient for Halo

Children's Medical Center of Dallas
4026 Prescott Ave, #2
Dallas, TX 75219

The process flowsheet and order form were developed to simplify the steps involved with patient preparation and ordering of a pediatric halotraction system.

Process for Obtaining Equipment and Preparing Patient for Halo

Patient identified
for Halo device

Patient, family, and staff informed of plan;
appropriate education provided to patient and family;
and child life involved in preparation

Halo sizing information sheet completed by staff
(see diagram/order form)

Completed Halo sizing form, faxed to neurosurgery office,
office called to notify that form has been sent, and
form placed in chart

Equipment ordered
(allow at least 24 hours for delivery)

Plan determined for placement by neurosurgery, including:
Approximate time and date for procedure
Level of sedation/analgesia required
Anesthesia required, if any placement (OR or floor)
Who will assist with the procedure
NPO status for child

Neurosurgery contacts appropriate persons
involved with Halo placement

If procedure to be done on the floor:
Gather other supplies for procedure:
  30 ml of 1% lidocaine with epinephrine
  CA monitor
  Betadine swabs
  "Surgical prep" razor to shave hair
  4 x 4 gauze
  (5) 10 ml syringes
  (5) 18 ga needles
  (5) 25 ga x 1.5 in needles

If procedure to be done in OR:
Neurosurgery will schedule

Necessary Halo Apparatus Sizing/Order Information

Complete the following information
on the attached form (see p. 287):

- Age
- Height
- Weight
- Head circumference (taken 1 cm above the eyebrow and 1 cm above the ear)
- Neck opening (diameter from one side of neck to the other, at base of neck)
- Circumferential measurement of chest at xiphoid process (pt relaxed—no breath holding)
- Length from shoulder to iliac crest (measured from median of clavicle)
- Length from shoulder to xiphoid process (measured from median of clavicle)
- Waist circumference
- Describe any medical devices in the chest or abdomen that must be considered for placement
- Describe any abnormal anatomy (e.g., large chest, barrel chest, exceptionally tall)

Request an "MRI-compatible" device.

FYI: CT/MRI Compatibility
A Halo device is MRI compatible if designated. The Halo will be "invisible." The Halo is safe and image compatible for CT. Ask the CT tech to "angle the approach" to get a better image.

HALO Sizing Information

Affix patient sticker here.

PLEASE <u>FAX THIS FORM</u> WHEN COMPLETE,
AND CALL TO NOTIFY THAT FORM WAS SENT.

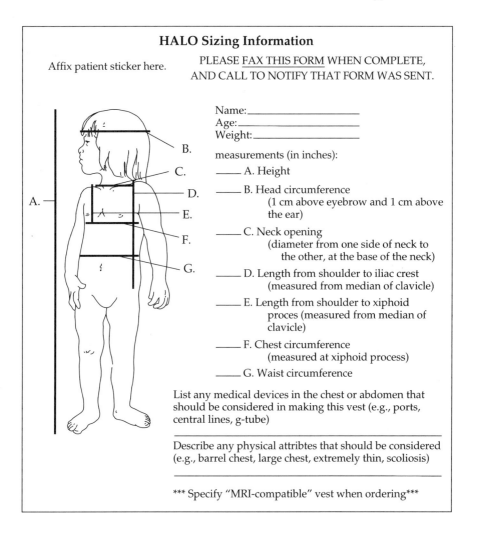

Name:_____
Age:_____
Weight:_____

measurements (in inches):

_____ A. Height

_____ B. Head circumference
(1 cm above eyebrow and 1 cm above
the ear)

_____ C. Neck opening
(diameter from one side of neck to
the other, at the base of the neck)

_____ D. Length from shoulder to iliac crest
(measured from median of clavicle)

_____ E. Length from shoulder to xiphoid
proces (measured from median of
clavicle)

_____ F. Chest circumference
(measured at xiphoid process)

_____ G. Waist circumference

List any medical devices in the chest or abdomen that
should be considered in making this vest (e.g., ports,
central lines, g-tube)
_____

Describe any physical attribtes that should be considered
(e.g., barrel chest, large chest, extremely thin, scoliosis)
_____

*** Specify "MRI-compatible" vest when ordering***

Known or Suspected Stroke Patients Algorithm

Janet R. Jenista, LCDR, NC, USN
School of Nursing, Emergency Care Clinical Track
University of Texas—Houston

This algorithm was developed by a graduate student emergency clinical nurse specialist for use in teaching emergency nurses the care of acute stroke patients.

Known or Suspected Stroke Patients Algorithm

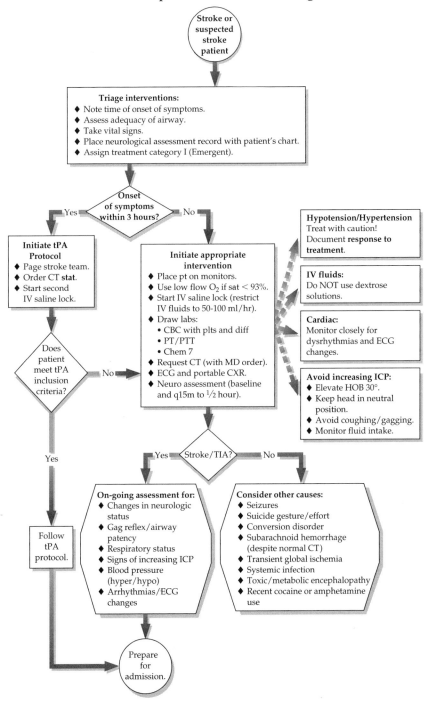

| Swallowing Screening Algorithm

Ruttonjee and Tang Shiu Kin Hospitals
266 Queen's Road East
Wanchai, Hong Kong

The Swallowing Screening Algorithm is commenced as soon as possible after admission, following the Speech Therapist's assessment. The Order Set is provided to doctors to facilitate immediate and effective interventions as soon as the patient is admitted.

Modified from Ruttonjee and Tang Shiu Kin Hospitals, Wanchai, Hong Kong. Used with permission.

Swallowing Screening Algorithm

Diagnosis: _____
Date of assessment: _____
Assessor's name: _____

Affix label on patient's particulars

*Please tick big and small boxes (☐ , ☐) as appropriate.

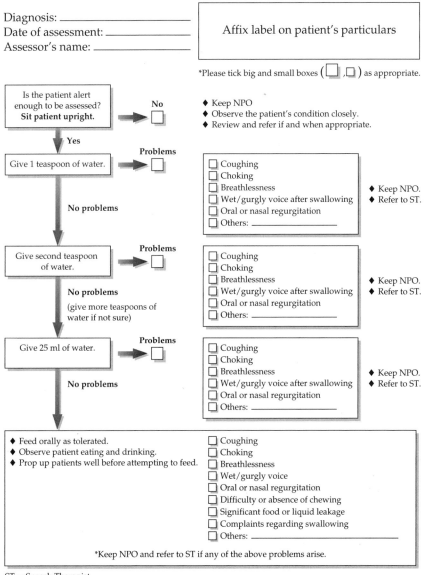

Is the patient alert enough to be assessed? Sit patient upright.

No → ☐

♦ Keep NPO
♦ Observe the patient's condition closely.
♦ Review and refer if and when appropriate.

Yes

Give 1 teaspoon of water.

Problems → ☐

☐ Coughing
☐ Choking
☐ Breathlessness
☐ Wet/gurgly voice after swallowing
☐ Oral or nasal regurgitation
☐ Others: _____

♦ Keep NPO.
♦ Refer to ST.

No problems

Give second teaspoon of water.

Problems → ☐

☐ Coughing
☐ Choking
☐ Breathlessness
☐ Wet/gurgly voice after swallowing
☐ Oral or nasal regurgitation
☐ Others: _____

♦ Keep NPO.
♦ Refer to ST.

No problems

(give more teaspoons of water if not sure)

Give 25 ml of water.

Problems → ☐

☐ Coughing
☐ Choking
☐ Breathlessness
☐ Wet/gurgly voice after swallowing
☐ Oral or nasal regurgitation
☐ Others: _____

♦ Keep NPO.
♦ Refer to ST.

No problems

♦ Feed orally as tolerated.
♦ Observe patient eating and drinking.
♦ Prop up patients well before attempting to feed.

☐ Coughing
☐ Choking
☐ Breathlessness
☐ Wet/gurgly voice
☐ Oral or nasal regurgitation
☐ Difficulty or absence of chewing
☐ Significant food or liquid leakage
☐ Complaints regarding swallowing
☐ Others: _____

*Keep NPO and refer to ST if any of the above problems arise.

ST = Speech Therapist

Lead-Specific Monitoring Algorithm

Andrew A. Galvin, LT, RN, MSN
School of Nursing, Emergency Care Clinical Track
University of Texas—Houston

This algorithm was developed by a graduate student emergency clinical nurse specialist for use in teaching emergency nurses appropriate selection of cardiac monitoring leads.

Lead-Specific Monitoring Algorithm

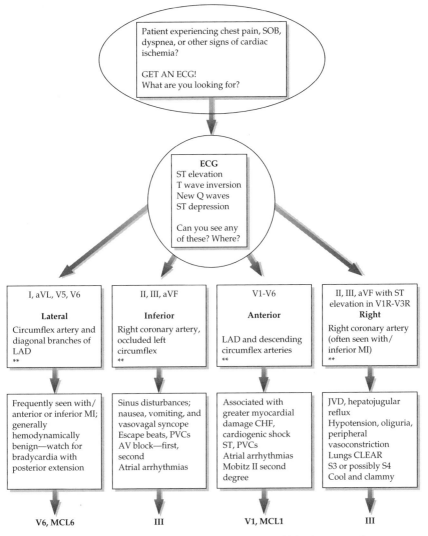

Patient experiencing chest pain, SOB, dyspnea, or other signs of cardiac ischemia?

GET AN ECG!
What are you looking for?

ECG
ST elevation
T wave inversion
New Q waves
ST depression

Can you see any of these? Where?

I, aVL, V5, V6	II, III, aVF	V1-V6	II, III, aVF with ST elevation in V1R-V3R
Lateral	**Inferior**	**Anterior**	**Right**
Circumflex artery and diagonal branches of LAD **	Right coronary artery, occluded left circumflex **	LAD and descending circumflex arteries **	Right coronary artery (often seen with/ inferior MI) **
Frequently seen with/ anterior or inferior MI; generally hemodynamically benign—watch for bradycardia with posterior extension	Sinus disturbances; nausea, vomiting, and vasovagal syncope Escape beats, PVCs AV block—first, second Atrial arrhythmias	Associated with greater myocardial damage CHF, cardiogenic shock ST, PVCs Atrial arrhythmias Mobitz II second degree	JVD, hepatojugular reflux Hypotension, oliguria, peripheral vasoconstriction Lungs CLEAR S3 or possibly S4 Cool and clammy
V6, MCL6	**III**	**V1, MCL1**	**III**

**Clinical signs and symptoms of myocardial ischemia, injury, and infarction may overlap.

| CHF Outpatient Management Algorithm

Borgess Medical Center
1521 Gull Road
Kalamazoo, Michigan 49001

The CHF Outpatient Management Algorithm is used in the physician's office to guide decision making regarding CHF patients. It defines the agreed-upon standard of care. The algorithms (and reference documents) are available in the office in a binder; charts are audited quarterly to determine areas for improvement. Aggregate results are incorporated into Health Alliance Outpatient Report Card for CHF, as well as provided to the individual practices.

CHF Outpatient Management Algorithm

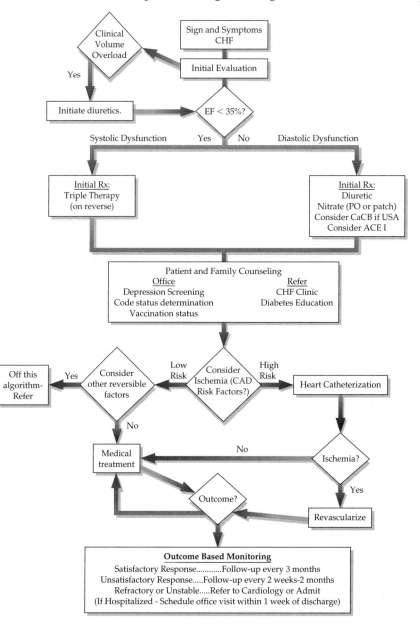

Thrombolytic Therapy for Acute Myocardial Infarction Protocol

Ruttonjee and Tang Shiu Kin Hospitals
Department of Medicine
266 Queen's Road East
Wanchai, Hong Kong

This protocol was developed to set the standard of care for delivery of thrombolytic therapy in acute myocardial infarction. It is used in conjunction with the acute myocardial infarction pathway (see p. 268).

Thrombolytic Therapy for Acute Myocardial Infarction Protocol

Inclusion Criteria
1. Chest pain or equivalent syndrome consistent with AMI ≤ 12 hrs from symptom onset

And

2. ECG changes:
ST elevation ≥ 1mm in ≥ 2 contiguous limb leads
or
ST elevation ≥ 2mm in ≥ 2 contiguous precordial leads
or
New BBB

Exclusion Criteria
A. Absolute contraindications:
1. Active internal bleeding
2. Known previous hemorrhagic CVA, CNS tumor, IC aneurysm, or AV malformation
3. Major trauma/surgery in past 2 months
4. Recent prolonged traumatic CPR (within 2 weeks)
5. Uncontrolled hypertension (> 200/120 mm Hg)
6. Suspected aortic dissection
7. Pregnancy

B. Relative contraindications:
1. Active peptic ulcer
2. History of CVA
3. Known bleeding disorders or current use of oral anticoagulant
4. Diabetic hemorrhagic retinopathy
5. Known advanced organ failure (liver or kidney)
6. Chronic severe hypertension (diastolic > 100 mm Hg)
7. Subclavian or internal venous cannulation

Considerations for Treatment
Consider rtPA over streptokinase in the following cases:
1. Previous allergy to streptokinase or prior exposure to streptokinase
2. Young patients with anterior MI
3. Early presentation (< 6 hours)
4. Hypotensive

Regimens
A. Accelerated rtPA with heparin infusion:
1. 15 mg IV bolus
2. 0.75 mg/kg over 30 minutes (total ≤ 50 mg)
3. 0.5 mg/kg over 60 minutes (total ≤ 35 mg)
4. Continue with heparin:
Load 3000 to 5000 units
Infuse 600-1000 units/hr
Aim at APTT = 60-85 seconds

B. Streptokinase infusion:
1. 1.5 megaunits in 100 ml normal saline IV infusion-60 minutes

Postthrombolytic Therapy Monitoring
1. Detect signs of allergic reaction (e.g., hypotension, anaphylaxis)
2. 12-lead ECG posttherapy then q8h prn
3. Record and report life-threatening arrhythmias
4. Monitor BP q1h and prn; continue cardiac monitoring.
5. Monitor neurologic state q1h × 6 hours then q4h × 24 hours for subtle signs of possible intracranial bleeding.
6. Assess degree/recurrence of chest pain (1-10 scale).
7. Assess effectiveness of thrombolytic therapy (see "Postthrombolytic Therapy Assessment Algorithm")

Bladder Training Protocol for Stroke Management

Ruttonjee and Tang Shiu Kin Hospitals
266 Queen's Road East
Wanchai, Hong Kong

This protocol was developed to guide the standardized assessment and management of bladder incontinence after stroke. It is used in conjunction with the stroke pathway.

Modified from Ruttonjee and Tang Shiu Kin Hospitals, Wanchai, Hong Kong. Used with permission.

**Bladder Training Protocol
for Stroke Management**

Inclusion Criteria
    FIM $\leq$ 5
Exclusion Criteria
    FIM > 5 (i.e., patients who are capable of self-care without assistance or supervision)

Procedure
1. Assess bladder management capacity—Bladder management includes complete and intentional control of the urinary bladder and, if necessary, use of equipment or agents for bladder control.[1]
2. Start patients use of the "Urinary Continence Chart" and "Intake and Output Chart."
3. Ensure fluid intake of 1.5 to 2 L/day throughout the day unless contraindicated.
4. Provide bedpans or urinals to patients whenever required.
5. Provide bedpans or urinals for patients to void every 2 hours.
6. If the patients can comply with the voiding schedule, increase voiding intervals by 1 hour each week until the patients can tolerate voiding every 4 to 6 hours.
7. Check residual urine if bladder distension is detected. Seek medical advice if retention of urine $\geq$ 350 ml.
8. If incidence of urinary incontinence is less than once a day, use diapers at night only.

---

[1] *Guide for the Uniform Data Set for Medical Rehabilitation, Adult FIM,* ed 4, 1993.

Renal Transplant Preoperative and Postoperative Physician's Orders

Dartmouth-Hitchcock Medical Center
1 Medical Center Drive
Lebanon, New Hampshire 03756

These preprinted preoperative and immediate postoperative standing orders are used in conjunction with the Renal Transplant Clinical Pathway (see p. 259).

ORDERED:		Medications, Treatments, and Diets
DATE	HOUR	

Admit: _____

Service/Attending: _____

Diagnosis: _____ Dialysis Type: _____

Allergies/ADRs: _____

☐ Initiate Renal Transplant Clinical Pathway
    ☐ VS per PACU with initial weight with bed scale.
    ☐ NPO except medications.
    ☐ Please place dual lumen central catheter if time and facility permit.
    ☐ CXR—check line placement if placed preop.
    ☐ Drain PD cath and send to OR dry.
    ☐ ECG.

☐ Labs: Type and cross four (4) units PRBCs—leukopoor/CMV negative.

☐ STAT labs: ☐ Lytes   ☐ CA ☐ BUN ☐ TP ☐ Mg
              ☐ ALB   ☐ Cr   ☐ CBC ☐ P04

☐ Other Labs/Tests: _____

☐ Viral Labs: ☐ EBV   ☐ HIV   ☐ CMV   ☐ VZV
             ☐ Herpes ☐ RPR ☐ Toxoplasmosis ☐ Hep C
             ☐ HbsAg ☐ HbsAb

Medications: Immunosuppression:
             Cyclosporine:
                 ☐ Neoral (microemulsion): _____
                 ☐ Sandimmune: _____
                 ☐ Other: _____
             ☐ Azathioprine mgs PO now
             ☐ Other: _____

             Antibiotic Prophylaxis: ☐ Cefazolin _____On call to OR___
                                 ☐ Other: _____

             Antiviral Prophylaxis: ☐ Acyclovir __800__ mg PO now
             (see protocol)   ☐ Gancyclovir _____ mg IV on
                                        call to OR

             Other (patient specific): ☐ Diltiazem CD _120__ mg PO now
                               ☐ Nizatidine _150__ mg PO now

             ☐ Other: _____ ☐ Other: _____

If patient has A-V fistula-no BP or blood drawing in _____ arm.

If using Quinton/Dialysis catheter, aspirate heparin each lumen prior to IV hook-up or blood drawing, following RN policy and procedure.

Physician Signature: _____ Beeper #: _____

(continued)

Dartmouth-Hitchcock Medical Center Mary Hitchcock Memorial Hospital Lebanon, NH 03756 Renal Transplant Postop PHYSICIAN'S ORDER SHEET—cont'd		Addressograph

ORDERED:	Medications,* Treatments, and Diets	
DATE	**HOUR**	

Diagnosis: End Stage Renal Disease 2⁰ _____
Procedure—Cadaveric/Living/Related Transplant

Ureteral Anastomosis:	Type: _____	
Ureteral Stent	☐ Yes	☐ No
Native Nephrectomy	☐ Yes	☐ No
Kidney Transplant	☐ Yes	☐ No

Condition: _____

Allergies/ADRs: _____

☐ No BP or blood draw in ————— arm.

☐ Initiate Renal Transplant Clinical Pathway.

☐ Nursing/PACU:
  • VS of 15 min until stabilized, then q1/2h until transfer
  • I&O q1/2h x 4 then q1h until discharge (call HO if urine <100 cc/hr)
  • Foley to gravity, routine Foley care
  • JP to bulb suction; attach to wall suction if >150 cc/hr
  • Peripheral vascular checks, pedal pulses x 2
  • Activity may elevate HOB

☐ Chest X-ray study (if not done preop for line placement)

☐ IV replacement: 1/2 NS 1 cc/1 cc urine output/hr, not to exceed 500 cc/hr

☐ IV maintenance: D5 1/2 NS C 50 cc/hr

☐ Labs upon arrival to PACU:

   Glucose, CBC, Lytes, BUN, Creatinine, PO_4, MG

☐ Nursing/4 West

   VS: q——   I&O:——   CVP if urine output <100 cc/hr O_2 2LNP prn
  • No BP or blood drawing in ————— arm
  • Daily AM weights (before 6 AM)
  • Diet: Clear liquids
  • Activity: May elevate HOB; OOB to chair within 24 hrs
  • Foley to gravity, routine Foley care
  • JP to bulb suction; attach to wall suction if >150 cc/hr
  • Peripheral vascular checks on arrival to floor

☐ IV replacement: 1/2 NS 1 cc/1 cc urine output/hr, not to exceed 500 cc/hr

☐ IV maintenance: D5 1/2 NS C 50 cc/hr

Labs:

☐ Daily labs STAT 5 AM: CBC, BUN, Creatinine, Lytes, Glucose, PO_4, MG

☐ LFTs, Ca, Alb, on ———————————————— (app. POD #3)

☐ Cyclosporine trough level on ————— (app. POD #5)

☐ Transplant ultrasound on —————

Medications (Doses Based on Renal Function):
  Immunosuppressive Medications:
    Cyclosporine:

      ☐ Neoral (microemulsion): _____
      ☐ Sandimmune: _____
      ☐ Other: _____

    ☐ Azathioprine: ——————————— mg/po
    ☐ Methylprednisolone: ——————————— mg/IV
    ☐ Mycophenolic acid: _____
    ☐ Other: _____
    ☐ Diltiazem CD 120 mg PO daily: _____

* A generic equivalent may be administered when a drug has been prescribed by brand name unless the order states to the contrary.

ORDERED:		Medications,* Treatments, and Diets
DATE	**HOUR**	

☐ Muromonab (OKT3): _____ mg/IVP
  Dose time over 1 min: _____

Premedication 1 hr prior to OKT3:
  ☐ Methylprednisolone: _____ mg/IVSS
  ☐ Acetaminophen: _____ mg PO/PR
  ☐ Diphenhydramine: _____ mg PO/IV

☐ Antithymocyte globulin (ATG) skin test 0.1 mcg ID now:
  Read skin test 20-30 min after application.

☐ ATG: _____ mg/IV
  Over 6 hrs start: _____

Premedication 1 hr prior to ATG:
  ☐ Acetaminophen (prn; temp >38.5°C): _____ mg PO/PR

Antibiotic Prophylaxis:
  ☐ Cefazolin: _____
  ☐ Other: _____

Antiviral Prophylaxis:
  ☐ Acyclovir: _____
  ☐ Gancyclovir: _____
  ☐ Other: _____

Antifungal Prophylaxis:
  ☐ Nystatin S/S 5 cc PO qid: _____
  ☐ Other: _____

Antihypertensive:
  ☐ Other: _____
  Nifedipine 10 mg PO q1h for BP >165/95 mm Hg prn: _____

☐ GI prophylaxis: _____
☐ Electrolyte replacement: _____

Diabetic Management: ☐ FS q__ h or_____
  ☐ Insulin (Reg Humulin): _____
  ☐ Sliding scale (Reg Humulin): _____
  ☐ Oral agent: _____
  ☐ Other: _____

Pain Management:
  ☐ See MS04 PCA sheet _____
  ☐ Other: _____

Bowel Management:
  ☐ Dulcolax 2 tabs PO bid: _____
  ☐ Other: _____

Time: _____   Date: _____

Print physician's name: _____   Beeper #: _____

Physician's signature: _____   Beeper #: _____

* A generic equivalent may be administered when a drug has been prescribed by brand name unless the order states to the contrary.

Preprocedure Orders for Cardiac Cath Lab (Adult)

Dartmouth-Hitchcock Medical Center
1 Medical Center Drive
Lebanon, New Hampshire 03756

This order set is used by house staff and attending physicians for patients preparing for cardiac catheterization, coronary angioplasty, coronary atherectomy, or coronary stent placement. It supports the interventions stated on the clinical pathway.

MARY HITCHCOCK MEMORIAL HOSPITAL
Lebanon, NH   03756

PHYSICIAN'S ORDER SHEET

(Addressograph)

ORDERED		Medications, Treatments, and Diets
Date	Hour	All Orders Applicable

PREPROCEDURE ORDERS FOR CARDIAC CATH LAB (ADULT)

Attending: _____

Resident: _____

Service: _____

Allergies/prior ADRs: _____

For _____ (procedure) on _____ (date) at _____ (time).

Laboratory work:

☐ PA and lateral chest x-ray study ☐ CBC, Lytes, BUN, Creatinine

☐ ECG ☐ Type and screen

☐ Fasting glucose by fingerstick AM of procedure (if diabetic)

☐ PT, PTT AM of procedure STAT

Other: _____

IV:

☐ For diagnostic cath, insert <u>one</u> 18-gauge IV catheter (unless present) in left arm. For planned or potential PTCA, insert <u>two</u> 18-gauge intravenous catheters, preferably in left arm. Cap with routine flushes.

☐ Infuse _____ ml of _____ (solution) at _____ ml/hr beginning at _____ (time) with macrodrip tubing, extension tubing, and regular bore SafSite T connector.

Medications:

Aspirin: ☐ Enteric coated 325 mg PO qd

☐ Soluble 325 mg PO or per NG tube qd

☐ Soluble 81 mg PO or per NG tube qd

If diabetic, insulin dose morning of procedure: _____

Other: _____

Premedicate on call to Cath Lab with:

☐ Diazepam _____ mg PO

☐ Diphenhydramine _____ mg PO

Other: _____

Void on call to Cath Lab.

Prepare as for OR except wear reading glasses, dentures, and hearing aid; do not wear snap gown.

☐ NPO after midnight; continue to take cardiac medications.

☐ Hold diuretic AM of cath.

Have PTCA patient complete patient admission survey; give patient copy of consent.

Physician's Signature	PRINT Name	Pager #

Postcoronary Artery Intervention Orders (Adult)

Dartmouth-Hitchcock Medical Center
1 Medical Center Drive
Lebanon, New Hampshire 03756

This standard order set is used by house staff, the physicians' assistants, and attending physicians for patients after coronary angioplasty, coronary atherectomy, or coronary stent placement. It supports the interventions stated on the clinical pathway.

MARY HITCHCOCK MEMORIAL HOSPITAL Lebanon, NH 03756 PHYSICIAN'S ORDER SHEET	Addressograph

ORDERED		Medications, Treatments, and Diets
Date	Hour	All Orders Applicable

POSTCORONARY ARTERY INTERVENTION ORDERS (ADULT)
Page 1 of 4
Attending: _____
Service: _____

Procedure performed: _____

Prior ADRs/allergies: _____

_____

Patient condition: _____

Call for problems associated with angioplasty: Dr. _____ at pager # _____

Diet: ☐ Liquids for first meal after stent. Follow with diet below as tolerated.

☐ NAS, low cholesterol; adjust diet per Sheath Removal Protocol; order finger food while patient in bed prn.

Other: _____

☐ Diet consult for discharge instruction in same diet as above.

Activity: ☐ **Early activity protocol:**
While sheaths in and for 6 hrs after sheaths out: complete bedrest with head of bed elevated to _____ °C and extremity below catheter site immobilized; then up to bathroom with assistance; then advanced activity as tolerated.

☐ **Delayed activity protocol:**
While sheaths in: complete bedrest with head of bed elevated ≤30° and extremity below cath site immobilized.

After sheaths out: complete bedrest for _____ hrs with head of bed elevated ≤30° and extremity below catheter site immobilized.

For next 24 hrs up to bedside chair; ambulate in room only; and bathroom privileges.

Then ambulate ad lib.

☐ Cardiac Rehab consult for (1) patient walking continuously for 5 min and taking 26 stairs up and down prior to discharge, (2) risk factor analysis and counseling, and (3) cardiac rehab follow-up.

Vital signs: ☐ Take vital signs according to Interventional Cardiology Procedures Protocol. Upon transfer from ASCU, measure pulse, respirations, and blood pressure q4h × 24 hrs and then every shift. Take temperature q8h.

_____
Physician's Signature

(continued)

MARY HITCHCOCK MEMORIAL HOSPITAL Lebanon, NH 03756 PHYSICIAN'S ORDER SHEET	Addressograph

<table>
<tr><td colspan="2">ORDERED</td><td>Medications, Treatments, and Diets</td></tr>
<tr><td>Date</td><td>Hour</td><td>All Orders Applicable</td></tr>
</table>

POSTCORONARY ARTERY INTERVENTION ORDERS (ADULT)—cont'd

Page 2 of 4

☐ ECG monitoring according to Interventional Cardiology Procedures Protocol

☐ I&O until AM and voiding without difficulty (ASCU only)

☐ Daily weights except while patient on bedrest

☐ Titrate oxygen to keep $SpO_2 \times 90\%$ on room air. Check SpO_2 per unit protocol.

Vascular sheaths:
Arterial: _____ Fr sheath in _____ artery
Venous: _____ Fr sheath in _____ vein
Other: _____ Fr sheath in _____ _____

Access site care:

☐ Assess access sites and peripheral circulation according to Interventional Cardiology Procedures Protocol. Upon transfer out of ASCU, assess every shift for 24 hrs and at discharge.

☐ Sandbag to _____ groin for 6 hrs after sheath removed.

☐ Protective device (e.g., sheet tuck, posey) to leg while arterial sheath in place and for 6 hrs after sheath removal if needed to restrict leg movement.

Sheath removal:

☐ Prior to sheath removal, hang 500 ml NS IV at K/O rate and administer the following medications:

☐ Morphine sulfate 2-4 mg × 1 IVP prn

☐ Midazolam 1-2 mg × 1 IVP prn

Other: _____

☐ Infiltrate the groin with 1% lidocaine for sheath removal.

Follow Sheath Removal Protocol checked below:

☐ **Early Sheath Removal Protocol:**

☐ Restart heparin at _____ hrs after sheath removal at last previous rate or at _____ units/hr. Continue adjustment according to Heparin Protocol orders.

☐ **AM Sheath Removal Protocol:**
Administer heparin IV overnight at:

☐ 1000 units/hr

☐ _____ units/hr (18 units/kg/hr)

☐ Restart heparin at _____ hrs after sheath removal at last previous rate or at _____ units/hr. Continue adjustment according to Heparin Protocol orders.

Physician's Signature _____

MARY HITCHCOCK MEMORIAL HOSPITAL Lebanon, NH 03756 PHYSICIAN'S ORDER SHEET	Addressograph

ORDERED		Medications, Treatments, and Diets
Date	Hour	All Orders Applicable

POSTCORONARY ARTERY INTERVENTION ORDERS (ADULT)
Page 3 of 4

Laboratory:

☐ CBC, Lytes, BUN, creatinine in AM

CBC qd ☐ or qod ☐ for patients on high intensity anticoagulation

☐ CPK and LDH (with isoenzymes if elevated) on arrival and in morning

☐ PTT and ACT per Sheath Removal Protocol; check first ACT at   hrs after heparin discontinued

☐ PTT after sheath removal according to Heparin Protocol orders

☐ Protime every morning (if on warfarin)

☐ Platelet count at   (2 hrs) and   (24 hrs) after abciximab bolus in Cath Lab; call physician if platelets <100,000

☐ STAT K$^+$ if diuresis >500 cc over 2 hrs and 1 hr after potassium replacement therapy completed

☐ ECG on arrival and in morning

Other:

Institute Bleeding Precautions for duration of hospital stay.

☐ Fluids to 1000 ml PO day of procedure.

Intravenous infusions:

☐ Maintenance: 1000 ml   (type) at   ml/hr ×   hours. When

☐ output > intake by 500 ml, administer bolus with 300 ml NS IV.

☐ IV nitroglycerin 50 mg in 250 ml NS. Infuse at   mcg/min; wean by   .

☐ IV abciximab (ReoPro) 9 mg in 250 ml NS; administer through a 0.22 micron non-protein-binding filter at ____ ml/hr until _____ (time) via dedicated IV line.

☐ Insert an 18G IV catheter for blood drawing and cap. Change the SafSite valve and flush after each blood draw (if on warfarin). If patient is receiving abciximab, draw all blood through this line after sheath removal for 24 hrs.

Avoid all venipunctures.

Other:

_____
Physician's Signature

(continued)

Addressograph

ORDERED		Medications, Treatments, and Diets
Date	Hour	All Orders Applicable

POSTCORONARY ARTERY INTERVENTION ORDERS (ADULT)—cont'd
Page 4 of 4

In the event of chest pain:

☐ Follow Interventional Cardiology Procedures Chest Pain Protocol.

☐ Administer nitroglycerin 0.4 mg SL; repeat q5min × 2 until angina is relieved.

☐ Increase nitroglycerin drip to _____ mcg/min or restart nitroglycerin at last documented rate.

☐ Restart heparin per physician's order.

Medications:

Aspirin: ☐ Enteric coated 325 mg PO qd

☐ Soluble 325 mg PO or per NG tube qd

☐ Soluble 81 mg PO or per NG tube qd

☐ Ticlopidine 250 mg PO bid

Warfarin: _____

Calcium channel blocker: _____

Analgesia: _____

Antianxiety: _____

Sleep: _____

GI prophylaxis: _____

Potassium supplementation: _____

☐ RBOs

☐ Mylanta II 10-15 ml PO q2-4h prn

Other: _____

_____

_____

_____

_____

_____

Perform emergency care according to the Interventional Cardiology Procedures Protocol.

Transfer patient from ASCU when meets discharge criteria.

_____	_____	_____
Physician's Signature	PRINT Name	Pager #

Heparin Protocol Orders (Adult) and Heparin Documentation Flowsheet

Dartmouth-Hitchcock Medical Center
1 Medical Center Drive
Lebanon, New Hampshire 03756

This standard order set was developed to encourage practitioners to use weight-based heparin dosing and to enable the RN to make the medication changes in a timely fashion. The nursing flow sheet is used to document all heparin administered in bolus and infusion forms at Inpatient Cardiac Services. It is also the tracking mechanism for recording the PTT values and subsequent medication changes.

<table>
<tr><td colspan="5">

MARY HITCHCOCK MEMORIAL HOSPITAL
Lebanon, NH   03756

CARDIAC SERVICES

PHYSICIAN'S ORDER SHEET

</td><td colspan="2">

Addressograph

</td></tr>
</table>

ORDERED		Medications, Treatments, and Diets
Date	Hour	All Orders Applicable

HEPARIN PROTOCOL ORDERS (ADULT)
Page 1 of 1

Prior ADRs/allergies: _____

_____

Heparin IV bolus: _____ units (80 units/kg to a maximum of 10,000 units[1])

Heparin 25,000 units in 500 cc D_5W as continuous infusion at _____ units/hr
(calculated as 18 units/kg/hr)[a]

☐   Adjust heparin according to following protocol starting 6 hrs after bolus:

APTT (sec)	BOLUS	STOP INFUSION	RATE CHANGE	REPEAT APTT[2]
<50	2000 U	No	Increase 200 units/hr	4 hrs
50-64	No	No	Increase 100 units/hr	4 hrs
65-85	No	No	No	6 or 24 hrs
86-100	No	No	Decrease 50 units/hr	6 hrs
101-120	No	30 min[3]	Decrease 100 units/hr	4 hrs
>120	No	60 min[3]	Decrease 150 units/hr	4 hrs

[1]Rasche R et al: The weight-based heparin dosing nomogram compared with a "standard care" nomogram, *Annals of Internal Medicine* 119:874, 1993.
[2]The interval between last heparin rate change and next APTT.
[3]If heparin is temporarily discontinued, be sure to restart drip on time.

Increase the interval between APTTs to 24 hrs (with usual morning blood draws) if:

☐   One APTT value is within therapeutic range.
☐   Two sequential APTT values drawn hours apart are within therapeutic range (coronary stent patient)

☐   Institute Bleeding Precautions.

Call physician if two consecutive boluses are given to patient according to above protocol.

If heparin is newly started, ask IV Team to place a second IV line dedicated to drawing blood.

Lab tests: ☐   PTT 6 hours after initial bolus (send STAT)
☐   PTT qd while on heparin (send STAT)
CBC while on heparin: ☐ qd   ☐ qod

_____

_____

_____	_____	_____
Physician's Signature	PRINT Name	Pager #

MARY HITCHCOCK MEMORIAL HOSPITAL
Lebanon, NH   03756

HEPARIN FLOW SHEET
Inpatient Cardiac Services

Addressograph

Date and time of MD order: _____ Secretary Initials: _____ RN Initials: _____

Initial heparin IV bolus: _____ units (80 units/kg to a maximum of 10,000 units)

Start heparin 25,000 units in 500 cc D_5W as continuous infusion at _____ units/hr (calculated as 18 units/kg/hr)

☐ Adjust heparin according to following protocol starting 6 hrs after bolus: D/C date: _____

APTT (sec)	BOLUS	STOP INFUSION	RATE CHANGE	REPEAT APTT[2]
<50	2000 U	No	Increase 200 units/hr	4 hrs
50-64	No	No	Increase 100 units/hr	4 hrs
65-85	No	No	No	6 or 24 hrs
86-100	No	No	Decrease 50 units/hr	6 hrs
101-120	No	30 min	Decrease 100 units/hr	4 hrs
>120	No	60 min	Decrease 150 units/hr	4 hrs

*The interval between PTTs may be increased to 24 hrs if:
• With a patient with coronary stent, two sequential PTT values require no rate adjustment.
• With other patients, one PTT value requires no rate adjustment.

Date	Time	PTT	IVP Bolus (units)	25,000 U in 500 cc D5W+ (↑↓)	IV Drip (units/hr)	(cc/hr)	Time of Day Drip Held	Next PTT Date	Next PTT Time	RN Initials

Transferred with heparin infusion at   units/hr.

Notes:

Elective Infrarenal Abdominal Aortic Aneurysm Repair Physician's Order Sheet

Dartmouth-Hitchcock Medical Center
1 Medical Center Drive
Lebanon, New Hampshire 03756

The order set is used with the Elective Infrarenal Abdominal Aortic Aneurysm Repair Critical Pathway (see p. 247) to complement care, expedite order entry, and ensure that practices are standardized.

Modified from Dartmouth-Hitchcock Medical Center, Lebanon, New Hampshire. Used with permission.

Darthmouth-Hitchcock Medical Center	
Mary Hitchcock Memorial Hospital Lebanon, NH 03756 Vascular Surgery PHYSICIAN'S ORDER SHEET Elective Infrarenal Abdominal Aortic Aneurysm Repair	Addressograph

ORDERED:		Medications,* Treatments, and Diets
DATE	**HOUR**	

Transfer to 4W s/p AAA repair   Vascular surgery staff physician: _____

Allergies/ADRs: _____

☐ Continue Abdominal Aortic Aneurysm Repair Critical Pathway

☐ Nursing:
   VS, peripheral vascular assessment per pathway
   Venodyne while in bed or chair ≥2 hours
   Respiratory assessment per pathway
   Titrate O_2 to maintain SpO_2 ≥90%
   Pulmonary toilet prn
   Weight qd
   I&O per pathway
   Foley care
   NGT ➝ LCS
   Maintain DSD for incisional drainage; may remove dressing if incision is dry and staples are intact
   Activity per pathway

IV Fluid: Rate: _____

☐ Cap heparin IV when tolerating liquids

Medications:

☐ Epidural per anesthesia
   When epidural removed:
      ☐ PCA per order sheet
      ☐ Percocet 1-2 PO q3-4h prn
      ☐ Other:

☐ Famotidine 20 mg IV bid until taking PO, then D/C

☐ ASA 325 mg PO qd when taking PO

☐ Restoril 15-30 mg PO qhs prn when taking PO

☐ Mylanta or ☐ Amphojel 30 cc PO q4h prn (specify) when taking PO

☐ For anxiety:

☐ For nausea:

☐ RBOs

Additional Medications:

☐ Diuretic: ×   days

☐ KCL supplement: ×   days

☐ Albuterol 0.83%, 3 ml solution for neb q2-6h prn

☐ Ipratropium 0.5 mg/2.5 ml solution for neb q2-6h prn

Labs:

☐ Daily Lytes, BUN/Cr   ×   days

☐ CBC, Lytes 2 days after transfer to 4W

Call HO if: HR >100, <50   Temp >38.5° C   RR >30
                 SBP >180, <100   Pulse ox <90%

Physician's Signature: Beeper #:

*A generic equivalent may be administered when a drug has been prescribed by brand name unless the order states to the contrary.

(continued)

Dartmouth-Hitchcock Medical Center
Mary Hitchcock Memorial Hospital
Lebanon, NH   03756

Vascular Surgery
PHYSICIAN'S ORDER SHEET
Elective Infrarenal Abdominal Aortic Aneurysm Repair—cont'd

Addressograph

ORDERED:		Medications,* Treatments, and Diets
DATE	**HOUR**	

Admit to ICU: Dr.   Vascular Surgery Staff Physician

Fellow/Chief: 3rd-Year Resident:

Attending CS: Team Color:

Allergies/ADRs:

Diagnosis: S/P AAA Repair:

☐   Implement Abdominal Aortic Aneurism Repair Critical Pathway

    Nursing: ☐ Vital signs, PA catheter, and A-line per ICU protocol
             Continuous ST segment monitoring
             Daily weights, routine Foley care, NPO except ice chips
             NG to LCS, flush 20 cc NS q4h and check pH
             Routine pulmonary toilet until extubated, then:
             Incentive spirometer; turn, cough, and deep breathe q1h while awake
             Lower extremity motor and sensory exam q1h × 4, then q2h × 8, then q8h
             Doppler ankle pressures on admission and qd
             Heme check: all stools
             Activity: bedrest overnight, OOB in morning
             Venodyne: start now

    Ventilator: ☐ Initial ventilation settings per CCS
              ☐ Evaluate for immediate extubation
              ☐ Standard ICU extubation protocol

    IV Fluid: ☐ D5LR at   cc/hr   ☐ Or:

    Call CCS if: Temp >38.5° C; RR >30, <12; SpO$_2$ <90%; Urine output <30 cc/hr
    Call CCS and VS: HR >100, <50; SBP >180, <100; ST change ≥2 mm
                 Cardiac index <2.0
                 Change in lower extremity motor, sensory, or Doppler exam
                 Heme (+) stools

    Medications: ☐ Vasoactive drips:
              ☐ Albuterol 0.83%, 3 ml solution for neb q6h and q2h prn
              ☐ Ipratropium 0.5 mg/2.5 ml solution for neb q6h and q2h prn
              ☐ Famotidine 20mg IV bid
               ☐ Mylanta or ☐ Amphojel 30-60 cc/NG prn pH <6.0
              ☐ Rx epidural for pain per APS
               ☐ Pain management if no epidural

    Antibiotics: ☐ Ancef 1 g q8h × 3 doses, start at   AM/PM
              ☐ ABX form
               ☐ Other:

    Cardiac Medications:
       For SBP × 180 call HO and start:
              ☐ Metoprolol 5 mg IV now and q2" prn   Or:

    Labs:
       Now: CBC, PT, PTT, Lytes, BUN, Creatinine, Glucose, Mg++, ABG
             ☐ Repeat CBC, K+ at   AM/PM   In AM: CBC, Lytes, BUN, Creatinine
             ☐ CPK and LDH with isoenzymes now and q8" × 3
    ECG: Now ☐ In AM   CXR: Now ☐ In AM

    Physician's Signature: Beeper #:

*A generic equivalent may be administered when a drug has been prescribed by brand name unless the order states to the contrary.

Page numbers in italics indicate boxes and
illustrations, page numbers followed by t
indicate tables.

Also from Tor Books

The SFWA Grand Masters, Volume One
(Robert A. Heinlein, Jack Williamson, Clifford D. Simak,
L. Sprague de Camp, and Fritz Leiber)
edited by Frederik Pohl

The SFWA GRAND MASTERS

VOLUME TWO

ANDRE NORTON

ARTHUR C. CLARKE

ISAAC ASIMOV

ALFRED BESTER

RAY BRADBURY

E D I T E D   B Y

FREDERIK POHL

TOR®

A TOM DOHERTY ASSOCIATES BOOK

NEW YORK

THE SFWA GRAND MASTERS: VOLUME TWO

Copyright © 2000 by Science Fiction and Fantasy Writers of America, Inc.

Edited by David G. Hartwell

A Tor Book
Published by Tom Doherty Associates, LLC
175 Fifth Avenue
New York, NY 10010

www.tor.com

Tor® is a registered trademark of Tom Doherty Associates, LLC.

Book design by Lisa Pifher

Library of Congress Cataloging-in-Publication Data

    The SFWA grand masters / edited by Frederik Pohl.
        p. cm.
    "A Tom Doherty Associates book."
    Contents: Andre Norton—Arthur C. Clarke—
Isaac Asimov—Alfred Bester—Ray Bradbury
    ISBN 0-312-86879-0 (hc)
    ISBN 0-312-86878-2 (pbk)
    1. Science fiction, American. I. Pohl, Frederik. II. Science Fiction Writers of America. III. Title: Grand masters.
PS648.S3 S44   2000
813'.0876208—dc21   99-21933
                                                      CIP

First Hardcover Edition: April 2000
First Trade Paperback Edition: April 2001

Printed in the United States of America

0 9 8 7 6 5 4 3 2 1

This book is dedicated to Damon Knight
who, all by himself, created
the Science Fiction Writers of America.

CONTENTS

INTRODUCTION

Science fiction has been around for a long time. How long, exactly, depends on how charitably one wants to define the term—as far back as the Roman Empire, if you're willing to admit *The Satyricon* of Petronius Arbiter and Lucian of Samosata's voyages to the Moon. Certainly Jonathan Swift wrote a kind of science fiction in *Gulliver's Travels* and so did Mary Wollstonecraft Shelley in *Frankenstein*; even more surely, Jules Verne and H. G. Wells were writing genuine science fiction a hundred years ago and more.

But in April 1926, there was a watershed event in the history of the field. Hugo Gernsback published his first issue of *Amazing Stories* and thus gave science fiction an identity of its own, a home and a name.

Actually the name he gave it wasn't "science fiction." Gernsback was a word-coiner, and he preferred to call it "scientifiction," but no matter. With a dedicated magazine of its own, science fiction became self-aware. The magazine attracted new readers; some new readers became new writers. When Doc Smith saw this new magazine on the stands, he pulled the manuscript of *The Skylark of Space* out of the desk drawer where it had languished since 1917, because he hadn't been able to find a good place to publish it, and at once the whole subgenre of space opera was born. By the early 1930s other magazines appeared, and a whole community of science fiction writers had taken form.

The early 1930s were not a particularly good time to be a writer of science fiction. Of the three existing magazines, two were bimonthly and none paid very much for the stories it bought. I once calculated that the average income for a science fiction writer in those days was not much more than $4 a week, and of academic respect for their work there was none.

By the time World War II had come and gone things had begun to improve for the new science fiction community. There were more of them now—a hundred or more men and women writing science fiction by then—and there were more markets, too. Several

dozen additional science fiction magazines had come along (and, mostly, gone away again). Science fiction, which had dealt with rockets and atomic energy and television, began to command a little more respect once these things had appeared in the real world. Anthologies of stories from the Good Old Days began to appear, so did book contracts and offers for radio dramatization of the stories, and now and then similar offers from the science fictiony new medium of TV itself and even, once in a great while, from the movies. And writers who for a generation had been cheerfully (or glumly) signing away all rights in return for their $50 short story checks suddenly became aware that these previously unconsidered "other rights" were worth trying to retain.

The time had come to do something about it.

In unity, the writers reasoned, there ought to be strength. So one evening around 1950, Fletcher Pratt invited fifteen or twenty other science fiction writers to his apartment on West Fifty-eighth Street in New York. The meeting had an agenda. Its purpose was to consider whether it was worth trying to form a science fiction writers' organization.

Nearly everyone present at once agreed that such an organization was worth having. Nearly no one agreed on just what form it should take.

In retrospect, that was inevitable. Science fiction writers were, and are, what science fiction writers were, and are.

What are they, exactly?

Why, it happens that I may be able to answer that for you. Some time ago a team of psychologists asked themselves that very question. To find the answer they embarked on a research project. They prepared a psychological evaluation questionnaire and sent it off to every science fiction writer they could find. From their answers the psychologists prepared a group personality profile and contrasted it with similar profiles from two other kinds of human beings—one a group of writers of another sort, the other not writers at all. They found that the three profiles were pretty similar in most respects. However, in one quality—technically they called it "adventurous versus withdrawn cyclothymia," but it translates to pure

stubbornness—the science fiction writers were right off the chart.

As a former editor, agent, and president of various science fiction writers' organizations, I can testify that this is a true bill. I think it may be an occupational trait. After all, to do his work a science fiction writer must turn her back on the real world around him and make up a whole new one of her own. To do that requires a considerable independence of mind, which is the "adventurous" part of the cyclothymia.

But whether that is the explanation or not, the phenomenon is real enough. By and large, science fiction writers are the nicest and smartest people you'd ever want to meet, but, boy, are they *stubborn*.

They gave an adequate demonstration of this trait at that meeting at Fletcher Pratt's apartment. After the first hour one writer stalked out because it sounded too much like a trade union to him, and he didn't want to join any confounded trade union. After the second hour another writer left because it didn't look like being *enough* of a trade union. At the end of the evening nothing had been resolved. So it was determined to meet again at some later date, when everybody had had a chance to think the matter through, and everyone went home. And that second meeting never occurred.

Over the next few years there were sporadic efforts to get something going, none of which got very far. Then, in the early 1960s, one writer, Damon Knight, took matters into his own hands. He announced the formation of the Science Fiction Writers of America. The question of exactly what it would do and how it would do it he left open, for the organization to decide for itself once it had come into being. He recruited a few of the writers he knew best, and set about signing up everyone else.

As it happened, I was editing a couple of science fiction magazines at the time. Every time a new issue appeared I would get from Damon a batch of letters addressed to each writer in the issue for me to forward. The letters invited the writer to join up, and, by gosh, a lot of them did.

That was pushing forty years ago, and now the Science Fiction Writers of America—later rechristened the Science Fiction and Fantasy Writers of America—is still going strong.

I can't say that it has ever really settled the question of what it should do. That is still debated constantly, and often vigorously, in its meetings and publications, but SFWA just goes on doing whatever seems necessary, regardless. It gives useful trade information to new writers. It investigates and acts on grievances. It provides an emergency fund to help writers in disastrous situations— actually, it is to benefit this fund with a share of the royalties that this particular series of anthologies was commissioned. It keeps its members informed of developments in their field of interest and gives them a forum to exchange their views.

And, once every year or so, it honors one of the great writers in its field by presenting him or her with what is called the Grand Master Award.

The Grand Master Award is given not for any single story but for a lifetime achievement in the fields of science fiction and fantasy. So far, fewer than twenty of them have ever been given. The first five recipients—Robert A. Heinlein, Jack Williamson, Clifford D. Simak, L. Sprague de Camp, and Fritz Leiber—were honored in the first volume of this series; the second five—Andre Norton, Isaac Asimov, Arthur C. Clarke, Alfred Bester, and Ray Bradbury—are herewith.

Enjoy their stories, please. And remember that this would not have happened if it hadn't been for the determination of that one stubborn individual, Damon Knight.

—Frederik Pohl

ANDRE NORTON

b. 1912

Andre Norton is unique among the winners of the Grand Master Award in two respects: first, in her gender—she is the only woman among the first fifteen Grand Masters—second, in the fact that she is the only one who made a distinguished career in science fiction and fantasy with almost no connection to the magazines. Her first published sf, "The People of the Crater," was for the short-lived *Fantasy Book* in 1947. But after that, with very few exceptions, it was novels all the way.

Alice Mary (now legally "Andre") Norton worked as a librarian in the Cleveland, Ohio, system, writing on the side as time permitted. Between 1934 and 1954 she published four novels that lay outside the sf-fantasy genre without making much of a stir. In 1952, however, she published her first sf novel, *Star Man's Son, 2250 A.D.* It was intended, and marketed, as a juvenile novel. So were many of her earlier novels, though they shared with the juvenile books of that other Grand Master, Robert A. Heinlein, the trait of being read avidly by a large number of adults as well. Like Heinlein's, her protagonists were usually young people, male or female, growing up in a spacefaring environment and conquering it. However, unlike Heinlein—and unlike nearly all of the other Grand Masters—Norton had no particular fondness for technology. Only Ray Bradbury shared with her the distaste for machines that marks Norton's work; when the human race turned to technology, Norton has said, we lost important parts of the living experience.

Perhaps for that reason there had always been strains of heroic fantasy in her science fiction, not unlike C. L. Moore's Jirel of Joiry

stories. From about 1970 on, the fantasy elements in her work won out, and she has written little on science fiction themes since.

Norton found her audience with her first science fiction novel, and it has stayed with her ever since. She left her job as a children's librarian in Cleveland and moved to Florida as a full-time writer. Some years later she relocated to Murfreesboro, Tennessee, and there she started a whole new project, this time not of her own writing. She called it "High Halleck."

Like several of the other Grand Masters, Norton felt that she had been fortunate in her life's calling and determined that it was worthwhile to try to give something back. That something is High Halleck—the complete title is High Halleck Genre Writers' Research and Reference Library—Norton's gift to the world of genre writers of all kinds.

Physically, High Halleck is in a large building adjacent to Norton's home in Murfreesboro, filled with reference books of all kinds. Norton's own work reflects the product of a good deal of careful research, and she has contributed to High Halleck the ten-thousand-volume reference library she herself accumulated over the years, along with early works of science fiction contributed by Forrest J. Ackerman; the late Robert Adams's collection of military materials, contributed by his widow; a "quite complete" (as Norton herself describes it) collection of early Gothic novels; along with Wiccan materials provided by an eighth-generation Welsh follower of the Wiccan beliefs . . . and, among much else, a pair of certified authentic witches' broomsticks. One major display is an outstanding assortment of fantasy art, but actually there is another interesting display outside the walls of the library. That is the city of Murfreesboro itself, of which the center section has been restored to what it was in the antebellum year of 1860.

"High Halleck," Norton writes, "is the product of many years of work and hoping." Because many of the materials are rare and sometimes quite fragile they can be consulted only on the premises themselves. But to use the materials, Norton says, any writer in any genre field "has merely to write and ask." (The address is High Halleck, 114 Eventide Drive, Murfreesboro TN 37130.)

Recommended Reading
by Andre Norton

Star Gate
The Beast Master
Secret of the Lost Race
Witch World
The Many Worlds of Andre Norton

MOUSETRAP

R emember that old adage about the man who built a better mousetrap and then could hardly cope with the business which beat a state highway to his door? I saw that happen once—on Mars.

Sam Levatts was politely introduced—for local color—by the tourist guides as a "desert spider." "Drunken bum" would have been the more exact term. He prospected over and through the dry lands out of Terraport and brought in Star Stones, Gormel ore, and like knickknacks to keep him sodden and mostly content. In his highly scented stupors he dreamed dreams and saw visions. At least his muttered description of the "lovely lady" was taken to be a vision, since there are no ladies in the Terraport dives he frequented and the females met there are far from lovely.

But Sam continued a peaceful dreamer until he met Len Collins and Operation Mousetrap began.

Every dumb tourist who steps into a scenic sandmobile at Terraport has heard of the "sand monsters." Those which still remain intact are now all the property of the tourist bureaus. And, brother, they're guarded as if they were a part of that cache of Martian royal jewels Black Spragg stumbled on twenty years ago. Because the monsters, which can withstand the dust storms, the extremes of desert cold and heat, crumble away if so much as a human fingertip is poked into their ribs.

Nowadays you are allowed to get within about twenty feet of the "Spider Man" or the "Armed Frog" and that's all. Try to edge a little closer and you'll get a shock that'll lay you flat on your back with your toes pointing Earthwards.

And, ever since the first monster went drifting off as a puff of dust under someone's hands, the museums back home have been adding to the cash award waiting for the fellow who can cement them for transportation. By the time Len Collins met Sam that award could be quoted in stellar figures.

Of course, all the bright boys in the glue, spray, and plastic business had been taking a crack at the problem for years. The frustrating answer being that when they stepped out of the rocket over here, all steamed up about the stickability of their new product, they had nothing to prove it on. Not one of the known monsters was available for testing purposes. Every one is insured, guarded, and under the personal protection of the Space Marines.

But Len Collins had no intention of trying to reach one of these treasures. Instead he drifted into Sam's favorite lapping ground and set them up for Levatts—three times in succession. At the end of half an hour Sam thought he had discovered the buddy of his heart. And on the fifth round he spilled his wild tale about the lovely lady who lived in the shelter of two red rocks—far away—a vague wave of the hand suggesting the general direction.

Len straightway became a lover of beauty panting to behold this supreme treat. And he stuck to Sam that night closer than a Moonman to his oxy-supply. The next morning they both disappeared from Terraport in a private sandmobile hired by Len.

Two weeks later Collins slunk into town again and booked passage back to New York. He clung to the port hotel, never sticking his head out of the door until it was time to scuttle to the rocket.

Sam showed up in the Flame Bird four nights later. He had a nasty sand burn down his jaw and he could hardly keep his feet for lack of sleep. He was also—for the first time in Martian history—cold and deadly sober. And he sat there all evening drinking nothing stronger than Sparkling Canal Water. Thereby shocking some kindred souls half out of their wits.

What TV guy doesn't smell a story in a quick change like that?

I'd been running the dives every night for a week—trying to pick up some local color for our six o'clock casting. And the most exciting and promising thing I had come across so far was Sam's sudden change of beverage. Strictly off the record—we cater to the family and tourist public mostly—I started to do a little picking and prying. Sam answered most of my feelers with grunts.

Then I hit pay dirt with the casual mention that the Three Planets Travel crowd had picked up another shocked cement dealer near their pet monster, "The Ant King." Sam rolled a mouthful of the Sparkling Water around his tongue, swallowed with a face to frighten all monsters, and asked a question of his own.

"Where do these here science guys think all the monsters come from?"

I shrugged. "No explanation that holds water. They can't examine them closely without destroying them. That's one reason for the big award awaiting any guy who can glue them together so they'll stand handling."

Sam pulled something from under the pocket flap of his spacealls. It was a picture, snapped in none too good a light, but clear enough.

Two large rocks curved toward each other to form an almost perfect archway and in the their protection stood a woman. At least her slender body had the distinctly graceful curves we have come to associate with the stronger half of the race. But she also had wings, outspread in a grand sweep as if she stood on tiptoe almost ready to take off. There were only the hints of features— that gave away the secret of what she really was—because none of the sand monsters ever showed clear features.

"Where—?" I began.

Sam spat. "Nowhere now." He was grim, and his features had tightened up. He looked about ten years younger and a darn sight tougher.

"I found her two years ago. And I kept going back just to look at her. She wasn't a monster like the rest of 'em. She was perfect. Then that—" Sam lapsed into some of the finest space-searing language I have ever been privileged to hear—"that Collins got me drunk enough to show him where she was. He knocked me out, sprayed her with his goo, and tried to load her into the back of the

'mobile. It didn't work. She held together for about five minutes and then—" He snapped his fingers. "Dust just like 'em all!"

I found myself studying the picture for a second time. And I was beginning to wish I had Collins alone for about three minutes or so. Most of the sand images I had seen I could cheerfully do without—they were all nightmare material. But, as Sam had pointed out, this was no monster. And it was the only one of its type I had ever seen or heard about. Maybe there might just be another somewhere—the desert dry lands haven't been one quarter explored.

Sam nodded as if he had caught that thought of mine right out of the smoky air.

"Won't do any harm to look. I've noticed one thing about all of the monsters—they are found only near the rocks. Red rocks like these," he tapped the snapshot, "that have a sort of blue-green moss growin' on 'em." His eyes focused on the wall but I had an idea that he was seeing beyond it, beyond all the sand barrier walls in Terraport, out into the dry lands. And I guessed that he wasn't telling all he knew—or suspected.

I couldn't forget that picture. The next night I was back at the Flame Bird. But Sam didn't show. Instead rumor had it that he had loaded up with about two months' supplies and had gone back to the desert. And that was the last I heard of him for weeks. Only, his winged woman had crept into my dreams and I hated Collins. The picture was something—but I would have given a month's credits—interstellar at that—to have seen the original.

During the next year Sam made three long trips out, keeping quiet about his discoveries, if any. He stopped drinking and he was doing better financially. Actually brought in two green Star Stones, the sale of which covered most of his expenses for the year. And he continued to take an interest in the monsters and the eternal quest for the fixative. Two of the rocket pilots told me that he was sending to Earth regularly for everything published on the subject.

Gossip had already labeled him "sand happy." I almost believed that after I met him going out of town one dawn. He was in his prospector's crawler and strapped up in plain sight on top of his water tanks was one of the damnedest contraptions I'd ever seen—a great big wire cage!

I did a double take at the thing when he slowed down to say good-by. He saw my bug-eyes and answered their protrusion with a grin, a wicked one.

"Gonna bring me back a sand mouse, fella. A smart man can learn a lot from just watchin' a sand mouse, he sure can!"

Martian sand mice may live in the sand—popularly they're supposed to eat and drink the stuff, too—but they are nowhere near like their Terran namesakes. And nobody with any brains meddles with a sand mouse. I almost dismissed Sam as hopeless then and there and wondered what form the final crack-up would take. But when he came back into town a couple of weeks later—minus the cage—he was still grinning. If Sam had held any grudge against me, I wouldn't have cared for that grin—not one bit!

Then Len Collins came back. And he started in right away at his old tricks—hanging around the dives listening to prospectors' talk. Sam had stayed in town and I caught up with them both at the Flame Bird, as thick as thieves over one table, Sam lapping up imported rye as if it were Canal Water and Len giving him cat-at-the-mouse-hole attention.

To my surprise Sam hailed me and pulled out a third stool at the table, insisting that I join them—much to Collins' annoyance. But I'm thick-skinned when I think I'm on the track of a story and I stuck. Stuck to hear Sam spill his big secret. He had discovered a new monster, one which so far surpassed the winged woman that they couldn't be compared. And Collins sat there licking his chops and almost drooling. I tried to shut Sam up—but I might as well have tried to can a dust storm. And in the end he insisted that I come along on their expedition to view this fabulous wonder. Well, I did.

We took a wind plane instead of a sandmobile. Collins was evidently in the chips and wanted speed. Sam piloted us. I noticed then, if Collins didn't, that Sam was a lot less drunk than he had been when he spilled his guts in the Flame Bird. And, noting that, I relaxed some—feeling a bit happier about the whole affair.

The red rocks we were hunting stood out like fangs—a whole row of them—rather nasty looking. From the air there was no sign of any image, but then those were mostly found in the shadow of

such rocks and might not be visible from above. Sam landed the plane and we slipped and slid through the shin-deep sand.

Sam was skidding around more than was necessary and he was muttering. Once he sang—in a rather true baritone—just playing the souse again. However, we followed along without question.

Collins dragged with him a small tank which had a hose attachment. And he was so eager that he fairly crowded on Sam's heels all the way. When at last Sam stopped short he slid right into him. But Sam apparently didn't even notice the bump. He was pointing ahead and grinning fatuously.

I looked along the line indicated by his finger, eager to see another winged woman or something as good. But there was nothing even faintly resembling a monster—unless you could count a lump of greenish stuff puffed up out of the sand a foot or so.

"Well, where is it?" Collins had fallen to one knee and had to put down his spray gun while he got up.

"Right there." Sam was still pointing to that greenish lump.

Collins' face had been wind-burned to a tomato red but now it darkened to a dusky purple as he stared at that repulsive hump.

"You fool!" Only he didn't say "fool." He lurched forward and kicked that lump, kicked it good and hard.

At the same time Sam threw himself flat on the ground and, having planted one of his oversize paws between my shoulders, took me with him. I bit into a mouthful of grit and sand and struggled wildly. But Sam's hand held me pinned tightly to the earth—as if I were a laboratory bug on a slide.

There was a sort of muffled exclamation, followed by an odd choking sound, from over by the rocks. But, in spite of my squirming, Sam continued to keep me more or less blindfolded. When he at last released me I was burning mad and came up with my fists ready. Only Sam wasn't there to land on. He was standing over by the rocks, his hands on his hips, surveying something with an open and proud satisfaction.

Because now there *was* a monster in evidence, a featureless anthropoidic figure of reddish stuff. Not as horrible as some I'd seen, but strange enough.

"Now—let's see if his goo does work this time!"

Sam took up the can briskly, pointed the hose tip at the monster, and let fly with a thin stream of pale bluish vapor, washing it all over that half-crouched thing.

"But—" I was still spitting sand between my teeth and only beginning to realize what must have happened. "Is that—that thing—"

"Collins? Yeah. He shouldn't have shown his temper that way. He kicked just once too often. That's what he did to her when she started to crumple, so I counted on him doing it again. Only, disturb one of those puff balls and get the stuff that's inside them on you and—presto—a monster! I got on to it when I was being chased by a sand mouse a couple of months back. The bugger got too close to one of those things—thinking more about dinner than danger, I guess—and whamoo! Hunted me up another mouse and another puff ball—just to be on the safe side. Same thing again. So—here we are! Say, Jim, I think this is going to work!" He had drawn one finger along the monster's outstretched arm and nothing happened. It still stood solid.

"Then all those monsters must once have been alive!" I shivered a little, remembering a few of them.

Sam nodded. "Maybe they weren't all natives of Mars—too many different kinds have been found. Terra was probably not the first to land a rocket here. Certainly the antmen and that big frog never lived together. Some day I'm going to get me a stellar ship and go out to look for the world my lady came from. This thin air could never have supported her wings.

"Now, Jim, if you'll just give me a hand, we'll get this work of art back to Terraport. How many million credits are the science guys offering if one is brought back in one piece?"

He was so businesslike about it that I simply did as he asked. And he collected from the scientists all right—collected enough to buy his stellar ship. He's out there now, prospecting along the Milky Way, hunting his winged lady. And the unique monster is in the Interplanetary Museum to be gaped at by all the tourists. Me—I avoid red rocks, green puff balls, and never, never kick at objects of my displeasure—it's healthier that way.

WERE-WRATH

Krobie meat! Krobie meat!

She who had once been the Lady Thra, and was now a brown bone of a woman as worn as one of the carrion birds she snarled at in a harsh whisper, dug her fist into the muck at the foot of the first forest tree. A sharp stone cut into her palm. She welcomed that pain as she made herself watch the scene in the valley below where a man kicked his way into death's peace.

Rinard, shy, slow spoken, hard of muscle if slightly dull of wit, was one of that fighting tail who had broken out of Lanfort at its taking, riding and fighting at her back. Now he, the last of them all, was gone at the hands of these haughty, cruel northerners who would have no more refugees to threaten their own private raids and wars. She was alone.

A black running hound on a blood-red banner—she would remember that. Oh, aye, she would hold that in mind and some day—her hand closed into a tight lock upon the stone, taking the hurt of it to seal the vow she made—though it was a vow she might have little chance to keep.

The forest was her only chance. They had cut her off from the open lands. It was both dark and thick and there were storm clouds gathering. She rose, settling her sword belt more easily, and shrugged the weight of her pack straight.

There were rumors that some made a living in this place of grim dark trees. But it was evil-mouthed by most. Still, she had seen greater evils caused by men with blood reek and fire, and the dusk ahead seemed to promise shelter.

Men were alien to this forest, that she had also heard. Well enough. In her heart she felt alien to her own kind; no beast could present a greater threat.

Her face was sharp featured beneath the shadow of a cap over-sewn with metal rings, and she had long forgot the luxury of clean linen. Her present world was a harsh one. But there was a path opening before her, a narrow slot marked here and there by paw or hoof, but with no trace of boot track.

The silence here brought odd thoughts to mind. This was a place in which to hide, aye, but one with a secret life of its own, so that now and then Thra glanced over a shoulder seeking something that she felt lurked and watched. Her uneasiness grew the stronger with every step she took as she listened keenly for sounds of pursuit.

Now the trail widened and, in spite of the clouds and the gloom beneath the trees, more light showed ahead. She came out into a glade where two of the giant trees had crashed and now lay together; the tangled mass of branches of the one twined beyond any freeing with the upturned roots of the other.

Backed against this root-branch maze was a hut rough and yet sturdy, part of it walled with stone, and its roof seeming strong enough for a storm shelter.

To her right a basin had been formed of the same stone and into that poured a gurgle of water, welcome to her dry throat and dusty body.

Screened by bushes, Thra studied the scene before her. There was a crude chimney on the cabin, but neither scent nor sign of smoke. Two dark slits, hardly wider than her own hand, flanked the bark-covered door—she sensed no life here.

A large butterfly spiraled down, its brilliant golden wings banded with sable. Suddenly out of a tangle of small plants sprang a gray beast, but its leap was not quick enough. Not until it landed, baffled of its prey, was Thra able to identify it as a cat.

The beast settled on the fallen trunk of the nearest tree and

elevated a hind leg to wash with the meticulous care of one uninterested in butterflies. Thra took an impulsive step into the open.
The cat looked well fed; its presence here argued habitation. Pausing in its washing the cat eyed her speculatively. Into Thra's
mind—

"Two-legs—a new two-legs—" There was critical appraisal in
that.

Nor was she completely startled by such an invasion. Since she
had entered the forest anything seemed possible. This place had its
own life. But—she wet her lips with the tip of her tongue—the
thought of addressing this furred creature as she might one of her
own kind was difficult to accept.

The cat looked from her to the cabin and back again before
she ventured hoarsely:

"Someone lives here?" To her own ears her voice was too loud.

"The den is empty—now."

Thra drew a deep breath. To be answered so! She advanced to
the side of the basin, went down on one knee, her right hand still
near her sword hilt, as she cupped water into the other, half lapped
at its freshness.

The cat continued to watch as she pulled forth her water bag,
dumped what remained of its murky contents and filled it anew.
Having made sure of that future supply, Thra settled herself cross-
legged to face the cat. There was a slumbrous content in this clearing which subtly eased both her mind and her body. She was aware
of herb scents borne by the rising wind and yawned—to catch
herself sharply.

Sorcery wooing her? She had fled too long from danger to trust
anything or anyone. Pulling to her feet, she went towards the cabin
still keeping eye on the cat.

Its gray body made no hostile move, the ears were not laid back
against the skull, no warning hiss sounded. Thra set hand to the
door on which no latch string dangled out in welcome. But, at the
pressure of her fingers it swung inward, moving easily.

In spite of the storm clouds the light of the clearing reached
now within, spreading before her like a carpet. A single room. To
her right was the rough fireplace. Boards formed a bunk place. Over
that was a shelf. There was also a box or coffer, a section of log

hollowed out. More shelves supported an array of mugs and bowls, some of wood, others lopsidedly made of fire-burned clay.

Yet there was another piece of furniture in the room and it was enough to center full attention. All the rest was ill made, without true craft, but this armoire might have come from a high lord's castle. Fashioned of reddish wood, it was carved with the skill of a master artist, following no general pattern, rather having a story deep chiseled in the wood. The carving hid the opening of the door, for she could discern neither crack nor hinge.

Twists of leaf garlands formed frames for squares, each of which embodied an intricate scene. Some of the tiny people so depicted were no taller than her fingernail. Here rode a company of men with hounds in the full cry of a hunt. While that which fled before them—

Thra stooped closer. Even in the cabin's gloom the carven pictures were visible. That which fled hunched its shoulder; the head did not seem altogether human in outline.

She shivered. There were old tales a-plenty in Greer. Men and women—in ancient days they were said to have shared lordship with . . . others. That which fled here, which was partly like unto herself—was also something else. Thra turned quickly to the next picture.

The squares *were* allied. Here that which ran had dropped to all fours, upper limbs had become shaggy, the hands were paws.

What of the upper panels? Thra straightened to look. There was one of a forest glade containing a pool beside which lounged a youth bare of body. He dabbled one hand, leaning over to gaze into the water's mirror. So skillful had been the craftsman who had wrought this that Thra never doubted he had taken for his model a living likeness. The scene was one of peace and content.

However, in the next square the head of the lounger was up as if startled, listening. In the next—the beginning of the hunt. Thra saw so well pictured the baying of hounds she could almost hear their cries—

"Found! Found! And away—!"

So the boy from the pool changed. Still, oddly, as Thra followed the pictured story from one square to the next, she found

nothing threatening or wrong in the alteration. Rather her sympathy was all for the pursued. He was the hunted—even as she had
been. She found herself scratching with a fingernail at the foremost
hound as if to claw it away.

Now she squatted on her heels the better to see the finish,
unaware that her heart was beating faster, her breath coming raggedly, as if she too ran that course.

A sharp hiss jerked her attention from the last scene to the
open door. The cat stood just within, staring in turn at the armoire.
Thra looked back to the cupboard. In the last square the runner
had thrown up a desperate forepaw to hook claws about a loop of
low hanging vine.

"Two legs," Thra spoke aloud, using the cat's designation, "or
four legs?"

"Both—neither—"

The answer was instant but one she could not understand. The
cat still watched the armoire.

"Both, yet neither?" Thra shifted to view the right hand side
of the armoire. Only there was no continuation of the hunt such
as she had expected to find.

Rather she looked at a small, deeply incised scene of a room,
as if she were a giantess spying through a window. Here was no
hunt, not even a peaceful lounger.

Instead, stretched on a bed was a woman, attendants gathered
about her. A maid fed wood to a fire on the hearth over which
hung a kettle. Such was the detail of the scene Thra could near
hear the bubbling of the water. What she saw was a bold representation of a birthing.

Quickly she sought the next square. Here the babe had safely
arrived, held up for the mother to view. Only there were expressions of aversion, horror, on the faces of all those gathered there,
even upon that of the mother.

A child so greeted—why? Thra hurriedly went to the next
square. A man was now present, by his ornamental robe one of
high degree. His face was stern set, and, plainly by his orders, one
of the nurses was placing the blanket-wrapped baby in a rush basket.

The fourth scene—another man, a huntsman by his clothing

and gear, was mounted on one of those ponies used for transport of game. This rider stooped to take the basket from the nurse, while the stern-faced man watched.

Now a forest—which suggested by the skill of the carver just such a one as held Thra now—dark and secret. Here was the hunter, leaning sidewise once more in his saddle to drop the basket into a stand of rank growth.

So far the story was plain enough. She had heard, even in the south where life had once been easier, old grim tales. Men did not slay those of their own blood, but a newborn babe conveniently left in a wild place—gone before being presented to the Kin—Yes, that might well have been done. She returned to that earlier scene—horror—truly that had been also in the mother's face. This babe must have been recognized at once as something monstrous.

Left abandoned, then what? Thra traced with her finger the vine wreathing the hunter at his cruel task. Some fault in the wood had here produced a streak of darker hue, and the artist had taken advantage of it to add to the somberness of the picture.

Then—next—from a bush showed a face, or was it a beast's eager muzzle?

Man or animal, or both together? Next, that lurker had come into the open and the mixture was plain. A furred, animal-like head with pricked and large pointed ears, supported on human shoulders giving away to a woman's full breasts.

She who advanced out of hiding appeared more human in the next scene, where she had gathered the babe to her so that a small eager mouth found one of her nipples. There was peace, joy, on the animal woman's near-human face.

In other scenes the baby grew with its foster mother, played, lived seemingly happy and content. Until in the last scene of all, a boy, at that age between youth and manhood, stood staring at a huddled body on the ground, a body from which stood a cruel arrow.

Thus he had been deprived of a mother and then—on the fore of the armoire—himself hunted. Thra was not aware that her jaw had set grimly nor that her hand had gone to sword hilt again. What of the panels on the other side? She hurried to look.

Here were the wreathing vines again, dividing the familiar

squares, but all of those were blank! Except for the very first one, where there were only scratches, perhaps marking out a general sketch of a scene yet to be completed. She squinted closely at those, feeling cheated of the rest of the tale. So much so that she thudded her fist home on the meaningless marks.

As flesh met wood there sounded a sharp sound and the well-concealed door of the armoire began to swing open, folding back.

Light! At first, bemused, Thra thought there must be a torch inside. Then she saw that the radiance issued from wooden walls which had been highly polished. To her nostrils came a clean scent such as she had once known to be used in the laying up of fine clothing.

The color of the inner wood was a clear ivory. There was no hint of mustiness or dust. Nor, on investigation, could she see any hinge or latch.

However, it was what hung within which caught her full attention. Two pegs set at her own shoulder height were there, one on either side. From one depended a sword. The hilt was plain of any gem setting, seemingly made of the same ivory which lined the cabinet. Its pommel was wrought into the head of a beast . . . such as was neither man nor animal. A plain scabbard shielded the blade, and the belt was of white leather studded with small yellow gems.

Against the opposite wall was looped a second belt. This was of sleek black fur, thick and plush, so shiny it might still be a part of the coat of some well-kept cleanly beast. It was near four fingers wide and, though it supported no weapon, there was a large clasp for its fastening made to match the head of the sword pommel. Save that this human-animal countenance was snarling, its open mouth revealing curved tusks ready to rend and tear.

Though the metal of the buckle was dark, other colors played across its surface: red, orange, like flames, icy blue, the gold of the sky at sunset.

Thra put out her hand, then snatched it back, for as her fingers passed within the armoire they tingled and smarted. There was some protection here she could not understand.

Power—the power of a blade which could become awesome when the hilt fitted a hand trained to wield such a weapon. The other—more power she did not understand, from which she shrank.

How long had these hung here waiting? And for whom?

The bare side of the armoire was frustrating. She shivered. It would have been better for her had she never stumbled upon such a mystery, even though the cabin was shelter. Still she was not uneasy enough, as yet, to leave that. There was—

Thra sought the right word—waiting! Aye, that was it! Here hung these waiting—but not for her. Someone else—who?

On impulse she looked to the cat. It no longer lounged at ease. The light from the open door of the cabin had grown less. Was this an early coming of evening or the storm at hand? The animal gazed into the open, the tip of its tail swinging slowly back and forth.

"Four-legs—" she began. Instantly the cat looked to her. "For whom do you wait?"

"Wait?" The cat's head lifted a fraction. "Two legs—four-legs—both pass in their time."

"But you remain?"

"I remain," the shared thought concurred.

There had been no cat picture in all that carving. Still, Thra was sure that the animal before her had some part in the mystery. The cabin looked long deserted—

"Who?" This time her voice sounded unnaturally loud, but not loud enough to drown out a roll of thunder. At least she would remain here until the storm was over. She shucked off her pack.

If she expected any answer to her half-question, she was to be disappointed. The cat withdrew, to face out again into the rain. Thra, used to making the most of any meager comfort, moved swiftly past the crouching animal to pull grass, breaking off small thornless branches to be dumped into the bed place. She would sleep this night in better ease than she had for some time.

There was even a stack of dusty wood lengths by the hearth and these she used for a fire. Honest flames leaping there banished some of the strangeness of the cabin. The roll of thunder grew louder, and there came a crack of lightning so near that the jagged light seemed about to probe inward to her.

Thra pushed the door shut as rain slanted across the floor. The fire provided only a palm-sized light, yet in the dusk the interior of the open armoire gave off a continuous glow.

The cat had not moved. Its head still pointed towards the door. While that feeling that she awaited some portentous happening fed Thra's uneasiness. To steady her thoughts, her shaking hands, she dug the last of her trail rations from her pack. Two journey cakes, now near stone-hard, were there. She hammered a piece from the larger with the pommel of her belt knife. Her other provision was a short stick of hard dried meat that she cut into thin slivers.

One of the clay pots from the shelf gave her a chance to crumble the cake and meat into some water, forming a mess she hoped to find more palatable than it looked. Thra spun out these preparations as long as she could, the cat paying no attention to her actions.

The storm continued to loose its fury. Thra heard a distant sound which must have marked the fall of another of the giant trees. She crowded closer to the fire, holding her sunbrowned hands to the flames, though she shivered more from what she guessed might happen than from any cold.

At last she drew both sword and knife and laid them close to hand, for the cat's doorwise stare added to her disquiet. Also she edged farther around that she, too, might watch that portal. Once she arose and strove to move the armoire itself for a barrier, but its weight was beyond her shifting.

She ate the unappetizing mush with her fingers, finding it no worse than much of the food she had eaten in the immediate past. Putting the bowl to one side she sat waiting, her hands loosely clasped about her knees. Unable to stand her own imaginings any longer she asked aloud:

"Who comes?"

For the first time the cat turned its eyes toward hers. "Long waited, perhaps come at last. Take you that sword, two-legs?" Distinctly it nodded towards the weapon hanging in the armoire.

"I hold by my own steel." She dropped hand to her blade. "What or who comes? Tell me, four-legs!"

The cat had turned its full attention to the armoire.

"There hangs power—"

"Still I hold by what I know!" Thra repeated. To be sitting thus, exchanging thoughts with a cat—had some fell fever fallen on her when she entered this misbegotten woodland, or was she

indeed ensorceled? Patience she had learned in a hard school during the past years and patience only might serve her now, until she discovered more.

That feeling of otherness which had been with her since she had come beneath these trees was growing sharper even though the storm seemed to be retreating. The cat showed no fear—perhaps that curiosity which men said was a strong trait in these beasts kept it here to watch her blunder into some web unknown to her.

Thra might not be forest-wise but she had stood sentry too many nights, every sense alert, to be mistaken now. Something was outside. There came a snuffling, faint but unmistakable, as if the nose of some creature swept close along the bottom crack of the door.

She arose, sword in hand, her dark brows a-scowl as she edged over to set her back to the armoire, ready to front whatever might force its way in. The lips in her gaunt face flattened against her teeth as if she could snarl like her furred companion. Yet the cat itself faced the door with no sign of anger or fear.

That snuffling ceased but, as surely as if she could see through the door, Thra believed the other still crouched there. Like the cat, it waited.

"You speak of power," she said. "Is it of claw and fang now out there?"

"Perhaps." To her astonishment the cat leaped straight for the armoire, brushing past her. Its teeth fastened upon the belt of fur, but all its energy could not pull that free from the peg on which it hung.

Hardly knowing whether she was reckless and foolhardy, or doing what was only right, Thra braved the warning prickle in her hand and reached inside to slip the strip free. It seemed to her that the fur arched upwards to meet her touch as might an animal seek a caress.

The belt fell, still held tight by the cat, and that animal backed away from the cupboard dragging it towards the door. Did it seek to deliver that prize to the lurker? With a stride Thra gained the door, her sword pointed at the cat.

"I do not know what game you would play," she said. "But here I am master—"

"You are but one sent." Words near as sharp as her own blade cut into her mind. "There is but one master!"

She could have easily spitted the animal, or kicked it aside. There was no good reason to let it outside to what waited. Save within her, brute force still did not entirely rule. So she slipped along the wall to be sheltered from the door as it opened, and then pushed, to let in a burst of rain-sweet wind.

From without sounded a strange cry, one which sent a chill along her half-crouched back. Thra wanted badly to see what stood there in the storm-dark but she did not move, only gripped her sword the more fiercely.

As if that sound were a summons, the cat, still trailing the belt from its jaws, sprang into the dark. Thra waited tensely. The light from the fire was small help and the edge of the door a screen.

Someone stepped within. She could strike now and make sure. Even as that thought came to her, the cat flashed once more into the full warmth of the fire, shaking itself vigorously.

Wet leather—her nose wrinkled at that acrid scent—also a strange musky odor as if he who wore such garments had lived unclean for a long time. For this was a man, not topping her in height more than an inch or so. He might be facing the cat and the fire, but Thra was sure he was well aware of just where she stood.

Aware but not alarmed. That realization awoke in her a spark of anger. Woman she might be, and wanderer without a following, but she was still a force to be reckoned with—as he would discover!

His arms hung loosely by his sides, there was no sword, not even the gleam of a knife-hilt at his belt. As her own, his clothing was leather but worse worn. On the shoulders tatters had peeled away, as they had also about his legs and thighs. His feet were bare, splotched with mud which he tracked on the floor.

Around his slender waist was the belt—its length of silky fur in contrast to the rest of him. For his hair was a tangle of greasy strings knotted with dried leaves and small twigs—he might have rooted in a thicket for weeks on end.

Thra fought to bring up her sword, aiming its point between those rack-thin shoulders. She had seen before men sunk to this extremity of neglect—many in the south. They could not be

trusted, nor could one call them beasts, for beasts were far more clean and merciful than such.

Still, though Thra was sure he knew she menaced him, he did not turn his head, but rather dropped to his bony knees before the hearth, raising both palms to the heat. She had a confused memory of how men had once knelt so in places of worship. Did this outcast then worship fire—or only what it signified—shelter, food, warmth—plunder?

That he continued to ignore her meant one of two things— that he was not alone, but the forerunner of a party of like out-casts—or that he possessed some means of defense which did not depend upon weapons.

Those outstretched hands, was there something odd about the nails—were they not unusually long and sharp? Thra wanted him to turn his head so that she might clearly see his features—hu-man—or strange?

The cat settled on the hearth, its back to the fire, tail curled over four paws. Thra could wait no longer; her voice was unnatu-rally loud in the room.

"Who are you?" She was not sure of her question until she had voiced that demand.

He glanced back over his shoulder at last, showing her three-quarters of his face. She had expected to see a tangle of beard as wild as the crop on his head, but his cheeks were smooth as a boy's, though weather-browned to a dark shade. There was an oddity about his features. Perhaps it lay in the slant-wise set of his brows, the narrow forward thrust of his chin. His frowsy hair grew down-ward in a peak between his eyes to nearly meet the brows.

Those eyes—green or yellow—or a mixture of both? Thra had never seen their like in the face of any man of Greer. While his mouth looked too wide, his lips were very dark red and glistening. Small points of teeth showed against those, almost as if he had fangs sprouting from his jaws.

Yet for all its alienness it was not a face to disgust one, nor did it bear the signs of degradation or idiotic mindlessness which she had expected to see. When he spoke his voice was not only low pitched, but calm, even gentle:

"You have my thanks, Lady of Laniat—"

Her sword quivered in her grip. Who in this northern land could still call her by that name? Was he some other refugee? Had she once met him long ago at some feastings? No. Once met this man could never be forgotten.

"There is no more Laniat—" she returned harshly. "But I have asked—who are you?"

His hands moved in a vague gesture she could not understand. "I do not know—"

Some drifter from a lost battle? She had heard of men head-wounded so they could not remember, but were afterwards like newborn children, having to learn again how to live.

"How came you here?"

At least he should be able to answer that, unless his wits were so disordered that even recent events were lost to him.

"I have always been—" His voice trailed away as he continued to regard her with a kind of eager curiosity. In his clear eyes she could detect nothing of a sleeping mind but rather eager intelligence.

Her sword point touched the pounded earth of the floor. In spite of his foul clothing and wild appearance, he had such a quiet air of certainty that he could be wearing a disguise.

His hands had gone now to his belt where he ran fingers back and forth across the sleek fur as one might caress a beloved animal—or reassure himself that a treasure long denied, long lost, had been safely returned.

"Always been?" Doggedly she kept to her point.

He nodded. An errant lock of hair fell across his face and he brushed it aside. Not soon enough. Thra held her breath for an instant. Just so—her eyes flickered to the door of the armoire and away again. No—this was no refugee from her own land. He was— She moved her shoulders along the wall, setting more of a distance between them.

"*What* are you?" Her voice was a whisper. Still, among the wild thoughts now churning in her mind there was no fear—rather wonder. This surely—grown somewhat older—was the youth of the carving—the one who had fled the hunters.

"Why do you ask that?" It was his voice which rang loud and sharp. "When you already know—if you allow yourself to face the

truth." His head inclined the slightest towards the open armoire door.

Thra moistened lips with tongue tip. "I have seen that." She, too, indicated the door. "You are like the hunted one. But—"

He raised hands from his belt, flexed his fingers full in the subdued glow of the fire. Those were claws with wet earth clinging to them, not overlong human nails.

"You have heard of my kind?"

Thra could not answer at once. What were old legends compared with this? Though the forest had such an ill name, her mind refused to connect such tales with this slender young man. Legend suggested that such as he were a dark menace of sorcery, yet in her there was no shrinking. She had met many of her own kind who carried with them a far greater stench of pure evil.

His lips drew back so those fang-sharp teeth showed clearly as he stood there straight and tall, as one facing an enemy about to make an assault on a poorly defended last redoubt.

"I am *were*." He might have been shouting a battle slogan against all the world which she represented.

Silence—so deep that she heard a leaf flutter across the floor inward from the open door. Once more his tongue swept across his lips. He looked almost sly—dangerous. Still within her she felt no menace and she held his gaze locked to hers.

"Do you understand, Lady Thra? Or are our kind not known in the south for the dreaded thrice-damned stock we are? Do you lack cursed forests there?"

Her sword point scratched a half-remembered protective pattern on the well packed earth. But what had such to do with turning aside the possible wrath of one who claimed his blood?

"You put your trust in steel?" Those slanting brows near vanished beneath the fringe of rough hair. "Ah, but steel, no matter how cunningly forged, cannot harm us. Though hounds may chase to pull us down, yet no true arrow nor spear can kill. We can feel pain but not death—save by silver. Silver or," his hands quivered, "fire."

"Still you warm yourself by that," Thra returned. "Is this not your home? Yet you bring your enemy fire into it."

His wide mouth stretched in a wry smile.

"You see me in a guise wherein fire is not master but servant. Ah, Grimclaw," he addressed the cat, "who have you summoned here? A lady who shows no fear, does not tremble nor look upon me as if I differed from those of her own kind, one who walks—"

"Two-legged?" Thra interrupted. "How is it that you greet me by my name, stranger? I am new come into these lands, only this day into your forest." She still held the thought that he might be one who had lost his wits from some battle injury.

"This is my talent—" Even as had the cat before him, he projected his unspoken answer into her mind.

That her thoughts could be so invaded was, to her, a kind of ravishment, such a blow as she had never taken before. She stiffened against showing outwardly her repugnance, but rage rose icily within her.

He no longer even looked in her direction; instead he moved a little closer to the armoire, gazing intently at the sword still hanging there. But if that weapon was his, as the belt seemed to be, he made no attempt to arm himself with it. Perhaps he had run four-legged so long that he clung to fangs and claws as his proper weapons.

"I have to thank you." Though he spoke aloud this time she thought that was a concession on his part. "I have been long afield and there are those to whom I am welcome prey. That you have brought me this much freedom," his fingers once more sought the circlet of fur about him, "is almost more than I had dared hope for. Perhaps there is some meaning in this. We are only the playthings of strange forces. And you chose a poor refuge here. Why, my lady?"

Need he ask, when he could read her mind and she could not shut him out? Thra longed to turn her sword on him—to banish so this—this *thing* who could know her in a way so unnatural. Was her every thought and feeling open to him now?

"I cannot enter where you hate—" His voice was low. "It was when I skulked outside and must know who or what waited here that I did that. We have our own oaths which we do not break!" There was high pride in him, such pride as matched her own and she felt herself responding when she did not want to yield. "Do you wish such an oath from me, lady?"

What did he awaken in her—feelings and beliefs she thought long slain? She shook her head, instead accepting this self-confessed

forest monster as she would one of her own rank in the old days.

"So—what brought you here?" He returned to his first question.

"A beast pack which marches under the banner of a running hound—" She spat forth the words and thumped the point of her sword into the earth. "My freedom was hard bought—the last of my liegemen hangs from a tree in the valley. Your lords hunt to ill deaths."

His eyes glowed flame-bright for an instant.

"A running hound—aye!" Once more his lips shaped a snarl which was feral. "Roth is abroad then or—" he scowled "—since time moves differently here within the wood and years sometimes speed by without noting—one of his get. They live with fear as their armor and their weapons, but lately they have not tried the forest ways. Perhaps now the hounds will course again—on *your* trail, lady!"

He showed no signs of uneasiness but rather spoke eagerly as if he looked forward to some contest.

"It might be so." She did not enlarge upon that, wondering if she would also be considered prey by some of the forest dwellers.

"This is a place of fear," he continued. "My brethren lair here, and yet even we do not know all the dark dangers which pad the trails." He weighed her with a bold and fierce gaze but she was not to be eyed down so. Instead she returned her sword to its sheath, showing him hands as bare as his own.

"Devils and dangers I have seen a-many and the worst of them are two-legged and name themselves men." She laughed harshly. "You have made free with my name; how then are you called?"

"I am Farne—and there is another name, only that your throat cannot voice. Grimclaw here is my marshal, the holder of my castle. I have not recently been resident in this part of my domain. Lady Thra, I offer you guest right."

He stooped to catch the lower end of one of the smaller branches half-consumed by the fire, holding it aloft so that flame sprouted from its tip as it might from a wax taper.

"I light you to your chamber," he began formally and then laughed. "I fear you shall have to take us as we are, which is in ill condition. But at least—" Still holding his improvised taper he

passed her to the door, to return a moment later swinging a brace of wood fowl by their feet.

"Even Roth might relish these—"

"Roth?" That was the second time he had mentioned that name. "His badge is the running hound? Roth of—" She waited.

"Farne." He had settled on his heels before the fire, drawing from a break between stones a knife with which he set about cleaning the fowl. "What is a name? It can be given to a thing, a place, a woman, a man. Those with the old knowledge claim that a name has power—that it can be used for or against that which bears it. But who truly knows?"

There was so much more she wanted to learn. What of the tale carved on the armoire of the babe abandoned in the wilds, the youth later hunted. Was it his story which was thus portrayed?

"The sword—" She pointed to that which hung in the cupboard. "Is that also of Farne?"

His head turned so suddenly she blinked and dropped hand to knife-hilt. Then he voiced a throaty sound like a growl, while the cat hissed. "What have you heard of Farne?"

"Nothing save your own words," she replied. "I saw the raiders at their work and lost a good friend to them. But yonder does hang a sword and its pommel is a head which is strange. While on two sides of that armoire is carven a tale clearly enough. Therefore I ask—does that blade fit your hand?"

"My heritage? Perhaps, lady, when the time is right. For now I wear that which is closer to me." He touched the furred belt. "That," he nodded to the sword, "has a purpose which will come." He arose from where he had set quarters of the fowls on improvised spits and went to the armoire.

"A purpose into which Farne enters?" Thra prodded him.

His shoulders tensed. She had a momentary feeling that this was all a dream. Then he caught at the door and with a sharp push sent it shut.

"Let it hang! I will not have it yet—perhaps never. There are traps and traps, and those who are hunted learn to sniff them out—or die."

Their meal was sizzling and he divided it fairly, laying it in the

bowls from the shelf. Thra licked fingers scorched by hot grease before she began avidly to chew the meat from the bones.

Night had come fully but Farne made no move to close the door. Also he paused now and then as if to listen. Perhaps his ears were better attuned to the normal forest sounds so he could detect the unusual. Thra heard the squalling cry of some furred hunter that had missed its prey, the hooting of an owl. And always there was the drip of moisture and the rustle of branch.

When he had finished Farne went to that crude tree-trunk box against the far wall, pawing through its contents to select an arm-load of fresh clothing. Saying nothing he went out into the night.

Thra licked her fingers well and fed wood to the fire. She was tired and this was shelter. She looked to that bunk she had filled with bedding. The cat was washing its face, though now and then its ears twitched as it picked up some sound.

There would soon be need for more wood if the fire was to burn through the night, but there was no use seeking that in the soaked outer world. Farne. A part of Thra wondered at her own calm acceptance of him. There were the old tales—she had heard more of them as she and Rinard had prowled closer to the forest.

They had been seeking greater knowledge of this very wood, as well as supplies, when they had been trapped in the raided village. Thra had thought Rinard close on her heels, but the poor fool had stood his ground, apparently believing that he served her so, as she had discovered too late. Rinard—forcibly she put him out of her mind now. Had the raiders sighted her, tracked her later?

"Hunters—" Thra was not even aware she said that aloud until the cat answered her.

"Not yet. But a hunt comes, yes. Those others seek always for *him!*"

"Often?" she pressed.

"Often enough. Until he chooses—" But there were no more mind words added to that. Thra felt that in another place a door had closed—firmly. She would learn no more—at least for now.

Those stories of the werefolk were awesome. And Farne might be only one of many. She shifted uneasily as the were appeared to materialize out of the dark. He was dressed in fresh leather as sleek as the belt he still wore. Twigs and mud had been brushed out of

his hair, the grime washed from his hands and face. He walked with assurance, and, with that same air of authority, he began to question Thra about the raid upon the village.

"It would seem that Roth, or he who holds the Hound rule now, grows overbold," Farne mused when she had done. "To this shelter—" he gestured with one hand, "you are welcome, rough though it is. But I would advise you not to remain here in the forest." He added that decisively and Thra knew resentment. There he stood fingering that belt of his and looking at her as if she were a green girl who had never heard an alarm bell.

"The forest—" He hesitated. "Oh, yes, there are those who *have* sought refuge here but mainly they are the unwary, the ignorant. Tomorrow I shall show you a trail leading westward out of Roth's way, and so see you free of this land. But tonight I have that which I must do." He turned on his heel and, with no other farewell, was gone again into the dark, the cat bounding after him.

Thra crouched in a dusk which was hardly thinned by the light of the dying fire. Her body ached with fatigue, her eyelids were heavy, yet in this place dared she yield to sleep? Tonight there was no Rinard to share the watch turn about.

She fed the last of the wood to the fire and lay down close to the hearth, drawing both sword and knife, to place them where her hand could fall easily. Thra closed her eyes knowing that, trust or no trust, she could not continue without rest.

However, she dreamed, and in that dream she fled, a hunted thing without any defense against the force on her trail. Yet within her rage flared so hot she felt as if her whole body was aflame. There arose before her a dark wall of vines so much interwoven and the terror of the chase flung her full at that. The vines writhed and wreathed, reached, clutched her in an unbreakable grip. She fought and tore at that growth, her hands rent in turn by thorns. Now she was held fast as the din of the hunt drew nearer and she heard a triumphant blast of horn.

Blast of horn! Thra opened her eyes—not upon a mass of imprisoning greenery, though the dream seemed still real for a second or two and her hands were up and out flailing the air. This was a dim and shadowed room—the only light, wan and limited, came through two narrow slits of windows.

As she pulled herself up, her body slick with sweat beneath her worn garments, she heard it clearly—a horn!

Hunters! On her own trail or merely loose in the forest? She dared not remain where she was lest she be trapped, yet to seek a path through the wood without a guide was also a lost cause.

She stumbled as she stooped for her weapons, and her hand, flung out to balance her, slapped the side of the armoire. For the second time the door swung open.

No furred belt—where was that now—and its wearer? But the sword—Her own blade would be the better for a smith's sharpening and it was well worn. Since Farne had chosen not to take this then why could she not arm herself the better?

Thra listened. The horn sounded once again and she could not deceive herself—its blatant blast was closer. She must be out and away. Slamming her own weapon into its sheath and kicking her pack towards the door, she reached for the armoire sword.

Her flesh tingled almost as if flames licked at her. But she had set the weapon swinging back and forth. Only, when she tried to grab for it her hand had no strength, fingers numb, with that numbness spreading up her wrist into her arm. She who had scoffed at tales of sorcery was helpless. Fear pushed her away from the slow swing of that sheathed blade.

A third call of the horn and now it was answered by a clear bay and then a second. Thra shivered. Men she could and had faced when necessity drove her to it, but hounds—with them she would have little chance. She swung around to survey the cabin. One entrance, those narrow slits of windows—it offered defense of a kind save there was no bar for the door and she had nothing to build a barricade. Only to venture out—with hounds ready to trail—

Knife, sword, she had no other weapons, she pushed aside the pack and shut the door. No bolt—it could be easily forced.

Thra fingered her knife. There was a way of escape if it came to a last desperate moment—by her own hand. To wait to be ravished by hound or huntsman, was that a coward's choice? How could she—?

A loud baying followed, with a note in that deep belling which startled her. Eagerness, such cry as a hound might give when its

prey was in sight. Yet that had not come from just without the cabin as she had expected, rather it was farther away—to the west. It was answered by a chorus of other cries trailing away from her. She hardly dared to believe that the hunt had turned. Now her shoulder grazed the armoire.

She stood before the deep carving of the door. The were who had fled—the hunters who followed. Farne's trail, had it this morning crossed hers, setting a counter scent to draw the hounds? She frowned, breathing a little faster as if, though she had not stirred from the cabin, she had indeed run a quarry's hard pace.

Farne—she did not doubt he had been hunted before. This was his country, he would know every rock, tree, shrub of it—be fully aware of any hole giving refuge. Yes, the sound was lessening—the hunt drew westward—she need only wait until she could hear no more and then head east.

Why had he done this? Had it been by chance? Somehow Thra doubted that as she reached for her pack again. By rights he owed her no favors. True, she had, by chance, opened the armoire and the cat had taken the belt—but was that so great a service—?

So far had her thoughts gone, when she was startled by what was no hound's triumphant bay—rather a deep throated howl. Not one of pain—rather anger and—fear!

It was drowned out almost instantly by the frenzied yapping of dogs and the shouts of men. Something—Farne?—was at bay. The shouting grew louder but she could not distinguish words. With bared sword in one hand she pulled open the cabin door.

Across the clearing leaped a flash of gray. The cat was within the hut before she truly saw it. Rearing up on its hind legs it pawed forcibly at the closed door of the armoire. Its ears were flat to its skull and it was snarling steadily. Now it turned its head a fraction as its eyes sought her.

"Trap!" The word sprang into her mind with the force of a blow.

That howl sounded again from the distance. Thra listened. This quarrel was none of hers. Farne, a were, was an enemy to her kind. That he had not harmed her—had offered the gesture of guesting rights—what difference did that make now? One sword against a hound pack and the men who followed it—what could that avail?

"Nothing—" she said aloud, to answer the pressure rising in her mind, what the cat would force upon her. "This is no ploy for me—"

There was no answer in words. Instead, for a moment which might have been lifted out of real time, she saw—not this hut, the furious cat—but rather another scene.

A net which writhed with the wild struggles of what it contained, a beast with a foam-flecked mouth which strove to snap at the cords which so bound it and who flinched from that weaving. Now she could see that it was no true net, rather hide strips interwoven with linked chains which had a silver glint.

Silver!

Memory stirred as that picture broke. What had Farne said— that silver was the bane of his kind.

"That is so!" She saw no prisoner now, rather the cat still reared against the cupboard, its claws busy striving to rip the wood apart.

Guessing the secret of the armoire from her two former experiences, Thra slapped the uncarven side and the door opened. The cat leaped, attempting to pull down the sword. But it could only set that swinging. Thra thrust the point of her own weapon within and caught the loop of the belt, pulling it towards her.

The sheathed blade slid down and the cat crouched before her snarling. Once free of the armoire the weapon appeared to draw light, and the eyes of the head which formed the pommel glinted as might the eyes of a living beast.

Thra let the weapon slide to the floor. She expected the cat to catch it up as it had the belt, but instead the animal stood guard, gazing straight at her.

"What would you have of me?" she demanded.

No reply flashed into her mind, no picture rose in answer. Once more the din of the hunt swelled—almost as if that was her reply.

"Take it if that is what is needed!" she urged.

The cat did not move. Though no words formed in Thra's mind there was a growing compulsion.

"No! Your Farne is no cup brother of mine, nor liegeman. What have I to do with him? One sword cannot stand against a hound pack and huntsmen. I shall not—"

Yet, even as she made that denial, there was rising in her some-

thing which she could not understand. Ensorcelment? She fought in vain but she stooped, utterly against her true will, to take up the sword belt.

The cat arose from its crouch and uttered what was undoubtedly a yowl of promised battle. It held her gaze for a long moment before it headed towards the door.

She turned as if another will possessed her, using her body awkwardly and against every instinct. Thra, her own sword drawn, the belt of the sheathed one in her other hand, followed the cat, at first stumblingly, and then with the even tread of one who goes to face some act of sworn duty.

Grimclaw sped ahead, not taking the faint path which had led her here but rounding one of the fallen trees and heading straight through the brush which filled the small clearing.

The clamor of the hunt had not dwindled. Apparently the hounds and their masters were not on the move. As she went in that direction Thra continued to fight the will—the thing which forced her to serve its purpose. Sweat gathered at the rim of her ring sewn cap, made tracks down her face.

She was one. Before her—how many? If she exhausted her strength in fighting this compulsion what might that cost her later? She abandoned the inner struggle, allowed that which possessed her full rein.

The din of the hounds slacked off but the voices of the men grew clearer. Someone was roaring orders to lower that, fasten this—get on with it.

Grimclaw stopped short to look back at her. Thra dropped to her knees and crawled forward through brush toward another clearing. With all the stealth she had learned during her wandering she covered that ground and used her sword tip to lift a branch of leafy shrub that she might see.

Five men, two of them now occupied with cuffing back the hounds and setting leashes to their collars. He who was doing the roaring stood to one side overlooking the labors of two of his fellows who were awkwardly striving to wind closer a net encompassing a still upright and struggling captive.

Thra recognized with an icy chill of full anger the badges these hunters wore—the running hound. But five of them and four

hounds—against her! She had no crossbow even, nothing except her sword—she could not attack these!

"Leave be!" ordered the roarer at last. He approached the captive to inspect the bonds tying the net to a tree. "The beast is well caught and my lord will want to see the rest of it. Jacon, get you to camp, you and Ruff taking those hounds. M'lord will not favor any who care not for *them*. And we do not know how many of such beasts slink hereabouts—"

" 'Twould be better to haul the were with us—" began one of those who had been busy by the tree.

Bull throat laughed. "It is well caught. M'lord truly had the proper secret for that after all these years. Silver they cannot break. See how it twists itself even now so that bare bits touch it not."

The prisoner so enfolded was writhing constantly, and, between the voices of the hounds being cuffed into order and those of the men, Thra caught desperate panting sounds which could only have come from the captive.

"Silver and—fire." There was brutal satisfaction in that strong voice. Aye, it was by *his* order that Rinard had been hung—with men shouting wagers on how long their captive would kick before death was merciful. Thra would have given all she possessed at that moment for a crossbow—he was so good a target standing there with his thumbs hooked in his belt, a grin stretching lips near hidden by a greasy beard. "There will be a handsome fire, perhaps of m'lord's own lighting—and good ale drunk this night!"

The two men he watched stepped back from their captive. In spite of the seeming helplessness of the netted creature, they appeared to have little liking for being near it. Thra started at a cold touch on her hand and was fearful that she might have so betrayed herself. It was Grimclaw.

"Behind—" The word blazed in her mind.

Behind what? It was hard to believe that those restless hounds had not already scented her or the cat. Away—get away before they too were trapped. Part of her mind seemed to scream that, but to no avail.

"Behind!" The cat's order was emphatic. It crouched upon its belly, one paw advanced gingerly to draw it forward and then the

other. So it angled away from her and the hounds. Also it was plain that she was expected to follow.

Thra hesitated. As she did so the man who had given the orders slouched across to stand by the netted creature. He leaned down to pick up an end of the rope which clearly showed the silver knotted in it. With evil deliberation he thrust this toward the captive, inserting the end through the mesh of the net.

She both heard and felt—the cry rang in her mind worse than a wound, and a searing pain stroked her left cheek, leaving stinging agony behind. What was aimed at the captive had also touched her.

On hands and knees, using all the skulker's skills she had learned, Thra followed the slinking cat. They moved away from the clearing even as the men led out the leashed hounds, but only so for a short distance before the cat made a deliberate turn to the left. "Behind" was plain now, they were heading to the rear of those trees where the net had been anchored. She had to bite down upon her lower lip, call upon full strength not to betray herself as the transferred torture of the captive continued to scorch her own flesh.

Grimclaw halted. There were no more spurts of pain, perhaps the hound master had tired of his game. She could hear a heavy breathing—perhaps from the prisoner.

Longing to be elsewhere Thra was still bound to obey that other will. Not too far away a twist of brown and silver was looped about an upstanding tree root—surely one of the anchors of the net.

With the blade of her own sword between her teeth, Thra reached for her belt knife. The rope was thick and she feared that, even if she could sever that, the metal within would not break. But as the strands parted, the silver did not seem so hard as she had feared—it must be unusually pure and so more workable. She pried and pulled loose an end, twisting that back and forth until it broke.

As the rope end swung free Grimclaw reached up and caught it between ready jaws, stretching it taut while Thra, with all the caution she could summon, started on the next.

"Two more—but two more!" No invasion of her thoughts by Grimclaw, that had come from the captive. Thra did not resent his

message, rather threw open her mind as well as she could for a picture of what must be done.

She followed the rope to her left—there was a second loop to be loosened, then hurriedly knotted about a branch to give the appearance of being untouched. She was sawing at the third when there came a shout in the clearing setting both Thra's hands to tear frenziedly at the bonds.

"Netted, by the Fangs of Rane! Netted as any beast!"

Gloating in that voice—and it was not the bull roar of the hunters' leader. Perhaps this was his lord.

"Were—" The tone of voice made the word an obscenity.

"Kinsman—" That answer was Farne's. She could never have mistaken his voice even though she had already been sure he was the captive.

"Beast—devil begotten—"

"Begotten by your blood, Kinsman—do *you* claim devil's blood?"

Thra laid hand to the last knot of rope and gave a jerk into which she put all the force she could summon. The silver mesh sawed at her fingers cruelly, but she twisted, not caring. As she fought, another voice broke in:

" 'Ware, m'lord. Perhaps there may be more of his breed nearby. On guard you dolts, on guard!"

The cord parted, leaving bleeding gouges in her fingers. She curled hand around sword hilt in spite of the pain. The sword she had dragged with her from the hut lay at her feet. Grimclaw burst from the bushes wild-eyed to stand before her.

"Give me the spell spear!" That was the lord's voice. "And you—stand near the brush on guard against any other devils this one may summon. Give me room for a cast now—"

Thra staggered back as a body swung at her. He who had been hanging in the net was free. And this was not the man who had left her in the hut but a furred, four-footed thing which had no right to run in a sane world.

Without thought Thra aimed a blow at the creature. Its yellow eyes blazed as it skidded to a halt and from the hairy throat came a deep warning growl.

Could it possess her by its will? Thra set her back to the broad

trunk of a tree. Between them lay the sword from the armoire. The yellow eyes shifted from her to that. The beast advanced a paw towards the belt and then drew back as if it, as well as silver, carried some malignant spell.

Then the lord of the hunters thrust through the brush, though he came warily, a spear held at ready. Farne, if indeed it was Farne, showed fangs. But the man's eyes flickered on to Thra. She had but a moment to duck sidewise before that spear thudded between her arm and her side. Instantly she scrambled on, seeking to set the tree between them.

"There be another! This one yet unwitched!"

The bushes in the direction Thra had headed tossed and crackled as someone forced a path through to bring them face to face. Farne moved—was before her again.

She steadied herself against the tree. Better take a spear through her here and now than fall helpless into their hands. She was already damned in their eyes and wanted to die cleanly.

The man now facing her was much younger than the leader of the hunters. Slim and agile, there was that about him which proclaimed some kinship with Farne when the latter walked two-legged. Only the eyes were different. Beneath the edging of a helm his were as blue and cold as winter ice.

He was also armed with a second spear, but now he pounded the butt of that into the forest muck and whipped out a sword of light colored metal. Was that also forged of silver?

He thought to take her alive then, perhaps for a fate like that promised Farne. Would his liegemen help to net her while she fought their lord?

"So this one does not run on all fours. What does such a devil know of skill with steel?"

"M'lord, watch yourself. These creatures deal in foul witchery—" that was the leader of the hunters. "They can make a man see what is not—"

Thra kept silent. If they believed her were, they would indeed be wary of ensorcelment and in their wariness might lie some small chance for her. Not, she knew grimly, that she would be fortunate to live through this encounter, but it was far better to die on steel.

"Watch *you* well!" ordered the lord. "Since this one would use

a blade, so shall I. Mayhap I can thus prove that such are not to be so dreaded as foolish tales would have us believe." He lunged at her with the confidence of one who has yet to meet his match.

Blade rang against blade. Thra saw a shift in those cold eyes. Had he truly thought to bring her down with that simple thrust? Was it ignorant self-confidence past belief, or knowledge that he had won many times before?

Her worn blade shivered with that contact and she feared meeting a second such blow would shatter that too often honed length. That other sword from the armoire, how far away now did it lie? She thought of Grimclaw—could the cat drag it to her? The cat had claimed the weapon from the cupboard yet her own hand had burned when she reached for it. Could one depend upon anything dark with witchery?

Thra fought defensively and kept the tree ever at her back. The point of that other weapon seemed to flicker in her very eyes and there was a sharp pain along her cheek. Where was Farne? She was sure he had been there at the beginning of this duel yet it would seem that the men had not sighted him—No time for that now—this battle was her own.

She fixed the picture of the sword in her mind. If Grimclaw read her thoughts now would he answer her? Then there was a flash of thought which did not seem aimed at her but did come like a third dancing blade to join the battle. Sword—to take the sword—to choose—

It was not her desire, something more powerful even than fear had awakened in her. There was denial, and anger, and yes, a touch of terror. The ancient enemy—the sword—No, rend, tear, take payment for the wrong thus. Fang right, claw right—those were best—always best!

There was no animal cry, but out of the bushes sprang a form which fastened upon one of the watching men. For only a second Thra spared a glance towards that struggle, heard sounds from others in the brush. Payment for that glance came with a blow upon her shoulder, which drove the mail painfully inward, bruising, though it did not cut the rings.

"Thus and thus—" He who fought sent the point again flickering into her face. She countered his stroke and her sword snapped,

leaving but a jagged fragment in her hand. He laughed then and moved in for the kill.

"Thus!" he cried for the third time and that was a sentence of death or so she hoped. Instead his blade cut painfully across her fingers so she dropped her hold on her broken weapon.

"What I promise I do. Do you take this one—" he turned his head a fraction to give that order.

Thra's knife came up toward her own throat. She was ready to press the point home when pain shot through her head and she would have fallen had not the tree supported her.

No pain of body—no—this was a deeper, stronger pain, such as her kind had never been meant to bear. She heard a voice cry aloud in torment and despair against a fate which could not be denied—but the voice was not hers.

Nor did Thra appear to suffer alone. The lord who had bested her staggered, his sword fell from his hand as he put both to his head. His mouth twisted in a wordless scream.

From where the brush had been beaten down by Farne's charge someone rose. He flung up his head, sending his hair back from his face, a face which wavered and changed even as they stared at him. Man not beast now, he leaped forward and in his hand was the other sword clear of its sheath, its blade giving off a reddish glow as if it were a shaft of Hell-fire.

There were cries. Men ran but Thra did not try to move and her knife was still ready in her hand.

The lord half-twisted to face the swordsman. He visibly drew a deep breath and stooped to seize again his own weapon as if he had already regained full control of body and mind. Of his followers only one flaccid body remained on the ground.

"Well met, ill met, Kinsman!" Farne smiled slowly. He stood waiting attack even as she had earlier done.

There was a wild rage in the other's eyes. Thra thought that for this lord of the hounds the whole world had suddenly narrowed to confrontation with this single man-beast.

The glow in Farne's blade spread. His fingers, locked about the hilt, reddened, the flush wreathed about his wrist, reached up his arm. In Thra a fire seemed to burn. She caught her breath and choked down a cry of agony. If this was the cost of using the

weapon to her who only stood aside, what must it be to Farne himself? For she was certain that what she felt was a reflection of what he now had to bear.

Instead he cried aloud on the edge of human rage yet still with an animal note. If the young lord thought that he faced easy meat he was made speedily aware of his mistake, for the fire blade kept play in a way which Thra with all her knowledge of weapons marveled to see.

Only for seconds she watched and then she remembered the others. What of the men who had gone with the hounds, the rest? No matter how skillful Farne might be he could not hope to stand against four or more of them. Dropping her sword shard she leaped for the body in the brush.

Red ruin above a torn throat, she looked no higher. But she had her hands on a spear haft. Above the clash of weapons behind her she heard a stifled moan.

There was a second man in the bushes. He half lay, stark faced, a mangled arm across his breast, staring at her wild-eyed as she came to him, his good hand awkwardly fumbling with a short hunting sword. She took that from him easily, wrenching it free, for her own arming.

While he spat meaningless words at her she staggered back, still afire, straight into the path of another running to the fight.

"Die, devil!"

She was still not at ready and he was about to cut her down when he shrieked aloud and threw up his hands, the wounded man echoing his cry. This pain in her head—she could hardly see. However on hands and knees Thra scrambled away as a heavy body crashed down. To make certain of his helplessness she brought the heavy pommel of the sword against the nape of his neck as his helm loosened and rolled away.

For a moment she simply crouched, sobbing for breath, hardly daring to believe she yet lived. The pain was now no longer a torment, rather a steady fire which strengthened her in a way she could not understand.

Out of a tangle of tall grass came Grimclaw. As he passed the legs of the man before her a paw aimed a quick blow, claws out.

Thra used the spear to aid her to her feet where those other two still fought with skill and desperation. Thrusting the hunting sword close to hand in the ground she stood with the spear at ready, to hold the lists. Grimclaw stationed himself beside her.

Mastery of steel—Thra knew that she watched two evenly matched fighting men of top skill. And they could almost have been brothers from one birthing. That strange cast of Farne's features had faded away. He was smiling slightly, yellow eyes alight—only the color differing from those of his enemy.

The blaze from his blade now formed a nebulous glow about his whole body, through which the sword moved like a darting tongue. Were they so evenly matched that they might fight forever without giving way? Thra could detect no sign of fatigue, no lightening of the clang of weapons.

She had no more than thought that when the flame wreathed blade appeared to turn of itself in Farne's hand. The weapon might command the man, not the man the weapon. There was a hard clang of sound and the lord's sword spun out of his grip to strike against the trunk of the tree where Thra had sheltered. He stood bare-handed, with no change of expression, as if he now awaited stoically that thrust at throat or breast which would put an end to him.

As the fire blade turned point down Farne caught and held those other chill eyes.

"Blood calls to blood," he said slowly.

The other's mouth contorted. He spat and the spittle flecked the trampled leaves by Farne's boots.

"Beast calls not to true man!" He flung up his head in harsh pride. "Kill if you will but think not that aught between us can ever be altered—runner in the night."

Farne swung the sword, not towards the other but as if he weighed something in his hand and that weight dragged heavy upon him. He shook his head.

"I run no more," he said slowly. "The choice has been forced upon me at last. I may well have lost more than I gain—"

"I do not understand you," broke in the other impatiently. "Kill me—you win nothing, beast—"

Farne, to Thra's surprise, nodded. "Nothing," he agreed. "Did you think I challenged your rulership with this?" Again he waved the sword.

That light which had blazed along it was gone. But the strangeness did not return to his face. Now he stepped back and away from the other.

"This much is true. You live, kinsman, by my leave."

The other scowled and took a step forward as if he wished to drag Farne down by strength alone.

"Also," once more the forest man shifted his grip on the sword, "I have at last come into my inheritance. No, kinsman, do not fear that you shall be dispossessed of your lands, your ill-ruled people— not yet. But the 'beast' you have been pleased to hunt is gone. Try your tricks again at your will, they shall net you naught. Take up your liegemen and get you gone. This forest has an ill name among your kind, that was not lightly earned nor shall it be forgotten."

Deliberately he sheathed the sword and held its belt in one hand. The other he put to the wide buckle of the furred belt.

As Farne's fingers touched that buckle it burst open. The metal over which the strange colors had played flaked away. Fur loosened from scaling hide and shifted through the air, the hide itself slipped and fell from about his body, to lie in bits upon the ground. Then he fastened the sword belt in its place.

The lord watched through narrowed eyes.

"You have given me quarter—I asked it not, nor shall I accept it!" His voice was harsh challenge.

"Accept or not as you wish." Farne shrugged. "You stand on land which I know and which knows me. I have made my choices—yours shall be yours only, and you will answer for them."

He turned his head to look to Thra. What he had just said, she thought, was meant in its latter part as much for her as for the lord.

She swallowed. Life was always choices and somehow she knew she faced a mighty one now. As she settled the sword she had taken into the empty scabbard at her belt she saw on the ground a wisp of dirty fur.

Two belts and a man, there was a meaning she could guess at. But in this forest one need not be surprised at anything. She made her choice.

As Farne moved forward she fell in at his right hand, Grimclaw padding into the shadow of the great trees at his left.

ALL CATS ARE GRAY

Steena of the Spaceways—that sounds just like a corny title for one of the Stellar-Vedo spreads. I ought to know; I've tried my hand at writing enough of them. Only this Steena was no glamorous babe. She was as colorless as a lunar planet—even the hair netted down to her skull had a sort of grayish cast, and I never saw her but once draped in anything but a shapeless and baggy gray spaceall.

Steena was strictly background stuff, and that is where she mostly spent her free hours—in the smelly, smoky, background corners of any stellar-port dive frequented by free spacers. If you really looked for her you could spot her—just sitting there listening to the talk—listening and remembering. She didn't open her own mouth often. But when she did, spacers had learned to listen. And the lucky few who heard her rare spoken words—these will never forget Steena.

She drifted from port to port. Being an expert operator on the big calculators, she found jobs wherever she cared to stay for a time. And she came to be something like the masterminded machines she tended—smooth, gray, without much personality of their own.

But it was Steena who told Bub Nelson about the Jovan moon rites—and her warning saved Bub's life six months later. It was Steena who identified the piece of stone Keene Clark was passing around a table one night, rightly calling it unworked Slitite. That

started a rush which made ten fortunes overnight for men who were down to their last jets. And, last of all, she cracked the case of the *Empress of Mars*.

All the boys who had profited by her queer store of knowledge and her photographic memory tried at one time or another to balance the scales. But she wouldn't take so much as a cup of canal water at their expense, let alone the credits they tried to push on her. Bub Nelson was the only one who got around her refusal. It was he who brought her Bat.

About a year after the Jovan affair, he walked into the Free Fall one night and dumped Bat down on her table. Bat looked at Steena and growled. She looked calmly back at him and nodded once. From then on they traveled together—the thin gray woman and the big gray tomcat. Bat learned to know the inside of more stellar bars than even most spacers visit in their lifetimes. He developed a liking for Vernal juice, drank it neat and quick, right out of the glass. And he was always at home on any table where Steena elected to drop him.

This is really the story of Steena, Bat, Cliff Moran, and the *Empress of Mars*, a story which is already a legend of the spaceways. And it's a damn good story, too. I ought to know, having framed the first version of it myself.

For I was there, right in the Rigel Royal, when it all began on the night that Cliff Moran blew in, looking lower than an antman's belly and twice as nasty. He'd had a spell of luck foul enough to twist a man into a slug snake, and we all knew that there was an attachment out for his ship. Cliff had fought his way up from the back courts of Venaport. Lose his ship and he'd slip back there— to rot. He was at the snarling stage that night when he picked out a table for himself and set out to drink away his troubles.

However, just as the first bottle arrived, so did a visitor. Steena came out of her corner, Bat curled around her shoulders stolewise, his favorite mode of travel. She crossed over and dropped down, without invitation, at Cliff's side. That shook him out of his sulks. Because Steena never chose company when she could be alone. If one of the man-stones on Ganymede had come stumping in, it wouldn't have made more of us look out of the corners of our eyes.

She stretched out one long-fingered hand, set aside the bottle

he had ordered, and said only one thing. "It's about time for the *Empress of Mars* to appear."

Cliff scowled and bit his lip. He was tough, tough as jet lining—you have to be granite inside and out to struggle up from Venaport to a ship command. But we could guess what was running through his mind at that moment. The *Empress of Mars* was just about the biggest prize a spacer could aim for. But in the fifty years she had been following her queer derelict orbit through space, many men had tried to bring her in—and none had succeeded.

A pleasure ship carrying untold wealth, she had been mysteriously abandoned in space by passengers and crew, none of whom had ever been seen or heard of again. At intervals thereafter she had been sighted, even boarded. Those who ventured into her either vanished or returned swiftly without any believable explanation of what they had seen—wanting only to get away from her as quickly as possible. But the man who could bring her in—or even strip her clean in space—that man would win the jackpot.

"All right!" Cliff slammed his fist on the table. "I'll try even that!"

Steena looked at him, much as she must have looked at Bat that day Bub Nelson brought him to her, and nodded. That was all I saw. The rest of the story came to me in pieces, months later and in another port half the system away.

Cliff took off that night. He was afraid to risk waiting—with a writ out that could pull the ship from under him. And it wasn't until he was in space that he discovered his passengers—Steena and Bat. We'll never know what happened then. I'm betting Steena made no explanation at all. She wouldn't.

It was the first time she had decided to cash in on her own tip and she was there—that was all. Maybe that point weighed with Cliff, maybe he just didn't care. Anyway, the three were together when they sighted the *Empress* riding, her deadlights gleaming, a ghost ship in night space.

She must have been an eerie sight because her other lights were on too, in addition to the red warnings at her nose. She seemed alive, a Flying Dutchman of space. Cliff worked his ship skillfully alongside and had no trouble in snapping magnetic lines to her lock. Some minutes later the three of them passed into her. There

was still air in her cabins and corridors, air that bore a faint corrupt taint which set Bat to sniffing greedily and could be picked up even by the less sensitive human nostrils.

Cliff headed straight for the control cabin, but Steena and Bat went prowling. Closed doors were a challenge to both of them and Steena opened each as she passed, taking a quick look at what lay within. The fifth door opened on a room which no woman could leave without further investigation.

I don't know what had been housed there when the *Empress* left port on her last lengthy cruise. Anyone really curious can check back on the old photo-reg cards. But there was a lavish display of silk trailing out of two travel kits on the floor, a dressing table crowded with crystal and jeweled containers, along with other lures for the female which drew Steena in. She was standing in front of the dressing table when she glanced into the mirror—glanced into it and froze.

Over her right shoulder she could see the spider-silk cover on the bed. Right in the middle of that sheer, gossamer expanse was a sparkling heap of gems, the dumped contents of some jewel case. Bat had jumped to the foot of the bed and flattened out as cats will, watching those gems, watching them and—something else!

Steena put out her hand blindly and caught up the nearest bottle. As she unstoppered it, she watched the mirrored bed. A gemmed bracelet rose from the pile, rose in the air and tinkled its siren song. It was as if an idle hand played. . . . Bat spat almost noiselessly. But he did not retreat. Bat had not yet decided his course.

She put down the bottle. Then she did something which perhaps few of the men she had listened to through the years could have done. She moved without hurry or sign of disturbance on a tour about the room. And, although she approached the bed, she did not touch the jewels. She could not force herself to do that. It took her five minutes to play out her innocence and unconcern. Then it was Bat who decided the issue.

He leaped from the bed and escorted something to the door, remaining a careful distance behind. Then he mewed loudly twice. Steena followed him and opened the door wider.

Bat went straight on down the corridor, as intent as a hound

on the warmest of scents. Steena strolled behind him, holding her pace to the unhurried gait of an explorer. What sped before them was invisible to her, but Bat was never baffled by it.

They must have gone into the control cabin almost on the heels of the unseen—if the unseen had heels, which there was good reason to doubt—for Bat crouched just within the doorway and refused to move on. Steena looked down the length of the instrument panels and officers' station seats to where Cliff Moran worked. Her boots made no sound on the heavy carpet, and he did not glance up but sat humming through set teeth, as he tested the tardy and reluctant responses to buttons which had not been pushed in years.

To human eyes they were alone in the cabin. But Bat still followed a moving something, which he had at last made up his mind to distrust and dislike. For now he took a step or two forward and spat—his loathing made plain by every raised hair along his spine. And in that same moment Steena saw a flicker—a flicker of vague outline against Cliff's hunched shoulders, as if the invisible one had crossed the space between them.

But why had it been revealed against Cliff and not against the back of one of the seats or against the panels, the walls of the corridor or the cover of the bed where it had reclined and played with its loot? What could Bat see?

The storehouse memory that had served Steena so well through the years clicked open a half-forgotten door. With one swift motion, she tore loose her spaceall and flung the baggy garment across the back of the nearest seat.

Bat was snarling now, emitting the throaty rising cry that was his hunting song. But he was edging back, back towards Steena's feet, shrinking from something he could not fight but which he faced defiantly. If he could draw it after him, past that dangling spaceall . . . He had to—it was their only chance!

"What the . . ." Cliff had come out of his seat and was staring at them.

What he saw must have been weird enough: Steena, bare-armed and bare-shouldered, her usually stiffly-netted hair falling wildly down her back; Steena watching empty space with narrowed eyes and set mouth, calculating a single wild chance. Bat, crouched

on his belly, was retreating from thin air step by step and wailing like a demon.

"Toss me your blaster." Steena gave the order calmly—as if they were still at their table in the Rigel Royal.

And as quietly, Cliff obeyed. She caught the small weapon out of the air with a steady hand—caught and leveled it.

"Stay where you are!" she warned. "Back, Bat, bring it back."

With a last throat-splitting screech of rage and hate, Bat twisted to safety between her boots. She pressed with thumb and forefinger, firing at the spaceall. The material turned to powdery flakes of ash—except for certain bits which still flapped from the scorched seat—as if something had protected them from the force of the blast. Bat sprang straight up in the air with a screech that tore their ears.

"What . . . ?" began Cliff again.

Steena made a warning motion with her left hand. *"Wait!"*

She was still tense, still watching Bat. The cat dashed madly around the cabin twice, running crazily with white-ringed eyes and flecks of foam on his muzzle. Then he stopped abruptly in the door-way, stopped and looked back over his shoulder for a long, silent moment. He sniffed delicately.

Steena and Cliff could smell it too now, a thick oily stench which was not the usual odor left by an exploding blaster shell.

Bat came back, treading daintily across the carpet, almost on the tips of his paws. He raised his head as he passed Steena, and then he went confidently beyond to sniff, to sniff and spit twice at the unburned strips of the spaceall. Having thus paid his respects to the late enemy, he sat down calmly and set to washing his fur with deliberation. Steena sighed once and dropped into the navigator's seat.

"Maybe now you'll tell me what in the hell's happened?" Cliff exploded as he took the blaster out of her hand.

"Gray," she said dazedly, "it must have been gray—or I couldn't have seen it like that. I'm color-blind, you see. I can see only shades of gray—my whole world is gray. Like Bat's—his world is gray, too—all gray. But he's been compensated, for he can see above and below our range of color vibrations, and apparently so can I!"

Her voice quavered, and she raised her chin with a new air

Cliff had never seen before—a sort of proud acceptance. She pushed back her wandering hair, but she made no move to imprison it under the heavy net again.

"That is why I saw the thing when it crossed between us. Against your spaceall it was another shade of gray—an outline. So I put out mine and waited for it to show against that—it was our only chance, Cliff.

"It was curious at first, I think, and it knew we couldn't see it— which is why it waited to attack. But when Bat's actions gave it away, it moved. So I waited to see that flicker against the spaceall, and then I let him have it. It's really very simple. . . ."

Cliff laughed a bit shakily. "But what *was* this gray thing? I don't get it."

"I think it was what made the *Empress* a derelict. Something out of space, maybe, or from another world somewhere." She waved her hands. "It's invisible because it's a color beyond our range of sight. It must have stayed in here all these years. And it kills—it must—when its curiosity is satisfied." Swiftly she described the scene, the scene in the cabin, and the strange behavior of the gem pile which had betrayed the creature to her.

Cliff did not return his blaster to its holder. "Any more of them aboard, d'you think?" He didn't look pleased at the prospect.

Steena turned to Bat. He was paying particular attention to the space between two front toes in the process of a complete bath. "I don't think so. But Bat will tell us if there are. He can see them clearly, I believe."

But there weren't any more and two weeks later, Cliff, Steena, and Bat brought the *Empress* into the lunar quarantine station. And that is the end of Steena's story because, as we have been told, happy marriages need no chronicles. Steena had found someone who knew of her gray world and did not find it too hard to share with her—someone besides Bat. It turned out to be a real love match.

The last time I saw her, she was wrapped in a flame-red cloak from the looms of Rigel and wore a fortune in Jovan rubies blazing on her wrists. Cliff was flipping a three figured credit bill to a waiter. And Bat had a row of Vernal juice glasses set up before him. Just a little family party out on the town.

SERPENT'S TOOTH

The haze was thinner than a drifting cloud, moving with the travelers . . . there was no rain here to temper the burning of the rough soil under Rentarn's bare and already scarred feet. Modic rode, even in this time and place he held to the dignity of a Seeker, but the trembling legs of the bony horse he bestrode (it was the worst mount of his train) threatened any moment to collapse, spilling rider on the ground. Only the Seeker's will kept the horse going along a wandering seam in the surface of the stones they had chanced upon an hour ago.

In Rentarn coiled and wove the old fears which had been bred in his kind for generations. He had been sure of disaster to come ever since this thin-faced man, with a jaw and nose which had the side view of a sword, had come to the village to demand, with a certainty overriding all other wills, a guide for journey west. Neither had Modic followed the rules of the Betweener village but had stabbed with a gloved forefinger at Rentarn and called for him. Though Sequine, the Speaker, had argued it was not the tall youth's turn.

Modic had only grinned fiercely and shaken his head when the first two drawn properly by lot came to him, saying that Rentarn looked sturdy enough to lead a Traveler into the Questionable Land. At last Sequine had shrugged and nodded. Each of them

knew sooner or later a guide found the Gate of Death. Now women and children hid in the mud-brick huts as all had heard of Betweeners slain for drunken amusement, or because would-be Seekers had been irritated by some small matter. From the moment Modic had made his choice they knew that it was Rentarn who must go. A half company of riders appearing on the bluff above had been an open warning for the clan village to obey Modic's desires.

"No knife." The Seeker had ridden closer to inspect the guide's equipment which Sequine's own son had brought forth. Modic kicked out as the boy passed him with such skill that the knife, a little loose in the scabbard, flew to strike against a hut wall.

"Leave it, you!" Modic moved his mount again until it stood between the Speaker and the boy. The Seeker said no more, but Rentarn nodded to the Speaker. "Obey . . . for the good of the clan."

In that last moment of boyhood the guide lost belief that truth and right were strong against any evil which might prevail. Now to be separated from his own people had only one meaning . . . this doom-faced warrior had a secret, and surely no one would live to betray its discovery. There were his men beyond; might he be able to get rid of them as easily?

"You pledge yourself . . ." That was no question. More like an order. Rentarn nodded. He could sense the tension seep out of the rest of the villagers. A bargain had been struck and surely this one, who knew so much of their customs, would now leave. It was unfortunate about Rentarn of course, but he had no kin here closer than a cousin, and between them had been many quarrels. What was the life of one man compared to all the village?

They had set out at the first color of sunrise and had kept plodding on straight into the heart of the vast waste. The now risen sun pressed a blanket of heat down upon them. They all carried water gourds which they had filled at the village spring. Yes, Rentarn thought, watching them when he believed Modic no longer checked upon him, these were indeed Seekers. Certainly they used water frugally at the rest stops Modic ordered each time the shadows of the towering stones standing here and there lengthened appreciatively. Also they watered their beasts, first giving them to drink

out of their helms and washing out the nostrils of each with a damp cloth. For themselves they allowed only what must have been a swallow or two.

Hereabouts the desert land was not still flat for there appeared a way which ran straight as if that had been cut by the force of man's desire for a road. Curiosity awakened in Rentarn. At the third stop he pretended to adjust the webbing which held his water gourd and packet of journey food, while, with his left hand, he stabbed one of his long and narrow fingers into the sand and gravel, far enough to scrape against the webbing of flesh which united all six fingers into a more solid fist. Underneath there was indeed a solid obstruction. Two of his middle fingers met a solid surface with bruising force.

Now he pulled his sun-resisting cloak higher on his shoulders and, through narrowed eyes, surveyed the country. Here stood a third hill, a mount of stone, partly seen there some summer dried shrubs . . . Yes! Rentarn's breath puffed against the edge of his cloak as straightaway he fought a sharp stab of emotion which he must not allow any of those about him to see.

Even the guides knew very little of this dreary world . . . save of the paths to which one or two bolder explorers might add a few new lengths several times in a lifetime. He knew that hill right enough . . . it marked the furthermost of his own rovings in this direction. Now, as he sighted it, he believed that this curious sand-covered cut ran directly towards that, as if the hill was indeed a marker on an ancient road.

It could lead where? Still aware of Modic he turned his head slowly, this time seemingly concentrating on the shoulder strapping of his supply net. He was somehow sure that he was right. They had camped on a portion of a forgotten road which ran straight ahead.

Rentarn's pointed tongue slid over his lower lip as if, like his very distant cousin of the true lizard breed, he could pick up scent impressions cast by man or animal.

One kept away from these roads. Such could be traced easily enough, but they led to the spirit places where the haze, such as they had traveled through earlier, thickened to give shelter to

things . . . things which he had heard described, legends of all guide villages. He slid his tongue out between his lips, startled past prudence into a grunt.

Could the Seeker know of this? Was he now aware that such roads led to the death light? A shadow fell across his face as he watched Modic, wondering for a moment of real fear if the man had guessed at his own discovery.

The Seeker dropped to the sand and crossed his legs, his hands playing with the hilt of his sword, drawing the blade out an inch or two from the scabbard and then thrusting it forcefully back again, as if he foresaw a need for its use. Rentarn had regained full control . . . he could hear the snick of the blade, however his narrow gaze was on Modic's face not the Seeker's hands. It was always the eyes into which one must look, Rentarn remembered clearly Sequine's warning. For it is by the changes in a man's eyes one could read the coming of violence.

"So," Modic's voice was hardly above a whisper, certainly it could not reach anyone farther away then Rentarn, "you have found it. Dig!" His lazy tone sharpened into an order, he motioned toward where the guide had been secretly delving. Obeying, Rentarn dug both-handed now. Within a number of breaths, lightly drawn breaths (lest he could take into him some danger of this place), he scooped out parched earth, throwing it to one side. He was right, it required very little in the way of labor to lay bare a section of a road of the waste devils . . . the black surface of it uncorroded by time and as smooth as his own scratched and bleeding skin.

Though Modic leaned more closely forward, Rentarn perceived he did not lose sight of the guide for more than half a breath at a time. "Right." When the Seeker spoke it seemed more to himself than to Rentarn. "The road to Lonscraft . . . at last!"

This time Rentarn's astonishment was rooted in fear. He jerked back his hands from hand contact with the damnable thing. Fighting to remain impassive, knowing within him that Modic was well aware of his inbred fear and was now studying the Betweener closely, a small evil smile about his lips.

"Ah, yes." The Seeker kept his voice low and confidential in tone, as if he and Rentarn shared some secret which was unknown

to the others. "This is the way to Lonscraft. Though that was not the name it bore in other days when the world was still all for men and not for sand-dwelling rats!"

He scrabbled inside his outer robe with his left hand, bringing out a small sheet of dull metal, near as thin as the skin of a ripe wavel. Still keeping one finger firmly on the edge of it he pushed the plate a little closer to Rentarn.

"Do you know the reading of maps, Guide, or do you only carry such information in your scaled head?" His slight smile now held no amusement, rather cruel, taunting humor.

So this one did not know of those treasure places located by villages . . . to which the youths went to learn . . . by heart and deep in the mind . . . the ancient roads and more than roads, the dangers and few secrets of the Sand Sea. One quick glance told Rentarn much. That which Modic held must have been graven by a master worker in metal. However only as far as the hillock behind them now did the lines assume any kinship with the records he himself had long ago memorized. This map displayed the warning blue of the Before Time road leading to a city of even darker blue, a color which seemed to pulsate in the light as if a breathing, and perhaps sentient, creature.

"Well, and what have you to say to this, Guide? I needed your steering to that hillock, knowing that what I sought lay beyond." Dry as it was, a droplet of saliva gathered at the corner of the Seeker's mouth, as he no longer gazed at Rentarn . . . rather at his map.

It was the colors which confused the sight, Rentarn decided. Certainly those lines did not really coil or quiver. From which clan had Modic stolen this record . . . one of the forbidden ones used to warn?

"It is true!" There was a sharp note in the man's voice as if Rentarn had openly questioned that fact. "Lonscraft lies awaiting us."

"That is a death place," Rentarn replied evenly. "He who rashly adventures into one of those gathers to him an ill for which there is no treatment. His skin rots upon his body, pain wrings him to death. There is nothing worth such a death . . . all the Betweeners know that."

Modic laughed, "Guide, you and your kind have been content

to exist for years on the border of this demon-haunted land with no reason for it. Every illness runs its course and then disappears. Have you not heard of the burning fever which may strike out of nowhere for a season and then be utterly gone ... or the Great Cough which has devastated whole cities, such as Quaadad, yet men may live there in comfort now. There is no death which lingers forever ... especially in a desert city where there is naught to feed its hunger. Long ago Lonscraft must have been deserted even by demons. Yet there still lies within its walls secrets. ..." The fingers of his hand clenched over the map as if he would pluck what he wished from the surface. "Riches beyond richness. Guide ... think on it!"

Riches, of course, were what had drawn this Seeker and his following of ragged men (who, nevertheless, carried well-kept arms) into the desert. How many such maps had been shown briefly to the Betweeners in the generations since they had begun their very cautious ventures into the parched land? Rentarn knew that it was not in the inner walls of Lonscraft which he himself feared, but perhaps the fact that he knew too much now. He guessed that Modic, on the threshold of what he thought an exciting and profitable discovery, would not parade and plume himself before his rag-tag crew. No, but he might talk freely before one who was destined never to come out of the Forgotten land. That sword which the Seeker held so tightly would put an end to any chance of another's betrayal. Not that Rentarn would fare better than any one of the men clinging to the shadows about them, seeking for some small answer to the burning of the sun. Murder was the practical move for Modic, and the Betweener already accepted the drastic end before him.

The Seeker would use him (in spite of that map) to follow the ancient way. ... He might even test the authenticity of legends by dispatching Rentarn alone into the midst of a dead city perhaps as bait to spring a trap.

One slight figure, cloaked against the heat, stood alone here. However, the death blow had not yet been openly delivered. Though every breath Rentarn drew brought him closer to that time of challenge.

Warnings known to his own kind worked in him. With those

a small spark of excitement flashed into life, turning his thoughts in another direction. If this Modic was right and he could win through to return with such knowledge for his own clan . . . ! Their own perilous situation might cease to be. There were other "cities" each reported to the Seeker . . . and the information was shared with two other villages within a three days' walking. No longer would they have to point these arrogant and cruel Seekers to the Dry Land, instead they would venture inward for their own loot and trade their findings openly at the Mus-fair, year's end. As long as Modic made no outward attack Rentarn would serve his own people, forcing into his memory a picture of here in relation to the hill point. However he must also watch for a chance of escape. It would indeed be strange . . . even without belief . . . that one of the guides could be tracked and captured traveling a country he knew well. Though he had kept his advance with Modic to a shambling trot which matched the pace of the bone rack of a horse . . . he could summon the speed of his far, far kin, tailed and going four-footed here. Let him but get Modic thoroughly interested in something other than himself . . . say, a forgotten treasure house . . . and Rentarn could slip away before anyone here could use lance or sword. The one thing he had to fear (bow bolts) was lacking among the troops.

He must play a perilous game. His thought, as well as his body, was intentionally slow.

"You seek a great treasure?" he asked, apparently taking no interest in the Seeker's hand upon the sword hilt.

Modic showed his yellow stained teeth in a wider grin.

"Treasure? Yes, but not perhaps quite as you and those . . ." he gestured to his men with his chin, "would so see it." Then he snapped his jaws shut and scowled at Rentarn and the others with narrow measurement, as if, of a sudden he regretted the revelation of even so little.

"You are a guide." He changed the subject abruptly. "Let us now see that vaunted power of such talent beyond the boundaries. Get me to Lonscraft or within sight of it before that sun is gone. He gave a quick glance over his shoulder as if to measure where in the sky the light-giving ball now rode.

"There are many cities . . ." Rentarn said quietly. "It can well

be that this trail," once more he patted the sand about that pocket in which lay the traces of the very ancient way, "could lead somewhere else than Lonscraft."

There came a sharp bark of laughter from the other. "No, it is here!" He had picked up his bit of engraved metal and thrust it back into hiding. "I have been long at this game, Guide, but not so long as to become weary and make such an error. Ten times over have I come across the Between lands . . . and more times than that have I listened to the tales told at Mus-fair. First, that hillock which you have found for us is pointing to Lonscraft."

Rentarn blinked, he had indeed believed that the Seeker was an old hand at the game of invading the uninvadable. But what could keep one of a sane mind so long at searching? It was true that the hill behind them was relatively unknown. He, himself, had chanced upon it only last season . . . it had been his first addition to the clan lore. However there were signs of others who visited there . . . horse dung dried into powder where the wind rolled it here and there, some scrapes on one of the upstanding stones which were too regular to be of natural fashioning and which Modic had studied with care as long as there was light enough to see both last night and again early this morning. Messages?

The clan no longer wrote such notes. He would report again what he had seen so that mention was made of it in the training of the young. Who needed scratches set on rocks when he could summon into memory . . . full and vivid as any picture . . . what he had seen over Modic's hunched shoulder?

The Seeker made no protest against Rentarn's watching. Though when one of his own men came near he had lashed out at him with a barbed tongue and an order which was to be obeyed.

Another reason for Rentarn to nourish his own belief that to find Lonscraft would mean his death. In fact he had wondered why that had not yet come. Modic had his road well ready to follow. What more did he want from Rentarn?

The Seeker swung around to give a hoarse, rallying cry which brought up the heads of his men, summoned their attention. He loped towards them at a curious one-sided, limping walk which was his pace when dismounted, meeting them part way. His own mount stood head hanging as others were saddled and made ready to ride.

Modic still bestrode the poorest of the lot, Rentarn noted, his eyes more than half shaded by wrinkled, greenish lids. Why such a choice, and why was Modic waving his men on that straight line which was the work of the ancients? Why would Modic share a treasure find with those ragged and brutish riders at all? Rentarn did not doubt in the least that Modic could have found some other track for them to follow. Yet he stood there, watching them ride on, as Rentarn rose to his feet behind him. They were indeed swinging into the trail Modic indicated. One, at least, had wit enough to be suspicious. He called out something in one of the complicated river languages, reining back his horse, his closest comrades drawing in about him.

"Na . . . Na . . ." Modic raised bare hands in a gesture meant to reassure, following his denial with a stream of speech, each word gliding close to the one before it so that Rentarn could not begin to pick out the few he knew . . . except one "treasure" . . . perhaps that was akin in meaning in every speech, because it was a universal cry to action. Though for a moment or two it looked as if this one rider was not easily convinced, though those who had gathered about him fell into eager talk with much gesturing of hands and licking of lips. At length he, too, grunted, the bush of filthy hair on his cheeks and chin stretching as he made a spitting motion into the sand. Though it was plain he had no excess liquid to so void.

Modic lingered, fussing with his horse's gear as if making sure all was in good order . . . in the mean time giving quick glances at the men riding, two together, down that defile which marked the road. As the last one passed another dune some distance away, he spoke again to Rentarn.

"What is the threat which keeps you and your kind from such places open for looting? I have seen pieces of ancient metal, gems, and even bits of carvings offered for sale. Yet upon the asking they will always say that such was found in some miserable small ruin. Have you never tried for Pospfer or Wejn or perhaps Slasta?"

Rentarn hoped he controlled his surprise well. Why did this Seeker mark down the three worst cities of the old tales, places where in lay death in waiting?

"Such are cursed," he replied shortly.

"The abodes of demons, eh?" Once again Modic showed his teeth in a grin. "How know you that it is not the dead themselves who rise to defend what they once held? What tales do your Speakers tell of these lands? That they were conquered one by one by a fearsome enemy? If that be so where is that enemy now? No tale of such an invasion has ever been told. Why strike your people at one portion of the land only?"

"These be the riddles all share, Seeker," answered Rentarn. He was on his feet, testing the cord of the net which held his supplies. "Legend says the death rode from the sky on a forked flame and where that touched the ground there was ruin and nothingness. . . . The dead do not live to fight for what was once theirs. But the breath of the dying clings to the cities. A man breathes in that which will shrivel his lungs, and stands against the unseen which will eat the flesh from his bones. Some times even now a reckless far rover dies so."

Modic fingered his bristled chin with two grimy fingers, staring after the disappearing men of his party.

"Breath of death . . ." he repeated slowly. "Then we shall at least prove that right or wrong." From one of his saddle bags he pulled two cloths, the metallic smell of leif about them both. One he tossed to Rentarn who automatically caught it. He watched Modic hang his cap on the saddle horn of his horse, shake out the material to pull it like a bag over his head. There were holes for eyes, and where the mouth would be a slit covered by a mesh woven of shining threads. Somewhat clumsily the guide followed the Seeker's action.

The heavy odor which appeared to waft from the material was so pungent that he began to cough and would have taken off the thing if Modic had not caught him by the wrist.

"Leave be, Betweener. That which you smell is a mighty spell against all which fills the air. I paid a full year of swording caravans to get those . . . and had a heavy argument into the bargain. There only lives one in the river land who makes such now. He works from a very old picture and notes of how it is done . . . and those he will share with none. Still Amers of Klydul, wearing one of these, did ride the streets of Maksheeff and returned alone of his company."

"To die ten days later screaming that a demon within him gnawed at his heart," replied Rentarn. "Yes, we have heard the full of that tale."

"Only his demon was a potion brewed by his own second wife, that she might set hand on what he had brought back but would show to no one, saying that it was worth the war ransom of at least five lords. Also he intended to take it to the Fire of Venex for an auction," Modic returned coolly. "It was not his travels which killed him . . . only his own foolish tongue for he told wide and far just what he had gained."

The last of the riders disappeared around an upstanding rock spur, and now Modic swung into the saddle and flicked his riding lash at Rentarn as a sharp-edged order to move. The guide was well able to match the ambling gait Modic's horse approved, it seemed that the Seeker must still be in quest of landmarks. However he and Rentarn followed the same path as those others.

Yet their rest had lasted longer than even Rentarn had noted. Now shadows crept out from the rocks and the chill of the open night, as the baking sun set, loosing winds which carried cold out of the western unknown. The far mountains were only distant blots against a graying sky. No guide had ever struck as far as to climb those. If ever a Seeker had gone there he had not returned. Rentarn pulled his cloak tidily about him and thought of the Seeker again and the tale which threatened all who were with him.

If Modic had even been to Maksheeff that was on a dream supplied by a night demon. Rentarn padded on tirelessly and thought of demons. During his own few years and his strikes into the Dry Country he had never seen a demon. Nor had anyone in his village back to the first foray accounts of their clan's coming, which Jawser the Blind kept counted in his bundle of remembering knots. Demons were talked of often . . . but they were never seen. Rentarn had come to think that they must be totally invisible. Yet the Speakers who had the freedom of Above and Below had not reported them either. Thus they indeed might . . . if they still existed . . . be able to shelter themselves on more than one level of dream seeing. That such would lurk in the dire, broken cities moldered half away by time was reasonable enough.

He felt a sickness gathering at the back of his mouth, born of

the stuff in which his mask was steeped. Now he tried to raise the banding from his throat and spat a glob of greenish phlegm to the rock beside him.

"Keep that mask on, you young fool!" Modic's words were muffled but could be heard. "See where we now stand, and you would give the ill which lies in waiting here a chance to get at you!"

The rock against which he spat he could see now through the dulling light of late afternoon, was not virgin stone but rather a tongue of what might be a buried building, pointed skyward. It was fashioned of small stones fitted together so that the cracks of their joining were difficult to see. On the other side of the road was a second such hill; the width between certainly measured a space of entrance which might once have stood as a gate to a road four or five times as wide as those which were known outside the Dry Land. Some of the sand was disturbed here, moved to show under red earth like unto any field where the keeps had little access to irrigation. Where this appeared it was churned and marked by the horsemen who had proceeded them.

Also they could hear voices from ahead where the piers of stone grew higher and even turned into a wall which ran true for more than just a stride or two. Modic's men were gathered there, all a-horse, gazing about them as if they were not really prepared for this. Ahead of them the walls arose abruptly. While there were cracks in them, they were not tumbled across the road. Those led to taller walls . . . to buildings like unto towers such as Rentarn had seen in ruin all along the border, as if erected hastily to help defend against what might come from the Dry Lands. These were broken here and there, after no regular pattern, by narrow slits which must have been intended to give watch sites for defenders.

Here, too, there was a difference. The sun had gone far enough down its sky trail now to lengthen shadows greatly. Only these were no honest shadows such as a man could trust with his eyes. For from those wall slots leaked a defused blue light, thin, hazelike, not unlike, save in color, to that haze which locked trails in the dawn hours.

The men had stopped where four roads came together and there was an open space centered by an oval which was curbed waist high, perhaps in order that none could fall within its circumference.

From that also curled, in wisps like the lazy curls of a smoking fire, bluish swirls.

One of the troopers had looked back to see the two of them. Now he gestured to the Seeker.

"Ho, Modic." They were not too far away for such a shout to carry, yet this greeting sounded as if it came from the other side of the sprawl of ruins, muddled and fuzzy. "Ho, Modic!"

It was plain to Rentarn that the Seeker was hesitating before, at last, he urged his sorry horse to amble on. Had the man actually sent this motley crew of his ahead to be picked off by any hidden enemy, thus securing his own entrance? Rentarn saw him raise his hand as if to pull off the odorous hood but he did not complete that gesture.

Before they had yet reached the party there shot, from the heart of the ruins, a shaft of light, rippling color . . . first the scarlet of man-blood, then the blue cast by the walls around. It reached up to the heavens, as if to provide a guide to a whole army of men even if they did not have the keen sight of the Betweeners. Having shot heavenwards, it now twisted to the left, whirled just above the roofs of the still standing buildings, moving so fast that it wove a great wheel of light. They might be standing again in full sun, save for the colors that touched them, first blue and then red and then blue again.

Having once established this circumference the haze descended again by sharp jerks until it engulfed the upper floors of the buildings and yet continued to descend.

Modic swung from his horse, grabbing hastily at his saddle bags and a coil of rope around the horn. The horse had lost its early lethargy. It tossed its head as Modic left the reins hanging and retreated before the next circling of the light as might a man, step by step, keeping its head forward and up, while it whinnied and snorted and than gave a sharp cry such as Rentarn had never heard issued from any mount before. Though he had not long to observe it, for Modic had caught his cloak-muffled arm in a grip which dug painfully into his flesh, and his light body was jerked by that hold into a pile of stone which was still connected to a standing wall on three sides. Then Modic flung himself down, perforce taking the guide with him, so they lay flattened on a stony pavement. The

eye holes of the mask so shortened Rentarn's vision that he could see nothing but a piece of wall, now red, now blue, and yet always bright at each viewing.

Perhaps he could not see, but hearing was not denied him. Horses screamed. There were other screams, too. With the sounding of each of those he could feel the pressure of Modic's hand still lying heavy upon him keeping him down. The Seeker was mouthing words in his own tongue in a steady litany. Rentarn recognized the name of one of the river land gods. Was Modic striving to make magic in a place already so ridden by the threat of evil? If so he was the greater fool, magic drew upon magic for feeding power, and somehow Rentarn believed that Modic's spell speaking would only encourage that which was on guard here.

So the guide waited, as they lay together under an overhang of an ancient building which was like a cave, for that which would also seek them out.

There was no more screaming from the horses. Once they heard a clatter of hooves showing that one of the mounts was less panicked, able to flee. There was instead a whimpering which tore at Rentarn's mind with the hurt and fear that it bore. Even that was done in time and yet they lay still. The colors no longer swept over the stone which was all Rentarn could watch. And humming, which he had not been really aware of until then, was gone. It was quiet enough so that he could hear the two deep breaths . . . almost like sobs . . . which Modic uttered as he took away his prisioning hand.

Rentarn edged as far as he could out of range of the Seeker's reach and sat up. There was still light overhead, but that was drawing together into the single beam which had first sent it forth. About them the full night was drawing in.

Modic raised up, not to his feet but instead crawled on hands and knees to an aperture through which he could see to where the men of his party had gathered. There he squatted while Rentarn leaned back against the wall, satisfying what had become a weakening hunger with a portion of journey rations he twisted off the tight cone of the stuff which he carried. He had no desire to view what must have been a battlefield of sorts. Now with his right hand he stroked the empty knife sheath at his belt. If he were to come

through this venture . . . alive . . . he would need a weapon of sorts. Perhaps Modic was saving him for a secondary sacrifice . . . Rentarn squared his shoulders back against the wall. The Seeker had now no followers, the guide was sure of that even though he had not looked beyond as Modic was doing. Certainly he had no armament which could stand against a circle of killing light. Modic was but a man without a following, no threat to Rentarn's clan. The guide's hand crept out of his cloak and he began to feel about him in the growing darkness. One finger suddenly smarted and instantly he was feeling along something which had a knife's shape right enough, but lacked the smoothness of metal, even though it was edged, as more delicate touch suggested. He still dared not look at what he had found, but continued to tug the object loose from where it had been planted almost straight up with only a finger's breadth or so of blade already uncovered. Wriggling it with care Rentarn kept his gaze on the Seeker, freeing the find by touch alone.

Modic, in this gloom, resembled a headless body for the bag mask covered his full head. He was breathing noisily . . . as might a man who had been running quite a distance. Then he spoke, in a very low voice, which was so muffled by the bag, Rentarn barely heard.

"The poor devils . . ."

Strange that he would mourn men he had sent to whatever frightening death the whirling colors had cloaked. Rentarn could never understand this man. If one of his own kind made an enemy, and that was seldom, for their barren life was precious to the Betweeners, none worked out such elaborate plot as this. Instead either of the two took their quarrel to the Speaker. There they talked, each telling what was in his mind and heart. Sometime it did lead to a battle with the hands and there would be hurts to tend. But death never entered in . . . that was too familiar a visitor on its own to be deliberately summoned.

Now Modic had stripped himself of his main threat, the men who rode in this train. There was certainly that between him and Rentarn which sooner or later would lead to open confrontation. The guide was not afraid but he accepted wariness to be a part of his thinking and planning from this time forth. He had freed the thing in the earth. Glancing up now and then to make sure that

Modic was paying no attention, he brought it forth, holding it under one of the flaps of his cloak to examine it more clearly.

It was, he believed, made of stone . . . but not the same as that which formed the buildings moldering around them. As long as his thin forearm it was a blade with a butt end surely intended for a hilt and a sharp point. The tip of that had been broken off, but the remained possessed a cutting edge. This was a shimmer of color. As the defense of the city had been red and blue interweaving, so this was a gray-white, in the depths of which showed gem beauty, red, golden, green, blue. Those colors moved when one turned the blade from side to side. Had Rentarn seen this cut into gem size, he would have believed he had a fortune in his hand. As it was he shoved it quickly back into full hiding. Hoping to have escaped Modic's eyes he slipped the blade into an inner loop of his cloak. However, as Rentarn dropped his fingers from the hilt, he was still aware of a tingling, a prickling. Modic had not moved. He had thrust head and shoulders as far as he could through the spy hole he had chosen. For a space there was quiet between them. Rentarn viewed the ruins about him, trying to guess what had been the original use of this now vanished building. At the same time, with the patience of a Xole caught waiting to make a heo prey he began a new search with his long prehensile toes trying to discover if any more treasure lay beneath the scum of wind-driven sand. His claws raked across the rock which appeared to be a flooring but each piece of that he so located was firm set and could not be lifted out. If another one of these gem-bladed knives awaited discovery it would take more time and perhaps a lot of extra digging to uncover it.

As Modic moved Rentarn ended such exploration. The Seeker drew back from his hole and untied his bag mask, signaling Rentarn to do likewise.

"There is naught to fear . . . for now!" Sweat had plastered his greasy hair flat to the skull, and small trickles of moisture made their way down, to drip from his square chin.

"You have been here before. . . ." Rentarn spoke aloud the suspicion which had been growing in him ever since the Seeker had waved on his men and taken a slower pace.

"No!" Modic sounded overly emphatic in that. "No!" His hand

went to the breast of his thigh-length overrobe where he had put the map stone for safe keeping. "No . . ."

Rentarn's tongue flicked out from between his jaws and in again. Once it was said that those of his blood could test the very air to sift truth from falsehood. If that gift had been lost they had other small ways of dealing with any double talk from strangers. Oddly enough Rentarn had to believe that Modic was now speaking the truth. Yet he was not ready to allow the Seeker to believe he had satisfied his unwilling companion by so much as that. And perhaps there was a frayed feeling of right within the man which brought out of him an explanation Rentarn was sure he had never meant to give.

Modic once more caressed his chin under the crust of sweat and plaster of sand, studying the guide narrowly. "The Old Ones, those who lived here," he made a gesture indicating the ruins, "had many secrets. Is not that the reason for both Seeker and Guide to come hither?"

Rentarn shook his head. "We wrest no secrets from the dead. . . ."

"The more fools you." Modic got to his feet, stretching arms and legs as if the time he spent at the spy hole had rendered him stiff. "If you seek not for treasures, why do you venture into this sin-damned land year after year? What brings you here?"

Rentarn once more flicked his tongue over his lower lip taking the grit of sand into his mouth. With it there seemed to come that sickening flavor with which the mask was imbued. He plucked that off and shook head and shoulder much as the Seeker had stretched. Then he deliberately wet a forefinger against his lips, used it to gather up some grains of sand from a nearby wall stone and licked that up. A moment later he spewed it forth.

"Now what do you do?" Modic wanted to know.

"There is salt in this earth. . . ." In turn Rentarn got to his feet and looked about the jumble of wall and piles of fallen stone.

"Salt!" Modic hooted with what he must consider laughter, still Rentarn slowly surveyed each standing wall, seeking something which was not there. "I asked you, Guide," the Seeker returned to the question, "what seek you within this desert if you come not to

plunder the towns? Do the demons walk only in those so you feel safe in the open . . . ?"

Rentarn's two strides took him even with and then past Modic. Now he needs must kneel to look upon what had so engrossed the Seeker. "We seek," his voice was absent in tone, for what he told was not secret . . . neither was it ever believed, "water."

"Water!" Modic's voice arose to a whoop. "Here in the dead sands you seek water? Be like you follow some old tale where some ancient evil one struck stone and it enclosed your precious water."

Rentarn did not turn his head, he found that he must crouch even lower to look through Modic's vantage point. "You have the truth of it, Seeker," he answered still absently. Then even forgot the man by his side when he looked out to where the horse and men had waited. Sun was gone, shadows were heavy. In his nostrils was the raw, sweet smell of blood, and he saw enough to near bring the scanty contents of his stomach up into his mouth. Bones . . . goblets of torn flesh. But the bones were the worst, for from the way they lay twisted and piled against each other he could believe that something might have stripped their bodies of flesh while yet they lived. There was a head which had rolled closer to his viewpoint and was exposing bone to chin and cheek and a mass tattered of flesh above. Yet by Hyqur, the Keeper of the Gates of Darkness, the flesh had not been devoured or even carried far. The still dripping chunks and strips lay within what once must have been a fountain, pulled into a pile as if laid out for a feast.

Modic's hand fell heavily on his shoulder. "Quiet as the sand when there is no puff of air to give it life." He was crouched beside Rentarn again, his mouth so close to the Betweener's leathery cheek that the foulness of his breath for an instant made Rentarn gag as he had from the mask. "There are those who come to feast at such a table. . . ."

"Yet," Rentarn dropped his own voice and half hissed, half whispered, "you have not been here before. Then how do you know what chances here? Let me guess, Seeker. You had full knowledge of that which killed and took precautions that you should not be among the slain by coming last. Why chose you . . ."

His question was interrupted by a soft sound like a heavy sigh such as a beast of burden might give when loosed of that burden,

the need for going on. The darkness was not quite as complete as it would have been outside the ruins. Rentarn was not sure just where the pale light came from, unless it was from the uncovered bones of the city itself. But he was able to see the outline of a horse's head against whitish block a little beyond them.

Modic chuckled. He might not have been viewing a fatal battlefield, but rather was anticipating some coming gift.

"So . . . SOOOO . . . sssoooo . . . Dus," again that whispering voice but he did not address Rentarn this time. The mount's ugly head swung in his direction and the horse took one step and then another as one answering a detested jerk upon dangling reins, edging by as far as it could from the horror about the pool.

"Never judge a mount by looks." Modic dug an elbow into Rentarn's ribs. "Dus has been a-questing before. But he has been thrice blessed by the Voice of Ugan and also endowed at birth with more brains than many a man! Ugly and spare he may look, but he is as fresh at the trail's ends as when he first stepped out. Ah!" Modic's first touch on the guide's arm became a grasp which twisted flesh and brought pain.

"Look you, Betweener! Here comes those to the banquet their protector has laid out for them!"

The horse had managed to reach their crowded hide just as his master spoke. The animal made no sound but his sweat was that of fear and it was rank in their small space. Giving voice to a harsh whinny Dus turned and pulled away. Modic did not appear to notice his going. Rentarn saw a dark shape detach itself from a fraction of wall to scuttle towards the basin of blood and flesh. It was only the first. However Rentarn was not to be turned by such a sight from his need for the truth.

"You know this place." He made a statement out of that, not a question. "Yet you swear you have never been here before."

"Nor have I, Betweener. But I have been to Lyrh and Kenzy. . . ." He spoke with pride in his voice. "Though never within these walls. Yet I saw a Seeker disappear into Lyrh with all his company. And he did not return, nor did any one or thing, save my fool Dus here, when the sun arose the next morning. There were sounds in a plenty during the night and they were not pleasant ones."

"If you were so near, how does it that you were not caught in the same trap?"

Again Modic chuckled. " 'Twas my own thinking which saved me there. I was well behind the Seeker, not a member of his crew, and when the killing light came I was beyond its radius. Also . . ." His hand strayed inside his robe again and Rentarn would swear that what he sought was that map. . . . "Also, I sat at the feet of many story tellers . . . in all the Down Lands. Some had one small bit to spew forth, some had nothing . . . but I listened with patience for more than a year. I even had such brought to tell to me alone. It was one of those, an ancient Speaker of your own kind, Betweener, who gave me the first clue." He settled back into the shadows and sat more at ease with his back against a broken wall. Yet he still spoke in so low a tone that Rentarn had trouble making sure of all the words.

"What do you know of the tale of Lonscraft, Betweener? Or is that legend so old it has dried up in all men's minds, to be blown away in an autumn tempest?"

Truth? Rentarn's tongue tasted the air. There were many foul and dangerous odors about but he could still pick up this Seeker. Modic told the truth, or what he believed to be the truth, or . . . at least a portion of it, destined to hook Rentarn to him.

"Lonscraft." He remembered back to days not so long ago when he had toiled over learning . . . names, places, events which had been the portion of the Betweeners lore for such a long time. "Lonscraft," he repeated, "is a tale. . . ."

"What are the past doings of us all but legends when time speeds further and further away from the event," Modic wanted to know. "Yes, there is the tale of Lonscraft . . . but it is worn ragged by passing through so many tellers, each changing a little to make it suit his or her own ideas of what was exciting, or fitting, or proper. Your people tell dark stories of the cities within this dead land, yet they learn its trails and mark its guide posts as if such acts are a matter of unchangeable law. You do believe yet, deep inside of you . . . there is a faint stirring when one calls the name of a vanished city. You have built up a number of taboos and most of them have truth in them. Your training tells you that death was here . . . and it was. Still you are not aware of what kind of death . . . only of its

shadow. But me, Modic," he thumped himself on the chest, "I allow no story to stand alone and be only half believed. Always have I sought for more. I heard of the woman Kasiu, she who was first wife to Amers. Her I hunted out and she was afraid, for there were many in her village who knew how much she hated her husband and who were skeptical of her story of Demons entering him when he came here. I made a bargain with her, that she could travel with my company down to the River towns and that she was grateful for, also she could not guess that more lay in her husband's journey bag upon his return than crumbs of food. But I learned where she had spilled the bag, so I found what I sought for what seems now half my life.

"There was the map and I hardly think truly that it was of his own making . . . it may be generations old. Also there were some guide scratches . . . look for yourself, Betweener."

Modic was holding out an oblong of slate painstakingly ground into a narrow slip. Rentarn accepted it gingerly, then might have gasped had his species been that of the Seeker. It was hot in his hand, not as something which had gathered body warmth from resting against flesh, but with a heat which radiated from it. He could have been holding an actual part of the sun's beam. To the sight in this part-dark it was bare, but when his fingers quested over it, ridges and curves lay plain against his skin. Deep in him was that first flutter of fear known when a thing which is thought to be without truth suddenly throws aside the cloak of falsehood. His lips shaped words which his voice whispered:

"In the ninth month when the Lords of the Three Lands strove together, there came out of the depths of the dead and riven land one who was veiled and lacking in speech. Yet no one raised hand to pull aside the veil and cloak, or spoke. Rather did they draw back away from this one who was not like unto others of the world.

"Then rose up Utyr of Lonscraft who was ever of hasty tongue and impatient hand. He spoke, saying that truth was to be known and if there was a message then let this one speak it forthwith.

"So that one from the dead land turned to Utyr and made certain gestures which no one understood, but which had an ill look to them. Utyr, though he shifted from one foot to the other as a person ill at ease, did not speak again. Nor did he give any

orders to his men as that shrouded one turned and walked from him. Those before the walker hunched to either side making a free path for the cloaked one. Thus the stranger came to the first opening of the broad marsh which was then to the gates of Lonscraft, that city being partly built on landing of stone long and deep set in unsteady earth. Going out upon one of the piers of the swift flying marsh boats, the stranger opened wide his cloak, which then hung in the air itself like wings. Although all the company stayed ashore and none could see what the cloak had hidden.

"But a hand flashed forth bearing such a weapon as no man had seen . . . white, and gold, blue, red and green, color followed color across its surface. Then the stranger whistled, a clear, sharp sound like the cry of some sea bird.

"Down one of the aisles of open water which served for the boats came that which those of the land had never seen. It was both a fish and a crawler upon the land for it showed stubbly legs. When it came to a belt of weed it climbed over that growth, not giving way to it.

"As for the staff, this flashed with color, mainly green, but also swirling red, blue, and gold.

"The head of the water one was held high above the surface, and from its mouth issued words which all man could hear but none could answer, for there was no understanding them. Then the voice grew louder, boomed and belled, until it filled the ears of all those in Lonscraft and there was no escaping it. Also it carried in it, even if one could not understand the words, a feeling of coming shadow and ill fortune. So that those waiting by Utyr drew sword or battle knife, even though no challenge had been offered.

"Utyr himself strode forward near enough to the stranger that he might grasp that one's shoulder if he wished; he even put forth his hand as if to do that very thing. Yet he did not complete that gesture for the thing in the water ceased upon an instant its calling and there was a strange and abiding silence which held for five breaths, perhaps more. Then he who stood at the pier's end turned slowly around so that those gathered there could see, that though he walked upright and cloaked as might a man of the city, he was not of their form nor wore any covering known to them. . . ."

"Yes," Modic broke in, "do your tellers of ancient tales say then what manner of creature this stranger was?"

Rentarn's tongue flicked out, he raised the water carrier to his wide mouth and took the smallest of sips, though that was enough to strengthen his voice.

"You have heard the same tale, Seeker . . . what manner of creature was this stranger?" prodded Modic.

Then he laughed. There was a shadow of contempt in his voice: "Go hunt out a quiet pool and look into it, Guide. There shall you see well what you wear . . . for the stranger was of your kin by blood."

What Rentarn might have replied to that was lost, for from the broken walls before them arose a keening cry, and straightway that was stifled in turn by cries and shouts of despair, horror and terror on the verge of madness. If some had escaped the massacre in the open they were now being dragged to their deaths.

So awesome was that chorus that Rentarn put his hands over his ears but found he could not shut out the sound which seemed to enter and pulsate in his body so he rocked a little forward and back as if he was shaken by something a great deal stronger than any sound, no matter how hideous.

A musky-sweet corruption of blood scent arose about him also. Thus he could believe that those scavengers of this ill-omened place gathered again for a feasting. There was movement behind him and he whirled to see something which slid through the black of shadow to advance past the end of a broken wall. From that spread the odor of horse sweat, Dus once more. The fear born in animal broke through the ugly spell which kept both travelers quiet. Modic did not move, but Rentarn stepped forward and caught again that trail of broken rein. By this he drew the bony horse to them.

Behind he heard once again Modic's chuckle as eerie as a madman's.

"Did I not say," Modic asked, "that Dus was one of the best of all that train? The rest stood pinned by fear until they met death, but this one fled, which is often the greater part of any valor, and note its coming does us also a service. For it would not venture to us now again if the way was not clear. Now yield your guideship

to me, Betweener, and we shall come out of this . . . but tell me first what sorcery your distant kin worked here which defeated Utyr, and with him many other lords of a land not then dead."

"That the tellers of tales never knew," Rentarn returned sharply.

The moans, screams, and cries of fear and torment had died away as if one by one those who voiced them were being silenced forever.

"And the water thing which came to his call? What was that, Betweener? Why during one day and night did all those who followed Utyr die? What death twisted and wrung their bodies, tore and shredded the very flesh which made them what they were?" Modic advanced a step or two, now facing Rentarn. There was a full moon and, as if he still clung to some ancient fear for all his brave talk, he was fingering the broken rein and standing close enough to the horse that he might be in the saddle and off before Rentarn could move.

The Betweener shrugged. "I know nothing of sorcelment or the plays of warlocks and Mages."

"Ha! And still those of the stranger's kin went out of the city untouched. None of them bore so much as a water bottle with them, bareheaded they went, unpursued and free. *That* is the ending of the tale they chant in the Down Lands. Eh, Guide, how fared them? Death did not claim *them*."

"I know no such ending of the legend," countered Rentarn. "When it is spoken among us death is universal."

Modic grinned evilly. "Do men, or Betweeners, ever really make that clear? Perhaps it is better to forget than to admit one has made some pact with that which should never have been thought of? Do we greet Betweeners with open arms and fair smiles to this day . . . even when they bring us those things we have need of? Why come you in parties of fighters if you are merchants with nothing to fear?"

Rentarn gestured with one hand as if brushing aside something worn threadbare, an action with its reason lost far back in time.

"Why do we stand here," he asked, "and talk of old tales and whether or not there was death of a city, a curse which grew out of Utyr's orders when he went desert raiding. Rather it would be

well for us now to be on our way before that guardian returns, to jealously remove us from its present lair."

"True, true. We shall go hence from here." Modic looked about him as if he stood in some noisome place. "But from Lonscraft we go not until . . ." He brought out of the bosom of his robe something which fitted into the hollow of his hand and which he handled as carefully as if he held a palm full of water which he must carry without its draining away. "Give me the map. . . ."

Rentarn handed him that oblong of stone which had the message on it near erased. With this firmly held in his left hand, Modic clapped his right hand about also. Though it looked to be a shard of dull gray, such as lay in the thousands along any trail, Modic was touching it to the map.

It was if he now held a coal, for there sprang up a steady red light in the stone. Modic's features twisted, his lips grimaced as if he did indeed carry a fire's heat against flesh. The fire was answered by a spark on the map, one which glowed as steadily as the Seeker's stone. Modic gave a half-stifled oath, his eyes wide and brightly open so that he would not lose a fraction of what he looked upon.

With the wane of the moon Modic stepped as forward boldly as he would have had it been day. For the lack of anything on which to base a protest, Rentarn followed after, leading the horse which plodded as if it had been sentenced to too heavy a task.

Lonscraft. In Rentarn's mind revolved the name of that ancient death of a city. So far the tale he himself had repeated had been exact . . . yet never had it told what manner of death was spewed forth by the marshes, or why it had not fallen upon those of Betweener blood, just those of Modic's species.

Still, in the many years since that time, perhaps too many to be told over without a knot string to aid, those who ventured into the Great Dry had died . . . one way or another. None had told what they had chanced upon which was so perilous an enemy. Lonscraft itself was the name which had been gasped by one of the earlier venturers as he died, tongue stricken save for that word.

They now angled well away from the open center about the dead pool where the others had died. The memory of the color which arose to slay, or else hold the intruders here until something more subtle had come seeking life and blood, haunted Rentarn. His

hand beneath his cloak sought out that piece of fire curling stone which he had found in the ruin. Yes, there was a brilliant swatch of color to match that which had flashed to kill on the rod or knife. With each step he took, he glanced sharply about and then at the blade. The star-dotted sky above the central buildings remained free of lighting or change. Though color still swirled within the pointless blade, it did not even reflect on the hand which held it. Still there was a feeling . . . Rentarn's head jerked as if that sudden thought had been a blow. Why did he come to imagine thus as he followed Modic through these ruins? Never before had he conceived of things which were not of the earth he knew.

Oh, there had been tales a-plenty concerning demons and creatures from other worlds (with hints that the meddling of some man or Betweener had opened forgotten gates), but always such had appeared or had happened to some guide or wanderer from another clan. One far away enough for the report to become muddled and overlaid with all the fears which were a part of their heritage.

He knew well that the men of the lower lands by the rivers had similar ghosts. Nor were there many who even dared to make a short essay into the Dry with or without a guide. Still there was about Modic now a kind of fever which darkened his skin even under the moon's glow, and made his journey one of erratic pauses and swifter advances, as if two desires warred violently within him, now this and now that taking command.

It was the horse who broke through the Seeker's tight absorption. Not uttering any sound, it drew back upon the rein, jerking its head as if to free itself. Bracing its spindly legs within a narrow way between two piles of rubble, it refused to advance.

Modic at once appeared fully awakened from his obsession. He stood dragging with all his force at the reins . . . the horse's head now stretched forward at a painful angle. It was the animal that struck first. It kicked out, though it was not facing Modic, and Rentarn, who had had no part in its pull forward, was the victim of that assault.

There was a keening wail . . . not from either man or beast in their struggle, nor from Rentarn either. The guide threw himself backward, not only to escape the hooves of the animal but in utter surprise . . . for the sound issued from the artifact he had found. Nor

did it emit a single note, rather a near scream which was suddenly cut off. Neither the horse nor Modic turned to see what had made that cry. Rather the horse sprung forward, near overrunning the man as it burst out of the narrow way between the two tottering pillars of rubble.

The light from the moon was gone. Clouds built up in the northern sky. Rentarn's instinct told him a storm was on the way. But that was of little importance when compared to this thing he had found. It was emitting a droning beat, broken now and then as if each portion of sound was a word of warning or a threat.

He could have turned in the moment and found his way out of this dead curl of broken walls and mounds of stone. The horse and Modic had vanished around a turn in the debris so that he could not be seen.

It was not curiosity, nor any sense of responsibility toward Modic, which brought him apart from the way where he had taken refuge some moments earlier. Seemingly of its own accord the hand holding the weapon (if weapon it was) shook free from his cloak without his willing it. The colors within were running as if he were turning the stone about in his hand. It was . . .

For a second, perhaps even less, he opened his eyes to their greatest extent. The thing was moving weapon-wise at last, though there was no enemy before him. His muscles responded as they never had to any journey knife or battle staff, thrusting and recovering with a knowledge which he knew he had never learned in any clan drill. His hand and arm might now be possessed by . . .

By the dead? In all the lore taught by his people there was no room for such an idea. One was born, lived, and when the time set had come, one died. Nor had the ken any tales of the walking of the dead, troubling from those who were past all of this world's sorrows, acts, thoughts. The dead spoke not . . . between them and the living there was not even the thinnest crack of a doorway.

It was not the dead suspicioned so to frighten some of the Seeker's people and be a part of the dangers of the Dry as far as they were concerned. The Betweeners hinted of dealing with dark powers. Demons . . . some of his kin, he knew, believed that there were unseen malignant forces at loose in ancient cities. This city . . .

Rentarn stopped short and stared unseeingly at the shard he

held. What of that story Modic had asked of him, a story long current among his own people? The cloaked one from out of the desert who had gone to the marsh pier and thereafter summoned a thing past any man's knowing.

Rentarn, still keeping the broken sliver in his hand under a flap of clothing, strode in the direction Modic and his mount had taken. Rounding a tall heap of debris he came abruptly into the open once more. There was just enough light to see a square ahead and the facades of the buildings forming its sides had apparently suffered less from whatever doom had erased Lonscraft. Directly across from him was a seemingly intact building which bore no signs of ruin at all. The wide doorway was above the level of the square so that a flight of broad steps led to its open doorway. Strangest of all in this desert country, there was a runnel which had cut its way through the steps, to a hole which gaped at ground level. Running water? No, the color was wrong. Each drop of that small flood was as scarlet as newly shed blood. While above its surface, back and forth, danced winged things which skimmed so closely to the small flood that they might have been swallowed up, yet always they coasted to safety beyond.

Modic had lost hold on the broken rein, the horse backed away from the steps and the liquid on them, showing the whites of its eyes, foam dripping from its nostrils to slime its nose and the bony expanse of its chest. It retreated from Modic, from the building. Then it swung half around and cantered awkwardly to Rentarn's left. Modic was pulling on the head-concealing mask that he had worn when they had entered Lonscraft. As he did so he walked as does one who bends his body against the force of a mountain wind, taking one slow step and then another. He gestured forceably with one arm as if to keep off an attack of flies. While in his other hand was that map which now was a fire to light the whole of the stairway. If that spark of light upon it had been fashioned to beckon, now surely it proclaimed to be nearly to the goal.

The smooth running rill was disturbed on the surface, now dimpled as if a shower fell upon it. The flies gathered in the upper air to become a black blot, still over the water but hovering above Modic as he climbed.

Rentarn shivered. He had known fear before, but it had always

been caused by things he understood . . . of one of the Vort beasts raiding the herds of the Betweeners . . . of the sickness which was supposed to strike anyone invading the old cities, of the ill will of his own clan should he break their few but skintight taboos (for that would unclan him and make him as one dead walking among the living). Now . . . this was like fronting a cold rage, an ire so great that his kin could not even sense more than a portion of it. Here lay in wait a will, a power, a brutal rule which shook him. Still the time had come . . . or he had come . . . too far past the borders of its control to struggle against it now.

A will, a power . . . he was caught up by sharp command as he came fully into the open passing the horse that now stood with drooping head as if the beast had lost all hope. This horse lived, so did Modic as he climbed from one step of the wide stair to the next. Still, though Rentarn began search with his own heightened guide's sense, he could trace back that bold assault against him to . . . nothing! There was no trace of man, of Betweener, of animal, of life as he knew it, aroused to draw him shivering towards the source. To that highly developed sense, trained to locate life, there came, at last, an answer from a source he had not expected.

From the broken tip of the many-colored blade sped a thin thread of red and blue, entwined one with the other. Those were the same colors as the light which had been thrown across the rubble-lined streets of Lonscraft . . . the fearsome alien weapon. What did Rentarn now hold? An artifact which was a dueling ground for bursts of killing color? By arousing his will, pitting his inner strength against that pull, the guide was able to linger on the second step, even as Modic reeled and wavered far closer to that aperture above which served as an ever open door.

Inch by inch Rentarn edged around to look back over the way he had come. The horse screamed and reared to strike out with its front feet as might a war-trained stallion. Around it ringed a crowd of shadows, curious moving bolts of darkness which never clearly showed themselves. Though there were a number of these remains gathered around the horse, others padded to the foot of the stair to form a double line of dark forms, though they avoided the running rill. Rentarn flicked out his tongue in their direction. Full of viciousness, yes, but these were not a true part of that which waited

within. However they now formed a guard wall against any retreat, and that could only mean that Modic and he were being edged towards another and doubtless more powerful enemy.

His foot touched on the next step. There was a crackling, the sound of something rolling back toward the waiting band. Rentarn saw a skull, polished enough to reflect the gleam of this alien light. He no longer watched the hunters, rather studied his footing. That remnant of his own species, or Modic's, was not alone. There lay a scattering of broken bones, some near reduced to powder, along each step.

He heard a thin, half-muffled cry which might have come from Modic, muffled as he was by mask. The Seeker tripped, fell to his knees on the last step, his shoulders shaking, his head turning from side to side as if so he tried to avoid blows. Some strong compulsion drew him on to crawl along the platform above as might a seriously injured animal seeking shelter. There was no cracking of splintering bones now, all sound had been absorbed by a deep hum which hurt Rentarn's ears, throbbed through his body. Two more strides brought the guide beside Modic. He reached down and hooked his fingers in the other's armpit, giving a steady pull, while the Seeker scrambled in the bones and flopped about, seeming unable regain to his feet.

"Up!" He was so near to Modic Rentarn believed that his words were not lost in that ever growing throb. "Up to your feet, Seeker. Would you meet battle on your knees, already so far spent as you seem?"

Modic turned his shaking head to look up at Rentarn dull eyed. Spittle ran from the corner of his mouth and with it a thread of blood from a lip he had bitten though. He showed no understanding, but some part of the guide's urgency must have reached him, as he swung around to clasp both of his sweat slicked hands on Rentarn's arm. Using that hold for leverage as he might a tree or rock pillar, he drew himself up, near oversetting Rentarn in the process, when for a moment or two he hung a dead weight on the other before regaining his feet.

The throbbing grew heavier, more assertive as if something ahead was impatient at their delay. As they moved forward, Modic,

still using Rentarn as a support, they were plunged into light . . . a blaze of blue. Modic halted, stopping Rentarn almost in midstride, to jerk at the edge of the mask the guide had worn into the city.

"Put on," he croaked hoarsely, his mouth close to the guide's nearest ear.

One-handed, for he could not put aside the gem light he held, the Betweener obediently pulled on the mask once again though he did not like the curtailment of sight which wearing it caused.

Only it was true that once he was again shrouded that blaze of raw light was subdued, and he could see enough to mark the fact they they were indeed in a palace or some incredibly rich shrine. The light might blot out a measure of response from the display of unbelievable wealth about them, but it could not utterly hide what was set in patterns on the walls, and not only on the walls. There were dunes and drifts of precious metals and gem stones across the floor, many of the pieces broken.

As they shuffled on they tramped on a medley of stones and metals of stones and metals such as could not be seen at a fair even if all which had ever changed hands there had been reassembled for one great showing.

There were weapons, too, swords and knives possessing hilts rich in jewels, strange other objects which were certainly not intended for adornment but which, if weapons, Rentarn did not recognize.

Here and there was a rack of bones . . . some draped with chains of office of the adornment of chief wives. Several of these lay broken across the things which Rentarn believed might be weapons.

Before them was still that blast of light which gave no hint of its source or purpose . . . unless that latter was death, which Rentarn could well believe. In his hands the colored spindle of stone quivered past all his endeavors to control it, but so far it had not broken free.

His tongue touched the rough stuff of the mask, the tip of it pointed through the hole which served for the mouth cutting and the opening for breathing. Deliberately he began to try to set the pace for himself, to be quickly forced into the maelstrom of color. It was a battle, and his uncovered skin pricked and stung. Modic

had again fallen to hands and knees. Even his head hung low so he did not watch the way ahead, he merely crawled toward the source of the light.

Rentarn was able to slow his advance though he could not tear himself free of the strong pull upon him. Still he quested with tongue tip, thrusting that even farther into the crackling air about. The light must have a source, and having a source it must be set, meant to protect it's own inner sanctum as he had seen its overflow light up the sky in the first coming of their party. Animal, biped, brain . . . thought process which?

His flesh was so seared by assault . . . what awaited him? For the first time . . . his Betweener-born organ for detection brought him no knowledge. There was nothing ahead, that sense insisted, but the light itself, and that was not tended by any living thing.

The way was growing narrower as the great room started to close in about them to form a corridor. Here the treasure was less visible. There were more skeletons, insignias of office mingled with brittle bones, and there were indeed weapons he knew, some lying half into the red flood of the stream from which he edged away as it began to flow widening more and more. The stench rising from it was choking. Rentarn coughed hollowly and leaned with one hand against the wall as he steadied himself against unseen gusts which struck him.

Modic halted. Then he hunched in a crouch, sweeping his hands from side to side about him though without seeming to see what lay there. By chance his fingers curved about one of the rod-like things which Rentarn believed was a weapon. Still not raising his head so that he might look at what he had found, the Seeker allowed the rod to slip through his fingers until a dark band meant for a grip was resting in his hold.

Rentarn was not prepared for what followed. Modic swung around, moving with the speed of a trained hand and foot warrior. The end of that rod pointed unerringly at Rentarn's middle, though the Seeker still did not lift his head.

No! Rentarn's sense had never proved to be deceptive but it had to be so now . . . it had to be! There was life in the other but it had dwindled down as might the last coal of a fire being fast smothered. In its place . . . the guide's tongue tip sent a thrill of

pain through his body, kept him pinned to the wall. There was life
ending . . . and nothing, nothing gathered beyond to take its place.
Yet Modic was on his knees, his head hanging forward nearly resting on his chest.

Not dead . . . possessed! Other evil tales from the wild slipped
into memory. The Seeker gave body room and aid to something
else. . . . Only, when Rentarn strove to touch that, to discover what
had chained the River worlder to such a trap, he could not pick
up anything save always the burning of the power.

Rentarn jerked his body to the left as that weapon pointed in
his direction. He felt the heat of a ray which burst at him. It was
gone as quickly as two breaths, though Modic still held it aimed at
the Betweener. Rentarn saw the other's hand tighten about the
band on the rod with full strength.

The shining length of his own find was ready. In its heart,
flaring from the butt to the broken point, was a rich roll of color.
That twisted as if to wrench itself free but Rentarn's six fingers held
tight. His whole body jerked as if the artifact from the city ruin
was a rope with him imprisoned in a loop. He flailed out with his
other arm, striving to keep his balance, and so struck against Modic.

Whether the unexpected contact between their bodies was the
reason or not, the Seeker staggered halfway around to bring up the
strange weapon. That gesture was never completed, for Modic's rod,
touching by chance the broken knife Rentarn unconciously advanced in defense, burst, scattering fragments which melted to drip
to the floor. Spots of dull dark blue fell smoking and glowing at
their cores. The Seeker lurched forward, his unsteady pace close to
a run, shouldering Rentarn aside. The guide went after him at a
speed which was nearly equal.

They came upon more skeletons. However the bones were scattered, no rack of them whole. Also they appeared as if they were
more recent than those in the hallway. Another Seeker band which
had reached this point before falling prey to an enemy they could
not sense? Rentarn wondered.

In the center of the large chamber beyond was a bank of chairs,
constructed, not of stone, but of some substance which glittered
with dancing lights. Before those bubbled a pool from which arose
the dread runnel of red they had companied with from without. It

appeared to Rentarn that small bursts of flame danced over surface just as had the black insects in the outer world.

At the entrance of the pool crouched something which was surely out of some nightmare of the damned. Rentarn, gazing at it with horror was near overborne. For it might be that one of his kin, larger, mad with blood lust, stared straight into his eyes as if the mask he still wore was transparent. The thing's mouth gaped wide and the pointed fangs within dripped glowing slime into the pool.

It was not dead. His own guide's sense told him rather it had never lived as he knew life. There was nothing at all Rentarn could detect from it. While in the seats . . .

Yes, there sat dead . . . six bodies, not riven and torn, not reduced to racks of bones. . . .

These were not Betweeners, nor Seekers, nor of any race Rentarn had knowledge of. What he could see of their skin (they wore wrappings which covered most of it) was a dark blue. The hands of each were spread out so the withered fingers could lie upon a series of buttons upon lap boards which perhaps kept each in his chair.

From this scene, the pool, and the long dead, there thrust upward a beam of light. Even as Rentarn sighted it that beam pulsed again and again and then vanished. He drew in breath and expelled it again in a hiss which near carried away his mask. The hands of the dead had moved . . . pressing certain of those buttons.

While the thing in the pool dropped its scaled muzzle into the slimy flood and drank—or seemed to do so. Yet that was impossible, Rentarn's senses still told him there was no life here. If there had ever been it was long since gone.

Modic scrambled along the edge of the pool. His head no longer hung down but his features were twisted in such an expression of rage as Rentarn had never seen.

The Seeker's mouth worked as he threw his mask into the pool, his eyes never leaving Rentarn's face. Now he half turned and sprang forward to the nearest of those seats. His hands closed upon the body there and he jerked it out of its perch to the floor, catching and holding the board as the body fell. Now he seated himself

where the corpse had been . . . his fingers also spanning the board of buttons.

His whole body shook as he flung up his head and brayed wild laughter, his attention on the thing which had drunk and again raised its head to stare at Rentarn.

"The hour is now!" Modic's voice seemed to fill the place. He might have been shouting with the full power of his lungs. "Let that which purifies go forth and . . ." His finger tips played a fluttering game on the board. "This is the hour," he repeated. "Broken was the pattern when these died." He glanced at his dead companions. "Some of their training lives on as was meant. They rule the world. . . ." He leaned forward a little, spittle flicks on his lips, and yet he grinned and the wild exultation was not gone from his eyes. . . .

He nodded toward that thing on opposite bank of the pool. "How go things with you, oh, Farguel? Yes, you are dead and gone but the treasure you gave us still does its duty. See this one of your kin . . . he knows not even now what he has found . . . the root of that which had made a desert of blooming land. Dead!" He pounded his hand on the arm of the chair in which he sat. "We died too soon!" Again his face twisted in that horrifying way, as much of a mask as the one he had flung from him.

"We will it not!" He pulled at his underrobe as if it had begun to choke him. "Dead, we shall take with us a dead world. Come, brothern from the outer stars. We shall move even as we have planned, for that one," he looked to Rentarn, "shall be food for Farguel. So fed life will return . . . is that not so? Have not I, Thebar, returned in the body of this rover . . . little by little he became me . . . first as a whisper of treasure, and, when he had taken that, a stronger vision and a stronger. Until he saw himself a conqueror and a king! And he had heard of this guide who knew the desert so well and would provide him with the means of coming. . . . Ah, brothern, rejoice that I was strong, that though I was what men called dead, I was not, only abiding deep within another body waiting.

"Did I not grow the stronger even as the chosen one began to come nearer? Did I not bid him send those fool beasts who followed him ahead that they might be harvested? Yes, the doing

was mine . . . and now I shall be even as he who once wore this body . . . Lord of the world . . . a world!"

Again he screeched with laughter, and now he beckoned to Rentarn "Come here, Betweener . . . look at Farguel who is what our voice called from the swamp!" He gestured to the thing which drank.

"Once all you and your kin were as he. That day shall come again. For it is my will and desire, and only what I wish shall ever more happen here. Look you . . . and die!"

Rentarn had seen men before who came raving from the wasteland. This talk of bodies and of kingdoms yet to come . . . those were only the dreams of a broken-headed man. Yet when he watched the sureness of Modic's fingers on the board he had taken from the dead there was something in the man as well as in this place which no Betweener had ever mentioned, which no legend enshrined from other years. Who were those from the past who Modic called upon? And this thing which had now lifted its head again from the deep red flood and stood, its jaws dripping red? The thing which had no life, or never had had, but which moved even as he watched, teetering a little with its forepaws near into the flood.

Farguel, Modic had named it. There was no such name in Betweener clans nor did any of his kin walk upon all fours. That huge head swung a little toward him, the mouth gaped as if the thing could wish him to it for feasting.

But there was something wrong with that mouth! Great forefangs promised death . . . in the strange light they changed in color with waves of blue, green, yellow, red running up and down. Yes, he could see now . . . one of these was missing. Without conscious thought Rentarn swung up the broken knife he had brought out of the ruins, comparing that to the dread fangs which the creature wore. It was certainly the truth . . . what he had must be a fang . . . but from what jaw had it been taken? This beast? Surely it depended too much on luck for that to be the truth and Rentarn's kind were suspicious of such a thing as luck.

"SSaaa . . ." The sound was a hissing mighty enough to be from the throat of a king serpent himself, another traveler's tale the core

of which perhaps to be found here. Rentarn blinked and blinked again.

That thing was changing form before his eyes. In the desert wind devils could raise whole phantom cities to delude a traveler. Yet never had they called her a Betweener. Guides were immune to that troubling of sight.

The legs of the thing were being drawn back into its bloated body. It now rested its belly flat.

"No!" Where Modic had sat voicing insane laughter, he now arose in the chair, clasping the board before him, his fingers thudding home with force on the buttons. "Farguel!" he screamed at the hunched shape of that thing. "Farguel, down with you to the battle even as we set together in thoughts of what must be done. Was it not I, Thebar, who drew you from the swamp to this city, who delivered to you those who were as the beasts, only food to nourish you? Remember, once you fought before and there were those who did not run and scream and strive to hide against that which allowed no hiding. Farguel, this two-legged meat standing here is such a one as those who drove you back, who starved you of food and drink, who made you what you are . . . for I think, Farguel, you are no longer the death hunter you were when we sealed our bargain. Kill this one, Farguel, and prove that you are again great and awesome, so that those sent to bear you down shall themselves die between your fangs. Kill, Farguel!"

Surely this thing, for all its alteration of shape, was not alive as he sensed life! Rentarn watched it coil its serpent shape and lift high that head now losing all resemblance to his own. It opened wide its mouth and a broken line of fangs was fully bared. Not alive, not alive . . . Rentarn held to that thought with all his strength of will.

Yet he could not judge whether it would answer Modic's order or not. His right hand still held in sight the fang, while the fingers of the other moved, writing on the air an unseen pattern. He had believed that such learning was a legend mumbled over by the old ones of the clans, and when he had been set to learning all that finger play he had done so believing it was only a part of his training.

The great head halted in its reach across the flood. Rentarn felt a blow on his shoulder hard enough to numb his arm and near send him sprawling forward into the stream. Modic's board of control lay but inches away on the very lip of the pool.

"Farguel, strike . . . there is no way he can . . ."

Modic was out of the seat, had sunk to his knees as he still held one arm over the chair and was manifestly trying to draw himself up again.

Rentarn watched the creature closely. Its head stretched even higher, supported by a long neck. The open mouth displayed the loss of a front fang.

"Farguel . . ." Modic's voice was harsh but faint as if that of the dead. Rentarn fell back a step as he sensed what was happening to the Seeker. Life was receding. No, now, returned again in a wave with a desperate surge. Was Modic making a supreme effort against another force?

"SSaaa . . ." hissing from the beast. Then a singsong of words from Modic. Only those words were not in any language that the guide could understand, drilled though as he was in the three major languages and numerous dialects of Between and River lands. There was an authority in that chant. Instinctively Rentarn reached for the knife he did not wear. The Seeker huddled again in the chair, his features strangely bloated as if he put on another type of mask.

Whatever he said was addressed, not to Rentarn, but to the thing by the stream. Modic raised his hands jerkily and outspread them again as if the button board still rested on his knees. Then, seeming to understand dimly that that was gone, he voiced a wailing cry, such a sound as Rentarn had never heard before, but the peril of which he could taste with his flickering tongue.

Modic did not face the guide but, at that moment, Rentarn's body throbbed as if that sound reached within him to the very bones, took command of him, flesh and blood. The head of the creature begun to swing again. Rentarn, in spite of his struggle to command himself, moved toward the lip of the pool. Also . . . his feet no longer obeyed his will, instead they carried him forward. Though the Betweeners no longer owned any god or goddess, they still believed in a force for good and one for evil. The Speakers had told of old days when certain strong people, both male and

female, reached such heights of control that they could command even stones to move. Those were of yesteryear and few believed their like might even have lived. Rather most Betweeners said inwardly that such were but creatures of legends cast into words by early Speakers to give the clans some fear of the unknown and thus limit their wandering.

"Essar, Roqued, Alsa . . ." To drown out Modic's call or summons without words Rentarn roared full throatedly those names of great bravery and supreme command. He bent his mind toward the battle with raw fear, worked for the control of his body. To that purpose he repeated the roll of Sacred Dead in a battle song. The serpent thing was moving. It drew back its head, tensed muscles, and then . . .

Like a journey staff used as a lance, the head flashed toward Rentarn. By the thickness of a bavard leaf only did it miss seizing upon him.

Modic shrilled that cry a second time. The sound got inside Rentarn's head to cause a new kind of pain. "Essar!" he shouted back, or did he?

Was it true that he was answered, or merely that the tone and pitch of his voice cut through the sound spell Modic was weaving? Rentarn might never know. Anymore than he could tell why and how the warmth in the broken length of colored fang ran up his arm, through him, banishing Modic's influence. Out of the far beginnings of his kind shot a thought that at first was a dim shadow, like a fear in night time, to set him moving.

"Alsa . . ." he said to himself. Modic was being answered by another effort of the serpent creature. Its head launched out a second time across the stream which divided them. The open jaws hung poised above him, ready to seize. Rentarn braced himself. Though the thing was near enough now that it could breathe upon him, there was no breath . . . but a faint odor he had smelled many time before, Lacseed oil such as filled any lamp.

The jaws closed in as Rentarn waited. His hand swung up. He thrust the butt end of the rod he had found into that open hollow in the jaw. It settled there, fastened tightly, now a part of the dreadful set of fangs.

Then . . . there was a flash of orange and green, followed by

streams of light. The snakey head rose high. It twisted. Something shaped like a door broken open in its side. One of the weighty feet snapped off.

The scent of oil was throat thickening as the creature threw itself backward, heaving and twisting violently. A shudder and the fearsome head broke loose to fly through the air and smash against one of the chairs of the dead. Bits of wire and small fragments of metal erupted out of the headless body.

That floundered forward into the stream. For a moment or two the water boiled up about it in a mighty sweep of the current. One of the great talons flairing outward caught upon the board of buttons which Modic had fingered. As the mutilated thing dropped, it drew that with it. There followed a flash so bright that Rentarn cupped his hands over smarting eyes, able to see nothing but the scarlet light. But he heard. This was no more wailing encouragement from the Seeker, rather explosions or giant crashs such as might come from the fall of a rock or of a great tree.

Another odor filled the stagnant air. Rentarn pressed the mask dizzly. What he smelled, what his tongue tasted was oil burning, but with that other stenches he could not name. He rubbed his eyes. The second lid there may have saved him from total blindness for he could see, hazily, yet enough to witness what had followed the destruction of the serpent-headed thing.

You could not say it was dead, for his senses still assured him that it had never lived. But the great head had rolled along the edge of the pool. Steam or mist arose from that sickeningly, making him flick his tongue back behind tight lips. A dark smoke rolled along the passage which carried the flood out of the pool. There were flames within that, burning with the same violent colors as had painted the sky when the first of the city's weapons had been launched.

Those flames were not alone. The mummified bodies in the chairs each became a candle set alight by the boards they held. From the heart of each of those pulsed tongues of fire, but these were white.

Modic still huddled in the chair. His body writhed from side to side as if he were caught in a trap and was fighting feebly for freedom. The Seeker's face had changed, it was the countenance

of a stranger, a stranger who could not believe in what was happening to him. He screamed a fountain of words, beating upon the arms of the chair with his fists.

The head of the snake thing had rolled to the foot of the first of the chairs. From it still spilled oily liquid which quickly drew sparks of fire. When the head thudded to a stop it was upright and those huge eyes stared at the funeral fire of the dead.

"Farguel!"

There was loss of all sanity in that whimper. Modic leaned forward to the next chair, paying no attention to the smoldering body it still supported.

He spewed forth more words in an erratic pattern which held ghosts of the ritual sounds of a curse or incantation. Then suddenly he stopped—his head shifted and he tried to raise his hands.

"Farguel . . ."

The head with a tangle of molten metal still trailing into the burning stream stared with its round eyes back at him. Modic looked shriveled, empty, as he might have been one of the dead who shared his perch. Rentarn tested the air once again.

That nameless will which he had felt—centering for a while in Modic—was gone. The man was now what he had always been, a Seeker, sly, treacherous, greedy. Only he was rapidly becoming less and less of a man. Flooding out of him, even as the molten metal had flowed from the serpent's head, was that other—that strength which was not his but an unknown other's.

He used the arms of his chair to lever himself to his feet and stood gazing about the whole of this chamber as might a child who had awakened from a dark dream. There was a looseness to his lips, his shoulders hunched as if he was awaiting some punishment. He said, not looking towards Rentarn, but as if he spoke to himself:

"He . . . he is gone." His hands clenched on the chest of his under robe. The edge of it was scorched and there was a small trail of smoke coming from it. "He is . . ." now he shook his head as if to dislodge some insect. For the first time he appeared to recognize Rentarn and there was bemusement on both his face and in the way he staggered as he arose from the seat.

He leaned forward to stare down at the serpent, shivering.

"Farguel . . . there is no way . . . no way! They believe in the

demons . . . we cleared the city so . . . and then . . ." He paused, looked at the dying embers which had been the bodies. "What do I say?" Modic drew a hand across his face and let it fall limply to his side. "I am not he . . . but he remains in a little here." Again his hand arose, to touch his head "To be a king . . . more than a king . . . to rule a world. That *he* might have done. . . ." Then Modic lapsed into silence.

For the first time Rentarn spoke, "Who was he, Seeker?"

"He was—one who waited—and waited—from our beginnings they came, all of them." He raised his hand a little to indicate the remains in the other chairs. "They made Farguel." His voice was stronger, as if some small thread of another still curled in his mind. "They would be rulers here and *he* was the greatest among them. But when those they awaited did not come, they put barriers about the cities they had taken and sat to wait. How long did *you* wait?" He addressed the nearest chair as if that still held a living man. "Too long, too long. They said then that they would set up the final guards and sleep as they sometimes did when they traveled among the stars. So it was decided. But not by *him!* He went hunting always, hunting for that which would awaken the rest, take from them dreams of stars that they would learn of this world and what could be done here.

"*He* sent out power to poison the land, to be another barrier behind which he remained to labor. . . ."

Another pause. Modic dug his fists hard against his temples. "Why do I remember, tell me that, Guide? He holds . . . still he holds . . . and he will . . . No." Before Rentarn could move, Modic, his voice shrilling upward, as it had during his frenzy of his possession, threw himself down and out. His body struck against the disintegrating head of the thing he had called Farguel. He did not scream again as he slid on and out into the fire which flowed with the stream.

Rentarn retreated swiftly to the far wall of the hall, then leaped toward the entrance of the corridor. As if the death of Modic was the last fuel, flames flared behind, reaching so that he had to beat the fire from the edge of his cloak. But that other will . . . that power which had measured him so hungrily was gone. There was no life any longer in this place.

The guide reached the outermost part of the great palace or temple. Flames sped in waves along the sluggish stream. Only that light which had touched the sky was gone. Here was only a dry emptiness, an absence of all life within the ruin.

That which Rentarn had sensed as shadows of terror was also gone. He stood, his chest heaving from his run. All the stream was now afire.

He glanced back just once at the palace from which he had escaped. His tongue flicked out . . . all life was not gone. There was a whinny. The horse showed himself within the core of a long gone building, picking his way toward the guide. Rentarn's mind filled with surprise, then content. He and this animal were alive. The flame which destroyed the dead—the last of that was licking at the pool, flickering as what had fueled it was eaten up.

"Come." The guide crossed to the horse who nuzzled at his shoulder and whinneyed louder than before. "Let us get out of this place, brother—for it is of long dead and should be left to them in peace."

He swung up into the saddle. Willingly the horse turned without urging, pacing along that road which had led to the heart of Lonscraft.

Rentarn would never understand all which had happened, but his flickering tongue assured him of safety—here was only tumbled stone, dust, and a sprung trap. The destruction of the creature (he had to think of that as having life even though he could not sense it) and of the will of that other unknown which Modic had brought to half life, had perhaps reversed the poison of this dust-dry land and all it held. However let that be proven at some later time, by those who were born to be Seekers. For himself now, he wanted no more of the Dry. Thus he threaded a way between the masses of stone rubble until he passed beyond the gate of Lonscraft which once was.

ARTHUR C. CLARKE

b. 1917

When Arthur Charles Clarke was a teenager in London, in the years before World War II, his nickname among his fellow science fiction fans was "Ego" Clarke. They didn't mean it as an insult. It was only their way of recognizing the fact that, from childhood on, Clarke had a high opinion of his own abilities. His opinion was right on target, too; it just took a while for the rest of the world to confirm it.

Like many other fans of the period, Clarke wasn't merely interested in reading and writing about the future. He wanted to make it happen, and he wanted it to happen *soon*. There was the matter of space travel, for instance.

It was perfectly obvious to young Arthur Clarke that if you simply built the right kind of rocket it would take you to the Moon—or, if you had a little more time, to pretty nearly anywhere else you wanted to go in the universe. All that was lacking to make this come about was money and a certain amount of engineering, plus the will to make it happen. To help find ways of supplying those needs, Clarke became a member of the brand-new British Interplanetary Society (still well and functioning, more than sixty years later), eventually becoming its secretary. World War II, however, called a recess to that sort of long-range rocket planning—that is, not counting what Werner von Braun was doing on the other side of the Channel.

The war didn't stop Clarke from thinking about space, though, and as it was drawing to a close he single-handedly invented the modern orbiting geosynchronous communications satellite, in a pa-

per published in a technical journal. The article clearly spelled out the technology for what has since become a megabillion-dollar industry. For some years in the sixties and seventies Clarke was wont to muse wistfully over how his fortunes might have fared if he had only thought to patent the idea, instead of giving it away. (Actually, not all that well. Patents have a finite life span. By the time all the ancillary technology to make communications satellites real came along, the patent would have expired anyway; such are the penalties of being ahead of one's time.)

Then Clarke found his true vocation. (One of them, anyway.) For the fun of it he wrote a science fiction story, "Rescue Party." He mailed it off to John Campbell on the chance it might make it into *Astounding*. It did, and the rest is history.

"Rescue Party" was an unusual first story. It was perfectly formed; it would have done credit to any of the best sf writers around, and it made the fans eager for more. Clarke didn't disappoint. Over the next few years he published a good many first-rate stories, culminating with the two novels that confirmed his reputation in science fiction, *Childhood's End* and *Against the Fall of Night*. (Curiously, Clarke wasn't satisfied with *Against the Fall of Night*. Not long afterward he rewrote it substantially and reissued it under the title of *The City and the Stars*. For a time the two different versions of the story were offered for sale side by side in the bookstores.)

Then Clarke's life moved to a new plateau. He had published a nonfiction book on space travel. The manuscript was given to Basil Davenport, powerful editor of the Book-of-the-Month Club and a closet science fiction fan; Davenport loved it, fought for it against considerable opposition from other BOMC editors and judges and managed to get it issued as a main selection of the club. This brought with it a paycheck orders of magnitude higher than any Clarke had seen before; more important, it made Clarke a familiar figure to the host of Book-of-the-Month Club members who had never previously given a thought to any science fiction writer.

Then, a decade or two later, along came Stanley Kubrick.

Kubrick was one of the most adventurous and idiosyncratic of movie moguls. It seemed to Kubrick that there was something that might make a great film somewhere in science fiction, some kind

of theme that went beyond the usual crop of quickies and Japanese monster movies. Kubrick didn't, however, know exactly what. More or less at random, he bought film rights on a cluster of four of Clarke's short stories, but the more he thought about them the more he realized that they weren't precisely what he wanted to film.

Then he and Clarke met. They talked about what a truly great science fiction film might be and decided that one of the four stories—"The Sentinel"—contained the germ of a filmable script. Kubrick gave the other three stories back to Clarke, and signed him up to collaborate on a scenario.

I wish I might have been a fly on the wall, to listen in on some of those endless story conferences. These were two men who, though alike in self-confidence and in limited tolerance for being told what to do by others, differed fundamentally in their approach to creation. Clarke's methodology was straightforward: get an idea, start writing, see where it takes you. Kubrick was a tinkerer: shoot a scene, look it over, shoot it again in a different way, or maybe throw it out and shoot something entirely different. When at last a script was agreed on and filmed, and the sets struck and Clarke allowed to go off to begin writing the novel version, Kubrick holed up and created the light show that ends the film all by himself— leaving Clarke with the problem of trying to describe, in comprehensible words, what Kubrick had been getting at with his fuzzy symbolism. (And all this time—years of it—Clarke had been so fully occupied with working with Kubrick that his production of saleable fiction had suffered. Publishers were waiting for the book, with large amounts of money ready to pour into Clarke's coffers— but none of it would pour until the book was finally finished and delivered.)

But then it was all done. The film was *2001: A Space Odyssey*, and Clarke was famous to the largest world yet.

2001 (Clarke said) elevated his financial status from the "rich poor" to the "poor rich." It made it possible for him to pick and choose among the things he might do with his writing time, so that (he also said) he could limit himself to projects which, (1) were worth doing for their own sake, (2) offered worthwhile rewards, and (3) were such that he was the person who could do them better than anyone else. It also made it possible for him to leave chilly

England and move to the sunny, lovely tropical island nation of Sri Lanka, which has been his home ever since.

In the summer of 1970 Arthur and I, with Brian Aldiss, Judith Merril, and a clutch of Soviet science fiction writers, spent a couple of weeks in a sort of Chautauqua tour of Japan, from Tokyo to the vacation resort of Lake Biwa. It was a relaxing trip with a lot of fun things going on between lecture appearances—for example, Arthur Clarke doing a hula for a fascinated audience of Japanese science fiction fans—but he wasn't entirely carefree. The Tamil insurgents were shooting up parts of Sri Lanka in their effort (still ongoing now) to attain independence, and sometimes they were coming close to his home. However, he was in good health and good spirits. The next time I saw him, in New York City a year or so later, not quite so much so.

Arthur had become a convert to the sport and science of scuba diving, for which there is no better place in the world than the waters around Sri Lanka. He dove every chance he got, wrote books on the subject, explored old wrecks and came up with fistsful of ancient silver coins, enjoyed every moment of it . . . but then there was a small sort of diving accident. It triggered some problems left over from childhood illnesses, and in New York he was having some difficulty in getting out of particularly deep chairs. It didn't get better. The problem kept recurring, ultimately putting him in a wheelchair. . . .

But not in the least slowing down his remarkable literary productivity. It turned out there were quite a few projects that met his strictures. The books kept pouring out, and so did such other ventures as Clarke's own syndicated TV series, *Arthur C. Clarke's Mysterious World*. All those activities brought rewards to match. Arthur Clarke became chancellor of Sri Lanka's university, a friend of the nation's president, the person journalists from all over the world called up for a reaction every time there was a news story concerning space or science. And in 1997 came the final accolade. Her Majesty, Queen Elizabeth II, knighted him for his accomplishments.

The only thing that surprised his many admirers was that it had taken so long to occur. But occur it did. The title was formally conferred upon him in person by HRH, the Prince of Wales, and now, and for all time to come, he is to be known as *Sir* Arthur Charles Clarke.

Recommended Reading
by Arthur C. Clarke

2001: A Space Odyssey
Childhood's End
Against the Fall of Night/The City and the Stars
A Meeting with Medusa
Rendezvous with Rama

RESCUE PARTY

Who *was to blame?* For three days Alveron's thoughts had come back to that question, and still he had found no answer. A creature of a less civilized or a less sensitive race would never have let it torture his mind, and would have satisfied himself with the assurance that no one could be responsible for the working of fate. But Alveron and his kind had been lords of the Universe since the dawn of history, since that far distant age when the Time Barrier had been folded round the cosmos by the unknown powers that lay beyond the Beginning. To them had been given all knowledge— and with infinite knowledge went infinite responsibility. If there were mistakes and errors in the administration of the Galaxy, the fault lay on the heads of Alveron and his people. And this was no mere mistake: it was one of the greatest tragedies in history.

The crew still knew nothing. Even Rugon, his closest friend and the ship's deputy captain, had been told only part of the truth. But now the doomed worlds lay less than a billion miles ahead. In a few hours, they would be landing on the third planet.

Once again Alveron read the message from Base: then, with a flick of a tentacle that no human eye could have followed, he pressed the "General Attention" button. Throughout the mile-long cylinder that was the Galactic Survey Ship S9000, creatures of

many races laid down their work to listen to the words of their captain.

"I know you have all been wondering," began Alveron, "why we were ordered to abandon our survey and to proceed at such an acceleration to this region of space. Some of you may realize what this acceleration means. Our ship is on its last voyage: the generators have already been running for sixty hours at Ultimate Overload. We will be very lucky if we return to Base under our own power.

"We are approaching a sun which is about to become a Nova. Detonation will occur in seven hours, with an uncertainty of one hour, leaving us a maximum of only four hours for exploration. There are ten planets in the system about to be destroyed—*and there is a civilization on the third.* That fact was discovered only a few days ago. It is our tragic mission to contact that doomed race, and if possible to save some of its members. I know that there is little we can do in so short a time with this single ship. No other machine can possibly reach the system before detonation occurs."

There was a long pause during which there could have been no sound or movement in the whole of the mighty ship as it sped silently towards the worlds ahead. Alveron knew what his companions were thinking and he tried to answer their unspoken question.

"You will wonder how such a disaster, the greatest of which we have any record, has been allowed to occur. On one point I can reassure you. The fault does not lie with the Survey.

"As you know, with our present fleet of under twelve thousand ships, it is possible to re-examine each of the eight thousand million solar systems in the Galaxy at intervals of about a million years. Most worlds change very little in so short a time as that.

"Less than four hundred thousand years ago, the survey ship S5060 examined the planets of the system we are approaching. It found intelligence on none of them, though the third planet was teeming with animal life and two other worlds had once been inhabited. The usual report was submitted and the system is due for its next examination in six hundred thousand years.

"It now appears that in that incredibly short period since the last survey, intelligent life has appeared in the system. The first intimation of this occurred when unknown radio signals were de-

tected on the planet Kulath in the system X29.35, Y34.76, Z27.93. Bearings were taken on them and they were found to come from the system ahead.

"Kulath is two hundred light-years from here, so those radio waves had been on their way for two centuries. Thus for at least that period of time a civilization has existed on one of these worlds—a civilization that can generate electromagnetic waves and all that that implies.

"An immediate telescopic examination of the system was made and it was then found that the sun was in the unstable prenova stage. Detonation might occur at any moment, and indeed might have done so while the light waves were on their way to Kulath.

"There was a slight delay while the supervelocity scanners on Kulath II were focused on to the system. They showed that the explosion had not yet occurred but was only a few hours away. If Kulath had been a fraction of a light-year further from this sun, we should never have known of its civilization until it had ceased to exist.

"The Administrator of Kulath contacted Sector Base immediately, and I was ordered to proceed to the system at once. Our object is to save what members we can of the doomed race, if indeed there are any left. But we have assumed that a civilization possessing radio could have protected itself against any rise of temperature that may have already occurred.

"This ship and the two tenders will each explore a section of the planet. Commander Torkalee will take Number One, Commander Orostron Number Two. They will have just under four hours in which to explore this world. At the end of that time, they *must* be back in the ship. It will be leaving then, with or without them. I will give the two commanders detailed instructions in the control room immediately.

"That is all. We enter the atmosphere in two hours."

On the world once known as Earth the fires were dying out: there was nothing left to burn. The great forests that had swept across the planet like a tidal wave with the passing of the cities were now no more than glowing charcoal and the smoke of their funeral pyres

still stained the sky. But the last hours were still to come, for the surface rocks had not yet begun to flow. The continents were dimly visible through the haze, but their outlines meant nothing to the watchers in the approaching ship. The charts they possessed were out of date by a dozen Ice Ages and more deluges than one.

The S9000 had driven past Jupiter and seen at once that no life could exist in those half-gaseous oceans of compressed hydrocarbons, now erupting furiously under the sun's abnormal heat. Mars and the outer planets they had missed, and Alveron realized that the worlds nearer the sun than Earth would be already melting. It was more than likely, he thought sadly, that the tragedy of this unknown race was already finished. Deep in his heart, he thought it might be better so. The ship could only have carried a few hundred survivors, and the problem of selection had been haunting his mind.

Rugon, Chief of Communications and Deputy Captain, came into the control room. For the last hour he had been striving to detect radiation from Earth, but in vain.

"We're too late," he announced gloomily. "I've monitored the whole spectrum and the ether's dead except for our own stations and some two-hundred-year-old programs from Kulath. Nothing in this system is radiating any more."

He moved towards the giant vision screen with a graceful flowing motion that no mere biped could ever hope to imitate. Alveron said nothing: he had been expecting this news.

One entire wall of the control room was taken up by the screen, a great black rectangle that gave an impression of almost infinite depth. Three of Rugon's slender control tentacles, useless for heavy work but incredibly swift at all manipulation, flickered over the selector dials and the screen lit up with a thousand points of light. The star field flowed swiftly past as Rugon adjusted the controls, bringing the projector to bear upon the sun itself.

No man of Earth would have recognized the monstrous shape that filled the screen. The sun's light was no longer: great violet-blue clouds covered half its surface and from them long streamers of flame were erupting into space. At one point an enormous prominence had reared itself out of the photosphere, far out even into the flickering veils of the corona. It was as though a tree of fire had

taken root in the surface of the sun—a tree that stood half a million miles high and whose branches were rivers of flame sweeping through space at hundreds of miles a second.

"I suppose," said Rugon presently, "that you are quite satisfied about the astronomers' calculations. After all—"

"Oh, we're perfectly safe," said Alveron confidently. "I've spoken to Kulath Observatory and they have been making some additional checks through our own instruments. That uncertainty of an hour includes a private safety margin which they won't tell me in case I feel tempted to stay any longer."

He glanced at the instrument board.

"The pilot should have brought us to the atmosphere now. Switch the screen back to the planet, please. Ah, there they go!"

There was a sudden tremor underfoot and a raucous clanging of alarms, instantly stilled. Across the vision screen two slim projectiles dived towards the looming mass of Earth. For a few miles they traveled together: then they separated, one vanishing abruptly as it entered the shadow of the planet.

Slowly the huge mother ship, with its thousand times greater mass, descended after them into the raging storms that already were tearing down the deserted cities of Man.

It was night in the hemisphere over which Orostron drove his tiny command. Like Torkalee, his mission was to photograph and record, and to report progress to the mother ship. The little scout had no room for specimens or passengers. If contact was made with the inhabitants of this world, the S9000 would come at once. There would be no time for parleying. If there was any trouble the rescue would be by force and the explanations could come later.

The ruined land beneath was bathed with an eerie, flickering light, for a great auroral display was raging over half the world. But the image on the vision screen was independent of external light, and it showed clearly a waste of barren rock that seemed never to have known any form of life. Presumably this desert land must come to an end somewhere. Orostron increased his speed to the highest value he dared risk in so dense an atmosphere.

The machine fled on through the storm, and presently the desert of rock began to climb towards the sky. A great mountain range lay ahead, its peaks lost in the smoke-laden clouds. Orostron di-

rected the scanners towards the horizon, and on the vision screen the line of mountains seemed suddenly very close and menacing. He started to climb rapidly. It was difficult to imagine a more un-promising land in which to find civilization and he wondered if it would be wise to change course. He decided against it. Five minutes later, he had his reward.

Miles below lay a decapitated mountain, the whole of its sum-mit sheared away by some tremendous feat of engineering. Rising out of the rock and straddling the artificial plateau was an intricate structure of metal girders, supporting masses of machinery. Orostron brought his ship to a halt and spiraled down towards the mountain.

The slight Doppler blur had now vanished, and the picture on the screen was clear-cut. The lattice-work was supporting some scores of great metal mirrors, pointing skyward at an angle of forty-five degrees to the horizontal. They were slightly concave, and each had some complicated mechanism at its focus. There seemed some-thing impressive and purposeful about the great array; every mirror was aimed at precisely the same spot in the sky—or beyond.

Orostron turned to his colleagues.

"It looks like some kind of observatory to me," he said. "Have you ever seen anything like it before?"

Klarten, a multitentacled, tripedal creature from a globular clus-ter at the edge of the Milky Way, had a different theory.

"That's communication equipment. Those reflectors are for fo-cusing electromagnetic beams. I've seen the same kind of installa-tion on a hundred worlds before. It may even be the station that Kulath picked up—though that's rather unlikely, for the beams would be very narrow from mirrors that size."

"That would explain why Rugon could detect no radiation be-fore we landed," added Hansur II, one of the twin beings from the planet Thargon.

Orostron did not agree at all.

"If that *is* a radio station, it must be built for interplanetary communication. Look at the way the mirrors are pointed. I don't believe that a race which has only had radio for two centuries can have crossed space. It took my people six thousand years to do it."

"We managed it in three," said Hansur II mildly, speaking a few seconds ahead of his twin. Before the inevitable argument could

develop, Klarten began to wave his tentacles with excitement. While the others had been talking, he had started the automatic monitor.

"Here it is! Listen!"

He threw a switch, and the little room was filled with a raucous whining sound, continually changing in pitch but nevertheless retaining certain characteristics that were difficult to define.

The four explorers listened intently for a minute; then Orostron said: "Surely that can't be any form of speech! No creature could produce sounds as quickly as that!"

Hansur I had come to the same conclusion.

"That's a television program. Don't you think so, Klarten?"

The other agreed.

"Yes, and each of those mirrors seems to be radiating a different program. I wonder where they're going? If I'm correct, one of the other planets in the system must lie along those beams. We can soon check that."

Orostron called the S9000 and reported the discovery. Both Rugon and Alveron were greatly excited, and made a quick check of the astronomical records.

The result was surprising—and disappointing. None of the other nine planets lay anywhere near the line of transmission. The great mirrors appeared to be pointing blindly into space.

There seemed only one conclusion to be drawn, and Klarten was the first to voice it.

"They *had* interplanetary communication," he said. "But the station must be deserted now, and the transmitters no longer controlled. They haven't been switched off, and are just pointing where they were left."

"Well, we'll soon find out," said Orostron. "I'm going to land."

He brought the machine slowly down to the level of the great metal mirrors, and past them until it came to rest on the mountain rock. A hundred yards away, a white stone building crouched beneath the maze of steel girders. It was windowless, but there were several doors in the wall facing them.

Orostron watched his companions climb into their protective suits and wished he could follow. But someone had to stay in the machine to keep in touch with the mother ship. Those were Al-

veron's instructions, and they were very wise. One never knew what would happen on a world that was being explored for the first time, especially under conditions such as these.

Very cautiously, the three explorers stepped out of the air lock and adjusted the antigravity field of their suits. Then, each with the mode of locomotion peculiar to his race, the little party went towards the building, the Hansur twins leading and Klarten following close behind. His gravity control was apparently giving trouble, for he suddenly fell to the ground, rather to the amusement of his colleagues. Orostron saw them pause for a moment at the nearest door—then it opened and they disappeared from sight.

So Orostron waited, with what patience he could, while the storm rose around him and the light of the aurora grew ever brighter in the sky. At the agreed times he called the mother ship and received brief acknowledgements from Rugon. He wondered how Torkalee was faring, halfway round the planet, but he could not contact him through the crash and thunder of solar interference.

It did not take Klarten and the Hansurs long to discover that their theories were largely correct. The building was a radio station, and it was deserted. It consisted of one tremendous room with a few small offices leading from it. In the main chamber, row after row of electrical equipment stretched into the distance; lights flickered and winked on hundreds of control panels, and a dull glow came from the elements in a great avenue of vacuum tubes.

But Klarten was not impressed. The first radio sets his race had built were now fossilized in strata a thousand million years old. Man, who had possessed electrical machines for only a few centuries, could not compete with those who had known them for half the lifetime of the Earth.

Nevertheless, the party kept their recorders running as they explored the building. There was still one problem to be solved. The deserted station was broadcasting programs—but where were they coming from? The central switchboard had been quickly located. It was designed to handle scores of programs simultaneously, but the source of those programs was lost in a maze of cables that vanished underground. Back in the S9000, Rugon was trying to analyze the broadcasts and perhaps his researchers would reveal

their origin. It was impossible to trace cables that might lead across continents.

The party wasted little time at the deserted station. There was nothing they could learn from it, and they were seeking life rather than scientific information. A few minutes later the little ship rose swiftly from the plateau and headed towards the plains that must lie beyond the mountains. Less than three hours were still left to them.

As the array of enigmatic mirrors dropped out of sight, Orostron was struck by a sudden thought. Was it imagination, or had they all moved through a small angle while he had been waiting, as if they were still compensating for the rotation of the Earth? He could not be sure, and he dismissed the matter as unimportant. It would only mean that the directing mechanism was still working, after a fashion.

They discovered the city fifteen minutes later. It was a great, sprawling metropolis, built around a river that had disappeared leaving an ugly scar winding its way among the great buildings and beneath bridges that looked very incongruous now.

Even from the air, the city looked deserted. But only two and a half hours were left—there was no time for further exploration. Orostron made his decision, and landed near the largest structure he could see. It seemed reasonable to suppose that some creatures would have sought shelter in the strongest buildings, where they would be safe until the very end.

The deepest coves—the heart of the planet itself—would give no protection when the final cataclysm came. Even if this race had reached the outer planets, its doom would only be delayed by the few hours it would take for the ravening wavefronts to cross the Solar System.

Orostron could not know that the city had been deserted not for a few days or weeks, but for over a century. For the culture of cities, which had outlasted so many civilizations, had been doomed at last when the helicopter brought universal transportation. Within a few generations the great masses of mankind, knowing that they could reach any part of the globe in a matter of hours, had gone back to the fields and forests for which they had always

longed. The new civilization had machines and resources of which earlier ages had never dreamed, but it was essentially rural and no longer bound to the steel and concrete warrens that had dominated the centuries before. Such cities that still remained were specialized centers of research, administration or entertainment; the others had been allowed to decay where it was too much trouble to destroy them. The dozen or so greatest of all cities, and the ancient university towns, had scarcely changed and would have lasted for many generations to come. But the cities that had been founded on steam and iron and surface transportation had passed with the industries that had nourished them.

And so while Orostron waited in the tender, his colleagues raced through endless empty corridors and deserted halls, taking innumerable photographs but learning nothing of the creatures who had used these buildings. There were libraries, meeting places, council rooms, thousands of offices—all were empty and deep with dust. If they had not seen the radio station on its mountain eyrie, the explorers could well have believed that this world had known no life for centuries.

Through the long minutes of waiting, Orostron tried to imagine where this race could have vanished. Perhaps they had killed themselves knowing that escape was impossible; perhaps they had built great shelters in the bowels of the planet, and even now were cowering in their millions beneath his feet, waiting for the end. He began to fear that he would never know.

It was almost a relief when at last he had to give the order for the return. Soon he would know if Torkalee's party had been more fortunate. And he was anxious to get back to the mother ship, for as the minutes passed the suspense had become more and more acute. There had always been the thought in his mind: "What if the astronomers of Kulath have made a mistake?" He would begin to feel happy when the walls of the S9000 were around him. He would be happier still when they were out in space and this ominous sun was shrinking far astern.

As soon as his colleagues had entered the air lock, Orostron hurled his tiny machine into the sky and set the controls to home on the S9000. Then he turned to his friends.

"Well, what have you found?" he asked.

Klarten produced a large roll of canvas and spread it out on the floor.

"This is what they were like," he said quietly. "Bipeds, with only two arms. They seem to have managed well, in spite of that handicap. Only two eyes as well, unless there are others in the back. We were lucky to find this; it's about the only thing they left behind."

The ancient oil painting stared stonily back at the three creatures regarding it so intently. By the irony of fate, its complete worthlessness had saved it from oblivion. When the city had been evacuated, no one had bothered to move Alderman John Richards, 1909–1974. For a century and a half he had been gathering dust while far away from the old cities the new civilization had been rising to heights no earlier culture had ever known.

"That was almost all we found," said Klarten. "The city must have been deserted for years. I'm afraid our expedition has been a failure. If there are any living beings on this world, they've hidden themselves too well for us to find them."

His commander was forced to agree.

"It was an almost impossible task," he said. "If we'd had weeks instead of hours we might have succeeded. For all we know, they may even have built shelters under the sea. No one seems to have thought of that."

He glanced quickly at the indicators and corrected the course.

"We'll be there in five minutes. Alveron seems to be moving rather quickly. I wonder if Torkalee has found anything?"

The S9000 was hanging a few miles above the seaboard of a blazing continent when Orostron homed upon it. The danger line was thirty minutes away and there was no time to lose. Skillfully, he maneuvered the little ship into its launching tube and the party stepped out of the air lock.

There was a small crowd waiting for them. That was to be expected, but Orostron could see at once that something more than curiosity had brought his friends here. Even before a word was spoken, he knew that something was wrong.

"Torkalee hasn't returned. He's lost his party and we're going to the rescue. Come along to the control room at once."

•   •   •

From the beginning, Torkalee had been luckier than Orostron. He had followed the zone of twilight, keeping away from the intolerable glare of the sun, until he came to the shores of an inland sea. It was a very recent sea, one of the latest of Man's works, for the land it covered had been desert less than a century before. In a few hours it would be desert again, for the water was boiling and clouds of steam were rising to the skies. But they could not veil the loveliness of the great white city that overlooked the tideless sea.

Flying machines were still parked neatly round the square in which Torkalee landed. They were disappointingly primitive, though beautifully finished, and depended on rotating airfoils for support. Nowhere was there any sign of life, but the place gave the impression that its inhabitants were not very far away. Lights were still shining from some of the windows.

Torkalee's three companions lost no time in leaving the machine. Leader of the party, by seniority of rank and race was T'sinadree, who like Alveron himself had been born on one of the ancient planets of the Central Suns. Next came Alarkane, from a race which was one of the youngest in the Universe and took a perverse pride in the fact. Last came one of the strange beings from the system of Palador. It was nameless, like all its kind, for it possessed no identity of its own, being merely a mobile but still dependent cell in the consciousness of its race. Though it and its fellows had long been scattered over the Galaxy in the exploration of countless worlds, some unknown link still bound them together as inexorably as the living cells in a human body.

When a creature of Palador spoke, the pronoun it used was always "We." There was not, nor could there ever be, any first person singular in the language of Palador.

The great doors of the splendid building baffled the explorers, though any human child would have known their secret. T'sinadree wasted no time on them but called Torkalee on his personal transmitter. Then the three hurried aside while their commander maneuvered his machine into the best position. There was a brief burst of intolerable flame; the massive steelwork flickered once at the edge of the visible spectrum and was gone. The stones were still

glowing when the eager party hurried into the building, the beams of their light projectors fanning before them.

The torches were not needed. Before them lay a great hall, glowing with light from lines of tubes along the ceiling. On either side, the hall opened out into long corridors, while straight ahead a massive stairway swept majestically towards the upper floors.

For a moment T'sinadree hesitated. Then, since one way was as good as another, he led his companions down the first corridor.

The feeling that life was near had now become very strong. At any moment, it seemed, they might be confronted by the creatures of this world. If they showed hostility—and they could scarcely be blamed if they did—the paralyzers would be used at once.

The tension was very great as the party entered the first room, and only relaxed when they saw that it held nothing but machines—row after row of them, now stilled and silent. Lining the enormous room were thousands of metal filing cabinets, forming a continuous wall as far as the eye could reach. And that was all; there was no furniture, nothing but the cabinets and the mysterious machines.

Alarkane, always the quickest of the three, was already examining the cabinets. Each held many thousand sheets of tough, thin material, perforated with innumerable holes and slots: The Paladorian appropriated one of the cards and Alarkane recorded the scene together with some close-ups of the machines. Then they left. The great room, which had been one of the marvels of the world, meant nothing to them. No living eye would ever again see that wonderful battery of almost human Hollerith analyzers and the five thousand million punched cards holding all that could be recorded of each man, woman and child on the planet.

It was clear that this building had been used very recently. With growing excitement, the explorers hurried on to the next room. This they found to be an enormous library, for millions of books lay all around them on miles and miles of shelving. Here, though the explorers could not know it, were the records of all the laws that Man had ever passed, and all the speeches that had ever been made in his council chambers.

T'sinadree was deciding his plan of action when Alarkane drew his attention to one of the racks a hundred yards away. It was half

empty, unlike all the others. Around it books lay in a tumbled heap on the floor, as if knocked down by someone in frantic haste. The signs were unmistakable. Not long ago, other creatures had been this way. Faint wheel marks were clearly visible on the floor to the acute sense of Alarkane, though the others could see nothing. Alarkane could even detect footprints, but knowing nothing of the creatures that had formed them he could not say which way they led.

The sense of nearness was stronger than ever now, but it was nearness in time, not in space. Alarkane voiced the thoughts of the party.

"Those books must have been valuable, and someone has come to rescue them—rather as an afterthought, I should say. That means there must be a place of refuge, possibly not very far away. Perhaps we may be able to find some other clues that will lead us to it."

T'sinadree agreed, but the Paladorian refused to be enthusiastic.

"That may be so," it said, "but the refuge may be anywhere on the planet, and we have just two hours left. Let us waste no more time if we hope to rescue these people."

The party hurried forward once more, pausing only to collect a few books that might be useful to the scientists at Base—though it was doubtful if they could ever be translated. They soon found that the great building was composed largely of small rooms, all showing signs of recent occupation. Most of them were in a neat and tidy condition, but one or two were very much the reverse. The explorers were particularly puzzled by one room—clearly an office of some kind—that appeared to have been completely wrecked. The floor was littered with papers, the furniture had been smashed, and smoke was pouring through the broken windows from the fires outside.

T'sinadree was rather alarmed.

"Surely no dangerous animal could have got into a place like this!" he exclaimed, fingering his paralyzer nervously.

Alarkane did not answer. He began to make that annoying sound which his race called "laughter." It was several minutes before he would explain what had amused him.

"I don't think any animal has done it," he said. "In fact, the explanation is very simple. Suppose you had been working all your life in this room, dealing with endless papers, year after year. And

suddenly, you are told that you will never see it again, that your work is finished, and that you can leave it forever. More than that—no one will come after you. *Everything* is finished. How would you make your exit, T'sinadree?"

The other thought for a moment.

"Well, I suppose I'd just tidy things up and leave. That's what seems to have happened in all the other rooms."

Alarkane laughed again.

"I'm quite sure you would. But some individuals have a different psychology. I think I should have liked the creature that used this room."

He did not explain himself further, and his two colleagues puzzled over his words for quite a while before they gave it up.

It came as something of a shock when Torkalee gave the order to return. They had gathered a great deal of information, but had found no clue that might lead them to the missing inhabitants of this world. That problem was as baffling as ever, and now it seemed that it would never be solved. There were only forty minutes left before the *S9000* would be departing.

They were halfway back to the tender when they saw the semicircular passage leading down into the depths of the building. Its architectural style was quite different from that used elsewhere, and the gently sloping floor was an irresistible attraction to creatures whose many legs had grown weary of the marble staircases which only bipeds could have built in such profusion. T'sinadree had been the worst sufferer, for he normally employed twelve legs and could use twenty when he was in a hurry—though no one had ever seen him perform this feat.

The party stopped dead and looked down the passageway with a single thought. A *tunnel, leading down into the depths of the earth.* At its end, they might yet find the people of this world and rescue some of them from their fate. For there was still time to call the mother ship if the need arose.

T'sinadree signaled to his commander and Torkalee brought the little machine immediately overhead. There might not be time for the party to retrace its footsteps through the maze of passages, so meticulously recorded in the Paladorian mind that there was no possibility of going astray. If speed were necessary, Torkalee could

blast his way through the dozen floors above their head. In any case, it should not take long to find what lay at the end of the passage.

It took only thirty seconds. The tunnel ended quite abruptly in a very curious cylindrical room with magnificently padded seats along the walls. There was no way out save that by which they had come and it was several seconds before the purpose of the chamber dawned on Alarkane's mind. It was a pity, he thought, that they would never have time to use this. The thought was suddenly interrupted by a cry from T'sinadree. Alarkane wheeled around, and saw that the entrance had closed silently behind them.

Even in that first moment of panic, Alarkane found himself thinking with some admiration: "Whoever they were, they knew how to build automatic machinery!"

The Paladorian was the first to speak. It waved one of its tendrils towards the seats.

"We think it would be best to be seated," it said. The multiplex mind of Palador had already analyzed the situation and knew what was coming.

They did not have long to wait before a low-pitched hum came from a grille overhead, and for the very last time in history a human, even if lifeless, voice was heard on Earth. The words were meaningless, though the trapped explorers could guess their message clearly enough.

"Choose your stations, please, and be seated."

Simultaneously, a wall panel at one end of the compartment glowed with light. On it was a simple map, consisting of a series of a dozen circles connected by a line. Each of the circles had writing alongside it, and beside the writing were two buttons of different colors.

Alarkane looked questiongly at his leader.

"Don't touch them," said T'sinadree. "If we leave the controls alone, the doors may open again."

He was wrong. The engineers who had designed the automatic subway had assumed that anyone who entered it would naturally wish to go somewhere. If they selected no intermediate station, their destination could only be the end of the line.

There was another pause while the relays and thyratrons waited

for their orders. In those thirty seconds, if they had known what to do, the party could have opened the doors and left the subway. But they did not know, and the machines geared to a human psychology acted for them.

The surge of acceleration was not very great; the lavish upholstery was a luxury, not a necessity. Only an almost imperceptible vibration told of the speed at which they were traveling through the bowels of the earth, on a journey the duration of which they could not even guess. And in thirty minutes, the S9000 would be leaving the Solar System.

There was a long silence in the speeding machine. T'sinadree and Alarkane were thinking rapidly. So was the Paladorian, though in a different fashion. The conception of personal death was meaningless to it, for the destruction of a single unit meant no more to the group mind than the loss of a nail-paring to a man. But it could, though with great difficulty, appreciate the plight of individual intelligences such as Alarkane and T'sinadree, and it was anxious to help them if it could.

Alarkane had managed to contact Torkalee with his personal transmitter, though the signal was very weak and seemed to be fading quickly. Rapidly he explained the situation, and almost at once the signals became clearer. Torkalee was following the path of the machine, flying above the ground under which they were speeding to their unknown destination. That was the first indication they had of the fact that they were traveling at nearly a thousand miles an hour, and very soon after that Torkalee was able to give the still more disturbing news that they were rapidly approaching the sea. While they were beneath the land, there was a hope, though a slender one, that they might stop the machine and escape. But under the ocean—not all the brains and the machinery in the great mother ship could save them. No one could have devised a more perfect trap.

T'sinadree had been examining the wall map with great attention. Its meaning was obvious, and along the line connecting the circles a tiny spot of light was crawling. It was already halfway to the first of the stations marked.

"I'm going to press one of those buttons," said T'sinadree at last. "It won't do any harm, and we may learn something."

"I agree. Which will you try first?"

"There are only two kinds, and it won't matter if we try the wrong one first. I suppose one is to start the machine and the other is to stop it."

Alarkane was not very hopeful.

"It started without any button pressing," he said. "I think it's completely automatic and we can't control it from here at all."

T'sinadree could not agree.

"These buttons are clearly associated with the stations, and there's no point in having them unless you can use them to stop yourself. The only question is, which is the right one?"

His analysis was perfectly correct. The machine could be stopped at any intermediate station. They had only been on their way ten minutes, and if they could leave now, no harm would have been done. It was just bad luck that T'sinadree's first choice was the wrong button.

The little light on the map crawled slowly through the illuminated circle without checking its speed. And at the same time Torkalee called from the ship overhead.

"You have just passed underneath a city and are heading out to sea. There cannot be another stop for nearly a thousand miles."

Alveron had given up all hope of finding life on this world. The S9000 had roamed over half the planet, never staying long in one place, descending ever and again in an effort to attract attention. There had been no response; Earth seemed utterly dead. If any of its inhabitants were still alive, thought Alveron, they must have hidden themselves in its depths where no help could reach them, though their doom would be none the less certain.

Rugon brought news of the disaster. The great ship ceased its fruitless searching and fled back through the storm to the ocean above which Torkalee's little tender was still following the track of the buried machine.

The scene was truly terrifying. Not since the days when Earth was born had there been such seas as this. Mountains of water were racing before the storm which had now reached velocities of many hundred miles an hour. Even at this distance from the mainland

the air was full of flying debris—trees, fragments of houses, sheets of metal, anything that had not been anchored to the ground. No airborne machine could have lived for a moment in such a gale. And ever and again even the roar of the wind was drowned as the vast water-mountains met head-on with a crash that seemed to shake the sky.

Fortunately, there had been no serious earthquakes yet. Far beneath the bed of the ocean, the wonderful piece of engineering which had been the world president's private vacuum-subway was still working perfectly, unaffected by the tumult and destruction above. It would continue to work until the last minute of the Earth's existence, which, if the astronomers were right, was not much more than fifteen minutes away—though precisely how much more, Alveron would have given a great deal to know. It would be nearly an hour before the trapped party could reach land and even the slightest hope of rescue.

Alveron's instructions had been precise, though even without them he would never have dreamed of taking any risks with the great machine that had been intrusted to his care. Had he been human, the decision to abandon the trapped members of his crew would have been desperately hard to make. But he came of a race far more sensitive than Man, a race that so loved the things of the spirit that long ago, and with infinite reluctance, it had taken over control of the Universe since only thus could it be sure that justice was being done. Alveron would need all his superhuman gifts to carry him through the next few hours.

Meanwhile, a mile below the bed of the ocean Alarkane and T'sinadree were very busy indeed with their private communicators. Fifteen minutes is not a long time in which to wind up the affairs of a lifetime. It is indeed, scarcely long enough to dictate more than a few of those farewell messages which at such moments are so much more important than all other matters.

All the while the Paladorian had remained silent and motionless, saying not a word. The other two, resigned to their fate and engrossed in their personal affairs, had given it no thought. They were startled when suddenly it began to address them in its peculiarly passionless voice.

"We perceive that you are making certain arrangements con-

cerning your anticipated destruction. That will probably be unnecessary. Captain Alveron hopes to rescue us if we can stop this machine when we reach land again."

Both T'sinadree and Alarkane were too surprised to say anything for a moment. Then the latter gasped, "How do you know?"

It was a foolish question for he remembered at once that there were several Paladorians—if one could use the phrase—in the S9000, and consequently their companion knew everything that was happening in the mother ship. So he did not wait for an answer but continued: "Alveron can't do that! He daren't take such a risk!"

"There will be no risk," said the Paladorian. "We have told him what to do. It is really very simple."

Alarkane and T'sinadree looked at their companion with something approaching awe, realizing now what must have happened. In moments of crisis, the single units comprising the Paladorian mind could link together in an organization no less close than that of any physical brain. At such moments they formed an intellect more powerful than any other in the Universe. All ordinary problems could be solved by a few hundred or thousand units. Very rarely millions would be needed, and on two historic occasions the billions of cells of the entire Paladorian consciousness had been welded together to deal with emergencies that threatened the race. The mind of Palador was one of the greatest mental resources of the Universe; its full force was seldom required, but the knowledge that it was available was supremely comforting to other races. Alarkane wondered how many cells had co-ordinated to deal with this particular emergency. He also wondered how so trivial an incident had ever come to its attention at all.

To that question he was never to know the answer, though he might have guessed it had he known that the chillingly remote Paladorian mind possessed an almost human streak of vanity. Long ago, Alarkane had written a book trying to prove that eventually all intelligent races would sacrifice individual consciousness and that one day only group minds would remain in the Universe. Palador, he had said, was the first of those ultimate intellects, and the vast, dispersed mind had not been displeased.

They had no time to ask any further questions before Alveron himself began to speak through their communicators.

"Alveron calling! We're staying on this planet until the detonation wave reaches it, so we may be able to rescue you. You're
heading towards a city on the coast which you'll reach in forty
minutes at your present speed. If you cannot stop yourselves then,
we're going to blast the tunnel behind and ahead of you to cut off
your power. Then we'll sink a shaft to get you out—the chief engineer says he can do it in five minutes with the main projectors.
So you should be safe within an hour, unless the sun blows up
before."

"And if that happens, you'll be destroyed as well! You mustn't
take such a risk!"

"Don't let that worry you; we're perfectly safe. When the sun
detonates, the explosion wave will take several minutes to rise to its
maximum. But apart from that, we're on the night side of the planet,
behind an eight-thousand-mile screen of rock. When the first warning of the explosion comes, we will accelerate out of the Solar System, keeping in the shadow of the planet. Under our maximum
drive, we will reach the velocity of light before leaving the cone
of shadow, and the sun cannot harm us then."

T'sinadree was still afraid to hope. Another objection came at
once into his mind.

"Yes, but how will you get any warning, here on the night side
of the planet?"

"Very easily," replied Alveron. "This world has a moon which
is now visible from this hemisphere. We have telescopes trained on
it. If it shows any sudden increase in brilliance, our main drive goes
on automatically and we'll be thrown out of the system."

The logic was flawless. Alveron, cautious as ever, was taking
no chances. It would be many minutes before the eight-thousand-
mile shield of rock and metal could be destroyed by the fires of the
exploding sun. In that time, the S9000 could have reached the
safety of the velocity of light.

Alarkane pressed the second button when they were still several miles from the coast. He did not expect anything to happen
then, assuming that the machine could not stop between stations.
It seemed too good to be true when, a few minutes later, the machine's slight vibration died away and they came to a halt.

The doors slid silently apart. Even before they were fully open,

the three had left the compartment. They were taking no more chances. Before them a long tunnel stretched into the distance rising slowly out of sight. They were starting along it when suddenly Alveron's voice called from the communicators.

"Stay where you are! We're going to blast!"

The ground shuddered once, and far ahead there came the rumble of falling rock. Again the earth shook—and a hundred yards ahead the passageway vanished abruptly. A tremendous vertical shaft had been cut clean through it.

The party hurried forward again until they came to the end of the corridor and stood waiting on its lip. The shaft in which it ended was a full thousand feet across and descended into the earth as far as the torches could throw their beams. Overhead, the storm clouds fled beneath a moon that no man would have recognized, so luridly brilliant was its disk. And, most glorious of all sights, the S9000 floated high above, the great projectors that had drilled this enormous pit still glowing cherry red.

A dark shape detached itself from the mother ship and dropped swiftly towards the ground. Torkalee was returning to collect his friends. A little later, Alveron greeted them in the control room. He waved to the great vision screen and said quietly:

"You see, we were only just in time."

The continent below them was slowly settling beneath the mile-high waves that were attacking its coasts. The last that anyone was ever to see of Earth was a great plain, bathed with the silver light of the abnormally brilliant moon. Across its face the waters were pouring in a glittering flood towards a distant range of mountains. The sea had won its final victory, but its triumph would be short-lived for soon sea and land would be no more. Even as the silent party in the control room watched the destruction below, the infinitely greater catastrophe to which this was only the prelude came swiftly upon them.

It was as though dawn had broken suddenly over this moonlit landscape. But it was not dawn: it was only the moon, shining with the brilliance of a second sun. For perhaps thirty seconds that awesome, unnatural light burnt fiercely on the doomed land beneath. Then there came a sudden flashing of indicator lights across the control board. The main drive was on. For a second Alveron

glanced at the indicators and checked their information. When he looked again at the screen, Earth was already gone.

The magnificent, desperately overstrained generators quietly died when the S9000 was passing the orbit of Persephone. It did not matter, the sun could never harm them now, and although the ship was speeding helplessly out into the lonely night of interstellar space, it would only be a matter of days before rescue came.

There was irony in that. A day ago, they had been the rescuers, going to the aid of a race that now no longer existed. Not for the first time Alveron wondered about the world that had just perished. He tried, in vain, to picture it as it had been in its glory, the streets of its cities thronged with life. Primitive though its people had been, they might have offered much to the Universe later in history. If only they could have made contact! Regret was useless: long before their coming, the people of this world must have buried themselves in its iron heart. And now they and their civilization would remain a mystery for the rest of time.

Alveron was glad when his thoughts were interrupted by Rugon's entrance. The chief of communications had been very busy ever since the take-off, trying to analyze the programs radiated by the transmitter Orostron had discovered. The problem was not a difficult one, but it demanded the construction of special equipment, and that had taken time.

"Well, what have you found?" asked Alveron.

"Quit a lot," replied his friend. "There's something mysterious here, and I don't understand it.

"It didn't take long to find how the vision transmissions were built up, and we've been able to convert them to suit our own equipment. It seems that there were cameras all over the planet, surveying points of interest. Some of them were apparently in cities, on the tops of very high buildings. The cameras were rotating continuously to give panoramic views. In the programs we've recorded there are about twenty different scenes.

"In addition, there are a number of transmissions of a different kind, neither sound nor vision. They seem to be purely scientific— possibly instrument readings or something of that sort. All these programs were going out simultaneously on different frequency bands.

"Now there must be a reason for all this. Orostron still thinks that the station simply wasn't switched off when it was deserted. But these aren't the sort of programs such a station would normally radiate at all. It was certainly used for interplanetary relaying—Klarten was quite right there. So these people must have crossed space, since none of the other planets had any life at the time of the last survey. Don't you agree?"

Alveron was following intently.

"Yes, that seems reasonable enough. But it's also certain that the beam was pointing to none of the other planets. I checked that myself."

"I know," said Rugon. "What I want to discover is why a giant interplanetary relay station is busily transmitting pictures of a world about to be destroyed—*pictures that would be of immense interest to scientists and astronomers*. Someone had gone to a lot of trouble to arrange all those panoramic cameras. I am convinced that those beams were going *somewhere*."

Alveron started up.

"Do you imagine that there might be an outer planet that hasn't been reported?" he asked. "If so, your theory's certainly wrong. The beam wasn't even pointing in the plane of the Solar System. And even if it were—just look at this."

He switched on the vision screen and adjusted the controls. Against the velvet curtain of space was hanging a blue-white sphere, apparently composed of many concentric shells of incandescent gas. Even though its immense distance made all movement invisible, it was clearly expanding at an enormous rate. At its center was a blinding point of light—the white dwarf star that the sun had now become.

"You probably don't realize just how big that sphere is," said Alveron. "Look at this."

He increased the magnification until only the center portion of the nova was visible. Close to its heart were two minute condensations, one on either side of the nucleus.

"Those are the two giant planets of the system. They have still managed to retain their existence—after a fashion. And they were several hundred million miles from the sun.

"The nova is still expanding—but it's already twice the size of the Solar System."

Rugon was silent for a moment.

"Perhaps you're right," he said, rather grudgingly. "You've disposed of my first theory. But you still haven't satisfied me."

He made several swift circuits of the room before speaking again. Alveron waited patiently, he knew the almost intuitive powers of his friend, who could often solve a problem when mere logic seemed insufficient.

Then, rather slowly, Rugon began to speak again.

"What do you think of this?" he said. "Suppose we've completely underestimated this people? Orostron did it once—he thought they could never have crossed space, since they'd only known radio for two centuries. Hansur II told me that. Well, Orostron was quite wrong. Perhaps we're all wrong. I've had a look at the material that Klarten brought back from the transmitter. He wasn't impressed by what he found, but it's a marvelous achievement for so short a time. There were devices in that station that belonged to civilizations thousands of years older. *Alveron, can we follow that beam to see where it leads?*"

Alveron said nothing for a full minute. He had been more than half expecting the question, but it was not an easy one to answer. The main generators had gone completely. There was no point in trying to repair them. But there was still power available, and while there was power, anything could be done in time. It would mean a lot of improvisation, and some difficult maneuvers, for the ship still had its enormous initial velocity. Yes, it could be done, and the activity would keep the crew from becoming further depressed, now that the reaction caused by the mission's failure had started to set in. The news that the nearest heavy repair ship could not reach them for three weeks had also caused a slump in morale.

The engineers, as usual, made a tremendous fuss. Again as usual, they did the job in half the time they had dismissed as being absolutely impossible. Very slowly, over many hours, the great ship began to discard the speed its main drive had given it in as many minutes. In a tremendous curve, millions of miles in radius, the *S9000* changed its course and the star fields shifted round it.

The maneuver took three days, but at the end of that time the ship was limping along a course parallel to the beam that had once come from Earth. They were heading out into emptiness, the blazing sphere that had been the sun dwindling slowly behind them. By the standards of interstellar flight, they were almost stationary.

For hours Rugon strained over his instruments, driving his detector beams far ahead into space. There were certainly no planets within many light-years; there was no doubt of that. From time to time Alveron came to see him and always he had to give the same reply: "Nothing to report." About a fifth of the time Rugon's intuition let him down badly; he began to wonder if this were such an occasion.

Not until a week later did the needles of the mass-detectors quiver feebly at the ends of their scales. But Rugon said nothing, not even to his captain. He waited until he was sure, and he went on waiting until even the short-range scanners began to react, and to build up the first faint pictures on the vision screen. Still he waited patiently until he could interpret the images. Then, when he knew that his wildest fancy was even less than the truth, he called his colleagues into the control room.

The picture on the vision screen was the familiar one of endless star fields, sun beyond sun to the very limits of the Universe. Near the center of the screen a distant nebula made a patch of haze that was difficult for the eye to grasp.

Rugon increased the magnification. The stars flowed out of the field; the little nebula expanded until it filled the screen and then— it was a nebula no longer. A simultaneous gasp of amazement came from all the company at the sight that lay before them.

Lying across league after league of space, ranged in a vast three dimensional array of rows and columns with the precision of a marching army, were thousands of tiny pencils of light. They were moving swiftly; the whole immense lattice holding its shape as a single unit. Even as Alveron and his comrades watched, the formation began to drift off the screen and Rugon had to recenter the controls.

After a long pause, Rugon started to speak.

"This is the race," he said softly, "that has only known radio for two centuries—the race that we believed had crept to die in

the heart of its planet. I have examined those images under the highest possible magnification.

"That is the greatest fleet of which there has ever been a record. Each of those points of light represents a ship larger than our own. Of course, they are very primitive—what you see on the screen are the jets of their rockets. Yes, they dared to use rockets to bridge interstellar space! You realize what that means. It would take them centuries to reach the nearest star. The whole race must have embarked on this journey in the hope that its descendants would complete it, generations later.

"To measure the extent of their accomplishment, think of the ages it took us to conquer space, and the longer ages still before we attempted to reach the stars. Even if we were threatened with annihilation, could we have done so much in so short a time? Remember, this is the youngest civilization in the Universe. Four hundred thousand years ago it did not even exist. What will it be a million years from now?"

An hour later, Orostron left the crippled mother ship to make contact with the great fleet ahead. As the little torpedo disappeared among the stars, Alveron turned to his friend and made a remark that Rugon was often to remember in the years ahead.

"I wonder what they'll be like?" he mused. "Will they be nothing but wonderful engineers, with no art or philosophy? They're going to have such a surprise when Orostron reaches them—I expect it will be rather a blow to their pride. It's funny how all isolated races think they're the only people in the Universe. But they should be grateful to us—we're going to save them a good many hundred years of travel."

Alveron glanced at the Milky Way, lying like a veil of silver mist across the vision screen. He waved towards it with a sweep of a tentacle that embraced the whole circle of the Galaxy, from the Central Planets to the lonely suns of the Rim.

"You know," he said to Rugon, "I feel rather afraid of these people. Suppose they don't like our little Federation?" He waved once more towards the star-clouds that lay massed across the screen, glowing with the light of their countless suns.

"Something tells me they'll be very determined people," he added. "We had better be polite to them. After all, we only outnumber them about a thousand million to one."

Rugon laughed at his captain's little joke.

Twenty years afterwards, the remark didn't seem so funny.

THE SECRET

Henry Cooper had been on the Moon for almost two weeks before he discovered that something was wrong. At first it was only an ill-defined suspicion, the sort of hunch that a hardheaded science reporter would not take too seriously. He had come here, after all, at the United Nations Space Administration's own request. UNSA had always been hot on public relations—especially just before budget time, when an overcrowded world was screaming for more roads and schools and sea farms, and complaining about the billions being poured into space.

So here he was, doing the lunar circuit for the second time, and beaming back two thousand words of copy a day. Although the novelty had worn off, there still remained the wonder and mystery of a world as big as Africa, thoroughly mapped, yet almost completely unexplored. A stone's throw away from the pressure domes, the labs, the spaceports, was a yawning emptiness that would challenge men for centuries to come.

Some parts of the Moon were almost too familiar, of course. Who had not seen that dusty scar in the Mare Imbrium, with its gleaming metal pylon and the plaque that announced in the three official languages of Earth:

ON THIS SPOT

AT 2001 UT

13 SEPTEMBER 1959

THE FIRST MAN-MADE OBJECT REACHED ANOTHER WORLD

Cooper had visited the grave of Lunik II—and the more famous tomb of the men who had come after it. But these things belonged to the past; already, like Columbus and the Wright brothers, they were receding into history. What concerned him now was the future.

When he had landed at Archimedes Spaceport, the Chief Administrator had been obviously glad to see him, and had shown a personal interest in his tour. Transportation, accommodation, and official guide were all arranged. He could go anywhere he liked, ask any questions he pleased. UNSA trusted him, for his stories had always been accurate, his attitude friendly. Yet the tour had gone sour; he did not know why, but he was going to find out.

He reached for the phone and said: "Operator? Please get me the Police Department. I want to speak to the Inspector General."

Presumably Chandra Coomaraswamy possessed a uniform, but Cooper had never seen him wearing it. They met, as arranged, at the entrance to the little park that was Plato City's chief pride and joy. At this time in the morning of the artificial twenty-four-hour "day" it was almost deserted, and they could talk without interruption.

As they walked along the narrow gravel paths, they chatted about old times, the friends they had known at college together, the latest developments in interplanetary politics. They had reached the middle of the park, under the exact center of the great blue-painted dome, when Cooper came to the point.

"You know everything that's happening on the Moon, Chandra," he said. "And you know that I'm here to do a series for UNSA—hope to make a book out of it when I get back to Earth. So why should people be trying to hide things from me?"

It was impossible to hurry Chandra. He always took his time to answer questions, and his few words escaped with difficulty around the stem of his hand-carved Bavarian pipe.

"What people?" he asked at length.

"You've really no idea?"

The Inspector General shook his head.

"Not the faintest," he answered; and Cooper knew that he was telling the truth. Chandra might be silent, but he would not lie.

"I was afraid you'd say that. Well, if you don't know any more than I do, here's the only clue I have—and it frightens me. Medical Research is trying to keep me at arm's length."

"Hmm," replied Chandra, taking his pipe from his mouth and looking at it thoughtfully.

"Is that all you have to say?"

"You haven't given me much to work on. Remember, I'm only a cop; I lack your vivid journalistic imagination."

"All I can tell you is that the higher I get in Medical Research, the colder the atmosphere becomes. Last time I was here, everyone was very friendly, and gave me some fine stories. But now, I can't even meet the Director. He's always too busy, or on the other side of the Moon. Anyway, what sort of man is he?"

"Dr. Hastings? Prickly little character. Very competent, but not easy to work with."

"What could he be trying to hide?"

"Knowing you, I'm sure you have some interesting theories."

"Oh, I thought of narcotics, and fraud, and political conspiracies—but they don't make sense, in these days. So what's left scares the hell out of me."

Chandra's eyebrows signaled a silent question mark.

"Interplanetary plague," said Cooper bluntly.

"I thought that was impossible."

"Yes—I've written articles myself proving that the life forms on other planets have such alien chemistries that they can't react with us, and that all our microbes and bugs took millions of years to adapt to our bodies. But I've always wondered if it was true. Suppose a ship has come back from Mars, say, with something *really* vicious—and the doctors can't cope with it?"

There was a long silence. Then Chandra said: "I'll start investigating. *I* don't like it either, for here's an item you probably don't know. There were three nervous breakdowns in the Medical Division last month—and that's very, very unusual."

He glanced at his watch, then at the false sky, which seemed so distant, yet which was only two hundred feet above their heads.

"We'd better get moving," he said. "The morning shower's due in five minutes."

The call came two weeks later, in the middle of the night—the real lunar night. By Plato City time, it was Sunday morning.

"Henry? Chandra here. Can you meet me in half an hour at air lock five? Good—I'll see you."

This was it, Cooper knew. Air lock five meant that they were going outside the dome. Chandra had found something.

The presence of the police driver restricted conversation as the tractor moved away from the city along the road roughly bulldozed across the ash and pumice. Low in the south, Earth was almost full, casting a brilliant blue-green light over the infernal landscape. However hard one tried, Cooper told himself, it was difficult to make the Moon appear glamorous. But nature guards her greatest secrets well; to such places men must come to find them.

The multiple domes of the city dropped below the sharply curved horizon. Presently, the tractor turned aside from the main road to follow a scarcely visible trail. Ten minutes later, Cooper saw a single glittering hemisphere ahead of them, standing on an isolated ridge of rock. Another vehicle, bearing a red cross, was parked beside the entrance. It seemed that they were not the only visitors.

Nor were they unexpected. As they drew up to the dome, the flexible tube of the air-lock coupling groped out toward them and snapped into place against their tractor's outer hull. There was a brief hissing as pressure equalized. Then Cooper followed Chandra into the building.

The air-lock operator led them along curving corridors and radial passageways toward the center of the dome. Sometimes they caught glimpses of laboratories, scientific instruments, computers—all perfectly ordinary, and all deserted on this Sunday morning. They must have reached the heart of the building, Cooper told himself when their guide ushered them into a large circular chamber and shut the door softly behind them.

It was a small zoo. All around them were cages, tanks, jars containing a wide selection of the fauna and flora of Earth. Waiting at its center was a short, gray-haired man, looking very worried, and very unhappy.

"Dr. Hastings," said Coomaraswamy, "meet Mr. Cooper." The Inspector General turned to his companion and added, "I've convinced the doctor that there's only one way to keep you quiet— and that's to tell you everything."

"Frankly," said Hastings, "I'm not sure if I give a damn any more." His voice was unsteady, barely under control, and Cooper thought, Hello! There's another breakdown on the way.

The scientist wasted no time on such formalities as shaking hands. He walked to one of the cages, took out a small bundle of fur, and held it toward Cooper.

"Do you know what this is?" he asked abruptly.

"Of course. A hamster—the commonest lab animal."

"Yes," said Hastings. "A perfectly ordinary golden hamster. Except that this one is five years old—like all the others in this cage."

"Well? What's odd about that?"

"Oh, nothing, nothing at all . . . except for the trifling fact that hamsters live for only two years. And we have some here that are getting on for ten."

For a moment no one spoke; but the room was not silent. It was full of rustlings and slitherings and scratchings, of faint whimpers and tiny animal cries. Then Cooper whispered: "My God— you've found a way of prolonging life!"

"No," retorted Hastings. "We've not found it. The Moon has given it to us . . . as we might have expected, if we'd looked in front of our noses."

He seemed to have gained control over his emotions—as if he was once more the pure scientist, fascinated by a discovery for its own sake and heedless of its implications.

"On Earth," he said, "we spend our whole lives fighting gravity. It wears down our muscles, pulls our stomachs out of shape. In seventy years, how many tons of blood does the heart lift through how many miles? And all that work, all that strain is reduced to a sixth here on the Moon, where a one-hundred-and-eighty-pound human weighs only thirty pounds."

"I see," said Cooper slowly. "Ten years for a hamster—and how long for a man?"

"It's not a simple law," answered Hastings. "It varies with the size and the species. Even a month ago, we weren't certain. But now we're quite sure of this: on the Moon, the span of human life will be at least two hundred years."

"And you've been trying to keep it secret!"

"You fool! Don't you understand?"

"Take it easy, Doctor—take it easy," said Chandra softly.

With an obvious effort of will, Hastings got control of himself again. He began to speak with such icy calm that his words sank like freezing raindrops into Cooper's mind.

"Think of them up there," he said, pointing to the roof, to the invisible Earth, whose looming presence no one on the Moon could ever forget. "Six billion of them, packing all the continents to the edges—and now crowding over into the sea beds. And here—" he pointed to the ground—"only a hundred thousand of *us*, on an almost empty world. But a world where we need miracles of technology and engineering merely to exist, where a man with an I.Q. of only a hundred and fifty can't even get a job.

"And now we find that we can live for two hundred years. Imagine how they're going to react to *that* news! This is your problem now, Mister Journalist; you've asked for it, and you've got it. Tell me this, please—I'd really be interested to know—*just how are you going to break it to them?*"

He waited, and waited. Cooper opened his mouth, then closed it again, unable to think of anything to say.

In the far corner of the room, a baby monkey started to cry.

REUNION

People of Earth, do not be afraid. We come in peace—and why not? For we are your cousins; we have been here before.

You will recognize us when we meet, a few hours from now. We are approaching the solar system almost as swiftly as this radio message. Already, your sun dominates the sky ahead of us. It is the sun our ancestors and yours shared ten million years ago. We are men, as you are; but you have forgotten your history, while we have remembered ours.

We colonized Earth, in the reign of the great reptiles, who were dying when we came and whom we could not save. Your world was a tropical planet then, and we felt that it would make a fair home for our people. We were wrong. Though we were masters of space, we knew so little about climate, about evolution, about genetics. . . .

For millions of summers—there were no winters in those ancient days—the colony flourished. Isolated though it had to be, in a universe where the journey from one star to the next takes years, it kept in touch with its parent civilization. Three or four times in every century, starships would call and bring news of the galaxy.

But two million years ago, Earth began to change. For ages it had been a tropical paradise; then the temperature fell, and the ice began to creep down from the poles. As the climate altered, so did the colonists. We realize now that it was a natural adaptation to

the end of the long summer, but those who had made Earth their home for so many generations believed that they had been attacked by a strange and repulsive disease. A disease that did not kill, that did no physical harm—but merely disfigured.

Yet some were immune; the change spared them and their children. And so, within a few thousand years, the colony had split into two separate groups—almost two separate species—suspicious and jealous of each other.

The division brought envy, discord, and, ultimately, conflict. As the colony disintegrated and the climate steadily worsened, those who could do so withdrew from Earth. The rest sank into barbarism.

We could have kept in touch, but there is so much to do in a universe of a hundred trillion stars. Until a few years ago, we did not know that any of you had survived. Then we picked up your first radio signals, learned your simple languages, and discovered that you had made the long climb back from savagery. We come to greet you, our long-lost relatives—and to help you.

We have discovered much in the eons since we abandoned Earth. If you wish us to bring back the eternal summer that ruled before the Ice Ages, we can do so. Above all, we have a simple remedy for the offensive yet harmless genetic plague that afflicted so many of the colonists.

Perhaps it has run its course—but if not, we have good news for you. People of Earth, you can rejoin the society of the universe without shame, without embarrassment.

If any of you are still white, we can cure you.

THE STAR

It is three thousand light-years to the Vatican. Once, I believed
that space could have no power over faith, just as I believed that
the heavens declared the glory of God's handiwork. Now I have
seen that handiwork, and my faith is sorely troubled. I stare at the
crucifix that hangs on the cabin wall above the Mark VI Computer,
and for the first time in my life I wonder if it is no more than an
empty symbol.

I have told no one yet, but the truth cannot be concealed. The
facts are there for all to read, recorded on the countless miles of
magnetic tape and the thousands of photographs we are carrying
back to Earth. Other scientists can interpret them as easily as I can,
and I am not one who would condone that tampering with the
truth which often gave my order a bad name in the olden days.

The crew are already sufficiently depressed: I wonder how they
will take this ultimate irony. Few of them have any religious faith,
yet they will not relish using this final weapon in their campaign
against me—that private, good-natured, but fundamentally serious,
war which lasted all the way from Earth. It amused them to have
a Jesuit as chief astrophysicist: Dr. Chandler, for instance, could
never get over it (why are medical men such notorious atheists?).
Sometimes he would meet me on the observation deck, where the
lights are always low so that the stars shine with undiminished

glory. He would come up to me in the gloom and stand staring out of the great oval port, while the heavens crawled slowly around us as the ship turned end over end with the residual spin we had never bothered to correct.

"Well, Father," he would say at last, "it goes on forever and forever, and perhaps *Something* made it. But how you can believe that Something has a special interest in us and our miserable little world—that just beats me." Then the argument would start, while the stars and nebulae would swing around us in silent, endless arcs beyond the flawlessly clear plastic of the observation port.

It was, I think, the apparent incongruity of my position that caused most amusement to the crew. In vain I would point to my three papers in the *Astrophysical Journal*, my five in the *Monthly Notices of the Royal Astronomical Society*. I would remind them that my order has long been famous for its scientific works. We may be few now, but ever since the eighteenth century we have made contributions to astronomy and geophysics out of all proportion to our numbers. Will my report on the Phoenix Nebula end our thousand years of history? It will end, I fear, much more than that.

I do not know who gave the nebula its name, which seems to me a very bad one. If it contains a prophecy, it is one that cannot be verified for several billion years. Even the word nebula is misleading: this is a far smaller object than those stupendous clouds of mist—the stuff of unborn stars—that are scattered throughout the length of the Milky Way. On the cosmic scale, indeed, the Phoenix Nebula is a tiny thing—a tenuous shell of gas surrounding a single star.

Or what is left of a star . . .

The Rubens engraving of Loyola seems to mock me as it hangs there above the spectrophotometer tracings. What would *you*, Father, have made of this knowledge that has come into my keeping, so far from the little world that was all the universe you knew? Would your faith have risen to the challenge, as mine has failed to do?

You gaze into the distance, Father, but I have traveled a distance beyond any that you could have imagined when you founded our order a thousand years ago. No other survey ship has been so far from Earth: we are at the very frontiers of the explored universe.

We set out to reach the Phoenix Nebula, we succeeded, and we are homeward bound with our burden of knowledge. I wish I could lift that burden from my shoulders, but I call to you in vain across the centuries and the light-years that lie between us.

On the book you are holding the words are plain to read. AD MAIOREM DEI GLORIAM, the message runs, but it is a message I can no longer believe. Would you still believe it, if you could see what we have found?

We knew, of course, what the Phoenix Nebula was. Every year, in our galaxy alone, more than a hundred stars explode, blazing for a few hours or days with thousands of times their normal brilliance before they sink back into death and obscurity. Such are the ordinary novae—the commonplace disasters of the universe. I have recorded the spectrograms and light curves of dozens since I started working at the Lunar Observatory.

But three or four times in every thousand years occurs something beside which even a nova pales into total insignificance.

When a star becomes a *supernova*, it may for a little while outshine all the massed suns of the galaxy. The Chinese astronomers watched this happen in A.D. 1054, not knowing what it was they saw. Five centuries later, in 1572, a supernova blazed in Cassiopeia so brilliantly that it was visible in the daylight sky. There have been three more in the thousand years that have passed since then.

Our mission was to visit the remnants of such a catastrophe, to reconstruct the events that led up to it, and, if possible, to learn its cause. We came slowly in through the concentric shells of gas that had been blasted out six thousand years before, yet were expanding still. They were immensely hot, radiating even now with a fierce violet light, but were far too tenuous to do us any damage. When the star had exploded, its outer layers had been driven upward with such speed that they had escaped completely from its gravitational field. Now they formed a hollow shell large enough to engulf a thousand solar systems, and at its center burned the tiny, fantastic object which the star had now become—a White Dwarf, smaller than the Earth, yet weighing a million times as much.

The glowing gas shells were all around us, banishing the normal

night of interstellar space. We were flying into the center of a cosmic bomb that had detonated millennia ago and whose incandescent fragments were still hurtling apart. The immense scale of the explosion, and the fact that the debris already covered a volume of space many billions of miles across, robbed the scene of any visible movement. It would take decades before the unaided eye could detect any motion in these tortured wisps and eddies of gas, yet the sense of turbulent expansion was overwhelming.

We had checked our primary drive hours before, and were drifting slowly toward the fierce little star ahead. Once it had been a sun like our own, but it had squandered in a few hours the energy that should have kept it shining for a million years. Now it was a shrunken miser, hoarding its resources as if trying to make amends for its prodigal youth.

No one seriously expected to find planets. If there had been any before the explosion, they would have been boiled into puffs of vapor, and their substance lost in the greater wreckage of the star itself. But we made the automatic search, as we always do when approaching an unknown sun, and presently we found a single small world circling the star at an immense distance. It must have been the Pluto of this vanished solar system, orbiting on the frontiers of the night. Too far from the central sun ever to have known life, its remoteness had saved it from the fate of all its lost companions.

The passing fires had seared its rocks and burned away the mantle of frozen gas that must have covered it in the days before the disaster. We landed, and we found the Vault.

Its builders had made sure that we should. The monolithic marker that stood above the entrance was now a fused stump, but even the first long-range photographs told us that here was the work of intelligence. A little later we detected the continent-wide pattern of radio-activity that had been buried in the rock. Even if the pylon above the Vault had been destroyed, this would have remained, an immovable and all but eternal beacon calling to the stars. Our ship fell toward this gigantic bull's-eye like an arrow into its target.

The pylon must have been a mile high when it was built, but now it looked like a candle that had melted down into a puddle of wax. It took us a week to drill through the fused rock, since we did

not have the proper tools for a task like this. We were astronomers, not archaeologists, but we could improvise. Our original purpose was forgotten: this lonely monument, reared with such labor at the greatest possible distance from the doomed sun, could have only one meaning. A civilization that knew it was about to die had made its last bid for immortality.

It will take us generations to examine all the treasures that were placed in the Vault. They had plenty of time to prepare, for their sun must have given its first warnings many years before the final denotation. Everything that they wished to preserve, all the fruit of their genius, they brought here to this distant world in the days before the end, hoping that some other race would find it and that they would not be utterly forgotten. Would we have done as well, or would we have been too lost in our own misery to give thought to a future we could never see or share?

If only they had had a little more time! They could travel freely enough between the planets of their own sun, but they had not yet learned to cross the interstellar gulfs, and the nearest solar system was a hundred light-years away. Yet even had they possessed the secret of the Transfinite Drive, no more than a few millions could have been saved. Perhaps it was better thus.

Even if they had not been so disturbingly human as their sculpture shows, we could not have helped admiring them and grieving for their fate. They left thousands of visual records and the machines for projecting them, together with elaborate pictorial instructions from which it will not be difficult to learn their written language. We have examined many of these records, and brought to life for the first time in six thousand years the warmth and beauty of a civilization that in many ways must have been superior to our own. Perhaps they only showed us the best, and one can hardly blame them. But their worlds were very lovely, and their cities were built with a grace that matches anything of man's. We have watched them at work and play, and listened to their musical speech sounding across the centuries. One scene is still before my eyes—a group of children on a beach of strange blue sand, playing in the waves as children play on Earth. Curious whiplike trees line the shore, and some very large animal is wading in the shadows yet attracting no attention at all.

And sinking into the sea, still warm and friendly and life-giving, is the sun that will soon turn traitor and obliterate all this innocent happiness.

Perhaps if we had not been so far from home and so vulnerable to loneliness, we should not have been so deeply moved. Many of us had seen the ruins of ancient civilizations on other worlds, but they had never affected us so profoundly. This tragedy was unique. It is one thing for a race to fail and die, as nations and cultures have done on Earth. But to be destroyed so completely in the full flower of its achievement, leaving no survivors—how could that be reconciled with the mercy of God?

My colleagues have asked me that, and I have given what answers I can. Perhaps you could have done better, Father Loyola, but I have found nothing in the *Exercitia Spiritualia* that helps me here. They were not an evil people: I do not know what gods they worshiped, if indeed they worshiped any. But I have looked back at them across the centuries, and have watched while the loveliness they used their last strength to preserve was brought forth again into the light of their shrunken sun. They could have taught us much: why were they destroyed?

I know the answers that my colleagues will give when they get back to Earth. They will say that the universe has no purpose and no plan, that since a hundred suns explode every year in our galaxy, at this very moment some race is dying in the depths of space. Whether that race has done good or evil during its lifetime will make no difference in the end: there is no divine justice, for there is no God.

Yet, of course, what we have seen proves nothing of the sort. Anyone who argues thus is being swayed by emotion, not logic. God has no need to justify His actions to man. He who built the universe can destroy it when He chooses. It is arrogance—it is perilously near blasphemy—for us to say what He may or may not do.

This I could have accepted, hard though it is to look upon whole worlds and peoples thrown into the furnace. But there comes a point when even the deepest faith must falter, and now, as I look at the calculations lying before me, I know I have reached that point at last.

We could not tell, before we reached the nebula, how long ago

the explosion took place. Now, from the astronomical evidence and the record in the rocks of that one surviving planet, I have been able to date it very exactly. I know in what year the light of this colossal conflagration reached our Earth. I know how brilliantly the supernova whose corpse now dwindles behind our speeding ship once shone in terrestrial skies. I know how it must have blazed low in the east before sunrise, like a beacon in that oriental dawn.

There can be no reasonable doubt: the ancient mystery is solved at last. Yet, oh God, there were so many stars you could have used. What was the need to give these people to the fire, that the symbol of their passing might shine above Bethlehem?

A MEETING WITH MEDUSA

---

1. A Day to Remember

The *Queen Elizabeth* was over three miles above the Grand Canyon, dawdling along at a comfortable hundred and eighty, when Howard Falcon spotted the camera platform closing in from the right. He had been expecting it—nothing else was cleared to fly at this altitude—but he was not too happy to have company. Although he welcomed any signs of public interest, he also wanted as much empty sky as he could get. After all, he was the first man in history to navigate a ship three-tenths of a mile long. . . .

So far, this first test flight had gone perfectly; ironically enough, the only problem had been the century-old aircraft carrier *Chairman Mao*, borrowed from the San Diego Naval Museum for support operations. Only one of *Mao's* four nuclear reactors was still operating, and the old battlewagon's top speed was barely thirty knots. Luckily, wind speed at sea level had been less than half this, so it had not been too difficult to maintain still air on the flight deck. Though there had been a few anxious moments during gusts, when the mooring lines had been dropped, the great dirigible had risen smoothly, straight up into the sky, as if on an invisible elevator. If all went well, *Queen Elizabeth IV* would not meet *Chairman Mao* again for another week.

Everything was under control; all test instruments gave normal readings. Commander Falcon decided to go upstairs and watch the rendezvous. He handed over to his second officer, and walked out into the transparent tubeway that led through the heart of the ship. There, as always, he was overwhelmed by the spectacle of the largest single space ever enclosed by man.

The ten spherical gas cells, each more than a hundred feet across, were ranged one behind the other like a line of gigantic soap bubbles. The tough plastic was so clear that he could see through the whole length of the array, and make out details of the elevator mechanism, more than a third of a mile from his vantage point. All around him, like a three-dimensional maze, was the structural framework of the ship—the great longitudinal girders running from nose to tail, the fifteen hoops that were the circular ribs of this sky-borne colossus, and whose varying sizes defined its graceful, stream-lined profile.

At this low speed, there was little sound—merely the soft rush of wind over the envelope and an occasional creak of metal as the pattern of stresses changed. The shadowless light from the rows of lamps far overhead gave the whole scene a curiously submarine quality, and to Falcon this was enhanced by the spectacle of the translucent gasbags. He had once encountered a squadron of large but harmless jellyfish, pulsing their mindless way above a shallow tropical reef, and the plastic bubbles that gave Queen Elizabeth her lift often reminded him of these—especially when changing pressures made them crinkle and scatter new patterns of reflected light.

He walked down the axis of the ship until he came to the forward elevator, between gas cells one and two. Riding up to the Observation Deck, he noticed that it was uncomfortably hot; and dictated a brief memo to himself on his pocket recorder. The Queen obtained almost a quarter of her buoyancy from the unlimited amounts of waste heat produced by her fusion power plant. On this lightly loaded flight, indeed, only six of ten gas cells contained helium; the remaining four were full of air. Yet she still carried two hundred tons of water as ballast. However, running the cells at high temperatures did produce problems in refrigerating the access ways; it was obvious that a little more work would have to be done there.

A refreshing blast of cooler air hit him in the face when he

stepped out onto the Observation Deck and into the dazzling sunlight streaming through the plexiglass roof. Half a dozen workmen, with an equal number of superchimp assistants, were busily laying the partly completed dance floor, while others were installing electric wiring and fixing furniture. It was a scene of controlled chaos, and Falcon found it hard to believe that everything would be ready for the maiden voyage, only four weeks ahead. Well, that was not *his* problem, thank goodness. He was merely the Captain, not the Cruise Director.

The human workers waved to him, and the "simps" flashed toothy smiles, as he walked through the confusion, into the already completed Skylounge. This was his favorite place in the whole ship, and he knew that once she was operating he would never again have it all to himself. He would allow himself just five minutes of private enjoyment.

He called the bridge, checked that everything was still in order, and relaxed into one of the comfortable swivel chairs. Below, in a curve that delighted the eye, was the unbroken silver sweep of the ship's envelope. He was perched at the highest point, surveying the whole immensity of the largest vehicle ever built. And when he had tired of that—all the way out to the horizon was the fantastic wilderness carved by the Colorado River in half a billion years of time.

Apart from the camera platform (it had now fallen back and was filming from amidships) he had the sky to himself. It was blue and empty, clear down to the horizon. In his grandfather's day, Falcon knew, it would have been streaked with vapor trails and stained with smoke. Both had gone: the aerial garbage had vanished with the primitive technologies that spawned it, and the long-distance transportation of this age arced too far beyond the stratosphere for any sight or sound of it to reach Earth. Once again, the lower atmosphere belonged to the birds and the clouds—and now to *Queen Elizabeth IV.*

It was true, as the old pioneers had said at the beginning of the twentieth century: this was the only way to travel—in silence and luxury, breathing the air around you and not cut off from it, near enough to the surface to watch the everchanging beauty of land and sea. The subsonic jets of the 1980s, packed with hundreds

of passengers seated ten abreast, could not even begin to match such comfort and spaciousness.

Of course, the *Queen* would never be an economic proposition, and even if her projected sister ships were built, only a few of the world's quarter of a billion inhabitants would ever enjoy this silent gliding through the sky. But a secure and prosperous global society could afford such follies and indeed needed them for their novelty and entertainment. There were at least a million men on Earth whose discretionary income exceeded a thousand new dollars a year, so the *Queen* would not lack for passengers.

Falcon's pocket communicator beeped. The copilot was calling from the bridge.

"O.K. for rendezvous, Captain? We've got all the data we need from this run, and the TV people are getting impatient."

Falcon glanced at the camera platform, now matching his speed a tenth of a mile away.

"O.K.," he replied. "Proceed as arranged. I'll watch from here."

He walked back through the busy chaos of the Observation Deck so that he could have a better view amidships. As he did so, he could feel the change of vibration underfoot; by the time he had reached the rear of the lounge, the ship had come to rest. Using his master key, he let himself out onto the small external platform flaring from the end of the deck; half a dozen people could stand here, with only low guardrails separating them from the vast sweep of the envelope—and from the ground, thousands of feet below. It was an exciting place to be, and perfectly safe even when the ship was traveling at speed, for it was in the dead air behind the huge dorsal blister of the Observation Deck. Nevertheless, it was not intended that the passengers would have access to it; the view was a little too vertiginous.

The covers of the forward cargo hatch had already opened like giant trap doors, and the camera platform was hovering above them, preparing to descend. Along this route, in the years to come, would travel thousands of passengers and tons of supplies. Only on rare occasions would the *Queen* drop down to sea level and dock with her floating base.

A sudden gust of cross wind slapped Falcon's cheek, and he tightened his grip on the guardrail. The Grand Canyon was a bad

place for turbulence, though he did not expect much at this altitude. Without any real anxiety, he focused his attention on the descending platform, now about a hundred and fifty feet above the ship. He knew that the highly skilled operator who was flying the remotely controlled vehicle had performed this simple maneuver a dozen times already; it was inconceivable that he would have any difficulties.

Yet he seemed to be reacting rather sluggishly. That last gust had drifted the platform almost to the edge of the open hatchway. Surely the pilot could have corrected before this. . . . Did he have a control problem? It was very unlikely; these remotes had multiple-redundancy, fail-safe takeovers, and any number of backup systems. Accidents were almost unheard of.

But there he went again, off to the left. Could the pilot be *drunk?* Improbable though that seemed, Falcon considered it seriously for a moment. Then he reached for his microphone switch.

Once again, without warning, he was slapped violently in the face. He hardly felt it, for he was staring in horror at the camera platform. The distant operator was fighting for control, trying to balance the craft on its jets—but he was only making matters worse. The oscillations increased—twenty degrees, forty, sixty, ninety. . . .

"Switch to automatic, you fool!" Falcon shouted uselessly into his microphone. "Your manual control's not working!"

The platform flipped over on its back. The jets no longer supported it, but drove it swiftly downward. They had suddenly become allies of the gravity they had fought until this moment.

Falcon never heard the crash, though he felt it; he was already inside the Observation Deck, racing for the elevator that would take him down to the bridge. Workmen shouted at him anxiously, asking what had happened. It would be many months before he knew the answer to that question.

Just as he was stepping into the elevator cage, he changed his mind. What if there was a power failure? Better be on the safe side, even if it took longer and time was the essence. He began to run down the spiral stairway enclosing the shaft.

Halfway down he paused for a second to inspect the damage. That damned platform had gone clear through the ship, rupturing two of the gas cells as it did so. They were still collapsing slowly, in great falling veils of plastic. He was not worried about the loss

of lift—the ballast could easily take care of that, as long as eight cells remained intact. Far more serious was the possibility of structural damage. Already he could hear the great latticework around him groaning and protesting under its abnormal loads. It was not enough to have sufficient lift; unless it was properly distributed, the ship would break her back.

He was just resuming his descent when a superchimp, shrieking with fright, came racing down the elevator shaft, moving with incredible speed, hand over hand, along the *outside* of the latticework. In its terror, the poor beast had torn off its company uniform, perhaps in an unconscious attempt to regain the freedom of its ancestors.

Falcon, still descending as swiftly as he could, watched its approach with some alarm. A distraught simp was a powerful and potentially dangerous animal, especially if fear overcame its conditioning. As it overtook him, it started to call out a string of words, but they were all jumbled together, and the only one he could recognize was a plaintive, frequently repeated "boss." Even now, Falcon realized, it looked toward humans for guidance. He felt sorry for the creature, involved in a manmade disaster beyond its comprehension, and for which it bore no responsibility.

It stopped opposite him, on the other side of the lattice; there was nothing to prevent it from coming through the open framework if it wished. Now its face was only inches from his, and he was looking straight into the terrified eyes. Never before had he been so close to a simp, and able to study its features in such detail. He felt that strange mingling of kinship and discomfort that all men experience when they gaze thus into the mirror of time.

His presence seemed to have calmed the creature. Falcon pointed up the shaft, back toward the Observation Deck, and said very clearly and precisely: "Boss—boss—go." To his relief, the simp understood; it gave him a grimace that might have been a smile, and at once started to race back the way it had come. Falcon had given it the best advice he could. If any safety remained aboard the *Queen*, it was in that direction. But his duty lay in the other.

He had almost completed his descent when, with a sound of rending metal, the vessel pitched nose down, and the lights went out. But he could still see quite well, for a shaft of sunlight streamed

through the open hatch and the huge tear in the envelope. Many years ago he had stood in a great cathedral nave watching the light pouring through the stained-glass windows and forming pools of multicolored radiance on the ancient flagstones. The dazzling shaft of sunlight through the ruined fabric high above reminded him of that moment. He was in a cathedral of metal, falling down the sky.

When he reached the bridge, and was able for the first time to look outside, he was horrified to see how close the ship was to the ground. Only three thousand feet below were the beautiful and deadly pinnacles of rock and the red rivers of mud that were still carving their way down into the past. There was no level area anywhere in sight where a ship as large as the *Queen* could come to rest on an even keel.

A glance at the display board told him that all the ballast had gone. However, rate of descent had been reduced to a few yards a second; they still had a fighting chance.

Without a word, Falcon eased himself into the pilot's seat and took over such control as still remained. The instrument board showed him everything he wished to know; speech was superfluous. In the background, he could hear the Communications Officer giving a running report over the radio. By this time, all the news channels of Earth would have been preempted, and he could imagine the utter frustration of the program controllers. One of the most spectacular wrecks in history was occurring—without a single camera to record it. The last moments of the *Queen* would never fill millions with awe and terror, as had those of the *Hindenburg*, a century and a half before.

Now the ground was only about seventeen hundred feet away, still coming up slowly. Though he had full thrust, he had not dared to use it, lest the weakened structure collapse; but now he realized that he had no choice. The wind was taking them toward a fork in the canyon, where the river was split by a wedge of rock like the prow of some gigantic, fossilized ship of stone. If she continued on her present course, the *Queen* would straddle that triangular plateau and come to rest with at least a third of her length jutting out over nothingness; she would snap like a rotten stick.

Far away, above the sound of straining metal and escaping gas, came the familiar whistle of the jets as Falcon opened up the lateral

thrusters. The ship staggered, and began to slew to port. The shriek of tearing metal was now almost continuous—and the rate of descent had started to increase ominously. A glance at the damage-control board showed that cell number five had just gone.

The ground was only yards away. Even now, he could not tell whether his maneuver would succeed or fail. He switched the thrust vectors over to vertical, giving maximum lift to reduce the force of impact.

The crash seemed to last forever. It was not violent—merely prolonged, and irresistible. It seemed that the whole universe was falling about them.

The sound of crunching metal came nearer, as if some great beast were eating its way through the dying ship.

Then floor and ceiling closed upon him like a vise.

2. "BECAUSE IT'S THERE"

"Why do you want to go to Jupiter?"

"As Springer said when he lifted for Pluto—'because it's there.'"

"Thanks. Now we've got *that* out of the way—the real reason."

Howard Falcon smiled, though only those who knew him well could have interpreted the slight, leathery grimace. Webster was one of them; for more than twenty years they had shared triumphs and disasters—including the greatest disaster of all.

"Well, Springer's cliché is still valid. We've landed on all the terrestrial planets, but none of the gas giants. They are the only real challenge left in the solar system."

"An expensive one. Have you worked out the cost?"

"As well as I can; here are the estimates. Remember, though— this isn't a one-shot mission, but a transportation system. Once it's proved out, it can be used over and over again. And it will open up not merely Jupiter, but all the giants."

Webster looked at the figures, and whistled.

"Why not start with an easier planet—Uranus, for example? Half the gravity, and less than half the escape velocity. Quieter weather, too—if that's the right word for it."

Webster had certainly done his homework. But that, of course, was why he was head of Long-Range Planning.

"There's very little saving—when you allow for the extra distance and the logistics problems. For Jupiter, we can use the facilities of Ganymede. Beyond Saturn, we'd have to establish a new supply base."

Logical, thought Webster; but he was sure that it was not the important reason. Jupiter was lord of the solar system; Falcon would be interested in no lesser challenge.

"Besides," Falcon continued, "Jupiter is a major scientific scandal. It's more than a hundred years since its radio storms were discovered, but we still don't know what causes them—and the Great Red Spot is as big a mystery as ever. That's why I can get matching funds from the Bureau of Astronautics. Do you know how many probes they have dropped into that atmosphere?"

"A couple of hundred, I believe."

"*Three* hundred and twenty-six, over the last fifty years—about a quarter of them total failures. Of course, they've learned a hell of a lot, but they've barely scratched the planet. Do you realize how *big it is?*"

"More than ten times the size of Earth."

"Yes, yes—but do you know what that really means?"

Falcon pointed to the large globe in the corner of Webster's office.

"Look at India—how small it seems. Well, if you skinned Earth and spread it out on the surface of Jupiter, it would look about as big as India does here."

There was a long silence while Webster contemplated the equation: Jupiter is to Earth as Earth is to India. Falcon had—deliberately, of course—chosen the best possible example. . . .

Was it already ten years ago? Yes, it must have been. The crash lay seven years in the past (*that* date was engraved on his heart), and those initial tests had taken place three years before the first and last flight of the *Queen Elizabeth.*

Ten years ago, then, Commander (no, Lieutenant) Falcon had invited him to a preview—a three-day drift across the northern plains of India, within sight of the Himalayas. "Perfectly safe," he

had promised. "It will get you away from the office—and will teach you what this whole thing is about."

Webster had not been disappointed. Next to his first journey to the Moon, it had been the most memorable experience of his life. And yet, as Falcon had assured him, it had been perfectly safe, and quite uneventful.

They had taken off from Srinagar just before dawn, with the huge silver bubble of the balloon already catching the first light of the Sun. The ascent had been made in total silence; there were none of the roaring propane burners that had lifted the hot-air balloons of an earlier age. All the heat they needed came from the little pulsed-fusion reactor, weighing only about two hundred and twenty pounds, hanging in the open mouth of the envelope. While they were climbing, its laser was zapping ten times a second, igniting the merest whiff of deuterium fuel. Once they had reached altitude, it would fire only a few times a minute, making up for the heat lost through the great gasbag overhead.

And so, even while they were almost a mile above the ground, they could hear dogs barking, people shouting, bells ringing. Slowly the vast, Sun-smitten landscape expanded around them. Two hours later, they had leveled out at three miles and were taking frequent draughts of oxygen. They could relax and admire the scenery; the on-board instrumentation was doing all the work—gathering the information that would be required by the designers of the still-unnamed liner of the skies.

It was a perfect day. The southwest monsoon would not break for another month, and there was hardly a cloud in the sky. Time seemed to have come to a stop; they resented the hourly radio reports which interrupted their reverie. And all around, to the horizon and far beyond, was that infinite, ancient landscape, drenched with history—a patchwork of villages, fields, temples, lakes, irrigation canals . . .

With a real effort, Webster broke the hypnotic spell of that ten-year-old memory. It had converted him to lighter-than-air flight—and it had made him realize the enormous size of India, even in a world that could be circled within ninety minutes. And yet, he repeated to himself, Jupiter is to Earth as Earth is to India. . . .

"Granted your argument," he said, "and supposing the funds are available, there's another question you have to answer. Why should you do better than the—what is it—three hundred and twenty-six robot probes that have already made the trip?"

"I am better qualified than they were—as an observer, and as a pilot. *Especially* as a pilot. Don't forget—I've more experience of lighter-than-air flight than anyone in the world."

"You could still serve as controller, and sit safely on Ganymede."

"*But that's just the point!* They've already done that. Don't you remember what killed the *Queen?*"

Webster knew perfectly well; but he merely answered: "Go on."

"*Time lag—time lag!* That idiot of a platform controller thought he was using a local radio circuit. But he'd been accidentally switched through a satellite—oh, maybe it wasn't his fault, but he should have noticed. That's a half-second time lag for the round trip. Even then it wouldn't have mattered flying in calm air. It was the turbulence over the Grand Canyon that did it. When the platform tipped, and he corrected for that—it had already tipped the other way. Ever tried to drive a car over a bumpy road with a half-second delay in the steering?"

"No, and I don't intend to try. But I can imagine it."

"Well, Ganymede is a million kilometers from Jupiter. That means a round-trip delay of six seconds. No, you need a controller on the spot—to handle emergencies in real time. Let me show you something. Mind if I use this?"

"Go ahead."

Falcon picked up a postcard that was lying on Webster's desk; they were almost obsolete on Earth, but this one showed a 3-D view of a Martian landscape, and was decorated with exotic and expensive stamps. He held it so that it dangled vertically.

"This is an old trick, but helps to make my point. Place your thumb and finger on either side, not quite touching. That's right."

Webster put out his hand, almost but not quite gripping the card.

"Now catch it."

Falcon waited for a few seconds; then, without warning, he let go of the card. Webster's thumb and finger closed on empty air.

"I'll do it again, just to show there's no deception. You see?"

Once again, the falling card had slipped through Webster's fingers.

"Now you try it on me."

This time, Webster grasped the card and dropped it without warning. It had scarcely moved before Falcon had caught it. Webster almost imagined he could hear a click, so swift was the other's reaction.

"When they put me together again," Falcon remarked in an expressionless voice, "the surgeons made some improvements. This is one of them—and there are others. I want to make the most of them. Jupiter is the place where I can do it."

Webster stared for long seconds at the fallen card, absorbing the improbable colors of the Trivium Charontis Escarpment. Then he said quietly: "I understand. How long do you think it will take?"

"With your help, plus the Bureau, plus all the science foundation we can drag in—oh, three years. Then a year for trials— we'll have to send in at least two test models. So, with luck—five years."

"That's about what I thought. I hope you get your luck; you've earned it. But there's one thing I won't do."

"What's that?"

"Next time you go ballooning, don't expect *me* as passenger."

3. THE WORLD OF THE GODS

The fall from Jupiter V to Jupiter itself takes only three and a half hours. Few men could have slept on so awesome a journey. Sleep was a weakness that Howard Falcon hated, and the little he still required brought dreams that time had not yet been able to exorcise. But he could expect no rest in the three days that lay ahead, and must seize what he could during the long fall down into that ocean of clouds, some sixty thousand miles below.

As soon as *Kon-Tiki* had entered her transfer orbit and all the computer checks were satisfactory, he prepared for the last sleep he might ever know. It seemed appropriate that at almost the same moment Jupiter eclipsed the bright and tiny Sun as he swept into

the monstrous shadow of the planet. For a few minutes a strange golden twilight enveloped the ship; then a quarter of the sky became an utterly black hole in space, while the rest was a blaze of stars. No matter how far one traveled across the solar system, *they* never changed; these same constellations now shone on Earth, millions of miles away. The only novelties here were the small, pale crescents of Callisto and Ganymede; doubtless there were a dozen other moons up there in the sky, but they were all much too tiny, and too distant, for the unaided eye to pick them out.

"Closing down for two hours," he reported to the mother ship, hanging almost a thousand miles above the desolate rocks of Jupiter V, in the radiation shadow of the tiny satellite. If it never served any other useful purpose, Jupiter V was a cosmic bulldozer perpetually sweeping up the charged particles that made it unhealthy to linger close to Jupiter. Its wake was almost free of radiation, and there a ship could park in perfect safety, while death sleeted invisibly all around.

Falcon switched on the sleep inducer, and consciousness faded swiftly out as the electric pulses surged gently through his brain. While *Kon-Tiki* fell toward Jupiter, gaining speed second by second in that enormous gravitational field, he slept without dreams. They always came when he awoke; and he had brought his nightmares with him from Earth.

Yet he never dreamed of the crash itself, though he often found himself again face to face with that terrified superchimp, as he descended the spiral stairway between the collapsing gasbags. None of the simps had survived; those that were not killed outright were so badly injured that they had been painlessly "euthed." He sometimes wondered why he dreamed only of this doomed creature— which he had never met before the last minutes of its life—and not of the friends and colleagues he had lost aboard the dying *Queen*.

The dreams he feared most always began with his first return to consciousness. There had been little physical pain; in fact, there had been no sensation of any kind. He was in darkness and silence, and did not even seem to be breathing. And—strangest of all—he could not locate his limbs. He could move neither his hands nor his feet, because he did not know where they were.

The silence had been the first to yield. After hours, or days, he had become aware of a faint throbbing, and eventually, after long thought, he deduced that this was the beating of his own heart. That was the first of his many mistakes.

Then there had been faint pinpricks, sparkles of light, ghosts of pressures upon still-unresponsive limbs. One by one his senses had returned, and pain had come with them. He had had to learn everything anew, recapitulating infancy and babyhood. Though his memory was unaffected, and he could understand words that were spoken to him, it was months before he was able to answer except by the flicker of an eyelid. He could remember the moments of triumph when he had spoken the first word, turned the page of a book—and, finally, learned to move under his own power. *That* was a victory indeed, and it had taken him almost two years to prepare for it. A hundred times he had envied that dead superchimp, but *he* had been given no choice. The doctors had made their decision—and now, twelve years later, he was where no human being had ever traveled before, and moving faster than any man in history.

Kon-Tiki was just emerging from shadow, and the Jovian dawn bridged the sky ahead in a titanic bow of light, when the persistent buzz of the alarm dragged Falcon up from sleep. The inevitable nightmares (he had been trying to summon a nurse, but did not even have the strength to push the button) swiftly faded from consciousness. The greatest—and perhaps last—adventure of his life was before him.

He called Mission Control, now almost sixty thousand miles away and falling swiftly below the curve of Jupiter, to report that everything was in order. His velocity had just passed thirty-one miles a second (*that* was one for the books) and in half an hour *Kon-Tiki* would hit the outer fringes of the atmosphere, as he started on the most difficult re-entry in the entire solar system. Although scores of probes had survived this flaming ordeal, they had been tough, solidly packed masses of instrumentation, able to withstand several hundred gravities of drag. *Kon-Tiki* would hit peaks of thirty g's, and would average more than ten, before she came to rest in the upper reaches of the Jovian atmosphere. Very carefully and thoroughly, Falcon began to attach the elaborate system of re-

straints that would anchor him to the walls of the cabin. When he had finished, he was virtually a part of the ship's structure.

The clock was counting backward; one hundred seconds to reentry. For better or worse, he was committed. In a minute and a half, he would graze the Jovian atmosphere, and would be caught irrevocably in the grip of the giant.

The countdown was three seconds late—not at all bad, considering the unknowns involved. From beyond the walls of the capsule came a ghostly sighing, which rose steadily to a high-pitched, screaming roar. The noise was quite different from that of a reentry on Earth or Mars; in this thin atmosphere of hydrogen and helium, all sounds were transformed a couple of octaves upward. On Jupiter, even thunder would have falsetto overtones.

With the rising scream came mounting weight; within seconds, he was completely immobilized. His field of vision contracted until it embraced only the clock and the accelerometer; fifteen g, and four hundred and eighty seconds to go. . . .

He never lost consciousness; but then, he had not expected to. *Kon-Tiki's* trail through the Jovian atmosphere must be really spectacular—by this time, thousands of miles long. Five hundred seconds after entry, the drag began to taper off: ten g, five g, two. . . . Then weight vanished almost completely. He was falling free, all his enormous orbital velocity destroyed.

There was a sudden jolt as the incandescent remnants of the heat shield were jettisoned. It had done its work and would not be needed again; Jupiter could have it now. He released all but two of the restraining buckles, and waited for the automatic sequencer to start the next, and most critical, series of events.

He did not see the first drogue parachute pop out, but he could feel the slight jerk, and the rate of fall diminished immediately. *Kon-Tiki* had lost all her horizontal speed and was going straight down at almost a thousand miles an hour. Everything depended on what happened in the next sixty seconds.

There went the second drogue. He looked up through the overhead window and saw, to his immense relief, that clouds of glittering foil were billowing out behind the falling ship. Like a great flower unfurling, the thousands of cubic yards of the balloon spread

out across the sky, scooping up the thin gas until it was fully inflated. *Kon-Tiki's* rate of fall dropped to a few miles an hour and remained constant. Now there was plenty of time; it would take him days to fall all the way down to the surface of Jupiter.

But he would get there eventually, even if he did nothing about it. The balloon overhead was merely acting as an efficient parachute. It was providing no lift; nor could it do so, while the gas inside and out was the same.

With its characteristic and rather disconcerting crack the fusion reactor started up, pouring torrents of heat into the envelope overhead. Within five minutes, the rate of fall had become zero; within six, the ship had started to rise. According to the radar altimeter, it had leveled out at about two hundred and sixty-seven miles above the surface—or whatever passed for a surface on Jupiter.

Only one kind of balloon will work in an atmosphere of hydrogen, which is the lightest of all gases—and that is a hot-hydrogen balloon. As long as the fuser kept ticking over, *Falcon* could remain aloft, drifting across a world that could hold a hundred Pacifics. After traveling over three hundred million miles, *Kon-Tiki* had at last begun to justify her name. She was an aerial raft, adrift upon the currents of the Jovian atmosphere.

Though a whole new world was lying around him, it was more than an hour before Falcon could examine the view. First he had to check all the capsule's systems and test its response to the controls. He had to learn how much extra heat was necessary to produce a desired rate of ascent, and how much gas he must vent in order to descend. Above all, there was the question of stability. He must adjust the length of the cables attaching his capsule to the huge, pear-shaped balloon, to damp out vibrations and get the smoothest possible ride. Thus far, he was lucky; at this level, the wind was steady, and the Doppler reading on the invisible surface gave him a ground speed of two hundred seventeen and a half miles an hour. For Jupiter, that was modest; winds of up to a thousand had been observed. But mere speed was, of course, unimportant; the real dan-

ger was turbulence. If he ran into that, only skill and experience and swift reaction could save him—and these were not matters that could yet be programed into a computer.

Not until he was satisfied that he had got the feel of his strange craft did Falcon pay any attention to Mission Control's pleadings. Then he deployed the booms carrying the instrumentation and the atmospheric samplers. The capsule now resembled a rather untidy Christmas tree, but still rode smoothly down the Jovian winds while it radioed its torrents of information to the recorders on the ship miles above. And now, at last, he could look around. . . .

His first impression was unexpected, and even a little disappointing. As far as the scale of things was concerned, he might have been ballooning over an ordinary cloudscape on Earth. The horizon seemed at a normal distance; there was no feeling at all that he was on a world eleven times the diameter of his own. Then he looked at the infrared radar, sounding the layers of atmosphere beneath him—and knew how badly his eyes had been deceived.

That layer of clouds apparently about three miles away was really more than thirty-seven miles below. And the horizon, whose distance he would have guessed at about one hundred and twenty-five, was actually eighteen hundred miles from the ship.

The crystalline clarity of the hydrohelium atmosphere and the enormous curvature of the planet had fooled him completely. It was even harder to judge distances here than on the Moon; everything he saw must be multiplied by at least ten.

It was a simple matter, and he should have been prepared for it. Yet somehow, it disturbed him profoundly. He did not feel that Jupiter was huge, but that *he* had shrunk—to a tenth of his normal size. Perhaps, with time, he would grow accustomed to the inhuman scale of this world; yet as he stared toward that unbelievably distant horizon, he felt as if a wind colder than the atmosphere around him was blowing through his soul. Despite all his arguments, this might never be a place for man. He could well be both the first and the last to descend through the clouds of Jupiter.

The sky above was almost black, except for a few wisps of ammonia cirrus perhaps twelve miles overhead. It was cold up there, on the fringes of space, but both pressure and temperature increased rapidly with depth. At the level where *Kon-Tiki* was drifting now,

it was fifty below zero, and the pressure was five atmospheres. Sixty-five miles farther down, it would be as warm as equatorial Earth, and the pressure about the same as at the bottom of one of the shallower seas. Ideal conditions for life. . . .

A quarter of the brief Jovian day had already gone; the sun was halfway up the sky, but the light on the unbroken cloudscape below had a curious mellow quality. That extra three hundred million miles had robbed the Sun of all its power. Though the sky was clear, Falcon found himself continually thinking that it was a heavily overcast day. When night fell, the onset of darkness would be swift indeed; though it was still morning, there was a sense of autumnal twilight in the air. But autumn, of course, was something that never came to Jupiter. There were no seasons here.

Kon-Tiki had come down in the exact center of the equatorial zone—the least colorful part of the planet. The sea of clouds that stretched out to the horizon was tinted a pale salmon; there were none of the yellows and pinks and even reds that banded Jupiter at higher altitudes. The Great Red Spot itself—most spectacular of all of the planet's features—lay thousands of miles to the south. It had been a temptation to descend there, but the south tropical disturbance was unusually active, with currents reaching over nine hundred miles an hour. It would have been asking for trouble to head into that maelstrom of unknown forces. The Great Red Spot and its mysteries would have to wait for future expeditions.

The Sun, moving across the sky twice as swiftly as it did on Earth, was now nearing the zenith and had become eclipsed by the great silver canopy of the balloon. Kon-Tiki was still drifting swiftly and smoothly westward at a steady two hundred and seventeen and a half, but only the radar gave any indication of this. Was it always as calm here? Falcon asked himself. The scientists who had talked learnedly of the Jovian doldrums, and had predicted that the equator would be the quietest place, seemed to know what they were talking about, after all. He had been profoundly skeptical of all such forecasts, and had agreed with one unusually modest researcher who had told him bluntly: "There are no experts on Jupiter." Well, there would be at least one by the end of this day.

If he managed to survive until then.

4. The Voices of the Deep

That first day, the Father of the Gods smiled upon him. It was as calm and peaceful here on Jupiter as it had been, years ago, when he was drifting with Webster across the plains of northern India. Falcon had time to master his new skills, until *Kon-Tiki* seemed an extension of his own body. Such luck was more than he had dared to hope for, and he began to wonder what price he might have to pay for it.

The five hours of daylight were almost over; the clouds below were full of shadows, which gave them a massive solidity they had not possessed when the Sun was higher. Color was swiftly draining from the sky, except in the west itself, where a band of deepening purple lay along the horizon. Above this band was the thin crescent of a closer moon, pale and bleached against the utter blackness beyond.

With a speed perceptible to the eye, the Sun went straight down over the edge of Jupiter, over eighteen hundred miles away. The stars came out in their legions—and there was the beautiful evening star of Earth, on the very frontier to twilight, reminding him how far he was from home. It followed the Sun down into the west. Man's first night on Jupiter had begun.

With the onset of darkness, *Kon-Tiki* started to sink. The balloon was no longer heated by the feeble sunlight and was losing a small part of its buoyancy. Falcon did nothing to increase lift; he had expected this and was planning to descend.

The invisible cloud deck was still over thirty miles below, and he would reach it about midnight. It showed up clearly on the infrared radar, which also reported that it contained a vast array of complex carbon compounds, as well as the usual hydrogen, helium, and ammonia. The chemists were dying for samples of that fluffy, pinkish stuff; though some atmospheric probes had already gathered a few grams, they had only whetted their appetites. Half the basic molecules of life were here, floating high above the surface of Jupiter. And where there was food, could life be far away? That was the question that, after more than a hundred years, no one had been able to answer.

The infrared was blocked by the clouds, but the microwave

radar sliced right through and showed layer after layer, all the way down to the hidden surface almost two hundred and fifty miles below. That was barred to him by enormous pressures and temperatures; not even robot probes had ever reached it intact. It lay in tantalizing inaccessibility at the bottom of the radar screen, slightly fuzzy, and showing a curious granular structure that his equipment could not resolve.

An hour after sunset, he dropped his first probe. It fell swiftly for about sixty miles, then began to float in the denser atmosphere, sending back torrents of radio signals, which he relayed to Mission Control. Then there was nothing else to do until sunrise, except to keep an eye on the rate of descent, monitor the instruments, and answer occasional queries. While she was drifting in this steady current, *Kon-Tiki* could look after herself.

Just before midnight, a woman controller came on watch and introduced herself with the usual pleasantries. Ten minutes later she called again, her voice at once serious and excited.

"Howard! Listen in on channel forty-six—high gain."

Channel forty-six? There were so many telemetering circuits that he knew the numbers of only those that were critical; but as soon as he threw the switch, he recognized this one. He was plugged in to the microphone on the probe, floating more than eighty miles below him in an atmosphere now almost as dense as water.

At first, there was only a soft hiss of whatever strange winds stirred down in the darkness of that unimaginable world. And then, out of the background noise, there slowly emerged a booming vibration that grew louder and louder, like the beating of a gigantic drum. It was so low that it was felt as much as heard, and the beats steadily increased their tempo, though the pitch never changed. Now it was a swift, almost infrasonic throbbing. Then, suddenly, in mid-vibration, it stopped—so abruptly that the mind could not accept the silence, but memory continued to manufacture a ghostly echo in the deepest caverns of the brain.

It was the most extraordinary sound that Falcon had ever heard, even among the multitudinous noises of Earth. He could think of no natural phenomenon that could have caused it; nor was it like the cry of any animal, not even one of the great whales. . . .

It came again, following exactly the same pattern. Now that

he was prepared for it, he estimated the length of the sequence; from first faint throb to final crescendo, it lasted just over ten seconds.

And this time there was a real echo, very faint and far away. Perhaps it came from one of the many reflecting layers, deeper in this stratified atmosphere; perhaps it was another, more distant source. Falcon waited for a second echo, but it never came.

Mission Control reacted quickly and asked him to drop another probe at once. With two microphones operating, it would be possible to find the approximate location of the sources. Oddly enough, none of *Kon-Tiki's* own external mikes could detect anything except wind noises. The boomings, whatever they were, must have been trapped and channeled beneath an atmospheric reflecting layer far below.

They were coming, it was soon discovered, from a cluster of sources about twelve hundred miles away. The distance gave no indication of their power; in Earth's oceans, quite feeble sounds could travel equally far. And as for the obvious assumption that living creatures were responsible, the Chief Exobiologist quickly ruled that out.

"I'll be very disappointed," said Dr. Brenner, "if there are no microorganisms or plants here. But nothing like animals, because there's no free oxygen. All biochemical reactions on Jupiter must be low-energy ones—there's just no way an active creature could generate enough power to function."

Falcon wondered if this was true; he had heard the argument before, and reserved judgment.

"In any case," continued Brenner, "some of those sound waves are a hundred yards long! Even an animal as big as a whale couldn't produce them. They *must* have a natural origin."

Yes, that seemed plausible, and probably the physicists would be able to come up with an explanation. What would a blind alien make, Falcon wondered, of the sounds he might hear when standing beside a stormy sea, or a geyser, or a volcano, or a waterfall? He might well attribute them to some huge beast.

About an hour before sunrise the voices of the deep died away, and Falcon began to busy himself with preparation for the dawn of his second day. *Kon-Tiki* was now only three miles above the near-

est cloud layer; the external pressure had risen to ten atmospheres, and the temperature was a tropical thirty degrees. A man could be comfortable here with no more equipment than a breathing mask and the right grade of heliox mixture.

"We've some good news for you," Mission Control reported, soon after dawn. "The cloud layer's breaking up. You'll have partial clearing in an hour—but watch out for turbulence."

"I've already noticed some," Falcon answered. "How far down will I be able to see?"

"At least twelve miles, down to the second thermocline. *That* cloud deck is solid—it never breaks."

And it's out of my reach, Falcon told himself; the temperature down there must be over a hundred degrees. This was the first time that any balloonist had ever had to worry, not about his ceiling, but about his basement!

Ten minutes later he could see what Mission Control had already observed from its superior vantage point. There was a change in color near the horizon, and the cloud layer had become ragged and humpy, as if something had torn it open. He turned up his little nuclear furnace and gave *Kon-Tiki* another three miles of altitude, so that he could get a better view.

The sky below was clearing rapidly, completely, as if something was dissolving the solid overcast. An abyss was opening before his eyes. A moment later he sailed out over the edge of a cloud canyon about twelve miles deep and six hundred miles wide.

A new world lay spread beneath him; Jupiter had stripped away one of its many veils. The second layer of clouds, unattainably far below, was much darker in color than the first. It was almost salmon pink, and curiously mottled with little islands of brick red. They were all oval-shaped, with their long axes pointing east-west, in the direction of the prevailing wind. There were hundreds of them, all about the same size, and they reminded Falcon of puffy little cumulus clouds in the terrestrial sky.

He reduced buoyancy, and *Kon-Tiki* began to drop down the face of the dissolving cliff. It was then that he noticed the snow.

White flakes were forming in the air and drifting slowly downward. Yet it was much too warm for snow—and, in any event, there was scarcely a trace of water at this altitude. Moreover, there was

no glitter or sparkle about these flakes as they went cascading down into the depths. When, presently, a few landed on an instrument boom outside the main viewing port, he saw that they were a dull, opaque white—not crystalline at all—and quite large—several inches across. They looked like wax, and Falcon guessed that this was precisely what they were. Some chemical reaction was taking place in the atmosphere around him, condensing out the hydro-carbons floating in the Jovian air.

About sixty miles ahead, a disturbance was taking place in the cloud layer. The little red ovals were being jostled around, and were beginning to form a spiral—the familiar cyclonic pattern so com-mon in the meteorology of Earth. The vortex was emerging with astonishing speed; if that was a storm ahead, Falcon told himself, he was in big trouble.

And then his concern changed to wonder—and to fear. What was developing in his line of flight was not a storm at all. Some-thing enormous—something scores of miles across—was rising through the clouds.

The reassuring thought that it, too, might be a cloud—a thun-derhead boiling up from the lower levels of the atmosphere—lasted only a few seconds. No; this was *solid*. It shouldered its way through the pink-and-salmon overcast like an iceberg rising from the deeps.

An *iceberg* floating on hydrogen? That was impossible, of course; but perhaps it was not too remote an analogy. As soon as he focused the telescope upon the enigma, Falcon saw that it was a whitish, crystalline mass, threaded with streaks of red and brown. It must be, he decided, the same stuff as the "snowflakes" falling around him—a mountain range of wax. And it was not, he soon realized, as solid as he had thought; around the edges it was con-tinually crumbling and reforming. . . .

"I know what it is," he radioed Mission Control, which for the last few minutes had been asking anxious questions. "It's a mass of bubbles—some kind of foam. Hydrocarbon froth. Get the chemists working on . . . *Just a minute!*"

"What is it?" called Mission Control. "What is it?"

He ignored the frantic pleas from space and concentrated all his mind upon the image in the telescope field. He had to be sure;

if he made a mistake, he would be the laughingstock of the solar system.

Then he relaxed, glanced at the clock, and switched off the nagging voice from Jupiter V.

"Hello, Mission Control," he said, very formally. "This is Howard Falcon aboard *Kon-Tiki*. Ephemeris Time nineteen hours twenty-one minutes fifteen seconds. Latitude zero degrees five minutes North. Longitude one hundred five degrees forty-two minutes, System One.

"Tell Dr. Brenner that there is life on Jupiter. And it's *big*. . . ."

5. THE WHEELS OF POSEIDON

"I'm very happy to be proved wrong," Dr. Brenner radioed back cheerfully. "Nature always has something up her sleeve. Keep the long-focus camera on target and give us the steadiest pictures you can."

The things moving up and down those waxen slopes were still too far away for Falcon to make out many details, and they must have been very large to be visible at all at such a distance. Almost black, and shaped like arrowheads, they maneuvered by slow undulations of their entire bodies, so that they looked rather like giant manta rays, swimming above some tropical reef.

Perhaps they were sky-borne cattle, browsing on the cloud pastures of Jupiter, for they seemed to be feeding along the dark, red-brown streaks that ran like dried-up river beds down the flanks of the floating cliffs. Occasionally, one of them would dive headlong into the mountain of foam and disappear completely from sight.

Kon-Tiki was moving only slowly with respect to the cloud layer below; it would be at least three hours before she was above those ephemeral hills. She was in a race with the Sun. Falcon hoped that darkness would not fall before he could get a good view of the mantas, as he had christened them, as well as the fragile landscape over which they flapped their way.

It was a long three hours. During the whole time, he kept the external microphones on full gain, wondering if here was the source

of that booming in the night. The mantas were certainly large enough to have produced it; when he could get an accurate measurement, he discovered that they were almost a hundred yards across the wings. That was three times the length of the largest whale—though he doubted if they could weigh more than a few tons.

Half an hour before sunset, Kon-Tiki was almost above the "mountains."

"No," said Falcon, answering Mission Control's repeated questions about the mantas, "they're still showing no reaction to me. I don't think they're intelligent—they look like harmless vegetarians. And even if they try to chase me, I'm sure they can't reach my altitude."

Yet he was a little disappointed when the mantas showed not the slightest interest in him as he sailed high above their feeding ground. Perhaps they had no way of detecting his presence. When he examined and photographed them through the telescope, he could see no signs of any sense organs. The creatures were simply huge black deltas, rippling over hills and valleys that, in reality, were little more substantial than the clouds of Earth. Though they looked solid, Falcon knew that anyone who stepped on those white mountains would go crashing through them as if they were made of tissue paper.

At close quarters he could see the myriads of cellules or bubbles from which they were formed. Some of these were quite large—a yard or so in diameter—and Falcon wondered in what witches' cauldron of hydrocarbons they had been brewed. There must be enough petrochemicals deep down in the atmosphere of Jupiter to supply all Earth's needs for a million years.

The short day had almost gone when he passed over the crest of the waxen hills, and the light was fading rapidly along their lower slopes. There were no mantas on this western side, and for some reason the topography was very different. The foam was sculptured into long, level terraces, like the interior of a lunar crater. He could almost imagine that they were gigantic steps leading down to the hidden surface of the planet.

And on the lowest of those steps, just clear of the swirling clouds that the mountain had displaced when it came surging sky-

ward, was a roughly oval mass, one or two miles across. It was difficult to see, since it was only a little darker than the gray-white foam on which it rested. Falcon's first thought was that he was looking at a forest of pallid trees, like giant mushrooms that had never seen the Sun.

Yes, it must be a forest—he could see hundreds of thin trunks, springing from the white waxy froth in which they were rooted. But the trees were packed astonishingly close together; there was scarcely any space between them. Perhaps it was not a forest, after all, but a single enormous tree—like one of the giant multi-trunked banyans of the East. Once he had seen a banyan tree in Java that was over six hundred and fifty yards across; this monster was at least ten times that size.

The light had almost gone. The cloudscape had turned purple with refracted sunlight, and in a few seconds that, too, would have vanished. In the last light of his second day on Jupiter, Howard Falcon saw—or thought he saw—something that cast the gravest doubts on his interpretation of the white oval.

Unless the dim light had totally deceived him, those hundreds of thin trunks were beating back and forth, in perfect synchronism, like fronds of kelp rocking in the surge.

And the tree was no longer in the place where he had first seen it.

"Sorry about this," said Mission Control, soon after sunset, "but we think Source Beta is going to blow within the next hour. Probability seventy percent."

Falcon glanced quickly at the chart. Beta—Jupiter latitude one hundred and forty degrees—was over eighteen thousand six hundred miles away and well below his horizon. Even though major eruptions ran as high as ten megatons, he was much too far away for the shock wave to be a serious danger. The radio storm that it would trigger was, however, quite a different matter.

The decameter outbursts that sometimes made Jupiter the most powerful radio source in the whole sky had been discovered back in the 1950s, to the utter astonishment of the astronomers. Now, more than a century later, their real cause was still a mystery. Only

the symptoms were understood; the explanation was completely unknown.

The "volcano" theory had best stood the test of time, although no one imagined that this word had the same meaning on Jupiter as on Earth. At frequent intervals—often several times a day—titanic eruptions occurred in the lower depths of the atmosphere, probably on the hidden surface of the planet itself. A great column of gas, more than six hundred miles high, would start boiling upward as if determined to escape into space.

Against the most powerful gravitational field of all the planets, it had no chance. Yet some traces—a mere few million tons—usually managed to reach the Jovian ionosphere; and when they did, all hell broke loose.

The radiation belts surrounding Jupiter completely dwarf the feeble Van Allen belts of Earth. When they are short-circuited by an ascending column of gas, the result is an electrical discharge millions of times more powerful than any terrestrial flash of lightning; it sends a colossal thunderclap of radio noise flooding across the entire solar system and on out to the stars.

It had been discovered that these radio outbursts came from four main areas of the planet. Perhaps there were weaknesses there that allowed the fires of the interior to break out from time to time. The scientists on Ganymede, largest of Jupiter's many moons, now thought that they could predict the onset of a decameter storm; their accuracy was about as good as a weather forecaster's of the early 1900s.

Falcon did not know whether to welcome or to fear a radio storm; it would certainly add to the value of the mission—if he survived it. His course had been planned to keep as far as possible from the main centers of disturbance, especially the most active one, Source Alpha. As luck would have it, the threatening Beta was the closest to him. He hoped that the distance, almost three-fourths the circumference of Earth, was safe enough.

"Probability ninety percent," said Mission Control with a distinct note of urgency. "And forget that hour. Ganymede says it may be any moment."

The radio had scarcely fallen silent when the reading on the magnetic field-strength meter started to shoot upward. Before it

could go off scale, it reversed and began to drop as rapidly as it had risen. Far away and thousands of miles below, something had given the planet's molten core a titanic jolt.

"There she blows!" called Mission Control.

"Thanks, I already know. When will the storm hit me?"

"You can expect onset in five minutes. Peak in ten."

Far around the curve of Jupiter, a funnel of gas as wide as the Pacific Ocean was climbing spaceward at thousands of miles an hour. Already the thunderstorms of the lower atmosphere would be raging around it—but they were nothing compared with the fury that would explode when the radiation belt was reached and began dumping its surplus electrons onto the planet. Falcon began to retract all the instrument booms that were extended out from the capsule. There were no other precautions he could take. It would be four hours before the atmospheric shock wave reached him— but the radio blast, traveling at the speed of light, would be here in a tenth of a second, once the discharge had been triggered.

The radio monitor, scanning back and forth across the spectrum, still showed nothing unusual, just the normal mush of background static. Then Falcon noticed that the noise level was slowly creeping upward. The explosion was gathering its strength.

At such a distance he had never expected to *see* anything. But suddenly a flicker as of far-off heat lightning danced along the eastern horizon. Simultaneously, half the circuit breakers jumped out of the main switchboard, the lights failed, and all communications channels went dead.

He tried to move, but was completely unable to do so. The paralysis that gripped him was not merely psychological; he seemed to have lost all control of his limbs and could feel a painful tingling sensation over his entire body. It was impossible that the electric field could have penetrated this shielded cabin. Yet there was a flickering glow over the instrument board, and he could hear the unmistakable crackle of a brush discharge.

With a series of sharp bangs, the emergency systems went into operation, and the overloads reset themselves. The lights flickered on again. And Falcon's paralysis disappeared as swiftly as it had come.

After glancing at the board to make sure that all circuits were

back to normal, he moved quickly to the viewing ports.

There was no need to switch on the inspection lamps—the cables supporting the capsule seemed to be on fire. Lines of light glowing an electric blue against the darkness stretched upward from the main lift ring to the equator of the giant balloon; and rolling slowly along several of them were dazzling balls of fire.

The sight was so strange and so beautiful that it was hard to read any menace in it. Few people, Falcon knew, had ever seen ball lightning from such close quarters—and certainly none had survived if they were riding a hydrogen-filled balloon back in the atmosphere of Earth. He remembered the flaming death of the *Hindenburg*, destroyed by a stray spark when she docked at Lakehurst in 1937; as it had done so often in the past, the horrifying old newsreel film flashed through his mind. But at least that could not happen here, though there was more hydrogen above his head than had ever filled the last of the Zeppelins. It would be a few billion years yet, before anyone could light a fire in the atmosphere of Jupiter.

With a sound like briskly frying bacon, the speech circuit came back to life.

"Hello, *Kon-Tiki*—are you receiving? Are you receiving?"

The words were chopped and badly distorted, but intelligible. Falcon's spirits lifted; he had resumed contact with the world of men.

"I receive you," he said. "Quite an electrical display, but no damage—so far."

"Thanks—thought we'd lost you. Please check telemetry channels three, seven, twenty-six. Also gain on camera two. And we don't quite believe the readings on the external ionization probes. . . ."

Reluctantly Falcon tore his gaze away from the fascinating pyrotechnic display around *Kon-Tiki*, though from time to time he kept glancing out of the windows. The ball lightning disappeared first, the fiery globes slowly expanding until they reached a critical size, at which they vanished in a gentle explosion. But even an hour later, there were still faint glows around all the exposed metal on the outside of the capsule; and the radio circuits remained noisy until well after midnight.

The remaining hours of darkness were completely uneventful—until just before dawn. Because it came from the east, Falcon assumed that he was seeing the first faint hint of sunrise. Then he realized that it was twenty minutes too early for this—and the glow that had appeared along the horizon was moving toward him even as he watched. It swiftly detached itself from the arch of stars that marked the invisible edge of the planet, and he saw that it was a relatively narrow band, quite sharply defined. The beam of an enormous searchlight appeared to be swinging beneath the clouds.

Perhaps sixty miles behind the first racing bar of light came another, parallel to it and moving at the same speed. And beyond that another, and another—until all the sky flickered with alternating sheets of light and darkness.

By this time, Falcon thought, he had been inured to wonders, and it seemed impossible that this display of pure, soundless luminosity could present the slightest danger. But it was so astonishing, and so inexplicable, that he felt cold, naked fear gnawing at his self-control. No man could look upon such a sight without feeling like a helpless pygmy in the presence of forces beyond his comprehension. Was it possible that, after all, Jupiter carried not only life but also intelligence? And, perhaps, an intelligence that only now was beginning to react to his alien presence?

"Yes, we see it," said Mission Control, in a voice that echoed his own awe. "We've no idea what it is. Stand by, we're calling Ganymede."

The display was slowly fading; the bands racing in from the far horizon were much fainter, as if the energies that powered them were becoming exhausted. In five minutes it was all over; the last faint pulse of light flickered along the western sky and then was gone. Its passing left Falcon with an overwhelming sense of relief. The sight was so hypnotic, and so disturbing, that it was not good for any man's peace of mind to contemplate it too long.

He was more shaken than he cared to admit. The electrical storm was something that he could understand; but *this* was totally incomprehensible.

Mission Control was still silent. He knew that the information banks up on Ganymede were now being searched as men and computers turned their minds to the problem. If no answer could be

found there, it would be necessary to call Earth; that would mean a delay of almost an hour. The possibility that even Earth might be unable to help was one that Falcon did not care to contemplate.

He had never before been so glad to hear the voice of Mission Control as when Dr. Brenner finally came on the circuit. The biologist sounded relieved, yet subdued—like a man who has just come through some great intellectual crisis.

"Hello, Kon-Tiki. We've solved your problem, but we can still hardly believe it.

"What you've been seeing is bioluminescence, very similar to that produced by microorganisms in the tropical seas of Earth. Here they're in the atmosphere, not the ocean, but the principle is the same."

"But the pattern," protested Falcon, "was so regular—so *artificial*. And it was hundreds of miles across!"

"It was even larger than you imagine; you observed only a small part of it. The whole pattern was over three thousand miles wide and looked like a revolving wheel. You merely saw the spokes, sweeping past you at about six-tenths of a mile a second. . . ."

"A *second!*" Falcon could not help interjecting. "No animals could move that fast!"

"Of course not. Let me explain. What you saw was triggered by the shock wave from Source Beta, moving at the speed of sound."

"But what about the pattern?" Falcon insisted.

"That's the surprising part. It's a very rare phenomenon, but identical wheels of light—except that they're a thousand times smaller—have been observed in the Persian Gulf and the Indian Ocean. Listen to this: British India Company's *Patna*, Persian Gulf, May 1880, 11:30 P.M.—'an enormous luminous wheel, whirling round, the spokes of which appeared to brush the ship along. The spokes were 200 or 300 yards long . . . each wheel contained about sixteen spokes. . . .' And here's one from the Gulf of Omar, dated May 23, 1906: 'The intensely bright luminescence approached us rapidly, shooting sharply defined light rays to the west in rapid succession, like the beam from the searchlight of a warship. . . . To the left of us, a gigantic fiery wheel formed itself, with spokes that reached as far as one could see. The whole wheel whirled around

for two or three minutes. . . .' The archive computer on Ganymede dug up about five hundred cases. It would have printed out the lot if we hadn't stopped it in time."

"I'm convinced—but still baffled."

"I don't blame you. The full explanation wasn't worked out until late in the twentieth century. It seems that these luminous wheels are the results of submarine earthquakes, and always occur in shallow waters where the shock waves can be reflected and cause standing wave patterns. Sometimes bars, sometimes rotating wheels—the 'Wheels of Poseidon,' they've been called. The theory was finally proved by making underwater explosions and photographing the results from a satellite. No wonder sailors used to be superstitious. Who would have believed a thing like *this?*"

So that was it, Falcon told himself. When Source Beta blew its top, it must have sent shock waves in all directions—through the compressed gas of the lower atmosphere, through the solid body of Jupiter itself. Meeting and crisscrossing, those waves must have canceled here, reinforced there; the whole planet must have rung like a bell.

Yet the explanation did not destroy the sense of wonder and awe; he would never be able to forget those flickering bands of light, racing through the unattainable depths of the Jovian atmosphere. He felt that he was not merely on a strange planet, but in some magical realm between myth and reality.

This was a world where absolutely *anything* could happen, and no man could possibly guess what the future would bring.

And he still had a whole day to go.

6. Medusa

When the true dawn finally arrived, it brought a sudden change of weather. *Kon-Tiki* was moving through a blizzard; waxen snowflakes were falling so thickly that visibility was reduced to zero. Falcon began to worry about the weight that might be accumulating on the envelope. Then he noticed that any flakes settling outside the windows quickly disappeared; *Kon-Tiki*'s continual outpouring of heat was evaporating them as swiftly as they arrived.

If he had been ballooning on Earth, he would also have worried about the possibility of collision. At least that was no danger here; any Jovian mountains were several hundred miles below him. And as for the floating islands of foam, hitting them would probably be like plowing into slightly hardened soap bubbles.

Nevertheless, he switched on the horizontal radar, which until now had been completely useless; only the vertical beam, giving his distance from the invisible surface, had thus far been of any value. Then he had another surprise.

Scattered across a huge sector of the sky ahead were dozens of large and brilliant echoes. They were completely isolated from one another and apparently hung unsupported in space. Falcon remembered a phrase the earliest aviators had used to describe one of the hazards of their profession: "clouds stuffed with rocks." That was a perfect description of what seemed to lie in the track of *Kon-Tiki*.

It was a disconcerting sight; then Falcon again reminded himself that nothing *really* solid could possibly hover in this atmosphere. Perhaps it was some strange meteorological phenomenon. In any case, the nearest echo was about a hundred and twenty-five miles.

He reported to Mission Control, which could provide no explanation. But it gave the welcome news that he would be clear of the blizzard in another thirty minutes.

It did not warn him, however, of the violent cross wind that abruptly grabbed *Kon-Tiki* and swept it almost at right angles to its previous track. Falcon needed all his skill and the maximum use of what little control he had over his ungainly vehicle to prevent it from being capsized. Within minutes he was racing northward at over three hundred miles an hour. Then, as suddenly as it had started, the turbulence ceased; he was still moving at high speed, but in smooth air. He wondered if he had been caught in the Jovian equivalent of a jet stream.

The snow storm dissolved; and he saw what Jupiter had been preparing for him.

Kon-Tiki had entered the funnel of a gigantic whirlpool, some six hundred miles across. The balloon was being swept along a curving wall of cloud. Overhead, the sun was shining in a clear sky; but far beneath, this great hole in the atmosphere drilled down to

unknown depths until it reached a misty floor where lightning flickered almost continuously.

Though the vessel was being dragged downward so slowly that
it was in no immediate danger, Falcon increased the flow of heat
into the envelope until *Kon-Tiki* hovered at a constant altitude.
Not until then did he abandon the fantastic spectacle outside and
consider again the problem of the radar.

The nearest echo was now only about twenty-five miles away.
All of them, he quickly realized, were distributed along the wall of
the vortex, and were moving with it, apparently caught in the
whirlpool like *Kon-Tiki* itself. He aimed the telescope along the
radar bearing and found himself looking at a curious mottled cloud
that almost filled the field of view.

It was not easy to see, being only a little darker than the whirling wall of mist that formed its background. Not until he had been
staring for several minutes did Falcon realize that he had met it
once before.

The first time it had been crawling across the drifting mountains of foam, and he had mistaken it for a giant, many-trunked
tree. Now at last he could appreciate its real size and complexity
and could give it a better name to fix its image in his mind. It did
not resemble a tree at all, but a jellyfish—a medusa, such as might
be met trailing its tentacles as it drifted along the warm eddies of
the Gulf Stream.

This medusa was more than a mile across and its scores of dangling tentacles were hundreds of feet long. They swayed slowly back
and forth in perfect unison, taking more than a minute for each
complete undulation—almost as if the creature was clumsily rowing
itself through the sky.

The other echoes were more distant medusae. Falcon focused
the telescope on half a dozen and could see no variations in shape
or size. They all seemed to be of the same species, and he wondered
just why they were drifting lazily around in this six-hundred-mile
orbit. Perhaps they were feeding upon the aerial plankton sucked
in by the whirlpool, as *Kon-Tiki* itself had been.

"Do you realize, Howard," said Dr. Brenner, when he had recovered from his initial astonishment, "that this thing is about a
hundred thousand times as large as the biggest whale? And even if

it's only a gasbag, it must still weigh a million tons! I can't even guess at its metabolism. It must generate megawatts of heat to maintain its buoyancy."

"But if it's just a gasbag, why is it such a damn good radar reflector?"

"I haven't the faintest idea. Can you get any closer?"

Brenner's question was not an idle one. If he changed altitude to take advantage of the differing wind velocities, Falcon could approach the medusa as closely as he wished. At the moment, however, he preferred his present twenty-five miles and said so, firmly.

"I see what you mean," Brenner answered, a little reluctantly. "Let's stay where we are for the present." That "we" gave Falcon a certain wry amusement; an extra sixty thousand miles made a considerable difference in one's point of view.

For the next two hours *Kon-Tiki* drifted uneventfully in the gyre of the great whirlpool, while Falcon experimented with filters and camera contrast, trying to get a clear view of the medusa. He began to wonder if its elusive coloration was some kind of camouflage; perhaps, like many animals of Earth, it was trying to lose itself against its background. That was a trick used by both hunters and hunted.

In which category was the medusa? That was a question he could hardly expect to have answered in the short time that was left to him. Yet just before noon, without the slightest warning, the answer came. . . .

Like a squadron of antique jet fighters, five mantas came sweeping through the wall of mist that formed the funnel of the vortex. They were flying in a V formation directly toward the pallid gray cloud of the medusa; and there was no doubt, in Falcon's mind, that they were on the attack. He had been quite wrong to assume that they were harmless vegetarians.

Yet everything happened at such a leisurely pace that it was like watching a slow-motion film. The mantas undulated along at perhaps thirty miles an hour; it seemed ages before they reached the medusa, which continued to paddle imperturbably along at an even slower speed. Huge though they were, the mantas looked tiny beside the monster they were approaching. When they flapped

down on its back, they appeared about as large as birds landing on a whale.

Could the medusa defend itself? Falcon wondered. He did not see how the attacking mantas could be in danger as long as they avoided those huge clumsy tentacles. And perhaps their host was not even aware of them; they could be insignificant parasites, tolerated as are fleas upon a dog.

But now it was obvious that the medusa was in distress. With agonizing slowness, it began to tip over like a capsizing ship. After ten minutes it had tilted forty-five degrees; it was also rapidly losing altitude. It was impossible not to feel a sense of pity for the beleaguered monster, and to Falcon the sight brought bitter memories. In a grotesque way, the fall of the medusa was almost a parody of the dying *Queen's* last moments.

Yet he knew that his sympathies were on the wrong side. High intelligence could develop only among predators—not among the drifting browsers of either sea or air. The mantas were far closer to him than was this monstrous bag of gas. And anyway, who could *really* sympathize with a creature a hundred thousand times larger than a whale?

Then he noticed that the medusa's tactics seemed to be having some effect. The mantas had been disturbed by its slow roll and were flapping heavily away from its back—like gorging vultures interrupted at mealtime. But they did not move very far, continuing to hover a few yards from the still-capsizing monster.

There was a sudden, blinding flash of light synchronized with a crash of static over the radio. One of the mantas, slowly twisting end over end, was plummeting straight downward. As it fell, a plume of black smoke trailed behind it. The resemblance to an aircraft going down in flames was quite uncanny.

In unison, the remaining mantas dived steeply away from the medusa, gaining speed by losing altitude. They had, within minutes, vanished back into the wall of cloud from which they had emerged. And the medusa, no longer falling, began to roll back toward the horizontal. Soon it was sailing along once more on an even keel, as if nothing had happened.

"Beautiful!" said Dr. Brenner, after a moment of stunned si-

lence. "It's developed electric defenses, like some of our eels and rays. But that must have been about a million volts! Can you see any organs that might produce the discharge? Anything looking like electrodes?"

"No," Falcon answered, after switching to the highest power of the telescope. "But here's something odd. Do you see this pattern? Check back on the earlier images. I'm sure it wasn't there before."

A broad, mottled band had appeared along the side of the medusa. It formed a startlingly regular checkerboard, each square of which was itself speckled in a complex subpattern of short horizontal lines. They were spaced at equal distances in a geometrically perfect array of rows and columns.

"You're right," said Dr. Brenner, with something very much like awe in his voice. "That's just appeared. And I'm afraid to tell you what I think it is."

"Well, I have no reputation to lose—at least as a biologist. Shall I give my guess?"

"Go ahead."

"That's a large meter-band radio array. The sort of thing they used back at the beginning of the twentieth century."

"I was afraid you'd say that. Now we know why it gave such a massive echo."

"But why has it just appeared?"

"Probably an aftereffect of the discharge."

"I've just had another thought," said Falcon, rather slowly. "Do you suppose it's *listening* to us?"

"On this frequency? I doubt it. Those are meter—no, *decameter* antennas—judging by their size. Hmm . . . that's an idea!"

Dr. Brenner fell silent, obviously contemplating some new line of thought. Presently he continued: "I bet they're tuned to the radio outbursts! That's something nature never got around to do on Earth. . . . We have animals with sonar and even electric senses, but nothing ever developed a radio sense. Why bother where there was so much light?

"But it's different here. Jupiter is *drenched* with radio energy. It's worth while using it—maybe even tapping it. That thing could be a floating power plant!"

A new voice cut into the conversation.

"Mission Commander here. This is all very interesting, but there's a much more important matter to settle. *Is it intelligent?* If so, we've got to consider the First Contact directives."

"Until I came here," said Dr. Brenner, somewhat ruefully, "I would have sworn that anything that could make a shortwave antenna system *must* be intelligent. Now, I'm not sure. This could have evolved naturally. I suppose it's no more fantastic than the human eye."

"Then we have to play safe and assume intelligence. For the present, therefore, this expedition comes under all the clauses of the Prime directive."

There was a long silence while everyone on the radio circuit absorbed the implications of this. For the first time in the history of space flight, the rules that had been established through more than a century of argument might have to be applied. Man had—it was hoped—profited from his mistakes on Earth. Not only moral considerations, but also his own self-interest demanded that he should not repeat them among the planets. It could be disastrous to treat a superior intelligence as the American settlers had treated the Indians, or as almost everyone had treated the Africans. . . .

The first rule was: keep your distance. Make no attempt to approach, or even to communicate, until "they" have had plenty of time to study you. Exactly what was meant by "plenty of time," no one had ever been able to decide. It was left to the discretion of the man on the spot.

A responsibility of which he had never dreamed had descended upon Howard Falcon. In the few hours that remained to him on Jupiter, he might become the first ambassador of the human race.

And *that* was an irony so delicious that he almost wished the surgeons had restored to him the power of laughter.

7. PRIME DIRECTIVE

It was growing darker, but Falcon scarcely noticed as he strained his eyes toward that living cloud in the field of the telescope. The wind that was steadily sweeping *Kon-Tiki* around the funnel of the great whirlpool had now brought him within twelve miles of the creature.

If he got much closer than six, he would take evasive action. Though he felt certain that the medusa's electric weapons were short-ranged, he did not wish to put the matter to the test. That would be a problem for future explorers, and he wished them luck.

Now it was quite dark in the capsule. That was strange, because sunset was still hours away. Automatically, he glanced at the horizontally scanning radar, as he had done every few minutes. Apart from the medusa he was studying, there was no other object within about sixty miles of him.

Suddenly, with startling power, he heard the sound that had come booming out of the Jovian night—the throbbing beat that grew more and more rapid, then stopped in mid-crescendo. The whole capsule vibrated with it like a pea in a kettledrum.

Falcon realized two things almost simultaneously during the sudden, aching silence. *This* time the sound was not coming from thousands of miles away, over a radio circuit. It was in the very atmosphere around him.

The second thought was even more disturbing. He had quite forgotten—it was inexcusable, but there had been other apparently more important things on his mind—that most of the sky above him was completely blanked out by *Kon-Tiki*'s gas-bag. Being lightly silvered to conserve its heat, the great balloon was an effective shield both to radar and to vision.

He had known this, of course; it had been a minor defect of the design, tolerated because it did not appear important. It seemed very important to Howard Falcon now—as he saw that fence of gigantic tentacles, thicker than the trunks of any tree, descending all around the capsule.

He heard Brenner yelling: "Remember the Prime directive! Don't alarm it!" Before he could make an appropriate answer that overwhelming drum beat started again and drowned all other sounds.

The sign of a really skilled test pilot is how he reacts not to foreseeable emergencies, but to ones that nobody could have anticipated. Falcon did not hesitate for more than a second to analyze the situation. In a lightning-swift movement, he pulled the rip cord.

That word was an archaic survival from the days of the first hydrogen balloons; on *Kon-Tiki*, the rip cord did not tear open the

gasbag, but merely operated a set of louvers around the upper curve of the envelope. At once the hot gas started to rush out; Kon-Tiki, deprived of her lift, began to fall swiftly in this gravity field two and a half times as strong as Earth's.

Falcon had a momentary glimpse of great tentacles whipping upward and away. He had just time to note that they were studded with large bladders or sacs, presumably to give them buoyancy, and that they ended in multitudes of thin feelers like the roots of a plant. He half expected a bolt of lightning—but nothing happened.

His precipitous rate of descent was slackening as the atmosphere thickened and the deflated envelope acted as a parachute. When Kon-Tiki had dropped about two miles, he felt that it was safe to close the louvers again. By the time he had restored buoyancy and was in equilibrium once more, he had lost another mile of altitude and was getting dangerously near his safety limit.

He peered anxiously through the overhead windows, though he did not expect to see anything except the obscuring bulk of the balloon. But he had sideslipped during his descent, and part of the medusa was just visible a couple of miles above him. It was much closer than he expected—and it was still coming down, faster than he would have believed possible.

Mission Control was calling anxiously. He shouted: "I'm O.K.—but it's still coming after me. I can't go any deeper."

That was not quite true. He could go a lot deeper—about one hundred and eighty miles. But it would be a one-way trip, and most of the journey would be of little interest to him.

Then, to his great relief, he saw that the medusa was leveling off, not quite a mile above him. Perhaps it had decided to approach this strange intruder with caution; or perhaps it, too, found this deeper layer uncomfortably hot. The temperature was over fifty degrees centigrade, and Falcon wondered how much longer his life-support system could handle matters.

Dr. Brenner was back on the circuit, still worrying about the Prime directive.

"Remember—it may only be inquisitive!" he cried, without much conviction. "Try not to frighten it!"

Falcon was getting rather tired of this advice and recalled a TV discussion he had once seen between a space lawyer and an astro-

naut. After the full implications of the Prime directive had been carefully spelled out, the incredulous spacer had exclaimed: "Then if there was no alternative, I must sit still and let myself be eaten?" The lawyer had not even cracked a smile when he answered: "That's an *excellent* summing up."

It had seemed funny at the time; it was not at all amusing now.

And then Falcon saw something that made him even more unhappy. The medusa was still hovering about a mile above him—but one of its tentacles was becoming incredibly elongated, and was stretching down toward *Kon-Tiki*, thinning out at the same time. As a boy he had once seen the funnel of a tornado descending from a storm cloud over the Kansas plains. The thing coming toward him now evoked vivid memories of that black, twisting snake in the sky.

"I'm rapidly running out of options," he reported to Mission Control. "I now have only a choice between frightening it—and giving it a bad stomach-ache. I don't think it will find *Kon-Tiki* very digestible, if that's what it has in mind."

He waited for comments from Brenner, but the biologist remained silent.

"Very well. It's twenty-seven minutes ahead of time, but I'm starting the ignition sequencer. I hope I'll have enough reserve to correct my orbit later."

He could no longer see the medusa; once more it was directly overhead. But he knew that the descending tentacle must now be very close to the balloon. It would take almost five minutes to bring the reactor up to full thrust. . . .

The fuser was primed. The orbit computer had not rejected the situation as wholly impossible. The air scoops were open, ready to gulp in tons of the surrounding hydrohelium on demand. Even under optimum conditions, this would have been the moment of truth—for there had been no way of testing how a nuclear ramjet would *really* work in the strange atmosphere of Jupiter.

Very gently something rocked *Kon-Tiki*. Falcon tried to ignore it.

Ignition had been planned at six miles higher, in an atmosphere of less than a quarter of the density and thirty degrees cooler. Too bad.

What was the shallowest dive he could get away with, for the

air scoops to work? When the ram ignited, he'd be heading toward Jupiter with two and a half g's to help him get there. Could he possibly pull out in time?

A large, heavy hand patted the balloon. The whole vessel bobbed up and down, like one of the yo-yo's that had just become the craze on Earth.

Of course, Brenner *might* be perfectly right. Perhaps it was just trying to be friendly. Maybe he should try to talk to it over the radio. Which should it be: "Pretty pussy"? "Down, Fido"? Or "Take me to your leader"?

The tritium-deuterium ratio was correct. He was ready to light the candle, with a hundred-million-degree match.

The thin tip of the tentacle came slithering around the edge of the balloon some sixty yards away. It was about the size of an elephant's trunk, and by the delicate way it was moving appeared to be almost as sensitive. There were little palps at its end, like questing mouths. He was sure that Dr. Brenner would be fascinated.

This seemed about as good a time as any. He gave a swift scan of the entire control board, started the final four-second ignition count, broke the safety seal, and pressed the JETTISON switch.

There was a sharp explosion and an instant loss of weight. *Kon-Tiki* was falling freely, nose down. Overhead, the discarded balloon was racing upward, dragging the inquisitive tentacle with it. Falcon had no time to see if the gasbag actually hit the medusa, because at that moment the ramjet fired and he had other matters to think about.

A roaring column of hot hydrohelium was pouring out of the reactor nozzles, swiftly building up thrust—but *toward* Jupiter, not away from it. He could not pull out yet, for vector control was too sluggish. Unless he could gain complete control and achieve horizontal flight within the next five seconds, the vehicle would dive too deeply into the atmosphere and would be destroyed.

With agonizing slowness—those five seconds seemed like fifty—he managed to flatten out, then pull the nose upward. He glanced back only once and caught a final glimpse of the medusa, many miles away. *Kon-Tiki*'s discarded gasbag had apparently escaped from its grasp, for he could see no sign of it.

Now he was master once more—no longer drifting helplessly

on the winds of Jupiter, but riding his own column of atomic fire back to the stars. He was confident that the ramjet would steadily give him velocity and altitude until he had reached near-orbital speed at the fringes of the atmosphere. Then, with a brief burst of pure rocket power, he would regain the freedom of space.

Halfway to orbit, he looked south and saw the tremendous enigma of the Great Red Spot—that floating island twice the size of Earth—coming up over the horizon. He stared into its mysterious beauty until the computer warned him that conversion to rocket thrust was only sixty seconds ahead. He tore his gaze reluctantly away.

"Some other time," he murmured.

"What's that?" said Mission Control. "What did you say?"

"It doesn't matter," he replied.

8. BETWEEN TWO WORLDS

"You're a hero now, Howard," said Webster, "not just a celebrity. You've given them something to think about—injected some excitement into their lives. Not one in a million will actually travel to the Outer Giants, but the whole human race will go in imagination. And that's what counts."

"I'm glad to have made your job a little easier."

Webster was too old a friend to take offense at the note of irony. Yet it surprised him. And this was not the first change in Howard that he had noticed since the return from Jupiter.

The Administrator pointed to the famous sign on his desk, borrowed from an impresario of an earlier age: ASTONISH ME!

"I'm not ashamed of my job. New knowledge, new resources—they're all very well. But men also need novelty and excitement. Space travel has become routine; you've made it a great adventure once more. It will be a long, long time before we get Jupiter pigeonholed. And maybe longer still before we understand those medusae. I still think that one *knew* where your blind spot was. Anyway, have you decided on your next move? Saturn, Uranus, Neptune—you name it."

"I don't know. I've thought about Saturn, but I'm not really

needed there. It's only one gravity, not two and a half like Jupiter. So men can handle it."

Men, thought Webster. He said "men." He's never done that before. And when did I last hear him use the word "we"? He's changing, slipping away from us. . . .

"Well," he said aloud, rising from his chair to conceal his slight uneasiness, "let's get the conference started. The cameras are all set up and everyone's waiting. You'll meet a lot of old friends."

He stressed the last word, but Howard showed no response. The leather mask of his face was becoming more and more difficult to read. Instead, he rolled back from the Administrator's desk, unlocked his undercarriage so that it no longer formed a chair, and rose on his hydraulics to his full seven feet of height. It had been good psychology on the part of the surgeons to give him that extra twelve inches, to compensate somewhat for all that he had lost when the *Queen* had crashed.

Falcon waited until Webster had opened the door, then pivoted neatly on his balloon tires and headed for it at a smooth and silent twenty miles an hour. The display of speed and precision was not flaunted arrogantly; rather, it had become quite unconscious.

Howard Falcon, who had once been a man and could still pass for one over a voice circuit, felt a calm sense of achievement—and, for the first time in years, something like peace of mind. Since his return from Jupiter, the nightmares had ceased. He had found his role at last.

He now knew why he had dreamed about that superchimp aboard the doomed *Queen Elizabeth*. Neither man nor beast, it was between two worlds; and so was he.

He alone could travel unprotected on the lunar surface. The life-support system inside the metal cylinder that had replaced his fragile body functioned equally well in space or under water. Gravity fields ten times that of Earth were an inconvenience, but nothing more. And no gravity was best of all. . . .

The human race was becoming more remote, the ties of kinship more tenuous. Perhaps these air-breathing, radiation-sensitive bundles of unstable carbon compounds had no right beyond the atmosphere; they should stick to their natural homes—Earth, Moon, Mars.

Some day the real masters of space would be machines, not men—and he was neither. Already conscious of his destiny, he took a somber pride in his unique loneliness—the first immortal midway between two orders of creation.

He would, after all, be an ambassador; between the old and the new—between the creatures of carbon and the creatures of metal who must one day supersede them.

Both would have need of him in the troubled centuries that lay ahead.

ISAAC ASIMOV

1920–1992

Isaac Asimov was born in Russia, in a small town near the city of Smolensk, but he didn't stay there. When he was three years old, his father sought a better life in America. The family emigrated to Brooklyn, New York, a borough from which Isaac hardly strayed for the next fifteen years of his life.

Although young Isaac was not geographically adventurous in the flesh, his mind wandered far from the little candy store his parents owned. Isaac was a reader. He read everything that came to his hand. (He was the only person I knew who had read the current edition of the *Encyclopedia Britannica* all the way through.) By his early teens his vicarious voyaging was spreading over galaxies, for he had found the reading he enjoyed most in the science fiction magazines.

From reading science fiction it was only a step to trying to write those stories for himself, and when he was seventeen he made the effort.

John Campbell's *Astounding* was the class magazine in the field, and Isaac aimed at the top. He was not an immediate success with Campbell. Campbell bounced his first couple of stories, "Marooned off Vesta" and "The Weapon Too Dreadful to Use," but they were not a total loss; Isaac promptly resubmitted them to the competing *Amazing Stories*, which snapped them up. But Isaac's diligence and talent won Campbell over, and before long he was a regular in *Astounding*. (Those two early rejections may have been a lucky break for Isaac. Bearing in mind Campbell's predilection for WASPish bylines, Isaac Asimov may narrowly have escaped being

persuaded to become something like "Anson MacIsaacs"—saved by the fact that by the time Campbell got around to buying something from him, Isaac already had an established presence under his own name.)

Isaac's family finally settled down at 174 Windsor Place in Brooklyn, where the candy store they operated was just a block or two from Brooklyn's wonderful Prospect Park. It happened that at the time I lived diagonally across the park, on St. John's Place. We had met as fellow sf fans and wannabee writers—members of that nest of wannabees, the fan club called the "Futurians." (A good many of us Futurian wannabees did in fact make it, including C. M. Kornbluth, Damon Knight, James Blish, Donald A. Wollheim, Robert A. W. Lowndes, and Judith Merril, among others.) It was no trouble for a teenager to stroll a mile or so across the park for a visit on a nice day—especially in my own case, since I had the extra incentive of getting a free malted milk at the candy store from Isaac's mother—and Isaac and I became good friends, staying that way for nearly sixty years.

The late 1930s were a busy time for Isaac. Candy stores are open for long hours. When Isaac's parents weren't in the store, Isaac or one of his siblings (sister Marcia, brother Stanley) had to take over. That chore was not always a dead loss for Isaac, because when business was slow he spent the time reading. Not all the reading was overtly recreational (although reading of all kinds was always recreational for Isaac), since by then he had entered Columbia University and had to study to prepare for his planned entry into medical school.

Medical school didn't happen for Isaac. Those were the days of a pervasive genteel anti-Semitism in American society. Some important people somewhere were of the opinion that there were more Jewish doctors than was appropriate, and so "Jewish quotas" were established in medical schools. Isaac didn't make the cut, and had ultimately to settle for a Ph.D in biochemistry instead of the M.D. he had wanted. Too bad for his possible future patients, because he would have made a fine doctor; not so bad for the rest of

us, because if Isaac had taken on the responsibilities of a physician, when would he have had time to write?

He did write. Found time somehow, kept it up. In those early years with Campbell at *Astounding* he began the continued works that are most closely associated with his name. First there were the "positronic robot" stories, later collected as *I, Robot* and half a dozen other volumes. Then some of that recreational reading produced a large dividend. Isaac had just finished *The Decline and Fall of the Roman Empire*, thought it suggested an interesting theme for science fiction stories, and wrote the novelette called *Foundation*.

Although I read nearly everything Isaac wrote until the 1950s, after which his massive production got hopelessly ahead of me, it is an odd fact that I never actually read the first few of the *Foundation* stories. I didn't have to. By then I had become a magazine editor on my own and had moved to Knickerbocker Village, down near the Manhattan Bridge in New York. On Sundays Isaac was likely to take the subway over for a visit. We'd go for a long walk—sometimes through nearby Chinatown, sometimes across the bridge to the Brooklyn side—and he would tell me the stories he had been writing. So when they came out in the magazines they were already old news to me.

When Isaac wrote his first robot story, he had no plans for a long-lasting series. It had simply occurred to him that a robot might make a good nursemaid for a small child, and so he wrote the story called "Robbie." Naturally he gave it first to Campbell, who bounced it at once. The trouble was, Campbell explained to Isaac, he hadn't really thought about what robots were actually going to be like. They couldn't just be clanking machines that did whatever their mechanical minds dictated. They had to be invested (the word *programmed* had not yet become fashionable) with certain basic constraints, else there was no telling what kind of trouble they might get into. Isaac took the point at once. The result was the famous "Three Laws of Robotics," which became gospel for all the robot stories which followed.

(Of course, that particular problem of self-willed robots has never arisen. No machine intelligence has yet shown any signs of enough self-awareness to need constraining. Actually, when the

great computer guru, Marvin Minsky, became a graduate student at MIT he remembered those stories, and so one of his first projects was to try to program the three laws into an actual computer. That turned out to be impossible, but in the process Minsky learned something about the nature of hierarchical programming.)

After Campbell bounced "Robbie," Isaac did what came naturally, he gave it to me for one of my new magazines, and I published it, changing the title to "Strange Playfellow." (Isaac hated the title change. Over the years I changed a lot of his titles, and he always hated it, and always had the last word. Every one of his stories got republished time and again, and he changed the titles back.)

Although from the beginning Isaac was part of that astonishing efflorescence of new writers that made up the golden age of *Astounding*, the place in the pantheon earned by his earliest stories was relatively inconspicuous. The thing that decisively marked him as a unique voice in that wonderful chorus wasn't a story at all; it was an "article" about a fascinating, but entirely imaginary, chemical compound called thiotimoline, which had the unique property of time-traveling by going into solution even before the solvent was added. The article was a splendid joke, taken as gospel by a few of the more credulous readers, denounced as irresponsible fraud by others, but enjoyed by just about all. From then on it was clear that this writer was something special.

During World War II Isaac remained a civilian, but became a part of that interesting research team at the Philadelphia Navy Yard that included our other Grand Masters, Heinlein and de Camp (see volume one). It wasn't until the war was over that the draft caught Isaac. He spent a few uncomfortable months in the Pacific (very nearly getting to be one of the soldiers ordered to witness some A-bomb tests), and got out to finish his pursuit of a doctorate and get back to writing.

One of the things he wrote was a short novel, on order for the magazine *Startling Stories*. It was called *Grow Old with Me* (from Robert Browning's poem, "Rabbi ben Ezra"), and the editor of *Startling* didn't like the title or, for that matter, the story itself. Although he had asked Isaac to write it, he rejected it outright.

It was then no longer possible for Isaac to turn his rejects over to me to publish in one of my magazines, because I hadn't returned to editing at that time. What I had done, though, was to become a literary agent.

Something new had been added to the field of science fiction publishing after World War II. Until then almost no American science fiction appeared in book form; if you didn't read the magazines, you didn't read American science fiction. But in the late 1940s a few fans began to set up their own little semiprofessional publishing companies, reprinting in volume form some of the great magazine serials of the past. As the salesmen for the big trade houses visited bookstores, they took note of this new publishing category that seemed to have an active market. When they got back from their sales trips, they told their home offices about it; and so a couple of the big New York publishers decided to experiment with a science fiction line. As an agent, I began doing business with some of them, and persuaded Isaac to take *Grow Old with Me* out of the file drawer and let me show it to Doubleday, who bought it, changing the title to *Pebble in the Sky*. (That title Isaac never changed back. Clearly, he was more afraid of Walter I. Bradbury, Doubleday's editor, than he had ever been of me.)

Thus began the long history of Isaac's career as Doubleday's— and maybe the world's—premier sf author. Isaac had contributed a section to a text on biochemistry a little earlier, but *Pebble in the Sky* was the first book of his own to see print. More than four hundred followed.

As writers go, Isaac Asimov was obsessed. I do not think the man ever saw a piece of paper he didn't want to write on. He wrote incessantly, wherever he was, all the time.

He and I cruised together once, on the Holland-American ship *Rotterdam*. It was a most memorable voyage, stopping at exotic ports in the Caribbean and pausing just off the coast of Cape Canaveral to observe the glorious night-time launch of *Apollo 17* to the Moon. Isaac showed up for meals and to watch with the rest of us as that wonderful plume of rocket fire leaped up from the launch pad and crossed the sky overhead, but that was about it. Every other time,

as I happened to pass his stateroom, I could hear the steady clickety-clack of his portable typewriter going inside.

It wasn't just science fiction that he wrote. Isaac had the wonderful trait of being able to read and absorb a score or a hundred books and journal articles, and then to pour the essence of them into one of his volumes explaining science—indeed, explaining *everything*—to his world of readers. He was a marvel. For a while he carried a jokey calling card, made for him by a friend, which described him simply as:

ISAAC ASIMOV
NATIONAL RESOURCE

And indeed he was.

Recommended Reading
by Isaac Asimov

Foundation
I, Robot
The Gods Themselves
Pebble in the Sky
I. Asimov

THE LAST QUESTION

The last question was asked for the first time, half in jest, on May 21, 2061, at a time when humanity first stepped into the light. The question came about as a result of a five-dollar bet over high-balls, and it happened this way:

Alexander Adell and Bertram Lupov were two of the faithful attendants of Multivac. As well as any human beings could, they knew what lay behind the cold, clicking, flashing face—miles and miles of face—of that giant computer. They had at least a vague notion of the general plan of relays and circuits that had long since grown past the point where any single human could possibly have a firm grasp of the whole.

Multivac was self-adjusting and self-correcting. It had to be, for nothing human could adjust and correct it quickly enough or even adequately enough. So Adell and Lupov attended the monstrous giant only lightly and superficially, yet as well as any men could. They fed it data, adjusted questions to its needs and translated the answers that were issued. Certainly they, and all others like them, were fully entitled to share in the glory that was Multivac's.

For decades, Multivac had helped design the ships and plot the trajectories that enabled man to reach the Moon, Mars, and Venus, but past that, Earth's poor resources could not support the ships. Too much energy was needed for the long trips. Earth exploited its

coal and uranium with increasing efficiency, but there was only so much of both.

But slowly Multivac learned enough to answer deeper questions more fundamentally, and on May 14, 2061, what had been theory, became fact.

The energy of the sun was stored, converted, and utilized directly on a planet-wide scale. All Earth turned off its burning coal, its fissioning uranium, and flipped the switch that connected all of it to a small station, one mile in diameter, circling the Earth at half the distance of the Moon. All Earth ran by invisible beams of sun-power.

Seven days had not sufficed to dim the glory of it and Adell and Lupov finally managed to escape from the public functions, and to meet in quiet where no one would think of looking for them, in the deserted underground chambers, where portions of the mighty buried body of Multivac showed. Unattended, idling, sorting data with contented lazy clickings, Multivac, too, had earned its vacation and the boys appreciated that. They had no intention, originally, of disturbing it.

They had brought a bottle with them, and their only concern at the moment was to relax in the company of each other and the bottle.

"It's amazing when you think of it," said Adell. His broad face had lines of weariness in it, and he stirred his drink slowly with a glass rod, watching the cubes of ice slur clumsily about. "All the energy we can possibly ever use for free. Enough energy, if we wanted to draw on it, to melt all Earth into a big drop of impure liquid iron, and still never miss the energy so used. All the energy we could ever use, forever and forever and forever."

Lupov cocked his head sideways. He had a trick of doing that when he wanted to be contrary, and he wanted to be contrary now, partly because he had had to carry the ice and glassware. "Not forever," he said.

"Oh, hell, just about forever. Till the sun runs down, Bert."

"That's not forever."

"All right, then. Billions and billions of years. Ten billion, maybe. Are you satisfied?"

Lupov put his fingers through his thinning hair as though to

reassure himself that some was still left and sipped gently at his own drink. "Ten billion years isn't forever."

"Well, it will last our time, won't it?"

"So would the coal and uranium."

"All right, but now we can hook up each individual spaceship to the Solar Station, and it can go to Pluto and back a million times without ever worrying about fuel. You can't do *that* on coal and uranium. Ask Multivac, if you don't believe me."

"I don't have to ask Multivac. I know that."

"Then stop running down what Multivac's done for us," said Adell, blazing up, "It did all right."

"Who says it didn't? What I say is that a sun won't last forever. That's all I'm saying. We're safe for ten billion years, but then what?" Lupov pointed a slightly shaky finger at the other. "And don't say we'll switch to another sun."

There was a silence for a while. Adell put his glass to his lips only occasionally, and Lupov's eyes slowly closed. They rested.

Then Lupov's eyes snapped open. "You're thinking we'll switch to another sun when ours is done, aren't you?"

"I'm not thinking."

"Sure you are. You're weak on logic, that's the trouble with you. You're like the guy in the story who was caught in a sudden shower and who ran to a grove of trees and got under one. He wasn't worried, you see, because he figured when one tree got wet through, he would just get under another one."

"I get it," said Adell. "Don't shout. When the sun is done, the other stars will be gone, too."

"Darn right they will," muttered Lupov. "It all had a beginning in the original cosmic explosion, whatever that was, and it'll all have an end when all the stars run down. Some run down faster than others. Hell, the giants won't last a hundred million years. The sun will last ten billion years and maybe the dwarfs will last two hundred billion for all the good they are. But just give us a trillion years and everything will be dark. Entropy has to increase to maximum, that's all."

"I know all about entropy," said Adell, standing on his dignity.

"The hell you do."

"I know as much as you do."

"Then you know everything's got to run down someday."

"All right. Who says they won't?"

"You did, you poor sap. You said we had all the energy we needed, forever. You said 'forever.' "

It was Adell's turn to be contrary. "Maybe we can build things up again someday," he said.

"Never."

"Why not? Someday."

"Never."

"Ask Multivac."

"*You* ask Multivac. I dare you. Five dollars says it can't be done."

Adell was just drunk enough to try, just sober enough to be able to phrase the necessary symbols and operations into a question which, in words, might have corresponded to this: Will mankind one day without the net expenditure of energy be able to restore the sun to its full youthfulness even after it had died of old age?

Or maybe it could be put more simply like this: How can the net amount of entropy of the universe be massively decreased?

Multivac fell dead and silent. The slow flashing of lights ceased, the distant sounds of clicking relays ended.

Then, just as the frightened technicians felt they could hold their breath no longer, there was a sudden springing to life of the teletype attached to that portion of Multivac. Five words were printed: INSUFFICIENT DATA FOR MEANINGFUL ANSWER.

"No bet," whispered Lupov. They left hurriedly.

By next morning, the two, plagued with throbbing head and cottony mouth, had forgotten the incident.

Jerrodd, Jerrodine, and Jerrodette I and II watched the starry picture in the visiplate change as the passage through hyperspace was completed in its non-time lapse. At once, the even powdering of stars gave way to the predominance of a single bright shining disk, the size of a marble, centered on the viewing-screen.

"That's X-23," said Jerrodd confidently. His thin hands clamped tightly behind his back and the knuckles whitened.

The little Jerrodettes, both girls, had experienced the hyper-

space passage for the first time in their lives and were self-conscious over the momentary sensation of inside-outness. They buried their giggles and chased one another wildly about their mother, screaming, "We've reached X-23—we've reached X-23—we've—"

"Quiet, children," said Jerrodine sharply. "Are you sure, Jerrodd?"

"What is there to be but sure?" asked Jerrodd, glancing up at the bulge of featureless metal just under the ceiling. It ran the length of the room, disappearing through the wall at either end. It was as long as the ship.

Jerrodd scarcely knew a thing about the thick rod of metal except that it was called a Microvac, that one asked it questions if one wished; that if one did not it still had its task of guiding the ship to a preordered destination; of feeding on energies from the various Subgalactic Power Stations; of computing the equations for the hyperspatial jumps.

Jerrodd and his family had only to wait and live in the comfortable residence quarters of the ship.

Someone had once told Jerrodd that the "ac" at the end of "Microvac" stood for "automatic computer" in ancient English, but he was on the edge of forgetting even that.

Jerrodine's eyes were moist as she watched the visiplate. "I can't help it. I feel funny about leaving Earth."

"Why, for Pete's sake?" demanded Jerrodd. "We had nothing there. We'll have everything on X-23. You won't be alone. You won't be a pioneer. There are over a million people on the planet already. Good Lord, our great-grandchildren will be looking for new worlds because X-23 will be overcrowded." Then, after a reflective pause, "I tell you, it's a lucky thing the computers worked out interstellar travel the way the race is growing."

"I know, I know," said Jerrodine miserably.

Jerrodette I said promptly, "Our Microvac is the best Microvac in the world."

"I think so, too," said Jerrodd, tousling her hair.

It was a nice feeling to have a Microvac of your own and Jerrodd was glad he was part of his generation and no other. In his father's youth, the only computers had been tremendous machines taking up a hundred square miles of land. There was only one to a

planet. Planetary ACs they were called. They had been growing in size steadily for a thousand years and then, all at once, came refinement. In place of transistors, had come molecular valves so that even the largest Planetary AC could be put into a space only half the volume of a spaceship.

Jerrodd felt uplifted, as he always did when he thought that his own personal Microvac was many times more complicated than the ancient and primitive Microvac that had first tamed the Sun, and almost as complicated as Earth's Planetary AC (the largest) that had first solved the problem of hyperspatial travel and had made trips to the stars possible.

"So many stars, so many planets," sighed Jerrodine, busy with her own thoughts. "I suppose families will be going to new planets forever, the way we are now."

"Not forever," said Jerrodd, with a smile. "It will all stop someday, but not for billions of years. Many billions. Even the stars run down, you know. Entropy must increase."

"What's entropy, Daddy?" shrilled Jerrodette II.

"Entropy, little sweet, is just a word which means the amount of running-down of the universe. Everything runs down, you know, like your little walkie-talkie robot, remember?"

"Can't you just put in a new power-unit, like with my robot?"

"The stars *are* the power-units, dear. Once they're gone, there are no more power-units."

Jerrodette I at once set up a howl. "Don't let them, Daddy. Don't let the stars run down."

"Now look what you've done," whispered Jerrodine, exasperated.

"How was I to know it would frighten them?" Jerrodd whispered back.

"Ask the Microvac," wailed Jerrodette I. "Ask him how to turn the stars on again."

"Go ahead," said Jerrodine. "It will quiet them down." (Jerrodette II was beginning to cry, also.)

Jerrodd shrugged. "Now, now, honeys. I'll ask Microvac. Don't worry, he'll tell us."

He asked the Microvac, adding quickly, "Print the answer."

Jerrodd cupped the strip of thin cellufilm and said cheerfully,

"See now, the Microvac says it will take care of everything when the time comes so don't worry."

Jerrodine said, "And now, children, it's time for bed. We'll be in our new home soon."

Jerrodd read the words on the cellufilm again before destroying it: INSUFFICIENT DATA FOR MEANINGFUL ANSWER.

He shrugged and looked at the visiplate, X-23 was just ahead.

VJ-23X of Lameth stared into the black depths of the three-dimensional, small-scale map of the Galaxy and said, "Are we ridiculous, I wonder, in being so concerned about the matter?"

MQ-17J of Nicron shook his head. "I think not. You know the Galaxy will be filled in five years at the present rate of expansion."

Both seemed in their early twenties, both were tall and perfectly formed.

"Still," said VJ-23X, "I hesitate to submit a pessimistic report to the Galactic Council."

"I wouldn't consider any other kind of report. Stir them up a bit. We've got to stir them up."

VJ-23X sighed. "Space is infinite. A hundred billion Galaxies are there for the taking. More."

"A hundred billion is not infinite and it's getting less infinite all the time. Consider! Twenty thousand years ago, mankind first solved the problem of utilizing stellar energy, and a few centuries later, interstellar travel became possible. It took mankind a million years to fill one small world and then only fifteen thousand years to fill the rest of the Galaxy. Now the population doubles every ten years—"

VJ-23X interrupted. "We can thank immortality for that."

"Very well. Immortality exists and we have to take it into account. I admit it has its seamy side, this immortality. The Galactic AC has solved many problems for us, but in solving the problem of preventing old age and death, it has undone all its other solutions."

"Yet you wouldn't want to abandon life, I suppose."

"Not at all," snapped MQ-17J, softening it at once to, "Not yet. I'm by no means old enough. How old are you?"

"Two hundred twenty-three. And you?"

"I'm still under two hundred. —But to get back to my point. Population doubles every ten years. Once this Galaxy is filled, we'll have filled another in ten years. Another ten years and we'll have filled two more. Another decade, four more. In a hundred years, we'll have filled a thousand Galaxies. In a thousand years, a million Galaxies. In ten thousand years, the entire known Universe. Then what?"

VJ-23X said, "As a side issue, there's a problem of transportation. I wonder how many sunpower units it will take to move Galaxies of individuals from one Galaxy to the next."

"A very good point. Already, mankind consumes two sunpower units per year."

"Most of it's wasted. After all, our own Galaxy alone pours out a thousand sunpower units a year and we only use two of those."

"Granted, but even with a hundred per cent efficiency, we only stave off the end. Our energy requirements are going up in a geometric progression even faster than our population. We'll run out of energy even sooner than we run out of Galaxies. A good point. A very good point."

"We'll just have to build new stars out of interstellar gas."

"Or out of dissipated heat?" asked MQ-17J, sarcastically.

"There may be some way to reverse entropy. We ought to ask the Galactic AC."

VJ-23X was not really serious, but MQ-17J pulled out his AC-contact from his pocket and placed it on the table before him.

"I've half a mind to," he said. "It's something the human race will have to face someday."

He stared somberly at his small AC-contact. It was only two inches cubed and nothing in itself, but it was connected through hyperspace with the great Galactic AC that served all mankind. Hyperspace considered, it was an integral part of the Galactic AC.

MQ-17J paused to wonder if someday in his immortal life he would get to see the Galactic AC. It was on a little world of its own, a spider webbing of force beams holding the matter within which surges of submesons took the place of the old clumsy molecular valves. Yet despite its sub-etheric workings, the Galactic AC was known to be a full thousand feet across.

MQ-17J asked suddenly of his AC-contact, "Can entropy ever be reversed?"

VJ-23X looked startled and said at once, "Oh, say, I didn't really mean to have you ask that."

"Why not?"

"We both know entropy can't be reversed. You can't turn smoke and ash back into a tree."

"Do you have trees on your world?" asked MQ-17J.

The sound of the Galactic AC startled them into silence. Its voice came thin and beautiful out of the small AC-contact on the desk. It said: THERE IS INSUFFICIENT DATA FOR A MEANINGFUL ANSWER.

VJ-23X said, "See!"

The two men thereupon returned to the question of the report they were to make to the Galactic Council.

Zee Prime's mind spanned the new Galaxy with a faint interest in the countless twists of stars that powdered it. He had never seen this one before. Would he ever see them all? So many of them, each with its load of humanity. —But a load that was almost a dead weight. More and more, the real essence of men was to be found out here, in space.

Minds, not bodies! The immortal bodies remained back on the planets, in suspension over the eons. Sometimes they roused for material activity but that was growing rarer. Few new individuals were coming into existence to join the incredibly mighty throng, but what matter? There was little room in the Universe for new individuals.

Zee Prime was roused out of his reverie upon coming across the wispy tendrils of another mind.

"I am Zee Prime," said Zee Prime. "And you?"

"I am Dee Sub Wun. Your Galaxy?"

"We call it only the Galaxy. And you?"

"We call ours the same. All men call their Galaxy their Galaxy and nothing more. Why not?"

"True. Since all Galaxies are the same."

"Not all Galaxies. On one particular Galaxy the race of man must have originated. That makes it different."

Zee Prime said, "On which one?"

"I cannot say. The Universal AC would know."

"Shall we ask him? I am suddenly curious."

Zee Prime's perceptions broadened until the Galaxies themselves shrank and became a new, more diffuse powdering on a much larger background. So many hundreds of billions of them, all with their immortal beings, all carrying their load of intelligences with minds that drifted freely through space. And yet one of them was unique among them all in being the original Galaxy. One of them had, in its vague and distant past, a period when it was the only Galaxy populated by man.

Zee Prime was consumed with curiosity to see this Galaxy and he called out: "Universal AC! On which Galaxy did mankind originate?"

The Universal AC heard, for on every world and throughout space, it had its receptors ready, and each receptor lead through hyperspace to some unknown point where the Universal AC kept itself aloof.

Zee Prime knew of only one man whose thoughts had penetrated within sensing distance of Universal AC, and he reported only a shining globe, two feet across, difficult to see.

"But how can that be all of Universal AC?" Zee Prime had asked.

"Most of it," had been the answer, "is in hyperspace. In what form it is there I cannot imagine."

Nor could anyone, for the day had long since passed, Zee Prime knew, when any man had any part of the making of a Universal AC. Each Universal AC designed and constructed its successor. Each, during its existence of a million years or more accumulated the necessary data to build a better and more intricate, more capable successor in which its own store of data and individuality would be submerged.

The Universal AC interrupted Zee Prime's wandering thoughts, not with words, but with guidance. Zee Prime's mentality was guided into the dim sea of Galaxies and one in particular enlarged into stars.

A thought came, infinitely distant, but infinitely clear. "THIS IS THE ORIGINAL GALAXY OF MAN."

But it was the same after all, the same as any other, and Zee Prime stifled his disappointment.

Dee Sub Wun, whose mind had accompanied the other, said suddenly, "And is one of these stars the original star of Man?"

The Universal AC said, "MAN'S ORIGINAL STAR HAS GONE NOVA. IT IS A WHITE DWARF."

"Did the men upon it die?" asked Zee Prime, startled and without thinking.

The Universal AC said, "A NEW WORLD, AS IN SUCH CASES WAS CONSTRUCTED FOR THEIR PHYSICAL BODIES IN TIME."

"Yes, of course," said Zee Prime, but a sense of loss overwhelmed him even so. His mind released its hold on the original Galaxy of Man, let it spring back and lose itself among the blurred pinpoints. He never wanted to see it again.

Dee Sub Wun said, "What is wrong?"

"The stars are dying. The original star is dead."

"They must all die. Why not?"

"But when all energy is gone, our bodies will finally die, and you and I with them."

"It will take billions of years."

"I do not wish it to happen even after billions of years. Universal AC! How may stars be kept from dying?"

Dee Sub Wun said in amusement, "You're asking how entropy might be reversed in direction."

And the Universal AC answered: "THERE IS AS YET INSUFFICIENT DATA FOR A MEANINGFUL ANSWER."

Zee Prime's thoughts fled back to his own Galaxy. He gave no further thought to Dee Sub Wun, whose body might be waiting on a Galaxy a trillion light-years away, or on the star next to Zee Prime's own. It didn't matter.

Unhappily, Zee Prime began collecting interstellar hydrogen out of which to build a small star of his own. If the stars must someday die, at least some could yet be built.

•   •   •

Man considered with himself, for in a way, Man, mentally, was one. He consisted of a trillion, trillion, trillion ageless bodies, each in its place, each resting quiet and incorruptible, each cared for by perfect automatons, equally incorruptible, while the minds of all the bodies freely melted one into the other, indistinguishable.

Man said, "The Universe is dying."

Man looked about at the dimming Galaxies. The giant stars, spendthrifts, were gone long ago, back in the dimmest of the dim far past. Almost all stars were white dwarfs, fading to the end.

New stars had been built of the dust between the stars, some by natural processes, some by Man himself, and those were going, too. White dwarfs might yet be crashed together and of the mighty forces so released, new stars built, but only one star for every thousand white dwarfs destroyed, and those would come to an end, too.

Man said, "Carefully husbanded, as directed by the Cosmic AC, the energy that is even yet left in all the Universe will last for billions of years."

"But even so," said Man, "eventually it will all come to an end. However it may be husbanded, however stretched out, the energy once expended is gone and cannot be restored. Entropy must increase forever to the maximum."

Man said, "Can entropy not be reversed? Let us ask the Cosmic AC."

The Cosmic AC surrounded them but not in space. Not a fragment of it was in space. It was in hyperspace and made of something that was neither matter nor energy. The question of its size and nature no longer had meaning in any terms that Man could comprehend.

"Cosmic AC," said Man, "how may entropy be reversed?"

The Cosmic AC said, "THERE IS AS YET INSUFFICIENT DATA FOR A MEANINGFUL ANSWER."

Man said, "Collect additional data."

The Cosmic AC said, "I WILL DO SO. I HAVE BEEN DOING SO FOR A HUNDRED BILLION YEARS. MY PREDECESSORS AND I HAVE BEEN ASKED THIS QUESTION MANY TIMES. ALL THE DATA I HAVE REMAINS INSUFFICIENT."

"Will there come a time," said Man, "when data will be sufficient or is the problem insoluble in all conceivable circumstances?"

The Cosmic AC said, "NO PROBLEM IS INSOLUBLE IN ALL CONCEIVABLE CIRCUMSTANCES."

Man said, "When will you have enough data to answer the question?"

The Cosmic AC said, "THERE IS AS YET INSUFFICIENT DATA FOR A MEANINGFUL ANSWER."

"Will you keep working on it?" asked Man.

The Cosmic AC said, "I WILL."

Man said, "We shall wait."

The stars and Galaxies died and snuffed out, and space grew black after ten trillion years of running down.

One by one Man fused with AC, each physical body losing its mental identity in a manner that was somehow not a loss but a gain.

Man's last mind paused before fusion, looking over a space that included nothing but the dregs of one last dark star and nothing besides but incredibly thin matter, agitated randomly by the tag ends of heat wearing out, asymptotically, to the absolute zero.

Man said, "AC, is this the end? Can this chaos not be reversed into the Universe once more? Can that not be done?"

AC said, "THERE IS AS YET INSUFFICIENT DATA FOR A MEANINGFUL ANSWER."

Man's last mind fused and only AC existed—and that in hyper-space.

Matter and energy had ended and with it space and time. Even AC existed only for the sake of the one last question that it had never answered from the time a half-drunken computer ten trillion years before had asked the question of a computer that was to AC far less than was a man to Man.

All other questions had been answered, and until this last question was answered also, AC might not release his consciousness.

All collected data had come to a final end. Nothing was left to be collected.

But all collected data had yet to be completely correlated and put together in all possible relationships.

A timeless interval was spent in doing that.

And it came to pass that AC learned how to reverse the direction of entropy.

But there was now no man to whom AC might give the answer of the last question. No matter. The answer—by demonstration—would take care of that, too.

For another timeless interval, AC thought how best to do this. Carefully, AC organized the program.

The consciousness of AC encompassed all of what had once been a Universe and brooded over what was now Chaos. Step by step, it must be done.

And AC said, "LET THERE BE LIGHT!"

And there was light—

IT'S SUCH A BEAUTIFUL DAY

On April 12, 2117, the field-modulator brake-valve in the Door belonging to Mrs. Richard Hanshaw depolarized for reasons unknown. As a result, Mrs. Hanshaw's day was completely upset and her son, Richard, Jr., first developed his strange neurosis.

It was not the type of thing you would find listed as a neurosis in the usual textbooks and certainly young Richard behaved, in most respects, just as a well-brought-up twelve-year-old in prosperous circumstances ought to behave.

And yet from April 12 on, Richard Hanshaw, Jr., could only with regret ever persuade himself to go through a Door.

Of all this, on April 12, Mrs. Hanshaw had no premonition. She woke in the morning (an ordinary morning) as her mekkano slithered gently into her room, with a cup of coffee on a small tray. Mrs. Hanshaw was planning a visit to New York in the afternoon and she had several things to do first that could not quite be trusted to a mekkano, so after one or two sips, she stepped out of bed.

The mekkano backed away, moving silently along the diamagnetic field that kept its oblong body half an inch above the floor, and moved back to the kitchen, where its simple computer was quite adequate to set the proper controls on the various kitchen appliances in order that an appropriate breakfast might be prepared.

Mrs. Hanshaw, having bestowed the usual sentimental glance

upon the cubograph of her dead husband, passed through the stages of her morning ritual with a certain contentment. She could hear her son across the hall clattering through his, but she knew she need not interfere with him. The mekkano was well adjusted to see to it, as a matter of course, that he was showered, that he had on a change of clothing, and that he would eat a nourishing breakfast. The tergoshower she had had installed the year before made the morning wash and dry so quick and pleasant that, really, she felt certain Dickie would wash even without supervision.

On a morning like this, when she was busy, it would certainly not be necessary for her to do more than deposit a casual peck on the boy's cheek before he left. She heard the soft chime the mekkano sounded to indicate approaching school time and she floated down the force-lift to the lower floor (her hair-style for the day only sketchily designed, as yet) in order to perform that motherly duty.

She found Richard standing at the door, with his text-reels and pocket projector dangling by their strap and a frown on his face.

"Say, Mom," he said, looking up, "I dialed the school's co-ords but nothing happens."

She said, almost automatically, "Nonsense, Dickie. I never heard of such a thing."

"Well, you try."

Mrs. Hanshaw tried a number of times. Strange, the school door was always set for general reception. She tried other co-ordinates. Her friends' Doors might not be set for reception, but there would be a signal at least, and then she could explain.

But nothing happened at all. The Door remained an inactive gray barrier despite all her manipulations. It was obvious that the Door was out of order—and only five months after its annual fall inspection by the company.

She was quite angry about it.

It *would* happen on a day when she had so much planned. She thought petulantly of the fact that a month earlier she had decided against installing a subsidiary Door on the ground that it was an unnecessary expense. How was she to know that Doors were getting to be so *shoddy*?

She stepped to the visiphone while the anger still burned in

her and said to Richard, "You just go down the road, Dickie, and use the Williamsons' Door."

Ironically, in view of later developments, Richard balked. "Aw, gee, Mom, I'll get dirty. Can't I stay home till the Door is fixed?"

And, as ironically, Mrs. Hanshaw insisted. With her finger on the combination board of the phone, she said, "You won't get dirty if you put flexies on your shoes, and don't forget to brush yourself well before you go into their house."

"But, golly—"

"No back-talk, Dickie. You've got to be in school. Just let me see you walk out of here. And quickly, or you'll be late."

The mekkano, an advanced model and very responsive, was already standing before Richard with flexies in one appendage.

Richard pulled the transparent plastic shields over his shoes and moved down the hall with visible reluctance. "I don't even know how to work this thing, Mom."

"You just push that button," Mrs. Hanshaw called. "The red button. Where it says 'For Emergency Use.' And don't dawdle. Do you want the mekkano to go along with you?"

"Gosh, no," he called back, morosely, "what do you think I am? A baby? Gosh!" His muttering was cut off by a slam.

With flying fingers, Mrs. Hanshaw punched the appropriate combination on the phone board and thought of the things she intended saying to the company about this.

Joe Bloom, a reasonable young man, who had gone through technology school with added training in force-field mechanics, was at the Hanshaw residence in less than half an hour. He was really quite competent, though Mrs. Hanshaw regarded his youth with deep suspicion.

She opened the movable house-panel when he first signaled and her sight of him was as he stood there, brushing at himself vigorously to remove the dust of the open air. He took off his flexies and dropped them where he stood. Mrs. Hanshaw closed the house-panel against the flash of raw sunlight that had entered. She found herself irrationally hoping that the step-by-step trip from the public Door had been an unpleasant one. Or perhaps that the public Door itself had been out of order and the youth had had to lug his tools even farther than the necessary two hundred yards. She wanted the

Company, or its representative at least, to suffer a bit. It would teach them what broken Doors meant.

But he seemed cheerful and unperturbed as he said, "Good morning, ma'am. I came to see about your Door."

"I'm glad someone did," said Mrs. Hanshaw, ungraciously. "My day is quite ruined."

"Sorry, ma'am. What seems to be the trouble?"

"It just won't work. Nothing at all happens when you adjust co-ords," said Mrs. Hanshaw. "There was no warning at all. I had to send my son out to the neighbors through that—that thing."

She pointed to the entrance through which the repair man had come.

He smiled and spoke out of the conscious wisdom of his own specialized training in Doors. "That's a door, too, ma'am. You don't give that kind a capital letter when you write it. It's a hand-door, sort of. It used to be the only kind once."

"Well, at least it works. My boy's had to go out in the dirt and germs."

"It's not bad outside today, ma'am," he said, with the connoisseur like air of one whose profession forced him into the open nearly every day. "Sometimes it *is* real unpleasant. But I guess you want I should fix this here Door, ma'am, so I'll get on with it."

He sat down on the floor, opened the large tool case he had brought in with him and in half a minute, by use of a point-demagnetizer, he had the control panel removed and a set of intricate vitals exposed.

He whistled to himself as he placed the fine electrodes of the field-analyzer on numerous points, studying the shifting needles on the dials. Mrs. Hanshaw watched him, arms folded.

Finally, he said, "Well, here's something," and with a deft twist, he disengaged the brake-valve.

He tapped it with a fingernail and said, "This here brake-valve is depolarized, ma'am. There's your whole trouble." He ran his finger along the little pigeonholes in his tool case and lifted out a duplicate of the object he had taken from the door mechanism. "These things just go all of a sudden. Can't predict it."

He put the control panel back and stood up. "It'll work now, ma'am."

He punched a reference combination, blanked it, then punched another. Each time, the dull gray of the Door gave way to a deep, velvety blackness. He said, "Will you sign here, ma'am? and put down your charge number, too, please? Thank you, ma'am."

He punched a new combination, that of his home factory, and with a polite touch of finger to forehead, he stepped through the Door. As his body entered the blackness, it cut off sharply. Less and less of him was visible and the tip of his tool case was the last thing that showed. A second after he had passed through completely, the Door turned back to dull gray.

Half an hour later, when Mrs. Hanshaw had finally completed her interrupted preparations and was fuming over the misfortune of the morning, the phone buzzed annoyingly and her real troubles began.

Miss Elizabeth Robbins was distressed. Little Dick Hanshaw had always been a good pupil. She hated to report him like this. And yet, she told herself, his actions were certainly queer. And she would talk to his mother, not to the principal.

She slipped out to the phone during the morning study period, leaving a student in charge. She made her connection and found herself staring at Mrs. Hanshaw's handsome and somewhat formidable head.

Miss Robbins quailed, but it was too late to turn back. She said, diffidently, "Mrs. Hanshaw, I'm Miss Robbins." She ended on a rising note.

Mrs. Hanshaw looked blank, then said, "Richard's teacher?" That, too, ended on a rising note.

"That's right. I called you, Mrs. Hanshaw," Miss Robbins plunged right into it, "to tell you that Dick was quite late to school this morning."

"He *was*? But that couldn't be. I saw him leave."

Miss Robbins looked astonished. She said, "You mean you saw him use the Door?"

Mrs. Hanshaw said quickly, "Well, no. Our Door was temporarily out of order. I sent him to a neighbor and he used that Door."

"Are you sure?"

"Of course I'm sure. I wouldn't lie to you."

"No, no, Mrs. Hanshaw. I wasn't implying that at all. I meant are you sure he found the way to the neighbor? He might have got lost."

"Ridiculous. We have the proper maps, and I'm sure Richard knows the location of every house in District A-3." Then, with the quiet pride of one who knows what is her due, she added, "Not that he ever needs to know, of course. The co-ords are all that are necessary at any time."

Miss Robbins, who came from a family that had always had to economize rigidly on the use of its Doors (the price of the power being what it was) and who had therefore run errands on foot until quite an advanced age, resented the pride. She said, quite clearly, "Well, I'm afraid, Mrs. Hanshaw, that Dick did not use the neighbor's Door. He was over an hour late to school and the condition of his flexies made it quite obvious that he tramped cross-country. They were *muddy*."

"*Muddy?*" Mrs. Hanshaw repeated the emphasis on the word. "What did he say? What was his excuse?"

Miss Robbins couldn't help but feel a little glad at the discomfiture of the other woman. She said, "He wouldn't talk about it. Frankly, Mrs. Hanshaw, he seems ill. That's why I called you. Perhaps you might want to have a doctor look at him."

"Is he running a temperature?" The mother's voice went shrill.

"Oh, no. I don't mean physically ill. It's just his attitude and the look in his eyes." She hesitated, then said with every attempt at delicacy, "I thought perhaps a routine checkup with a psychic probe—"

She didn't finish. Mrs. Hanshaw, in a chilled voice and with what was as close to a snort as her breeding would permit, said, "Are you implying that Richard is *neurotic*?"

"Oh, no, Mrs. Hanshaw, but—"

"It certainly sounded so. The idea! He has always been perfectly healthy. I'll take this up with him when he gets home. I'm sure there's a perfectly normal explanation which he'll give to *me*."

The connection broke abruptly, and Miss Robbins felt hurt and uncommonly foolish. After all she had only tried to help, to fulfill what she considered an obligation to her students.

She hurried back to the classroom with a glance at the metal face of the wall clock. The study period was drawing to an end. English Composition next.

But her mind wasn't completely on English Composition. Automatically, she called the students to have them read selections from their literary creations. And occasionally she punched one of those selections on tape and ran it through the small vocalizer to show the students how English *should* be read.

The vocalizer's mechanical voice, as always, dripped perfection, but, again as always, lacked character. Sometimes, she wondered if it was wise to try to train the students into a speech that was divorced from individuality and geared only to a mass-average accent and intonation.

Today, however, she had no thought for that. It was Richard Hanshaw she watched. He sat quietly in his seat, quite obviously indifferent to his surroundings. He was lost deep in himself and just not the same boy he had been. It was obvious to her that he had had some unusual experience that morning and, really, she was right to call his mother, although perhaps she ought not to have made the remark about the probe. Still it was quite the thing these days. All sorts of people get probed. There wasn't any disgrace attached to it. Or there shouldn't be, anyway.

She called on Richard, finally. She had to call twice, before he responded and rose to his feet.

The general subject assigned had been: "If you had your choice of traveling on some ancient vehicle, which would you choose, and why?" Miss Robbins tried to use the topic every semester. It was a good one because it carried a sense of history with it. It forced the youngster to think about the manner of living of people in past ages.

She listened while Richard Hanshaw read in a low voice.

"If I had my choice of ancient vehicles," he said, pronouncing the "h" in vehicles, "I would choose the stratoliner. It travels slow like all vehicles but it is clean. Because it travels in the stratosphere, it must be all enclosed so that you are not likely to catch disease. You can see the stars if it is night time almost as good as in a planetarium. If you look down you can see the Earth like a map or maybe see clouds—" He went on for several hundred more words.

She said brightly when he had finished reading, "It's pronounced vee-ick-ulls, Richard. No 'h.' Accent on the first syllable. And you don't say 'travels slow' or 'see good.' What do you say, class?"

There was a small chorus of responses and she went on, "That's right. Now what is the difference between an adjective and an adverb? Who can tell me?"

And so it went. Lunch passed. Some pupils stayed to eat; some went home. Richard stayed. Miss Robbins noted that, as usually he didn't.

The afternoon passed, too, and then there was the final bell and the usual upsurging hum as twenty-five boys and girls rattled their belongings together and took their leisurely place in line.

Miss Robbins clapped her hands together. "Quickly, children. Come, Zelda, take your place."

"I dropped my tape-punch, Miss Robbins," shrilled the girl, defensively.

"Well, pick it up, pick it up. Now children, be brisk, be brisk."

She pushed the button that slid a section of the wall into a recess and revealed the gray blankness of a large Door. It was not the usual Door that the occasional student used in going home for lunch, but an advanced model that was one of the prides of this well-to-do private school.

In addition to its double width, it possessed a large and impressively gear-filled "automatic serial finder" which was capable of adjusting the Door for a number of different co-ordinates at automatic intervals.

At the beginning of the semester, Miss Robbins always had to spend an afternoon with the mechanic, adjusting the device for the coordinates of the homes of the new class. But then, thank goodness, it rarely needed attention for the remainder of the term.

The class lined up alphabetically, first girls, then boys. The Door went velvety black and Hester Adams waved her hand and stepped through. "By-y-y—"

The "bye" was cut off in the middle, as it almost always was.

The Door went gray, then black again, and Theresa Cantrocchi went through. Gray, black, Zelda Charlowicz. Gray, black, Patricia Coombs. Gray, black, Sara May Evans.

The line grew smaller as the Door swallowed them one by one, depositing each in her home. Of course, an occasional mother forgot to leave the house Door on special reception at the appropriate time and then the school Door remained gray. Automatically, after a minute-long wait, the Door went on to the next combination in line and the pupil in question had to wait till it was all over, after which a phone call to the forgetful parent would set things right. This was always bad for the pupils involved, especially the sensitive ones who took seriously the implication that they were little thought of at home. Miss Robbins always tried to impress this on visiting parents, but it happened at least once every semester just the same.

The girls were all through now. John Abramowitz stepped through and then Edwin Byrne—

Of course, another trouble, and a more frequent one was the boy or girl who got into line out of place. They *would* do it despite the teacher's sharpest watch, particularly at the beginning of the term when the proper order was less familiar to them.

When that happened, children would be popping into the wrong houses by the half-dozen and would have to be sent back. It always meant a mixup that took minutes to straighten out and parents were invariably irate.

Miss Robbins was suddenly aware that the line had stopped. She spoke sharply to the boy at the head of the line.

"Step through, Samuel. What are you waiting for?"

Samuel Jones raised a complacent countenance and said, "It's not my combination, Miss Robbins."

"Well, whose is it?" She looked impatiently down the line of five remaining boys. Who was out of place?

"It's Dick Hanshaw's, Miss Robbins."

"Where is he?"

Another boy answered, with the rather repulsive tone of self-righteousness all children automatically assume in reporting the deviations of their friends to elders in authority, "He went through the fire door, Miss Robbins."

"What?"

The schoolroom Door had passed on to another combination and Samuel Jones passed through. One by one, the rest followed.

Miss Robbins was alone in the classroom. She stepped to the fire door. It was a small affair, manually operated, and hidden behind a bend in the wall so that it would not break up the uniform structure of the room.

She opened it a crack. It was there as a means of escape from the building in case of fire, a device which was enforced by an anachronistic law that did not take into account the modern methods of automatic fire-fighting that all public buildings used. There was nothing outside, but the—outside. The sunlight was harsh and a dusty wind was blowing.

Miss Robbins closed the door. She was glad she had called Mrs. Hanshaw. She had done her duty. More than ever, it was obvious that something was wrong with Richard. She suppressed the impulse to phone again.

Mrs. Hanshaw did not go to New York that day. She remained home in a mixture of anxiety and an irrational anger, the latter directed against the impudent Miss Robbins.

Some fifteen minutes before school's end, her anxiety drove her to the Door. Last year she had had it equipped with an automatic device which activated it to the school's co-ordinates at five of three and kept it so, barring manual adjustment, until Richard arrived.

Her eyes were fixed on the Door's dismal gray (why couldn't an inactive force-field be any other color, something more lively and cheerful?) and waited. Her hands felt cold as she squeezed them together.

The Door turned black at the precise second but nothing happened. The minutes passed and Richard was late. Then quite late. Then very late.

It was a quarter of four and she was distracted. Normally, she would have phoned the school, but she couldn't, she couldn't. Not after that teacher had deliberately cast doubts on Richard's mental well-being. How could she?

Mrs. Hanshaw moved about restlessly, lighting a cigarette with fumbling fingers, then smudging it out. Could it be something quite normal? Could Richard be staying after school for some reason?

Surely he would have told her in advance. A gleam of light struck her; he knew she was planning to go to New York and might not be back till late in the evening—

No, he would surely have told her. Why fool herself?

Her pride was breaking. She would have to call the school, or even (she closed her eyes and teardrops squeezed through between the lashes) the police.

And when she opened her eyes, Richard stood before her, eyes on the ground and his whole bearing that of someone waiting for a blow to fall.

"Hello, Mom."

Mrs. Hanshaw's anxiety transmuted itself instantly (in a manner known only to mothers) into anger. "Where have you been, Richard?"

And then, before she could go further into the refrain concerning careless, unthinking sons and broken-hearted mothers, she took note of his appearance in greater detail, and gasped in utter horror.

She said, "You've been in the open."

Her son looked down at his dusty shoes (minus flexies), at the dirt marks that streaked his lower arms and at the small, but definite tear in his shirt. He said, "Gosh, Mom, I just thought I'd—" and he faded out.

She said, "Was there anything wrong with the school Door?"

"No, Mom."

"Do you realize I've been worried sick about you?" She waited vainly for an answer. "Well, I'll talk to you afterward, young man. First, you're taking a bath, and every stitch of your clothing is being thrown out. Mekkano!"

But the mekkano had already reacted properly to the phrase "taking a bath" and was off to the bathroom in its silent glide.

"You take your shoes off right here," said Mrs. Hanshaw, "then march after mekkano."

Richard did as he was told with a resignation that placed him beyond futile protest.

Mrs. Hanshaw picked up the soiled shoes between thumb and forefinger and dropped them down the disposal chute which hummed in faint dismay at the unexpected load. She dusted her

hands carefully on a tissue which she allowed to float down the chute after the shoes.

She did not join Richard at dinner but let him eat in the worse-than-lack-of-company of the mekkano. This, she thought, would be an active sign of her displeasure and would do more than any amount of scolding or punishment to make him realize that he had done wrong. Richard, she frequently told herself, was a sensitive boy.

But she went up to see him at bedtime.

She smiled at him and spoke softly. She thought that would be the best way. After all, he had been punished already.

She said, "What happened today, Dickie-boy?" She had called him that when he was a baby and just the sound of the name softened her nearly to tears.

But he only looked away and his voice was stubborn and cold. "I just don't like to go through those darn Doors, Mom."

"But why ever not?"

He shuffled his hands over the filmy sheet (fresh, clean, antiseptic and, of course, disposable after each use) and said, "I just don't like them."

"But then how do you expect to go to school, Dickie?"

"I'll get up early," he mumbled.

"But there's nothing wrong with Doors."

"Don't like 'em." He never once looked up at her.

She said, despairingly, "Oh, well, you have a good sleep and tomorrow morning you'll feel much better."

She kissed him and left the room, automatically passing her hand through the photo-cell beam and in that manner dimming the room lights.

But she had trouble sleeping herself that night. Why should Dickie dislike Doors so suddenly? They had never bothered him before. To be sure, the Door had broken down in the morning but that should make him appreciate them all the more.

Dickie was behaving so unreasonably.

Unreasonably? That reminded her of Miss Robbins and her diagnosis and Mrs. Hanshaw's soft jaw set in the darkness and privacy of her bedroom. Nonsense! The boy was upset and a night's sleep was all the therapy he needed.

But the next morning when she arose, her son was not in the house. The mekkano could not speak but it could answer questions with gestures of its appendages equivalent to a yes or no, and it did not take Mrs. Hanshaw more than half a minute to ascertain that the boy had arisen thirty minutes earlier than usual, skimped his shower, and darted out of the house.

But not by way of the Door.

Out the other way—through the door. Small "d."

Mrs. Hanshaw's visiphone signaled genteelly at 3:10 P.M. that day. Mrs. Hanshaw guessed the caller and having activated the receiver, saw that she had guessed correctly. A quick glance in the mirror to see that she was properly calm after a day of abstracted concern and worry and then she keyed in her own transmission.

"Yes, Miss Robbins," she said coldly.

Richard's teacher was a bit breathless. She said, "Mrs. Hanshaw, Richard has deliberately left through the fire door although I told him to use the regular Door. I do not know where he went."

Mrs. Hanshaw said, carefully, "He left to come home."

Miss Robbins looked dismayed, "Do you approve of this?"

Pale-faced, Mrs. Hanshaw set about putting the teacher in her place. "I don't think it is up to you to criticize. If my son does not choose to use the Door, it is his affair and mine. I don't think there is any school ruling that would force him to use the Door, is there?" Her bearing quite plainly intimated that if there were she would see to it that it was changed.

Miss Robbins flushed and had time for one quick remark before contact was broken. She said, "I'd have him probed. I really would."

Mrs. Hanshaw remained standing before the quartzinium plate, staring blindly at its blank face. Her sense of family placed her for a few moments quite firmly on Richard's side. Why *did* he have to use the Door if he chose not to? And then she settled down to wait and pride battled the gnawing anxiety that something after all was wrong with Richard.

He came home with a look of defiance on his face, but his mother, with a strenuous effort at self-control, met him as though nothing were out of the ordinary.

For weeks, she followed that policy. It's nothing, she told herself. It's a vagary. He'll grow out of it.

It grew into an almost normal state of affairs. Then, too, every once in a while, perhaps three days in a row, she would come down to breakfast to find Richard waiting sullenly at the Door, then using it when school time came. She always refrained from commenting on the matter.

Always, when he did that, and especially when he followed it up by arriving home via the Door, her heart grew warm and she thought, "Well, it's over." But always with the passing of one day, two or three, he would return like an addict to his drug and drift silently out by the door—small "d"—before she woke.

And each time she thought despairingly of psychiatrists and probes, and each time the vision of Miss Robbins' low-bred satisfaction at (possibly) learning of it, stopped her, although she was scarcely aware that that was the true motive.

Meanwhile, she lived with it and made the best of it. The mekkano was instructed to wait at the door—small "d"—with a Tergo kit and a change of clothing. Richard washed and changed without resistance. His underthings, socks and flexies were disposable in any case, and Mrs. Hanshaw bore uncomplainingly the expense of daily disposal of shirts. Trousers she finally allowed to go a week before disposal on condition of rigorous nightly cleansing.

One day she suggested that Richard accompany her on a trip to New York. It was more a vague desire to keep him in sight than part of any purposeful plan. He did not object. He was even happy. He stepped right through the Door, unconcerned. He didn't hesitate. He even lacked the look of resentment he wore on those mornings he used the Door to go to school.

Mrs. Hanshaw rejoiced. This could be a way of weaning him back into Door usage, and she racked her ingenuity for excuses to make trips with Richard. She even raised her power bill to quite unheard-of heights by suggesting, and going through with, a trip to Canton for the day in order to witness a Chinese festival.

That was on a Sunday, and the next morning Richard marched directly to the hole in the wall he always used. Mrs. Hanshaw, having wakened particularly early, witnessed that. For once, badg-

ered past endurance, she called after him plaintively, "Why not the Door, Dickie?"

He said, briefly, "It's all right for Canton," and stepped out of the house.

So that plan ended in failure. And then, one day, Richard came home soaking wet. The mekkano hovered about him uncertainly and Mrs. Hanshaw, just returned from a four-hour visit with her sister in Iowa, cried, "Richard Hanshaw!"

He said, hang-dog fashion, "It started raining. All of a sudden, it started raining."

For a moment, the word didn't register with her. Her own school days and her studies of geography were twenty years in the past. And then she remembered and caught the vision of water pouring recklessly and endlessly down from the sky—a mad cascade of water with no tap to turn off, no button to push, no contact to break.

She said, "And you stayed out in it?"

He said, "Well, gee, Mom, I came home fast as I could. I didn't know it was going to rain."

Mrs. Hanshaw had nothing to say. She was appalled and the sensation filled her too full for words to find a place.

Two days later, Richard found himself with a running nose, and a dry, scratchy throat. Mrs. Hanshaw had to admit that the virus of disease had found a lodging in her house, as though it were a miserable hovel of the Iron Age.

It was over that that her stubbornness and pride broke and she admitted to herself that, after all, Richard had to have psychiatric help.

Mrs. Hanshaw chose a psychiatrist with care. Her first impulse was to find one at a distance. For a while, she considered stepping directly into the San Francisco Medical Center and choosing one at random.

And then it occurred to her that by doing that she would become merely an anonymous consultant. She would have no way of obtaining any greater consideration for herself than would be forthcoming to any public-Door user of the city slums. Now if she remained in her own community, her word would carry weight—

She consulted the district map. It was one of that excellent

series prepared by Doors, Inc., and distributed free of charge to their clients. Mrs. Hanshaw couldn't quite suppress that little thrill of civic pride as she unfolded the map. It wasn't a fine-print directory of Door co-ordinates only. It was an actual map, with each house carefully located.

And why not? District A-3 was a name of moment in the world, a badge of aristocracy. It was the first community on the planet to have been established on a completely Doored basis. The first, the largest, the wealthiest, the best-known. It needed no factories, no stores. It didn't even need roads. Each house was a little secluded castle, the Door of which had entry anywhere the world over where other Doors existed.

Carefully, she followed down the keyed listing of the five thousand families of District A-3. She knew it included several psychiatrists. The learned professions were well represented in A-3.

Doctor Hamilton Sloane was the second name she arrived at and her finger lingered upon the map. His office was scarcely two miles from the Hanshaw residence. She liked his name. The fact that he lived in A-3 was evidence of worth. And he was a neighbor, practically a neighbor. He would understand that it was a matter of urgency—and confidential.

Firmly, she put in a call to his office to make an appointment.

Doctor Hamilton Sloane was a comparatively young man, not quite forty. He was of good family and he had indeed heard of Mrs. Hanshaw.

He listened to her quietly and then said, "And this all began with the Door breakdown."

"That's right, Doctor."

"Does he show any fear of the Doors?"

"Of course not. What an idea!" She was plainly startled.

"It's possible, Mrs. Hanshaw, it's possible. After all, when you stop to think of how a Door works it is rather a frightening thing, really. You step into a Door, and for an instant your atoms are converted into field-energies, transmitted to another part of space and reconverted into matter. For that instant you're not alive."

"I'm sure no one thinks of such things."

"But your son may. He witnessed the breakdown of the Door. He may be saying to himself, 'What if the Door breaks down just as I'm half-way through?'"

"But that's nonsense. He still uses the Door. He's even been to Canton with me; Canton, China. And as I told you, he uses it for school about once or twice a week."

"Freely? Cheerfully?"

"Well," said Mrs. Hanshaw, reluctantly, "he does seem a bit put out by it. But really, Doctor, there isn't much use talking about it, is there? If you would do a quick probe, see where the trouble was," and she finished on a bright note, "why, that would be all. I'm sure it's quite a minor thing."

Dr. Sloane sighed. He detested the word "probe" and there was scarcely any word he heard oftener.

"Mrs. Hanshaw," he said patiently, "there is no such thing as a quick probe. Now I know the mag-strips are full of it and it's a rage in some circles, but it's much overrated."

"Are you serious?"

"Quite. The probe is very complicated and the theory is that it traces mental circuits. You see, the cells of the brains are interconnected in a large variety of ways. Some of those interconnected paths are more used than others. They represent habits of thought, both conscious and unconscious. Theory has it that these paths in any given brain can be used to diagnose mental ills early and with certainty."

"Well, then?"

"But subjection to the probe is quite a fearful thing, especially to a child. It's a traumatic experience. It takes over an hour. And even then, the results must be sent to the Central Psychoanalytical Bureau for analysis, and that could take weeks. And on top of all that, Mrs. Hanshaw, there are many psychiatrists who think the theory of probe-analyses to be most uncertain."

Mrs. Hanshaw compressed her lips. "You mean nothing can be done."

Dr. Sloane smiled. "Not at all. There were psychiatrists for centuries before there were probes. I suggest that you let me talk to the boy."

"Talk to him? Is that all?"

"I'll come to you for background information when necessary, but the essential thing, I think, is to talk to the boy."

"Really, Dr. Sloane, I doubt if he'll discuss the matter with you. He won't talk to me about it and I'm his mother."

"That often happens," the psychiatrist assured her. "A child will sometimes talk more readily to a stranger. In any case, I cannot take the case otherwise."

Mrs. Hanshaw rose, not at all pleased. "When can you come, Doctor?"

"What about this coming Saturday? The boy won't be in school. Will you be busy?"

"We will be ready."

She made a dignified exit. Dr. Sloane accompanied her through the small reception room to his office Door and waited while she punched the co-ordinates of her house. He watched her pass through. She became a half-woman, a quarter-woman, an isolated elbow and foot, a nothing.

It *was* frightening.

Did a Door ever break down during passage, leaving half a body here and half there? He had never heard of such a case, but he imagined it could happen.

He returned to his desk and looked up the time of his next appointment. It was obvious to him that Mrs. Hanshaw was annoyed and disappointed at not having arranged for a psychic probe treatment.

Why, for God's sake? Why should a thing like the probe, an obvious piece of quackery in his own opinion, get such a hold on the general public? It must be part of this general trend toward machines. Anything man can do, machines can do better. Machines! More machines! Machines for anything and everything! O tempora! O mores!

Oh, hell!

His resentment of the probe was beginning to bother him. Was it a fear of technological unemployment, a basic insecurity on his part, a mechanophobia, if that was the word—

He made a mental note to discuss this with his own analyst.

Dr. Sloane had to feel his way. The boy wasn't a patient who had come to him, more or less anxious to talk, more or less anxious to be helped.

Under the circumstances it would have been best to keep his first meeting with Richard short and noncommittal. It would have been sufficient merely to establish himself as something less than a total stranger. The next time he would be someone Richard had seen before. The time after he would be an acquaintance, and after that a friend of the family.

Unfortunately, Mrs. Hanshaw was not likely to accept a long-drawn-out process. She would go searching for a probe and, of course, she would find it.

And harm the boy. He was certain of that.

It was for that reason he felt he must sacrifice a little of the proper caution and risk a small crisis.

An uncomfortable ten minutes had passed when he decided he must try. Mrs. Hanshaw was smiling in a rather rigid way, eyeing him narrowly, as though she expected verbal magic from him. Richard wriggled in his seat, unresponsive to Dr. Sloane's tentative comments, overcome with boredom and unable not to show it.

Dr. Sloane said, with casual suddenness, "Would you like to take a walk with me, Richard?"

The boy's eyes widened and he stopped wriggling. He looked directly at Dr. Sloane. "A walk, sir?"

"I mean, outside."

"Do you go—outside?"

"Sometimes. When I feel like it."

Richard was on his feet, holding down a squirming eagerness. "I didn't think anyone did."

"I do. And I like company."

The boy sat down, uncertainly. "Mom?"

Mrs. Hanshaw had stiffened in her seat, her compressed lips radiating horror, but she managed to say, "Why certainly, Dickie. But watch yourself."

And she managed a quick and baleful glare at Dr. Sloane.

•   •   •

In one respect, Dr. Sloane had lied. He did not go outside "sometimes." He hadn't been in the open since early college days. True, he had been athletically inclined (still was to some extent) but in his time the indoor ultraviolet chambers, swimming pools, and tennis courts had flourished. For those with the price, they were much more satisfactory than the outdoor equivalents, open to the elements as they were, could possibly be. There was no occasion to go outside.

So there was a crawling sensation about his skin when he felt wind touch it, and he put down his flexied shoes on bare grass with a gingerly movement.

"Hey, look at that." Richard was quite different now, laughing, his reserve broken down.

Dr. Sloane had time only to catch a flash of blue that ended in a tree. Leaves rustled and he lost it.

"What was it?"

"A bird," said Richard. "A blue kind of bird."

Dr. Sloane looked about him in amazement. The Hanshaw residence was on a rise of ground, and he could see for miles. The area was only lightly wooded and between clumps of trees, grass gleamed brightly in the sunlight.

Colors set in deeper green made red and yellow patterns. They were flowers. From the books he had viewed in the course of his lifetime and from the old video shows, he had learned enough so that all this had an eerie sort of familiarity.

And yet the grass was so trim, the flowers so patterned. Dimly, he realized he had been expecting something wilder. He said, "Who takes care of all this?"

Richard shrugged. "I dunno. Maybe the mekkanos do it."

"Mekkanos?"

"There's loads of them around. Sometimes they got a sort of atomic knife they hold near the ground. It cuts the grass. And they're always fooling around with the flowers and things. There's one of them over there."

It was a small object, half a mile away. Its metal skin cast back highlights as it moved slowly over the gleaming meadow, engaged in some sort of activity that Dr. Sloane could not identify.

Dr. Sloane was astonished. Here it was a perverse sort of estheticism, a kind of conspicuous consumption—

"What's that?" he asked suddenly.

Richard looked. He said, "That's a house. Belongs to the Froehlichs. Co-ordinates, A-3, 23, 461. That little pointy building over there is the public Door."

Dr. Sloane was staring at the house. Was that what it looked like from the outside? Somehow he had imagined something much more cubic, and taller.

"Come along," shouted Richard, running ahead.

Dr. Sloane followed more sedately. "Do you know all the houses about here?"

"Just about."

"Where is A-23, 26, 475?" It was his own house, of course.

Richard looked about. "Let's see. Oh, sure, I know where it is—you see that water there?"

"Water?" Dr. Sloane made out a line of silver curving across the green.

"Sure. Real water. Just sort of running over rocks and things. It keeps running all the time. You can get across it if you step on the rocks. It's called a river."

More like a creek, thought Dr. Sloane. He had studied geography, of course, but what passed for the subject these days was really economic and cultural geography. Physical geography was almost an extinct science except among specialists. Still, he knew what rivers and creeks were, in a theoretical sort of way.

Richard was still talking. "Well, just past the river, over that hill with the big clump of trees and down the other side a way is A-23, 26, 475. It's a light green house with a white roof."

"It is?" Dr. Sloane was genuinely astonished. He hadn't known it was green.

Some small animal disturbed the grass in its anxiety to avoid the oncoming feet. Richard looked after it and shrugged. "You can't catch them. I tried."

A butterfly flitted past, a wavering bit of yellow. Dr. Sloane's eyes followed it.

There was a low hum that lay over the fields, interspersed with an occasional harsh, calling sound, a rattle, a twittering, a chatter

that rose, then fell. As his ear accustomed itself to listening, Dr.
Sloane heard a thousand sounds, and none were man-made.

A shadow fell upon the scene, advancing toward him, covering
him. It was suddenly cooler and he looked upward, startled.

Richard said, "It's just a cloud. It'll go away in a minute—looka
these flowers. They're the kind that smell."

They were several hundred yards from the Hanshaw residence.
The cloud passed and the sun shone once more. Dr. Sloane looked
back and was appalled at the distance they had covered. If they
moved out of sight of the house and if Richard ran off, would he
be able to find his way back?

He pushed the thought away impatiently and looked out toward the line of water (nearer now) and past it to where his own
house must be. He thought wonderingly: Light green?

He said, "You must be quite an explorer."

Richard said, with a shy pride, "When I go to school and come
back, I always try to use a different route and see new things."

"But you don't go outside every morning, do you? Sometimes
you use the Doors, I imagine."

"Oh, sure."

"Why is that, Richard?" Somehow, Dr. Sloane felt there might
be significance in that point.

But Richard quashed him. With his eyebrows up and a look of
astonishment on his face, he said, "Well, gosh, some mornings it
rains and I *have* to use the Door. I hate that, but what can you do?
About two weeks ago, I got caught in the rain and I—" he looked
about him automatically, and his voice sank to a whisper "—caught
a cold, and wasn't Mom upset, though."

Dr. Sloane sighed. "Shall we go back now?"

There was a quick disappointment on Richard's face. "Aw,
what for?"

"You remind me that your mother must be waiting for us."

"I guess so." The boy turned reluctantly.

They walked slowly back. Richard was saying, chattily, "I wrote
a composition at school once about how if I could go on some
ancient vehicle" (he pronounced it with exaggerated care) "I'd go
in a stratoliner and look at stars and clouds and things. Oh, boy, I
was sure nuts."

"You'd pick something else now?"

"You bet. I'd go in an aut'm'bile, real slow. Then I'd see everything there was."

Mrs. Hanshaw seemed troubled, uncertain. "You don't think it's abnormal, then, Doctor?"

"Unusual, perhaps, but not abnormal. He likes the outside."

"But how can he? It's so dirty, so unpleasant."

"That's a matter of individual taste. A hundred years ago our ancestors were all outside most of the time. Even today, I dare say there are a million Africans who have never seen a Door."

"But Richard's always been taught to behave himself the way a decent person in District A-3 is supposed to behave," said Mrs. Hanshaw, fiercely. "Not like an African or—or an ancestor."

"That may be part of the trouble, Mrs. Hanshaw. He feels this urge to go outside and yet he feels it to be wrong. He's ashamed to talk about it to you or to his teacher. It forces him into sullen retreat and it could eventually be dangerous."

"Then how can we persuade him to stop?"

Dr. Sloane said, "Don't try. Channel the activity instead. The day your Door broke down, he was forced outside, found he liked it, and that set a pattern. He used the trip to school and back as an excuse to repeat that first exciting experience. Now suppose you agree to let him out of the house for two hours on Saturdays and Sundays. Suppose he gets it through his head that after all he can go outside without necessarily having to go anywhere in the process. Don't you think he'll be willing to use the Door to go to school and back thereafter? And don't you think that will stop the trouble he's now having with his teacher and probably with his fellow-pupils?"

"But then will matters remain so? Must they? Won't he ever be normal again?"

Dr. Sloane rose to his feet. "Mrs. Hanshaw, he's as normal as need be right now. Right now, he's tasting the joys of the forbidden. If you cooperate with him, show that you don't disapprove, it will lose some of its attraction right there. Then, as he grows older, he will become more aware of the expectations and demands of soci-

ety. He will learn to conform. After all, there is a little of the rebel in all of us, but it generally dies down as we grow old and tired. Unless, that is, it is unreasonably suppressed and allowed to build up pressure. Don't do that. Richard will be all right."

He walked to the Door.

Mrs. Hanshaw said, "And you don't think a probe will be necessary, Doctor?"

He turned and said vehemently, "No, definitely not! There is nothing about the boy that requires it. Understand? Nothing."

His fingers hesitated an inch from the combination board and the expression on his face grew lowering.

"What's the matter, Dr. Sloane?" asked Mrs. Hanshaw.

But he didn't hear her because he was thinking of the Door and the psychic probe and all the rising, choking tide of machinery. There is a little of the rebel in all of us, he thought.

So he said in a soft voice, as his hand fell away from the board and his feet turned away from the Door, "You know, it's such a beautiful day that I think I'll walk."

STRIKEBREAKER

E lvis Blei rubbed his plump hands and said, "Self-containment is the word." He smiled uneasily as he helped Steven Lamorak of Earth to a light. There was uneasiness all over his smooth face with its small wide-set eyes.

Lamorak puffed smoke appreciatively and crossed his lanky legs.

His hair was powered with gray and he had a large and powerful jawbone. "Home grown?" he asked, staring critically at the cigarette. He tried to hide his own disturbance at the other's tension.

"Quite," said Blei.

"I wonder," said Lamorak, "that you have room on your small world for such luxuries."

(Lamorak thought of his first view of Elsevere from the spaceship visiplate. It was a jagged, airless planetoid, some hundred miles in diameter—just a dust-gray rough-hewn rock, glimmering dully in the light of its sun, 200,000,000 miles distant. It was the only object more than a mile in diameter that circled that sun, and now men had burrowed into that miniature world and constructed a society in it. And he himself, as a sociologist, had come to study the world and see how humanity had made itself fit into that queerly specialized niche.)

Blei's polite fixed smile expanded a hair. He said, "We are not a small world, Dr. Lamorak; you judge us by two-dimensional stan-

dards. The surface area of Elsevere is only three quarters that of the State of New York, but that's irrelevant. Remember, we can occupy, if we wish, the entire interior of Elsevere. A sphere of fifty miles radius has a volume of well over half a million cubic miles. If all of Elsevere were occupied by levels fifty feet apart, the total surface area within the planetoid would be 56,000,000 square miles, and that is equal to the total land area of Earth. And none of these square miles, Doctor, would be unproductive."

Lamorak said, "Good Lord," and stared blankly for a moment. "Yes, of course you're right. Strange I never thought of it that way. But then, Elsevere is the only thoroughly exploited asteroid world in the Galaxy; the rest of us simply can't get away from thinking of two-dimensional surfaces, as you pointed out. Well, I'm more than ever glad that your Council has been so cooperative as to give me a free hand in this investigation of mine."

Blei nodded convulsively at that.

Lamorak frowned slightly and thought: He acts for all the world as though he wished I had not come. Something's wrong.

Blei said, "Of course, you understand that we are actually much smaller than we could be; only minor portions of Elsevere have as yet been hollowed out and occupied. Nor are we particularly anxious to expand, except very slowly. To a certain extent we are limited by the capacity of our pseudo-gravity engines and Solar energy converters."

"I understand. But tell me, Councillor Blei—as a matter of personal curiosity, and not because it is of prime importance to my project—could I view some of your farming and herding levels first? I am fascinated by the thought of fields of wheat and herds of cattle inside a planetoid."

"You'll find the cattle small by your standards, Doctor, and we don't have much wheat. We grow yeast to a much greater extent. But there will be some wheat to show you. Some cotton and rice, too. Even fruit trees."

"Wonderful. As you say, self-containment. You recirculate everything, I imagine."

Lamorak's sharp eyes did not miss the fact that this last remark twinged Blei. The Elseverian's eyes narrowed to slits that hid his expression.

He said, "We must recirculate, yes. Air, water, food, minerals—everything that is used up—must be restored to its original state; waste products are reconverted to raw materials. All that is needed is energy and we have enough of that. We don't manage with one hundred percent efficiency, of course; there is a certain seepage. We import a small amount of water each year; and if our needs grow, we may have to import some coal and oxygen."

Lamorak said, "When can we start our tour, Councillor Blei?"

Blei's smile lost some of its negligible warmth. "As soon as we can, Doctor. There are some routine matters that must be arranged."

Lamorak nodded, and having finished his cigarette, stubbed it out.

Routine matters? There was none of this hesitancy during the preliminary correspondence. Elsevere had seemed proud that its unique asteroid existence had attracted the attention of the Galaxy.

He said, "I realize I would be a disturbing influence in a tightly knit society," and watched grimly as Blei leaped at the explanation and made it his own.

"Yes," said Blei, "we feel marked off from the rest of the Galaxy. We have our own customs. Each individual Elseverian fits into a comfortable niche. The appearance of a stranger without fixed caste is unsettling."

"The caste system does involve a certain inflexibility."

"Granted," said Blei quickly, "but there is also a certain self-assurance. We have firm rules of intermarriage and rigid inheritance of occupation. Each man, woman, and child knows his place, accepts it, and is accepted in it; we have virtually no neurosis or mental illness."

"And are there no misfits?" asked Lamorak.

Blei shaped his mouth as though to say no, then clamped it suddenly shut, biting the word into silence; a frown deepened on his forehead. He said, at length, "I will arrange for the tour, Doctor. Meanwhile, I imagine you would welcome a chance to freshen up and to sleep."

They rose together and left the room, Blei politely motioning the Earthman to precede him out the door.

•   •   •

Lamorak felt oppressed by the vague feeling of crisis that had pervaded his discussion with Blei.

The newspaper reinforced that feeling. He read it carefully before getting into bed, with what was at first merely a clinical interest. It was an eight-page tabloid of synthetic paper. One quarter of its items consisted of "personals": births, marriages, deaths, record quotas, expanding habitable volume (not area! three dimensions!). The remainder included scholarly essays, educational material, and fiction. Of news, in the sense to which Lamorak was accustomed, there was virtually nothing.

One item only could be so considered and that was chilling in its incompleteness.

It said, under a small headline: DEMANDS UNCHANGED: *There has been no change in his attitude of yesterday. The Chief Councillor, after a second interview, announced that his demands remain completely unreasonable and cannot be met under any circumstances.*

Then, in parenthesis, and in different type, there was the statement: *The editors of this paper agree that Elsevere cannot and will not jump to his whistle, come what may.*

Lamorak read it over three times. *His* attitude. *His* demands. *His* whistle.

Whose?

He slept uneasily, that night.

He had no time for newspapers in the days that followed; but spasmodically, the matter returned to his thoughts.

Blei, who remained his guide and companion for most of the tour, grew ever more withdrawn.

On the third day (quite artificially clock-set in an Earthlike twenty-four-hour pattern), Blei stopped at one point, and said, "Now this level is devoted entirely to chemical industries. That section is not important—"

But he turned away a shade too rapidly, and Lamorak seized his arm. "What are the products of that section?"

"Fertilizers. Certain organics," said Blei stiffly.

Lamorak held him back, looking for what sight Blei might be evading. His gaze swept over the close-by horizons of lined rock and the buildings squeezed and layered between the levels.

Lamorak said, "Isn't that a private residence there?"

Blei did not look in the indicated direction.

Lamorak said, "I think that's the largest one I've seen yet. Why is it here on a factory level?" That alone made it noteworthy. He had already seen that the levels on Elsevere were divided rigidly among the residential, the agricultural, and the industrial.

He looked back and called, "Councillor Blei!"

The councillor was walking away and Lamorak pursued him with hasty steps. "Is there something wrong, sir?"

Blei muttered, "I am rude, I know. I am sorry. There are matters that prey on my mind—" He kept up his rapid pace.

"Concerning *his* demands."

Blei came to a full halt. "What do *you* know about that?"

"No more than I've said. I read that much in the newspaper."

Blei muttered something to himself.

Lamorak said, "Ragusnik? What's that?"

Blei sighed heavily. "I suppose you ought to be told. It's humiliating, deeply embarrassing. The Council thought that matters would certainly be arranged shortly and that your visit need not be interfered with, that you need not know or be concerned. But it is almost a week now. I don't know what will happen and, appearances notwithstanding, it might be best for you to leave. No reason for an Outworlder to risk death."

The Earthman smiled incredulously. "Risk death? In this little world, so peaceful and busy. I can't believe it."

The Elseverian councillor said, "I can explain. I think it best I should." He turned his head away. "As I told you, everything on Elsevere must recirculate. You understand that."

"Yes."

"That includes—uh, human wastes."

"I assumed so," said Lamorak.

"Water is reclaimed from it by distillation and absorption. What remains is converted into fertilizer for yeast use; some of it

is used as a source of fine organics and other by-products. These factories you see are devoted to this."

"Well?" Lamorak had experienced a certain difficulty in the drinking of water when he first landed on Elsevere, because he had been realistic enough to know what it must be reclaimed from; but he had conquered the feeling easily enough. Even on Earth, water was reclaimed by natural processes from all sorts of unpalatable substances.

Blei, with increasing difficulty, said, "Igor Ragusnik is the man who is in charge of the industrial processes immediately involving the wastes. The position has been in his family since Elsevere was first colonized. One of the original settlers was Mikhail Ragusnik and he—he—"

"Was in charge of waste reclamation."

"Yes. Now that residence you singled out is the Ragusnik residence; it is the best and most elaborate on the asteroid. Ragusnik gets many privileges the rest of us do not have; but, after all—" Passion entered the Councillor's voice with great suddenness. "We cannot *speak* to him."

"What?"

"He demands full social equality. He wants his children to mingle with ours, and our wives to visit—Oh!" It was a groan of utter disgust.

Lamorak thought of the newspaper item that could not even bring itself to mention Ragusnik's name in print, or to say anything specific about his demands. He said, "I take it he's an outcast because of his job."

"Naturally. Human wastes and—" Words failed Blei. After a pause, he said more quietly, "As an Earthman, I suppose you don't understand."

"As a sociologist, I think I do." Lamorak thought of the Untouchables in ancient India, the ones who handled corpses. He thought of the position of swineherds in ancient Judea.

He went on, "I gather Elsevere will not give in to those demands."

"Never," said Blei, energetically. "Never."

"And so?"

"Ragusnik has threatened to cease operations."

"Go on strike, in other words."

"Yes."

"Would that be serious?"

"We have enough food and water to last quite a while; reclamation is not essential in that sense. But the wastes would accumulate; they would infect the asteroid. After generations of careful disease control, we have low natural resistance to germ diseases. Once an epidemic started—and one would—we would drop by the hundred."

"Is Ragusnik aware of this?"

"Yes, of course."

"Do you think he is likely to go through with his threat, then?"

"He is mad. He has already stopped working; there has been no waste reclamation since the day before you landed." Blei's bulbous nose sniffed at the air as though it already caught the whiff of excrement.

Lamorak sniffed mechanically at that, but smelled nothing.

Blei said, "So you see why it might be wise for you to leave. We are humiliated, of course, to have to suggest it."

But Lamorak said, "Wait; not just yet. Good Lord, this is a matter of great interest to me professionally. May I speak to the Ragusnik?"

"On no account," said Blei, alarmed.

"But I would like to understand the situation. The sociological conditions here are unique and not to be duplicated elsewhere. In the name of science—"

"How do you mean, speak? Would image-reception do?"

"Yes."

"I will ask the Council," muttered Blei.

They sat about Lamorak uneasily, their austere and dignified expressions badly marred with anxiety. Blei, seated in the midst of them, studiously avoided the Earthman's eyes.

The Chief Councillor, gray-haired, his face harshly wrinkled, his neck scrawny, said in a soft voice, "If in any way you can per-

suade him, sir, out of your own convictions, we will welcome that. In no case, however, are you to imply that we will, in any way, yield."

A gauzy curtain fell between the Council and Lamorak. He could make out the individual councillors still, but now he turned sharply toward the receiver before him. It glowed to life.

A head appeared in it, in natural color and with great realism. A strong dark head, with massive chin faintly stubbled, and thick, red lips set into a firm horizontal line.

The image said, suspiciously, "Who are you?"

Lamorak said, "My name is Steven Lamorak; I am an Earthman."

"An Outworlder?"

"That's right. I am visiting Elsevere. You are Ragusnik?"

"Igor Ragusnik, at your service," said the image, mockingly. "Except that there is no service and will be none until my family and I are treated like human beings."

Lamorak said, "Do you realize the danger that Elsevere is in? The possibility of epidemic disease?"

"In twenty-four hours, the situation can be made normal, if they allow me humanity. The situation is theirs to correct."

"You sound like an educated man, Ragusnik."

"So?"

"I am told you're denied no material comforts. You are housed and clothed and fed better than anyone on Elsevere. Your children are the best educated."

"Granted. But all by servo-mechanism. And motherless girl-babies are sent us to care for until they grow to be our wives. And they die young for loneliness. Why?" There was sudden passion in his voice. "Why must we live in isolation as if we were all monsters, unfit for human beings to be near? Aren't we human beings like others, with the same needs and desires and feelings. Don't we perform an honorable and useful function?"

There was a rustling of sighs from behind Lamorak. Ragusnik heard it, and raised his voice. "I see you of the Council behind there. Answer me: Isn't it an honorable and useful function? It is *your*

waste made into food for you. Is the man who purifies corruption worse than the man who produces it?—Listen, Councillors, I will not give in. Let all of Elsevere die of disease—including myself and my son, if necessary—but I will not give in. My family will be better dead of disease, than living as now."

Lamorak interrupted. "You've led this life since birth, haven't you?"

"And if I have?"

"Surely you're used to it."

"Never. Resigned, perhaps. My father was resigned, and I was resigned for a while; but I have watched my son, my only son, with no other little boy to play with. My brother and I had each other, but my son will never have anyone, and I am no longer resigned. I am through with Elsevere and through with talking."

The receiver went dead.

The Chief Councillor's face had paled to an aged yellow. He and Blei were the only ones of the group left with Lamorak. The Chief Councillor said, "The man is deranged; I do not know how to force him."

He had a glass of wine at his side; as he lifted it to his lips, he spilled a few drops that stained his white trousers with purple splotches.

Lamorak said, "Are his demands so unreasonable? Why can't he be accepted into society?"

There was momentary rage in Blei's eyes. "A dealer in excrement." Then he shrugged. "You are from Earth."

Incongruously, Lamorak thought of another unacceptable, one of the numerous classic creations of the medieval cartoonist, Al Capp. The variously named "inside man at the skonk works."

He said, "Does Ragusnik really deal with excrement? I mean, is there physical contact? Surely, it is all handled by automatic machinery."

"Of course," said the Chief Councillor.

"Then exactly what is Ragusnik's function?"

"He manually adjusts the various controls that assure the proper functioning of the machinery. He shifts units to allow repairs to be made; he alters functional rates with the time of day; he varies end production with demand." He added sadly, "If we had the space to

make the machinery ten times as complex, all this could be done automatically; but that would be such needless waste."

"But even so," insisted Lamorak, "all Ragusnik does he does simply by pressing buttons or closing contacts or things like that."

"Yes."

"Then his work is no different from any Elseverian's."

Blei said, stiffly, "You don't understand."

"And for that you will risk the death of your children?"

"We have no other choice," said Blei. There was enough agony in his voice to assure Lamorak that the situation was torture for him, but that he had no other choice indeed.

Lamorak shrugged in disgust. "Then break the strike. Force him."

"How?" said the Chief Councillor. "Who would touch him or go near him? And if we kill him by blasting from a distance, how will that help us?"

Lamorak said, thoughtfully, "Would you know how to run his machinery?"

The Chief Councillor came to his feet. "I?" he howled.

"I don't mean *you*," cried Lamorak at once. "I used the pronoun in its indefinite sense. Could *someone* learn how to handle Ragusnik's machinery?"

Slowly, the passion drained out of the Chief Councillor. "It is in the handbooks, I am certain—though I assure you I have never concerned myself with it."

"Then couldn't someone learn the procedure and substitute for Ragusnik until the man gives in?"

Blei said, "Who would agree to do such a thing? Not I, under any circumstances."

Lamorak thought fleetingly of Earthly taboos that might be almost as strong. He thought of cannibalism, incest, a pious man cursing God. He said, "But you must have made provision for vacancy in the Ragusnik job. Suppose he died."

"Then his son would automatically succeed to his job, or his nearest other relative," said Blei.

"What if he had no adult relatives? What if all his family died at once?"

"That has never happened; it will never happen."

The Chief Councillor added, "If there were danger of it, we might, perhaps, place a baby or two with the Ragusniks and have it raised to the profession."

"Ah. And how would you choose that baby?"

"From among children of mothers who died in childbirth, as we choose the future Ragusnik bride."

"Then choose a substitute Ragusnik now, by lot," said Lamorak.

The Chief Councillor said. "No! Impossible! How can you suggest that? If we select a baby, that baby is brought up to the life; it knows no other. At this point, it would be necessary to choose an adult and subject him to Ragusnik-hood. No, Dr. Lamorak, we are neither monsters nor abandoned brutes."

No use, thought Lamorak helplessly. No use, unless—

He couldn't bring himself to face that unless just yet.

That night, Lamorak slept scarcely at all. Ragusnik asked for only the basic elements of humanity. But opposing that were thirty thousand Elseverians who faced death.

The welfare of thirty thousand on one side; the just demands of one family on the other. Could one say that thirty thousand who would support such injustice deserved to die? Injustice by what standards? Earth's? Elsevere's? And who was Lamorak that he should judge?

And Ragusnik? He was willing to let thirty thousand die, including men and women who merely accepted a situation they had been taught to accept and could not change if they wished to. And children who had nothing at all to do with it.

Thirty thousand on one side; a single family on the other.

Lamorak made his decision in something that was almost despair; in the morning he called the Chief Councillor.

He said, "Sir, if you can find a substitute, Ragusnik will see that he has lost all chance to force a decision in his favor and will return to work."

"There can be no substitute," sighed the Chief Councillor; "I have explained that."

"No substitute among the Elseverians, but I am not an Elseverian; it doesn't matter to me. I will substitute."

They were excited, much more excited than Lamorak himself. A dozen times they asked him if he was serious.

Lamorak had not shaved, and he felt sick. "Certainly, I'm serious. And any time Ragusnik acts like this, you can always import a substitute. No other world has the taboo and there will always be plenty of temporary substitutes available if you pay enough."

(He was betraying a brutally exploited man, and he knew it. But he told himself desperately: *Except for ostracism, he's very well treated. Very well.*)

They gave him the handbooks and he spent six hours, reading and rereading. There was no use asking questions. None of the Elseverians knew anything about the job, except for what was in the handbook; and all seemed uncomfortable if the details were as much as mentioned.

"Maintain zero reading of galvanometer A-2 at all times during red signal of the Lunge-howler," read Lamorak. "Now what's a Lunge-howler?"

"There will be a sign," muttered Blei, and the Elseverians looked at each other hang-dog and bent their heads to stare at their fingerends.

They left him long before he reached the small rooms that were the central headquarters of generations of working Ragusniks, serving their world. He had specific instructions concerning which turnings to take and what level to reach, but they hung back and let him proceed alone.

He went through the rooms painstakingly, identifying the instruments and controls, following the schematic diagrams in the handbook.

There's a Lunge-howler, he thought, with gloomy satisfaction.

The sign did indeed say so. It had a semicircular face bitten into holes that were obviously designed to glow in separate colors. Why a "howler" then?

He didn't know.

Somewhere, thought Lamorak, *somewhere wastes are accumulating pushing against gears and exits, pipelines and stills, waiting to be handled in half a hundred ways. Now they just accumulate.*

Not without a tremor, he pulled the first switch as indicated by the handbook in its directions for "Initiation." A gentle murmur of life made itself felt through the floors and walls. He turned a knob and lights went on.

At each step, he consulted the handbook, though he knew it by heart; and with each step, the rooms brightened and the dial-indicators sprang into motion and a humming grew louder.

Somewhere deep in the factories, the accumulated wastes were being drawn into the proper channels.

A high-pitched signal sounded and startled Lamorak out of his painful concentration. It was the communications signal and Lamorak fumbled his receiver into action.

Ragusnik's head showed, startled; then slowly, the incredulity and outright shock faded from his eyes. "*That's* how it is, then."

"I'm not an Elseverian, Ragusnik; I don't mind doing this."

"But what business is it of yours? Why do you interfere?"

"I'm on your side, Ragusnik, but I must do this."

"Why, if you're on my side? Do they treat people on your world as they treat me here?"

"Not any longer. But even if you are right, there are thirty thousand people on Elsevere to be considered."

"They would have given in; you've ruined my only chance."

"They would *not* have given in. And in a way, you've won; they know now that you're dissatisfied. Until now, they never dreamed a Ragusnik could be unhappy, that he could make trouble."

"What if they know? Now all they need do is hire an Out-worlder anytime."

Lamorak shook his head violently. He had thought this through

in these last bitter hours. "The fact that they know means that the Elseverians will begin to think about you; some will begin to won-der if it's right to treat a human so. And if Outworlders are hired, they'll spread the word that this goes on upon Elsevere and Galactic public opinion will be in your favor."

"And?"

"Things will improve. In your son's time, things will be much better."

"In my son's time," said Ragusnik, his cheeks sagging. "I might have had it now. Well, I lose. I'll go back to the job."

Lamorak felt an overwhelming relief. "If you'll come here now, sir, you may have your job and I'll consider it an honor to shake your hand."

Ragusnik's head snapped up and filled with a gloomy pride. "You call me 'sir' and offer to shake my hand. Go about your busi-ness, Earthman, and leave me to my work, for I would not shake yours."

Lamorak returned the way he had come, relieved that the crisis was over, and profoundly depressed, too.

He stopped in surprise when he found a section of corridor cordoned off, so he could not pass. He looked about for alternate routes, then startled at a magnified voice above his head. "Dr. La-morak, do you hear me? This is Councillor Blei."

Lamorak looked up. The voice came over some sort of public address system, but he saw no sign of an outlet.

He called out, "Is anything wrong? Can you hear me?"

"I hear you."

Instinctively, Lamorak was shouting. "Is anything wrong? There seems to be a block here. Are there complications with Ragusnik?"

"Ragusnik has gone to work," came Blei's voice. "The crisis is over, and you must make ready to leave."

"Leave?"

"Leave Elsevere; a ship is being made ready for you now."

"But wait a bit." Lamorak was confused by this sudden leap of events. "I haven't completed my gathering of data."

Blei's voice said, "This cannot be helped. You will be directed

to the ship and your belongings will be sent after you by servo-mechanisms. We trust—we trust—"

Something was becoming clear to Lamorak. "You trust *what?*"

"We trust you will make no attempt to see or speak directly to any Elseverian. And of course we hope you will avoid embarrassment by not attempting to return to Elsevere at any time in the future. A colleague of yours would be welcome if further data concerning us is needed."

"I understand," said Lamorak, tonelessly. Obviously, he had himself become a Ragusnik. He had handled the controls that in turn had handled the wastes; he was ostracized. He was a corpse-handler, a swineherd, an inside man at the skonk works.

He said, "Good-bye."

Blei's voice said, "Before we direct you, Dr. Lamorak—on behalf of the Council of Elsevere, I thank you for your help in this crisis."

"You're welcome," said Lamorak, bitterly.

THE MARTIAN WAY

1

From the doorway of the short corridor between the only two rooms in the travel-head of the spaceship, Mario Esteban Rioz watched sourly as Ted Long adjusted the video dials painstakingly. Long tried a touch clockwise, then a touch counter. The picture was lousy.

Rioz knew it would stay lousy. They were too far from Earth and at a bad position facing the Sun. But then Long would not be expected to know that. Rioz remained standing in the doorway for an additional moment, head bent to clear the upper lintel, body turned half sidewise to fit the narrow opening. Then he jerked into the galley like a cork popping out of a bottle.

"What are you after?" he asked.

"I thought I'd get Hilder," said Long.

Rioz propped his rump on the corner of a table shelf. He lifted a conical can of milk from the companion shelf just above his head. Its point popped under pressure. He swirled it gently as he waited for it to warm.

"What for?" he said. He upended the cone and sucked noisily.

"Thought I'd listen."

"I think it's a waste of power."

Long looked up, frowning. "It's customary to allow free use of personal video sets."

"Within reason," retorted Rioz.

Their eyes met challengingly. Rioz had the rangy body, the gaunt, cheek-sunken face that was almost the hallmark of the Martian Scavenger, those Spacers who patiently haunted the space routes between Earth and Mars. Pale blue eyes were set keenly in the brown, lined face which, in turn, stood darkly out against the white surrounding syntho-fur that lined the upturned collar of his leathtic space jacket.

Long was altogether paler and softer. He bore some of the marks of the Grounder, although no second-generation Martian could be a Grounder in the sense that Earthmen were. His own collar was thrown back and his dark brown hair freely exposed.

"What do you call within reason?" demanded Long.

Rioz's thin lips grew thinner. He said, "Considering that we're not even going to make expenses this trip, the way it looks, any power drain at all is outside reason."

Long said, "If we're losing money, hadn't you better get back to your post? It's your watch."

Rioz grunted and ran a thumb and forefinger over the stubble on his chin. He got up and trudged to the door, his soft, heavy boots muting the sound of his steps. He paused to look at the thermostat, then turned with a flare of fury.

"I *thought* it was hot. Where do you think you are?"

Long said, "Forty degrees isn't excessive."

"For you it isn't, maybe. But this is space, not a heated office at the iron mines." Rioz swung the thermostat control down to minimum with a quick thumb movement. "Sun's warm enough."

"The galley isn't on Sunside."

"It'll percolate through, damn it."

Rioz stepped through the door and Long stared after him for a long moment, then turned back to the video. He did not turn up the thermostat.

The picture was still flickering badly, but it would have to do. Long folded a chair down out of the wall. He leaned forward, waiting through the formal announcement, the momentary pause before

the slow dissolution of the curtain, the spotlight picking out the well-known bearded figure which grew as it was brought forward until it filled the screen.

The voice, impressive even through the flutings and croakings induced by the electron storms of twenty millions of miles, began, "Friends! My fellow citizens of Earth . . ."

2

Rioz's eye caught the flash of the radio signal as he stepped into the pilot room. For one moment, the palms of his hands grew clammy when it seemed to him that it was a radar pip; but that was only his guilt speaking. He should not have left the pilot room while on duty theoretically, though all Scavengers did it. Still, it was the standard nightmare, this business of a strike turning up during just those five minutes when one knocked off for a quick coffee because it seemed certain that space was clear. And the nightmare had been known to happen, too.

Rioz threw in the multiscanner. It was a waste of power, but while he was thinking about it, he might as well make sure.

Space was clear except for the far-distant echoes from the neighboring ships on the scavenging line.

He hooked up the radio circuit, and the blond, long-nosed head of Richard Swenson, copilot of the next ship on the Mars-ward side, filled it.

"Hey, Mario," said Swenson.

"Hi. What's new?"

There was a second and a fraction of pause between that and Swenson's next comment, since the speed of electromagnetic radiation is not infinite.

"What a day I've *had*."

"Something happened?" Rioz asked.

"I had a strike."

"Well, good."

"Sure, if I'd roped it in," said Swenson morosely.

"What happened?"

"Damn it, I headed in the wrong direction."

Rioz knew better than to laugh. He said, "How did you do that?"

"It wasn't my fault. The trouble was the shell was moving way out of the ecliptic. Can you imagine the stupidity of a pilot who can't work the release maneuver decently? How was I to know? I got the distance of the shell and let it go at that. I just assumed its orbit was in the usual trajectory family. Wouldn't you? I started along what I thought was a good line of intersection and it was five minutes before I noticed the distance was still going up. The pips were taking their sweet time returning. So then I took the angular projections of the thing, and it was too late to catch up with it."

"Any of the other boys getting it?"

"No. It's 'way out of the ecliptic and'll keep on going forever. That's not what bothers me so much. It was only an inner shell. But I hate to tell you how many tons of propulsion I wasted getting up speed and then getting back to station. You should have heard Canute."

Canute was Richard Swenson's brother and partner.

"Mad, huh?" said Rioz.

"Mad? Like to have killed me! But then we've been out five months now and it's getting kind of sticky. You know."

"I know."

"How are you doing, Mario?"

Rioz made a spitting gesture. "About that much this trip. Two shells in the last two weeks and I had to chase each one for six hours."

"Big ones?"

"Are you kidding? I could have scaled them down to Phobos by hand. This is the worst trip I've ever had."

"How much longer are you staying?"

"For my part, we can quit tomorrow. We've only been out two months and it's got so I'm chewing Long out all the time."

There was a pause over and above the electromagnetic lag.

Swenson said, "What's he like, anyway? Long, I mean."

Rioz looked over his shoulder. He could hear the soft, crackly mutter of the video in the galley. "I can't make him out. He says

to me about a week after the start of the trip, 'Mario, why are you a Scavenger?' I just look at him and say, 'To make a living. Why do you suppose?' I mean, what the hell kind of a question is that? Why is anyone a Scavenger?

"Anyway, he says, 'That's not it, Mario.' *He's* telling *me*, you see. He says, 'You're a Scavenger because this is part of the Martian way.'"

Swenson said, "And what did he mean by that?"

Rioz shrugged. "I never asked him. Right now he's sitting in there listening to the ultramicrowave from Earth. He's listening to some Grounder called Hilder."

"Hilder? A Grounder politician, an Assemblyman or something, isn't he?"

"That's right. At least, I think that's right. Long is always doing things like that. He brought about fifteen pounds of books with him, all about Earth. Just plain dead weight, you know."

"Well, he's your partner. And talking about partners, I think I'll get back on the job. If I miss another strike, there'll be murder around here."

He was gone and Rioz leaned back. He watched the even green line that was the pulse scanner. He tried the multiscanner a moment. Space was still clear.

He felt a little better. A bad spell is always worse if the Scavengers all about you are pulling in shell after shell, if the shells go spiraling down the Phobos scrap forges with everyone's brand welded on except your own. Then, too, he had managed to work off some of his resentment toward Long.

It was a mistake teaming up with Long. It was always a mistake to team up with a tenderfoot. They thought what you wanted was conversation, especially Long, with his eternal theories about Mars and its great new role in human progress. That was the way he said it—Human Progress: the Martian Way; the New Creative Minority. And all the time what Rioz wanted wasn't talk, but a strike, a few shells to call their own.

At that, he hadn't any choice, really. Long was pretty well known down on Mars and made good pay as a mining engineer. He was a friend of Commissioner Sankov and he'd been out on one or two short scavenging missions before. You can't turn a fellow

down flat before a tryout, even though it did look funny. Why should a mining engineer with a comfortable job and good money want to muck around in space?

Rioz never asked Long that question. Scavenger partners are forced too close together to make curiosity desirable, or sometimes even safe. But Long talked so much that he answered the question.

"I had to come out here, Mario," he said. "The future of Mars isn't in the mines; it's in space."

Rioz wondered how it would be to try a trip alone. Everyone said it was impossible. Even discounting lost opportunities when one man had to go off watch to sleep or attend to other things, it was well known that one man alone in space would become intolerably depressed in a relatively short while.

Taking a partner along made a six-month trip possible. A regular crew would be better, but no Scavenger could make money on a ship large enough to carry one. The capital it would take in propulsion alone!

Even two didn't find it exactly fun in space. Usually you had to change partners each trip and you could stay out longer with some than with others. Look at Richard and Canute Swenson. They teamed up every five or six trips because they were brothers. And yet whenever they did, it was a case of constantly mounting tension and antagonism after the first week.

Oh, well. Space was clear. Rioz would feel a little better if he went back in the galley and smoothed down some of the bickering with Long. He might as well show he was an old spacehand who took the irritations of space as they came.

He stood up, walked the three steps necessary to reach the short, narrow corridor that tied together the two rooms of the spaceship.

3

Once again Rioz stood in the doorway for a moment, watching. Long was intent on the flickering screen.

Rioz said gruffly, "I'm shoving up the thermostat. It's all right— we can spare the power."

Long nodded. "If you like."

Rioz took a hesitant step forward. Space was clear, so to hell with sitting and looking at a blank, green, pipless line. He said, "What's the Grounder been talking about?"

"History of space travel mostly. Old stuff, but he's doing it well. He's giving the whole works—color cartoons, trick photography, stills from old films, everything."

As if to illustrate Long's remarks, the bearded figure faded out of view, and a cross-sectional view of a spaceship flitted onto the screen. Hilder's voice continued, pointing out features of interest that appeared in schematic color. The communications system of the ship outlined itself in red as he talked about it, the storerooms, the proton micropile drive, the cybernetic circuits . . .

Then Hilder was back on the screen. "But this is only the travel-head of the ship. What moves it? What gets it off the Earth?"

Everyone knew what moved a spaceship, but Hilder's voice was like a drug. He made spaceship propulsion sound like the secret of the ages, like an ultimate revelation. Even Rioz felt a slight tingling of suspense, though he had spent the greater part of his life aboard ship.

Hilder went on. "Scientists call it different names. They call it the Law of Action and Reaction. Sometimes they call it Newton's Third Law. Sometimes they call it Conservation of Momentum. But we don't have to call it any name. We can just use our common sense. When we swim, we push water backward and move forward ourselves. When we walk, we push back against the ground and move forward. When we fly a gyro-flivver, we push air backward and move forward.

"Nothing can move forward unless something else moves backward. It's the old principle of "You can't get something for nothing."

"Now imagine a spaceship that weighs a hundred thousand tons lifting off Earth. To do that, something else must be moved downward. Since a spaceship is extremely heavy, a great deal of material must be moved downward. So much material, in fact, that there is no place to keep it all aboard ship. A special compartment must be built behind the ship to hold it."

Again Hilder faded out and the ship returned. It shrank and a truncated cone appeared behind it. In bright yellow, words appeared

within it: MATERIAL TO BE THROWN AWAY.

"But now," said Hilder, "the total weight of the ship is much greater. You need still more propulsion and still more."

The ship shrank enormously to add on another larger shell and still another immense one. The ship proper, the travel-head, was a little dot on the screen, a glowing red dot.

Rioz said, "Hell, this is kindergarten stuff."

"Not to the people he's speaking to, Mario," replied Long. "Earth isn't Mars. There must be billions of Earth people who've never even seen a spaceship; don't know the first thing about it."

Hilder was saying, "When the material inside the biggest shell is used up, the shell is detached. It's thrown away, too."

The outermost shell came loose, wobbled about the screen.

"Then the second one goes," said Hilder, "and then, if the trip is a long one, the last is ejected."

The ship was just a red dot now, with three shells shifting and moving, lost in space.

Hilder said, "These shells represent a hundred thousand tons of tungsten, magnesium, aluminum, and steel. They are gone forever from Earth. Mars is ringed by Scavengers, waiting along the routes of space travel, waiting for the cast-off shells, netting and branding them, saving them for Mars. Not one cent of payment reaches Earth for them. They are salvage. They belong to the ship that finds them."

Rioz said, "We risk our investment and our lives. If we don't pick them up, no one gets them. What loss is that to Earth?"

"Look," said Long, "he's been talking about nothing but the drain that Mars, Venus, and the Moon put on Earth. This is just another item of loss."

"They'll get their return. We're mining more iron every year."

"And most of it goes right back into Mars. If you can believe his figures, Earth has invested two hundred billion dollars in Mars and received back about five billion dollars' worth of iron. It's put five hundred billion dollars into the Moon and gotten back a little over twenty-five billion dollars of magnesium, titanium, and assorted light metals. It's put fifty billion dollars into Venus and gotten back nothing. And that's what the taxpayers of Earth are really interested in—tax money out; nothing in."

The screen was filled, as he spoke, with diagrams of the Scavengers on the route to Mars; little, grinning caricatures of ships, reaching out wiry, tenuous arms that groped for the tumbling, empty shells, seizing and snaking them in, branding them MARS PROPERTY in glowing letters, then scaling them down to Phobos.

Then it was Hilder again. "They tell us eventually they will return it all to us. Eventually! Once they are a going concern! We don't know when that will be. A century from now? A thousand years? A million? 'Eventually.' Let's take them at their word. Someday they will give us back all our metals. Someday they will grow their own food, use their own power, live their own lives.

"But one thing they can never return. Not in a hundred million years. *Water!*

"Mars has only a trickle of water because it is too small. Venus has no water at all because it is too hot. The Moon has none because it is too hot and too small. So Earth must supply not only drinking water and washing water for the Spacers, water to run their industries, water for the hydroponic factories they claim to be setting up—but even water to throw away by the millions of tons.

"What is the propulsive force that spaceships use? What is it they throw out behind so that they can accelerate forward? Once it was the gases generated from explosives. That was very expensive. Then the proton micropile was invented—a cheap power source that could heat up any liquid until it was a gas under tremendous pressure. What is the cheapest and most plentiful liquid available? Why, water, of course.

"Each spaceship leaves Earth carrying nearly a million tons—not pounds, *tons*—of water, for the sole purpose of driving it into space so that it may speed up or slow down.

"Our ancestors burned the oil of Earth madly and willfully. They destroyed its coal recklessly. We despise and condemn them for that, but at least they had this excuse—they thought that when the need arose, substitutes would be found. And they were right. We have our plankton farms and our proton micropiles.

"But there is no substitute for water. None! There never can be. And when our descendants view the desert we will have made of Earth, what excuse will they find for us? When the droughts come and grow—"

Long leaned forward and turned off the set. He said, "That bothers me. The damn fool is deliberately—What's the matter?"

Rioz had risen uneasily to his feet. "I ought to be watching the pips."

"The hell with the pips." Long got up likewise, followed Rioz through the narrow corridor, and stood just inside the pilot room. "If Hilder carries this through, if he's got the guts to make a real issue out of it—Wow!"

He had seen it too. The pip was a Class A, racing after the outgoing signal like a greyhound after a mechanical rabbit.

Rioz was babbling, "Space was clear, I tell you, clear. For Mars' sake, Ted, don't just freeze on me. See if you can spot it visually."

Rioz was working speedily and with an efficiency that was the result of nearly twenty years of scavenging. He had the distance in two minutes. Then, remembering Swenson's experience, he measured the angle of declination and the radial velocity as well.

He yelled at Long, "One point seven six radians. You can't miss it, man."

Long held his breath as he adjusted the vernier. "It's only half a radian off the Sun. It'll only be crescent-lit."

He increased magnification as rapidly as he dared, watching for the one "star" that changed position and grew to have a form, revealing itself to be no star.

"I'm starting, anyway," said Rioz. "We can't wait."

"I've got it. I've got it." Magnification was still too small to give it a definite shape, but the dot Long watched was brightening and dimming rhythmically as the shell rotated and caught sunlight on cross sections of different sizes.

"Hold on."

The first of many fine spurts of steam squirted out of the proper vents, leaving long trails of microcrystals of ice gleaming mistily in the pale beams of the distant Sun. They thinned out for a hundred miles or more. One spurt, then another, then another, as the Scavenger ship moved out of its stable trajectory and took up a course tangential to that of the shell.

"It's moving like a comet at perihelion!" yelled Rioz. "Those damned Grounder pilots knock the shells off that way on purpose. I'd like to—"

He swore his anger in a frustrated frenzy as he kicked steam backward and backward recklessly, till the hydraulic cushioning of his chair had soughed back a full foot and Long had found himself all but unable to maintain his grip on the guardrail.

"Have a heart," he begged.

But Rioz had his eye on the pips. "If you can't take it, man, stay on Mars!" The steam spurts continued to boom distantly.

The radio came to life. Long managed to lean forward through what seemed like molasses and closed contact. It was Swenson, eyes glaring.

Swenson yelled, "Where the hell are you guys going? You'll be in my sector in ten seconds."

Rioz said, "I'm chasing a shell."

"In *my* sector?"

"It started in mine and you're not in position to get it. Shut off that radio, Ted."

The ship thundered through space, a thunder that could be heard only within the hull. And then Rioz cut the engines in stages large enough to make Long flail forward. The sudden silence was more ear-shattering than the noise that had preceded it.

Rioz said, "All right. Let me have the 'scope."

They both watched. The shell was a definite truncated cone now, tumbling with slow solemnity as it passed along among the stars.

"It's a Class A shell, all right," said Rioz with satisfaction. A giant among shells, he thought. It would put them into the black.

Long said, "We've got another pip on the scanner. I think it's Swenson taking after us."

Rioz scarcely gave it a glance. "He won't catch us."

The shell grew larger still, filling the visiplate.

Rioz's hands were on the harpoon lever. He waited, adjusted the angle microscopically twice, played out the length allotment. Then he yanked, tripping the release.

For a moment, nothing happened. Then a metal mesh cable snaked out onto the visiplate, moving toward the shell like a striking cobra. It made contact, but it did not hold. If it had, it would have snapped instantly like a cobweb strand. The shell was turning with a rotational momentum amounting to thousands of tons. What

the cable did do was to set up a powerful magnetic field that acted as a brake on the shell.

Another cable and another lashed out. Rioz sent them out in an almost heedless expenditure of energy.

"I'll get this one! By Mars, I'll get this one!"

With some two dozen cables stretching between ship and shell, he desisted. The shell's rotational energy, converted by braking into heat, had raised its temperature to a point where its radiation could be picked up by the ship's meters.

Long said, "Do you want me to put our brand on?"

"Suits me. But you don't have to if you don't want to. It's my watch."

"I don't mind."

Long clambered into his suit and went out the lock. It was the surest sign of his newness to the game that he could count the number of times he had been out in space in a suit. This was the fifth time.

He went out along the nearest cable, hand over hand, feeling the vibration of the mesh against the metal of his mitten.

He burned their serial number in the smooth metal of the shell. There was nothing to oxidize the steel in the emptiness of space. It simply melted and vaporized, condensing some feet away from the energy beam, turning the surface it touched into a gray, powdery dullness.

Long swung back toward the ship.

Inside again, he took off his helmet, white and thick with frost that collected as soon as he had entered.

The first thing he heard was Swenson's voice coming over the radio, almost unrecognizable in his rage: ". . . straight to the Commissioner. Damn it, there are rules to this game!"

Rioz sat back, unbothered. "Look, it hit my sector. I was late spotting it and I chased it into yours. You couldn't have gotten it with Mars for a backstop. That's all there is to it—You back, Long?"

He cut contact.

The signal button raged at him, but he paid no attention.

"He's going to the Commissioner?" Long asked.

"Not a chance. He just goes on like that because it breaks the

monotony. He doesn't mean anything by it. He knows it's our shell. And how do you like that hunk of stuff, Ted?"

"Pretty good."

"Pretty good? It's terrific! Hold on. I'm setting it swinging."

The side jets spat steam and the ship started a slow rotation about the shell. The shell followed it. In thirty minutes, they were a gigantic bola spinning in emptiness. Long checked the *Ephemeris* for the position of Deimos.

At a precisely calculated moment, the cables released their magnetic field and the shell went streaking off tangentially in a trajectory that would, in a day or so, bring it within pronging distance of the shell stores on the Martian satellite.

Rioz watched it go. He felt good. He turned to Long. "This is one fine day for us."

"What about Hilder's speech?" asked Long.

"What? Who? Oh, that. Listen, if I had to worry about every thing some damned Grounder said, I'd never get any sleep. Forget it."

"I don't think we should forget it."

"You're nuts. Don't bother me about it, will you? Get some sleep instead."

4

Ted Long found the breadth and height of the city's main thoroughfare exhilarating. It had been two months since the Commissioner had declared a moratorium on scavenging and had pulled all ships out of space, but this feeling of a stretched-out vista had not stopped thrilling Long. Even the thought that the moratorium was called pending a decision on the part of Earth to enforce its new insistence on water economy, by deciding upon a ration limit for scavenging, did not cast him entirely down.

The roof of the avenue was painted a luminous light blue, perhaps as an old-fashioned imitation of Earth's sky, Ted wasn't sure. The walls were lit with the store windows that pierced them.

Off in the distance, over the hum of traffic and the sloughing

noise of people's feet passing him, he could hear the intermittent blasting as new channels were being bored into Mars' crust. All his life he remembered such blastings. The ground he walked on had been part of solid, unbroken rock when he was born. The city was growing and would keep on growing—if Earth would only let it.

He turned off at a cross street, narrower, not quite as brilliantly lit, shop windows giving way to apartment houses, each with its row of lights along the front façade. Shoppers and traffic gave way to slower-paced individuals and to squawling youngsters who had as yet evaded the maternal summons to the evening meal.

At the last minute, Long remembered the social amenities and stopped off at a corner water store.

He passed over his canteen. "Fill 'er up."

The plump storekeeper unscrewed the cap, cocked an eye into the opening. He shook it a little and let it gurgle. "Not much left," he said cheerfully.

"No," agreed Long.

The storekeeper trickled water in, holding the neck of the canteen close to the hose tip to avoid spillage. The volume gauge whirred. He screwed the cap back on.

Long passed over the coins and took his canteen. It clanked against his hip now with a pleasing heaviness. It would never do to visit a family without a full canteen. Among the boys, it didn't matter. Not as much, anyway.

He entered the hallway of No. 27, climbed a short flight of stairs, and paused with his thumb on the signal.

The sound of voices could be heard plainly.

One was a woman's voice, somewhat shrill. "It's all right for you to have your Scavenger friends here, isn't it? I'm supposed to be thankful you manage to get home two months a year. Oh, it's quite enough that you spend a day or two with me. After that, it's the Scavengers again."

"I've been home for a long time now," said a male voice, "and this is business. For Mars' sake, let up, Dora. They'll be here soon."

Long decided to wait a moment before signaling. It might give them a chance to hit a more neutral topic.

"What do I care if they come?" retorted Dora. "Let them hear

me. And I'd just as soon the Commissioner kept the moratorium on permanently. You hear me?"

"And what would we live on?" came the male voice hotly. "You tell me that."

"I'll tell you. You can make a decent, honorable living right here on Mars, just like everybody else. I'm the only one in this apartment house that's a Scavenger widow. That's what I am—a widow. I'm worse than a widow, because if I were a widow, I'd at least have a chance to marry someone else—What did you say?"

"Nothing. Nothing at all."

"Oh, I know what you said. Now listen here, Dick Swenson—"

"I only said," cried Swenson, "that now I know why Scavengers usually don't marry."

"You shouldn't have either. I'm tired of having every person in the neighborhood pity me and smirk and ask when you're coming home. Other people can be mining engineers and administrators and even tunnel borers. At least tunnel borers' wives have a decent homelife and their children don't grow up like vagabonds. Peter might as well not have a father—"

A thin boy-soprano voice made its way through the door. It was somewhat more distant, as though it were in another room. "Hey, Mom, what's a vagabond?"

Dora's voice rose a notch. "Peter! You keep your mind on your homework."

Swenson said in a low voice, "It's not right to talk this way in front of the kid. What kind of notions will he get about me?"

"Stay home then and teach him better notions."

Peter's voice called out again. "Hey, Mom, I'm going to be a Scavenger when I grow up."

Footsteps sounded rapidly. There was a momentary hiatus in the sounds, then a piercing, "Mom! Hey, Mom! Leggo my ear! What did I do?" and a snuffling silence.

Long seized the chance. He worked the signal vigorously.

Swenson opened the door, brushing down his hair with both hands.

"Hello, Ted," he said in a subdued voice. Then loudly, "Ted's here, Dora. Where's Mario, Ted?"

Long said, "He'll be here in a while."

Dora came bustling out of the next room, a small, dark woman with a pinched nose, and hair, just beginning to show touches of gray, combed off the forehead.

"Hello, Ted. Have you eaten?"

"Quite well, thanks. I haven't interrupted you, have I?"

"Not at all. We finished ages ago. Would you like some coffee?"

"I think so." Ted unslung his canteen and offered it.

"Oh, goodness, that's all right. We've plenty of water."

"I insist."

"Well, then—"

Back into the kitchen she went. Through the swinging door, Long caught a glimpse of dishes sitting in Secoterg, the "waterless cleaner that soaks up and absorbs grease and dirt in a twinkling. One ounce of water will rinse eight square feet of dish surface clean as clean. Buy Secoterg. Secoterg just cleans it right, makes your dishes shiny bright, does away with water waste—"

The tune started whining through his mind and Long crushed it with speech. He said, "How's Pete?"

"Fine, fine. The kid's in the fourth grade now. You know I don't get to see him much. Well, sir, when I came back last time, he looked at me and said . . ."

It went on for a while and wasn't too bad as bright sayings of bright children as told by dull parents go.

The door signal burped and Mario Rioz came in, frowning and red.

Swenson stepped to him quickly. "Listen, don't say anything about shell-snaring. Dora still remembers the time you fingered a Class A shell out of my territory and she's in one of her moods now."

"Who the hell wants to talk about shells?" Rioz slung off a fur-lined jacket, threw it over the back of the chair, and sat down.

Dora came through the swinging door, viewed the newcomer with a synthetic smile, and said, "Hello, Mario. Coffee for you, too?"

"Yeah," he said, reaching automatically for his canteen.

"Just use some more of my water, Dora," said Long quickly. "He'll owe it to me."

"Yeah," said Rioz.

"What's wrong, Mario?" asked Long.

Rioz said heavily, "Go on. Say you told me so. A year ago when Hilder made that speech, you told me so. Say it."

Long shrugged.

Rioz said, "They've set up the quota. Fifteen minutes ago the news came out."

"Well?"

"Fifty thousand tons of water per trip."

"What?" yelled Swenson, burning. "You can't get off Mars with fifty thousand!"

"That's the figure. It's a deliberate piece of gutting. No more scavenging."

Dora came out with the coffee and set it down all around.

"What's all this about no more scavenging?" She sat down very firmly and Swenson looked helpless.

"It seems," said Long, "that they're rationing us at fifty thousand tons and that means we can't make any more trips."

"Well, what of it?" Dora sipped her coffee and smiled gaily. "If you want my opinion, it's a good thing. It's time all you Scavengers found yourselves nice, steady jobs here on Mars. I mean it. It's no life to be running all over space—"

"Please, Dora," said Swenson.

Rioz came close to a snort.

Dora raised her eyebrows. "I'm just giving my opinions."

Long said, "Please feel free to do so. But I would like to say something. Fifty thousand is just a detail. We know that Earth—or at least Hilder's party—wants to make political capital out of a campaign for water economy, so we're in a bad hole. We've got to get water somehow or they'll shut us down altogether, right?"

"Well, sure," said Swenson.

"But the question is how, right?"

"If it's only getting water," said Rioz in a sudden gush of words, "there's only one thing to do and you know it. If the Grounders won't give us water, we'll take it. The water doesn't belong to them just because their fathers and grandfathers were too damned sick-yellow ever to leave their fat planet. Water belongs to people wherever they are. We're people and the water's ours, too. We have a right to it."

"How do you propose taking it?" asked Long.

"Easy! They've got oceans of water on Earth. They can't post a guard over every square mile. We can sink down on the night side of the planet any time we want, fill our shells, then get away. How can they stop us?"

"In half a dozen ways, Mario. How do you spot shells in space up to distances of a hundred thousand miles? One thin metal shell in all that space. How? By radar. Do you think there's no radar on Earth? Do you think that if Earth ever gets the notion we're engaged in waterlegging, it won't be simple for them to set up a radar network to spot ships coming in from space?"

Dora broke in indignantly. "I'll tell you one thing, Mario Rioz. My husband isn't going to be part of any raid to get water to keep up his scavenging with."

"It isn't just scavenging," said Mario. "Next they'll be cutting down on everything else. We've got to stop them now."

"But we don't need their water, anyway," said Dora. "We're not the Moon or Venus. We pipe enough water down from the polar caps for all we need. We have a water tap right in this apartment. There's one in every apartment on this block."

Long said, "Home use is the smallest part of it. The mines use water. And what do we do about the hydroponic tanks?"

"That's right," said Swenson. "What about the hydroponic tanks, Dora? They've got to have water and it's about time we arranged to grow our own fresh food instead of having to live on the condensed crud they ship us from Earth."

"Listen to him," said Dora scornfully. "What do you know about fresh food? You've never eaten any."

"I've eaten more than you think. Do you remember those carrots I picked up once?"

"Well, what was so wonderful about them? If you ask me, good baked protomeal is much better. And healthier, too. It just seems to be the fashion now to be talking fresh vegetables because they're increasing taxes for these hydroponics. Besides, all this will blow over."

Long said, "I don't think so. Not by itself, anyway. Hilder will probably be the next Coordinator, and then things may really get bad. If they cut down on food shipments, too—"

"Well, then," shouted Rioz, "what do we do? I still say take it! Take the water!"

"And I say we can't do that, Mario. Don't you see that what you're suggesting is the Earth way, the Grounder way? You're trying to hold on to the umbilical cord that ties Mars to Earth. Can't you get away from that? Can't you see the Martian way?"

"No, I can't. Suppose you tell me."

"I will, if you'll listen. When we think about the Solar System, what do we think about? Mercury, Venus, Earth, Moon, Mars, Phobos, and Deimos. There you are—seven bodies, that's all. But that doesn't represent one per cent of the Solar System. We Martians are right at the edge of the other ninety-nine per cent. Out there, farther from the Sun, there's unbelievable amounts of water!"

The others stared.

Swenson said uncertainly, "You mean the layers of ice on Jupiter and Saturn?"

"Not that specifically, but it is water, you'll admit. A thousand-mile-thick layer of water is a lot of water."

"But it's all covered up with layers of ammonia or—or something, isn't it?" asked Swenson. "Besides, we can't land on the major planets."

"I know that," said Long, "but I haven't said that was the answer. The major planets aren't the only objects out there. What about the asteroids and the satellites? Vesta is a two-hundred-mile-diameter asteroid that's hardly more than a chunk of ice. One of the moons of Saturn is mostly ice. How about that?"

Rioz said, "Haven't you ever been in space, Ted?"

"You know I have. Why do you ask?"

"Sure, I know you have, but you still talk like a Grounder. Have you thought of the distances involved? The average asteroid is a hundred twenty million miles from Mars at the closest. That's twice the Venus-Mars hop and you know that hardly any liners do even that in one jump. They usually stop off at Earth or the Moon. After all, how long do you expect anyone to stay in space, man?"

"I don't know. What's your limit?"

"You know the limit. You don't have to ask me. It's six months. That's handbook data. After six months, if you're still in space you're psychotherapy meat. Right, Dick?"

Swenson nodded.

"And that's just the asteroids," Rioz went on. "From Mars to Jupiter is three hundred thirty million miles, and to Saturn it's seven hundred million. How can anyone handle that kind of distance? Suppose you hit standard velocity or, to make it even, say you get up to a good two hundred kilomiles an hour. It would take you—let's see, allowing time for acceleration and deceleration—about six or seven months to get to Jupiter and nearly a year to get to Saturn. Of course, you could hike the speed to a million miles an hour, theoretically, but where would you get the water to do that?"

"Gee," said a small voice attached to a smutty nose and round eyes. "Saturn!"

Dora whirled in her chair. "Peter, march right back into your room."

"Aw, Ma."

"Don't 'Aw, Ma' me." She began to get out of the chair, and Peter scuttled away.

Swenson said, "Say, Dora, why don't you keep him company for a while? It's hard to keep his mind on homework if we're all out here talking."

Dora sniffed obstinately and stayed put. "I'll sit right here until I find out what Ted Long is thinking of. I tell you right now I don't like the sound of it."

Swenson said nervously, "Well, never mind Jupiter and Saturn. I'm sure Ted isn't figuring on that. But what about Vesta? We could make it in ten or twelve weeks there and the same back. And two hundred miles in diameter. That's four million cubic miles of ice!"

"So what?" said Rioz. "What do we do on Vesta? Quarry the ice? Set up mining machinery? Say, do you know how long that would take?"

Long said, "I'm talking about Saturn, not Vesta."

Rioz addressed an unseen audience. "I tell him seven hundred million miles and he keeps on talking."

"All right," said Long, "suppose you tell me how you know we can only stay in space six months, Mario?"

"It's common knowledge, damn it."

"Because it's in the *Handbook of Space Flight*. It's data compiled

by Earth scientists from experience with Earth pilots and spacemen. You're still thinking Grounder style. You won't think the Martian way."

"A Martian may be a Martian, but he's still a man."

"But how can you be so blind? How many times have you fellows been out for over six months without a break?"

Rioz said, "That's different."

"Because you're Martians? Because you're professional Scavengers?"

"No. Because we're not on a flight. We can put back for Mars any time we want to."

"But you *don't* want to. That's my point. Earthmen have tremendous ships with libraries of films, with a crew of fifteen plus passengers. Still, they can only stay out six months maximum. Martian Scavengers have a two-room ship with only one partner. But we can stick it out more than six months."

Dora said, "I suppose you want to stay in a ship for a year and go to Saturn."

"Why not, Dora?" said Long. "We can do it. Don't you see we can? Earthmen can't. They've got a real world. They've got open sky and fresh food, all the air and water they want. Getting into a ship is a terrible change for them. More than six months is too much for them for that very reason. Martians are different. We've been living on a ship our entire lives.

"That's all Mars is—a ship. It's just a big ship forty-five hundred miles across with one tiny room in it occupied by fifty thousand people. It's closed in like a ship. We breathe packaged air and drink packaged water, which we repurify over and over. We eat the same food rations we eat aboard ship. When we get into a ship; it's the same thing we've known all our lives. We can stand it for a lot more than a year if we have to."

Dora said, "Dick, too?"

"We all can."

"Well, Dick can't. It's all very well for you, Ted Long, and this shell stealer here, this Mario, to talk about jaunting off for a year. You're not married. Dick is. He has a wife and he has a child and that's enough for him. He can just get a regular job right here on Mars. Why, my goodness, suppose you go to Saturn and find there's

no water there. How'll you get back? Even if you had water left, you'd be out of food. It's the most ridiculous thing I ever heard of."

"No. Now listen," said Long tightly. "I've thought this thing out. I've talked to Commissioner Sankov and he'll help. But we've got to have ships and men. I can't get them. The men won't listen to me. I'm green. You two are known and respected. You're veterans. If you back me, even if you don't go yourselves, if you'll just help me sell this thing to the rest, get volunteers—"

"First," said Rioz grumpily, "you'll have to do a lot more explaining. Once we get to Saturn, where's the water?"

"That's the beauty of it," said Long. "That's why it's got to be Saturn. The water there is just floating around in space for the taking."

5

When Hamish Sankov had come to Mars, there was no such thing as a native Martian. Now there were two-hundred-odd babies whose grandfathers had been born on Mars—native in the third generation.

When he had come as a boy in his teens, Mars had been scarcely more than a huddle of grounded space ships connected by sealed underground tunnels. Through the years, he had seen buildings grow and burrow widely, thrusting blunt snouts up into the thin, unbreathable atmosphere. He had seen huge storage depots spring up into which spaceships and their loads could be swallowed whole. He had seen the mines grow from nothing to a huge gouge in the Martian crust, while the population of Mars grew from fifty to fifty thousand.

It made him feel old, these long memories—they and the even dimmer memories induced by the presence of this Earthman before him. His visitor brought up those long-forgotten scraps of thought about a soft-warm world that was as kind and gentle to mankind as the mother's womb.

The Earthman seemed fresh from that womb. Not very tall, not very lean; in fact, distinctly plump. Dark hair with a neat little wave in it, a neat little mustache, and neatly scrubbed skin. His

clothing was right in style and as fresh and neatly turned as plastek could be.

Sankov's own clothes were of Martian manufacture, serviceable and clean, but many years behind the times. His face was craggy and lined, his hair was pure white, and his Adam's apple wobbled when he talked.

The Earthman was Myron Digby, member of Earth's General Assembly. Sankov was Martian Commissioner.

Sankov said, "This all hits us hard, Assemblyman."

"It's hit most of us hard, too, Commissioner."

"Uh-huh. Can't honestly say then that I can make it out. Of course, you understand, I don't make out that I can understand Earth ways, for all that I was born there. Mars is a hard place to live, Assemblyman, and you have to understand that. It takes a lot of shipping space just to bring us food, water, and raw materials so we can live. There's not much room left for books and news films. Even video programs can't reach Mars, except for about a month when Earth is in conjunction, and even then nobody has much time to listen.

"My office gets a weekly summary film from Planetary Press. Generally, I don't have time to pay attention to it. Maybe you'd call us provincial, and you'd be right. When something like this happens, all we can do is kind of helplessly look at each other."

Digby said slowly, "You can't mean that your people on Mars haven't heard of Hilder's anti-Waster campaign."

"No, can't exactly say that. There's a young Scavenger, son of a good friend of mine who died in space—" Sankov scratched the side of his neck doubtfully—"who makes a hobby out of reading up on Earth history and things like that. He catches video broadcasts when he's out in space and he listened to this man Hilder. Near as I can make out, that was the first talk Hilder made about Wasters.

"The young fellow come to me with that. Naturally, I didn't take him very serious. I kept an eye on the Planetary Press films for a while after that, but there wasn't much mention of Hilder and what there was made him out to look pretty funny."

"Yes, Commissioner," said Digby, "it all seemed quite a joke when it started."

Sankov stretched out a pair of long legs to one side of his desk and crossed them at the ankles. "Seems to me it's still pretty much of a joke. What's his argument? We're using up water. Has he tried looking at some figures? I got them all here. Had them brought to me when this committee arrived.

"Seems that Earth has four hundred million cubic miles of water in its oceans and each cubic mile weighs four and a half billion tons. That's a lot of water. Now we use some of that heap in space flight. Most of the thrust is inside Earth's gravitational field, and that means the water thrown out finds its way back to the oceans. Hilder doesn't figure that in. When he says a million tons of water is used up per flight, he's a liar. It's less than a hundred thousand tons.

"Suppose, now, we have fifty thousand flights a year. We don't, of course; not even fifteen hundred. But let's say there are fifty thousand. I figure there's going to be considerable expansion as time goes on. With fifty thousand flights, one cubic mile of water would be lost to space each year. That means that in a million years, Earth would *lose one quarter of one per cent* of its total water supply!"

Digby spread his hands, palms upward, and let them drop. "Commissioner, Interplanetary Alloys has used figures like that in their campaign against Hilder, but you can't fight a tremendous, emotion-filled drive with cold mathematics. This man Hilder has invented a name, 'Wasters.' Slowly he has built this name up into a gigantic conspiracy; a gang of brutal, profit-seeking wretches raping Earth for their own immediate benefit.

"He has accused the government of being riddled with them, the Assembly of being dominated by them, the press of being owned by them. None of this, unfortunately, seems ridiculous to the average man. He knows all too well what selfish men can do to Earth's resources. He knows what happened to Earth's oil during the Time of Troubles, for instance, and the way topsoil was ruined.

"When a farmer experiences a drought, he doesn't care that the amount of water lost in space flight isn't a droplet in a fog as far as Earth's overall water supply is concerned. Hilder has given him something to blame and that's the strongest possible consolation for disaster. He isn't going to give that up for a diet of figures."

Sankov said, "That's where I get puzzled. Maybe it's because I

don't know how things work on Earth, but it seems to me that there aren't just droughty farmers there. As near as I could make out from the news summaries, these Hilder people are a minority. Why is it Earth goes along with a few farmers and some crackpots that egg them on?"

"Because, Commissioner, there are such things as worried human beings. The steel industry sees that an era of space flight will stress increasingly the light, nonferrous alloys. The various miners' unions worry about extraterrestrial competition. Any Earthman who can't get aluminum to build a prefab is certain that it is because the aluminum is going to Mars. I know a professor of archaeology who's an anti-Waster because he can't get a government grant to cover his excavations. He's convinced that all government money is going into rocketry research and space medicine, and he resents it."

Sankov said, "That doesn't sound like Earth people are much different from us here on Mars. But what about the General Assembly? Why do they have to go along with Hilder?"

Digby smiled sourly. "Politics isn't pleasant to explain. Hilder introduced this bill to set up a committee to investigate waste in space flight. Maybe three-fourths or more of the General Assembly was against such an investigation as an intolerable and useless extension of bureaucracy—which it is. But then how could any legislator be against a mere investigation of waste? It would sound as though he had something to fear or to conceal. It would sound as though he were himself profiting from waste. Hilder is not in the least afraid of making such accusations, and whether true or not, they would be a powerful factor with the voters in the next election. The bill passed.

"And then there came the question of appointing the members of the committee. Those who were against Hilder shied away from membership, which would have meant decisions that would be continually embarrassing. Remaining on the sidelines would make one that much less a target for Hilder. The result is that I am the only member of the committee who is outspokenly anti-Hilder and it may cost me reelection."

Sankov said, "I'd be sorry to hear that, Assemblyman. It looks as though Mars didn't have as many friends as we thought we had.

We wouldn't like to lose one. But if Hilder wins out—what's he after, anyway?"

"I should think," said Digby, "that that is obvious. He wants to be the next Global Coordinator."

"Think he'll make it?"

"If nothing happens to stop him, he will."

"And then what? Will he drop this Waster campaign then?"

"I can't say. I don't know if he's laid his plans past the Coordinacy. Still, if you want my guess, he couldn't abandon the campaign and maintain his popularity. It's gotten out of hand."

Sankov scratched the side of his neck. "All right. In that case, I'll ask you for some advice. What can we folks on Mars do? You know Earth. You know the situation. We don't. Tell us what to do."

Digby rose and stepped to the window. He looked out upon the low domes of other buildings; red, rocky, completely desolate plain in between; a purple sky and a shrunken sun.

He said without turning, "Do you people really like it on Mars?"

Sankov smiled. "Most of us don't exactly know any other world, Assemblyman. Seems to me Earth would be something queer and uncomfortable to them."

"But wouldn't Martians get used to it? Earth isn't hard to take after this. Wouldn't your people learn to enjoy the privilege of breathing air under an open sky? You once lived on Earth. You remember what it was like."

"I sort of remember. Still, it doesn't seem to be easy to explain. Earth is just there. It fits people and people fit it. People take Earth the way they find it. Mars is different. It's sort of raw and doesn't fit people. People got to make something out of it. They got to build a world, and not take what they find. Mars isn't much yet, but we're building, and when we're finished, we're going to have just what we like. It's sort of a great feeling to know you're building a world. Earth would be kind of unexciting after that."

The Assemblyman said, "Surely the ordinary Martian isn't such a philosopher that he's content to live this terribly hard life for the sake of a future that must be hundreds of generations away."

"No-o, not just like that." Sankov put his right ankle on his left knee and cradled it as he spoke. "Like I said, Martians are a lot like Earthmen, which means they're sort of human beings, and

human beings don't go in for philosophy much. Just the same, there's something to living in a growing world, whether you think about it much or not.

"My father used to send me letters when I first came to Mars. He was an accountant and he just sort of stayed an accountant. Earth wasn't much different when he died from what it was when he was born. He didn't see anything happen. Everyday was like every other day, and living was just a way of passing time until he died.

"On Mars, it's different. Every day there's something new—the city's bigger, the ventilation system gets another kick, the water lines from the poles get slicked up. Right now, we're planning to set up a news-film association of our own. We're going to call it Mars Press. If you haven't lived when things are growing all about you, you'll never understand how wonderful it feels.

"No, Assemblyman, Mars is hard and tough and Earth is a lot more comfortable, but seems to me if you take our boys to Earth, they'll be unhappy. They probably wouldn't be able to figure out why, most of them, but they'd feel lost; lost and useless. Seems to me lots of them would never make the adjustment."

Digby turned away from the window and the smooth, pink skin of his forehead was creased into a frown. "In that case, Commissioner, I am sorry for you. For all of you."

"Why?"

"Because I don't think there's anything your people on Mars can do. Or the people on the Moon or Venus. It won't happen now; maybe it won't happen for a year or two, or even five years. But pretty soon you'll all have to come back to Earth, unless—"

Sankov's white eyebrows bent low over his eyes. "Well?"

"Unless you can find another source of water besides the planet Earth."

Sankov shook his head. "Don't seem likely, does it?"

"Not very."

"And except for that, seems to you there's no chance?"

"None at all."

Digby said that and left, and Sankov stared for a long time at nothing before he punched a combination of the local communi-line.

After a while, Ted Long looked out at him.

Sankov said, "You were right, son. There's nothing they can do. Even the ones that mean well see no way out. How did you know?"

"Commissioner," said Long, "when you've read all you can about the Time of Troubles, particularly about the twentieth century, nothing political can come as a real surprise."

"Well, maybe. Anyway, son, Assemblyman Digby is sorry for us, quite a piece sorry, you might say, but that's all. He says we'll have to leave Mars—or else get water somewhere else. Only he thinks that we can't get water somewhere else."

"You know we can, don't you, Commissioner?"

"I know we *might*, son. It's a terrible risk."

"If I find enough volunteers, the risk is our business."

"How is it going?"

"Not bad. Some of the boys are on my side right now. I talked Mario Rioz into it, for instance, and you know he's one of the best."

"That's just it—the volunteers will be the best men we have. I hate to allow it."

"If we get back, it will be worth it."

"If! It's a big word, son."

"And a big thing we're trying to do."

"Well, I gave my word that if there was no help on Earth, I'll see that the Phobos water hole lets you have all the water you'll need. Good luck."

6

Half a million miles above Saturn, Mario Rioz was cradled on nothing and sleep was delicious. He came out of it slowly and for a while, alone in his suit, he counted the stars and traced lines from one to another.

At first, as the weeks flew past, it was scavenging all over again, except for the gnawing feeling that every minute meant an additional number of thousands of miles away from all humanity. That made it worse.

They had aimed high to pass out of the ecliptic while moving through the Asteroid Belt. That had used up water and had prob-

ably been unnecessary. Although tens of thousands of worldlets look as thick as vermin in two-dimensional projection upon a photographic plate, they are nevertheless scattered so thinly through the quadrillions of cubic miles that make up their conglomerate orbit that only the most ridiculous of coincidences would have brought about a collision.

Still, they passed over the Belt and someone calculated the chances of collision with a fragment of matter large enough to do damage. The value was so low, so impossibly low, that it was perhaps inevitable that the notion of the "space-float" should occur to someone.

The days were long and many, space was empty, only one man was needed at the controls at any one time. The thought was a natural.

First, it was a particularly daring one who ventured out for fifteen minutes or so. Then another who tried half an hour. Eventually, before the asteroids were entirely behind, each ship regularly had its off-watch member suspended in space at the end of a cable.

It was easy enough. The cable, one of those intended for operations at the conclusion of their journey, was magnetically attached at both ends, one to the space suit to start with. Then you clambered out the lock onto the ship's hull and attached the other end there. You paused awhile, clinging to the metal skin by the electromagnets in your boots. Then you neutralized those and made the slightest muscular effort.

Slowly, ever so slowly, you lifted from the ship and even more slowly the ship's larger mass moved an equivalently shorter distance downward. You floated incredibly, weightlessly, in solid, speckled black. When the ship had moved far enough away from you, your gauntleted hand, which kept touch upon the cable, tightened its grip slightly. Too tightly, and you would begin moving back toward the ship and it toward you. Just tightly enough, and friction would halt you. Because your motion was equivalent to that of the ship, it seemed as motionless below you as though it had been painted against an impossible background while the cable between you hung in coils that had no reason to straighten out.

It was a half ship to your eye. One half was lit by the light of the feeble Sun, which was still too bright to look at directly without

the heavy protection of the polarized space-suit visor. The other half was black on black, invisible.

Space closed in and it was like sleep. Your suit was warm, it renewed its air automatically, it had food and drink in special containers from which it could be sucked with a minimal motion of the head, it took care of wastes appropriately. Most of all, more than anything else, there was the delightful euphoria of weightlessness.

You never felt so well in your life. The days stopped being too long, they weren't long enough, and there weren't enough of them.

They had passed Jupiter's orbit at a spot some thirty degrees from its then position. For months, it was the brightest object in the sky, always excepting the glowing white pea that was the Sun. At its brightest, some of the Scavengers insisted they could make out Jupiter as a tiny sphere, one side squashed out of true by the night shadow.

Then over a period of additional months it faded, while another dot of light grew until it was brighter than Jupiter. It was Saturn, first as a dot of brilliance, then as an oval, glowing splotch.

("Why oval?" someone asked, and after a while, someone else said, "The rings, of course," and it was obvious.)

Everyone space-floated at all possible times toward the end, watching Saturn incessantly.

("Hey, you jerk, come on back in, damn it. You're on duty." "Who's on duty? I've got fifteen minutes more by my watch." "You set your watch back. Besides, I gave you twenty minutes yesterday." "You wouldn't give two minutes to your grandmother." "Come on in, damn it, or I'm coming out anyway." "All right, I'm coming. Holy howlers, what a racket over a lousy minute." But no quarrel could possibly be serious, not in space. It felt too good.)

Saturn grew until at last it rivaled and then surpassed the Sun. The rings, set at a broad angle to their trajectory of approach, swept grandly about the planet, only a small portion being eclipsed. Then, as they approached, the span of the rings grew still wider, yet narrower as the angle of approach constantly decreased.

The larger moons showed up in the surrounding sky like serene fireflies.

Mario Rioz was glad he was awake so that he could watch again.

Saturn filled half the sky, streaked with orange, the night shadow cutting it fuzzily nearly one quarter of the way in from the right. Two round little dots in the brightness were shadows of two of the moons. To the left and behind him (he could look over his left shoulder to see, and as he did so, the rest of his body inched slightly to the right to conserve angular momentum) was the white diamond of the Sun.

Most of all he liked to watch the rings. At the left, they emerged from behind Saturn, a tight, bright triple band of orange light. At the right, their beginnings were hidden in the night shadow, but showed up closer and broader. They widened as they came, like the flare of a horn, growing hazier as they approached, until, while the eye followed them, they seemed to fill the sky and lose themselves.

From the position of the Scavenger fleet just inside the outer rim of the outermost ring, the rings broke up and assumed their true identity as a phenomenal cluster of solid fragments rather than the tight, solid band of light they seemed.

Below him, or rather in the direction his feet pointed, some twenty miles away, was one of the ring fragments. It looked like a large, irregular splotch, marring the symmetry of space, three quarters in brightness and the night shadow cutting it like a knife. Other fragments were farther off, sparkling like star dust, dimmer and thicker, until, as you followed them down, they became rings once more.

The fragments were motionless, but that was only because the ships had taken up an orbit about Saturn equivalent to that of the outer edge of the rings.

The day before, Rioz reflected, he had been on that nearest fragment, working along with more than a score of others to mold it into the desired shape. Tomorrow he would be at it again.

Today—today he was space-floating.

"Mario?" The voice that broke upon his earphones was questioning.

Momentarily Rioz was flooded with annoyance. Damn it, he wasn't in the mood for company.

"Speaking," he said.

"I thought I had your ship spotted. How are you?"

"Fine. That you, Ted?"

"That's right," said Long.

"Anything wrong on the fragment?"

"Nothing. I'm out here floating."

"You?"

"It gets me, too, occasionally. Beautiful, isn't it?"

"Nice," agreed Rioz.

"You know, I've read Earth books—"

"Grounder books, you mean." Rioz yawned and found it difficult under the circumstances to use the expression with the proper amount of resentment.

"—and sometimes I read descriptions of people lying on grass," continued Long. "You know that green stuff like thin, long pieces of paper they have all over the ground down there, and they look up at the blue sky with clouds in it. Did you ever see any films of that?"

"Sure. It didn't attract me. It looked cold."

"I suppose it isn't, though. After all, Earth is quite close to the Sun, and they say their atmosphere is thick enough to hold the heat. I must admit that personally I would hate to be caught under open sky with nothing on but clothes. Still, I imagine they like it."

"Grounders are nuts!"

"They talk about the trees, big brown stalks, and the winds, air movements, you know."

"You mean drafts. They can keep that, too."

"It doesn't matter. The point is they describe it beautifully, almost passionately. Many times I've wondered, 'What's it really like? Will I ever feel it or is this something only Earthmen can possibly feel?' I've felt so often that I was missing something vital. Now I know what it must be like. It's this. Complete peace in the middle of a beauty-drenched universe."

Rioz said, "They wouldn't like it. The Grounders, I mean. They're so used to their own lousy little world they wouldn't appreciate what it's like to float and look down on Saturn." He flipped his body slightly and began swaying back and forth about his center of mass, slowly, soothingly.

Long said, "Yes, I think so too. They're slaves to their planet. Even if they come to Mars, it will only be their children that are free. There'll be starships someday; great, huge things that can carry thousands of people and maintain their self-contained equilibrium for decades, maybe centuries. Mankind will spread through the whole Galaxy. But people will have to live their lives out on shipboard until new methods of interstellar travel are developed, so it will be Martians, not planet-bound Earthmen, who will colonize the Universe. That's inevitable. It's got to be. It's the Martian way."

But Rioz made no answer. He had dropped off to sleep again, rocking and swaying gently, half a million miles above Saturn.

7

The work shift of the ring fragment was the tail of the coin. The weightlessness, peace, and privacy of the space-float gave place to something that had neither peace nor privacy. Even the weightlessness, which continued, became more a purgatory than a paradise under the new conditions.

Try to manipulate an ordinarily nonportable heat projector. It could be lifted despite the fact that it was six feet high and wide and almost solid metal, since it weighed only a fraction of an ounce. But its inertia was exactly what it had always been, which meant that if it wasn't moved into position very slowly, it would just keep on going, taking you with it. Then you would have to hike the pseudo-grav field of your suit and come down with a jar.

Keralski had hiked the field a little too high and he came down a little too roughly, with the projector coming down with him at a dangerous angle. His crushed ankle had been the first casualty of the expedition.

Rioz was swearing fluently and nearly continuously. He continued to have the impulse to drag the back of his hand across his forehead in order to wipe away the accumulating sweat. The few times that he had succumbed to the impulse, metal had met silicone with a clash that rang loudly inside his suit, but served no useful purpose. The desiccators within the suit were sucking at maximum and, of course, recovering the water and restoring ion-exchanged

liquid, containing a careful proportion of salt, into the appropriate receptacle.

Rioz yelled, "Damn it, Dick, wait till I give the word, will you?"

And Swenson's voice rang in his ears, "Well, how long am I supposed to sit here?"

"Till I say," replied Rioz.

He strengthened pseudo-grav and lifted the projector a bit. He released pseudo-grav, ensuring that the projector would stay in place for minutes even if he withdrew support altogether. He kicked the cable out of the way (it stretched beyond the close "horizon" to a power source that was out of sight) and touched the release.

The material of which the fragment was composed bubbled and vanished under its touch. A section of the lip of the tremendous cavity he had already carved into its substance melted away and a roughness in its contour had disappeared.

"Try it now," called Rioz.

Swenson was in the ship that was hovering nearly over Rioz's head.

Swenson called, "All clear?"

"I told you to go ahead."

It was a feeble flicker of steam that issued from one of the ship's forward vents. The ship drifted down toward the ring fragment. Another flicker adjusted a tendency to drift sidewise. It came down straight.

A third flicker to the rear slowed it to a feather rate.

Rioz watched tensely. "Keep her coming. You'll make it. You'll make it."

The rear of the ship entered the hole, nearly filling it. The bellying walls came closer and closer to its rim. There was a grinding vibration as the ship's motion halted.

It was Swenson's turn to curse. "It doesn't fit," he said.

Rioz threw the projector groundward in a passion and went flailing up into space. The projector kicked up a white crystalline dust all about it, and when Rioz came down under pseudo-grav, he did the same.

He said, "You went in on the bias, you dumb Grounder."

"I hit it level, you dirt-eating farmer."

Backward-pointing side jets of the ship were blasting more

strongly than before, and Rioz hopped to get out of the way.

The ship scraped up from the pit, then shot into space half a mile before forward jets could bring it to a halt.

Swenson said tensely, "We'll spring half a dozen plates if we do this once again. Get it right, will you?"

"I'll get it right. Don't worry about it. Just you come in right."

Rioz jumped upward and allowed himself to climb three hundred yards to get an overall look at the cavity. The gouge marks of the ship were plain enough. They were concentrated at one point halfway down the pit. He would get that.

It began to melt outward under the blaze of the projector.

Half an hour later the ship snuggled neatly into its cavity, and Swenson, wearing his space suit, emerged to join Rioz.

Swenson said, "If you want to step in and climb out of the suit I'll take care of the icing."

"It's all right," said Rioz. "I'd just as soon sit here and watch Saturn."

He sat down at the lip of the pit. There was a six-foot gap between it and the ship. In some places about the circle, it was two feet; in a few places, even merely a matter of inches. You couldn't expect a better fit out of handwork. The final adjustment would be made by steaming ice gently and letting it freeze into the cavity between the lip and the ship.

Saturn moved visibly across the sky, its vast bulk inching below the horizon.

Rioz said, "How many ships are left to put in place?"

Swenson said, "Last I heard, it was eleven. We're in now, so that means only ten. Seven of the ones that are placed are iced in. Two or three are dismantled."

"We're coming along fine."

"There's plenty to do yet. Don't forget the main jets at the other end. And the cables and the power lines. Sometimes I wonder if we'll make it. On the way out, it didn't bother me so much, but just now I was sitting at the controls and I was saying, 'We won't make it. We'll sit out here and starve and die with nothing but Saturn over us.' It makes me feel—"

He didn't explain how it made him feel. He just sat there.

Rioz said, "You think too damn much."

"It's different with you," said Swenson. "I keep thinking of Pete—and Dora."

"What for? She said you could go, didn't she? The Commissioner gave her that talk on patriotism and how you'd be a hero and set for life once you got back, and she said you could go. You didn't sneak out the way Adams did."

"Adams is different. That wife of his should have been shot when she was born. Some women can make hell for a guy, can't they? She didn't want him to go—but she'd probably rather he didn't come back if she can get his settlement pay."

"What's your kick, then? Dora wants you back, doesn't she?"

Swenson sighed. "I never treated her right."

"You turned over your pay, it seems to me. I wouldn't do that for any woman. Money for value received, not a cent more."

"Money isn't it. I get to thinking out here. A woman likes company. A kid needs his father. What am I doing 'way out here?"

"Getting set to go home."

"Ah-h, you don't understand."

8

Ted Long wandered over the ridged surface of the ring fragment with his spirits as icy as the ground he walked on. It had all seemed perfectly logical back on Mars, but that was Mars. He had worked it out carefully in his mind in perfectly reasonable steps. He could still remember exactly how it went.

It didn't take a ton of water to move a ton of ship. It was not mass equals mass, but mass times velocity equals mass times velocity. It didn't matter, in other words, whether you shot out a ton of water at a mile a second or a hundred pounds of water at twenty miles a second. You got the same final velocity out of the ship.

That meant the jet nozzles had to be made narrower and the steam hotter. But then drawbacks appeared. The narrower the nozzle, the more energy was lost in friction and turbulence. The hotter the steam, the more refractory the nozzle had to be and the shorter its life. The limit in that direction was quickly reached.

Then, since a given weight of water could move considerably

more than its own weight under the narrow-nozzle conditions, it paid to be big. The bigger the water-storage space, the larger the size of the actual travel-head, even in proportion. So they started to make liners heavier and bigger. But then the larger the shell, the heavier the bracings, the more difficult the weldings, the more exacting the engineering requirements. At the moment, the limit in that direction had been reached also.

And then he had put his finger on what had seemed to him to be the basic flaw—the original unswervable conception that the fuel had to be placed *inside* the ship; the metal had to be built to encircle a million tons of water.

Why? Water did not have to be water. It could be ice, and ice could be shaped. Holes could be melted into it. Travel-heads and jets could be fitted into it. Cables could hold travel-heads and jets stiffly together under the influence of magnetic field-force grips.

Long felt the trembling of the ground he walked on. He was at the head of the fragment. A dozen ships were blasting in and out of sheaths carved in its substance, and the fragment shuddered under the continuing impact.

The ice didn't have to be quarried. It existed in proper chunks in the rings of Saturn. That's all the rings were—pieces of nearly pure ice, circling Saturn. So spectroscopy stated and so it had turned out to be. He was standing on one such piece now, over two miles long, nearly one mile thick. It was almost half a billion tons of water, all in one piece, and he was standing on it.

But now he was face to face with the realities of life. He had never told the men just how quickly he had expected to set up the fragment as a ship, but in his heart, he had imagined it would be two days. It was a week now and he didn't dare to estimate the remaining time. He no longer even had any confidence that the task was a possible one. Would they be able to control jets with enough delicacy through leads slung across two miles of ice to manipulate out of Saturn's dragging gravity?

Drinking water was low, though they could always distill more out of the ice. Still, the food stores were not in a good way either.

He paused, looked up into the sky, eyes straining. *Was* the

object growing larger? He ought to measure its distance. Actually, he lacked the spirit to add that trouble to the others. His mind slid back to greater immediacies.

Morale, at least, was high. The men seemed to enjoy being out Saturn-way. They were the first humans to penetrate this far, the first to pass the asteroids, the first to see Jupiter like a glowing pebble to the naked eye, the first to see Saturn—like that.

He didn't think fifty practical, case-hardened, shell-snatching Scavengers would take time to feel that sort of emotion. But they did. And they were proud.

Two men and a half-buried ship slid up the moving horizon as he walked.

He called crisply, "Hello, there!"

Rioz answered, "That you, Ted?"

"You bet. Is that Dick with you?"

"Sure. Come on, sit down. We were just getting ready to ice in and we were looking for an excuse to delay."

"I'm not," said Swenson promptly. "When will we be leaving, Ted?"

"As soon as we get through. That's no answer, is it?"

Swenson said dispiritedly, "I suppose there isn't any other answer."

Long looked up, staring at the irregular bright splotch in the sky.

Rioz followed his glance. "What's the matter?"

For a moment, Long did not reply. The sky was black otherwise and the ring fragments were an orange dust against it. Saturn was more than three fourths below the horizon and the rings were going with it. Half a mile away a ship bounded past the icy rim of the planetoid into the sky, was orange-lit by Saturnlight, and sank down again.

The ground trembled gently.

Rioz said, "Something bothering you about the Shadow?"

They called it that. It was the nearest fragment of the rings, quite close considering that they were at the outer rim of the rings, where the pieces spread themselves relatively thin. It was perhaps twenty miles off, a jagged mountain, its shape clearly visible.

"How does it look to you?" asked Long.

Rioz shrugged. "Okay, I guess. I don't see anything wrong."

"Doesn't it seem to be getting larger?"

"Why should it?"

"Well, doesn't it?" Long insisted.

Rioz and Swenson stared at it thoughtfully.

"It does look bigger," said Swenson.

"You're just putting the notion into our minds," Rioz argued. "If it were getting bigger, it would be coming closer."

"What's impossible about that?"

"These things are on stable orbits."

"They were when we came here," said Long. "There, did you feel that?"

The ground had trembled again.

Long said, "We've been blasting this thing for a week now. First, twenty-five ships landed on it, which changed its momentum right there. Not much, of course. Then we've been melting parts of it away and our ships have been blasting in and out of it—all at one end, too. In a week, we may have changed its orbit just a bit. The two fragments, this one and the Shadow, might be converging."

"It's got plenty of room to miss us in." Rioz watched it thoughtfully. "Besides, if we can't even tell for sure that it's getting bigger, how quickly can it be moving? Relative to us, I mean."

"It doesn't have to be moving quickly. Its momentum is as large as ours, so that, however gently it hits, we'll be nudged completely out of our orbit, maybe in toward Saturn, where we don't want to go. As a matter of fact, ice has a very low tensile strength, so that both planetoids might break up into gravel."

Swenson rose to his feet. "Damn it, if I can tell how a shell is moving a thousand miles away, I can tell what a mountain is doing twenty miles away." He turned toward the ship.

Long didn't stop him.

Rioz said, "There's a nervous guy."

The neighboring planetoid rose to zenith, passed overhead, began sinking. Twenty minutes later, the horizon opposite that portion behind which Saturn had disappeared burst into orange flame as its bulk began lifting again.

Rioz called into his radio, "Hey, Dick, are you dead in there?"

"I'm checking," came the muffled response.

"Is it moving?" asked Long.

"Yes."

"Toward us?"

There was a pause. Swenson's voice was a sick one. "On the nose, Ted. Intersection of orbits will take place in three days."

"You're crazy!" yelled Rioz.

"I checked four times," said Swenson.

Long thought blankly, What do we do now?

9

Some of the men were having trouble with the cables. They had to be laid precisely; their geometry had to be very nearly perfect for the magnetic field to attain maximum strength. In space, or even in air, it wouldn't have mattered. The cables would have lined up automatically once the juice went on.

Here it was different. A gouge had to be plowed along the planetoid's surface and into it the cable had to be laid. If it were not lined up within a few minutes of arc of the calculated direction, a torque would be applied to the entire planetoid, with consequent loss of energy, none of which could be spared. The gouges then had to be redriven, the cables shifted and iced into the new positions.

The men plodded wearily through the routine.

And then the word reached them:

"All hands to the jets!"

Scavengers could not be said to be the type that took kindly to discipline. It was a grumbling, growling, muttering group that set about disassembling the jets of the ships that yet remained intact, carrying them to the tail end of the planetoid, grubbing them into position, and stringing the leads along the surface.

It was almost twenty-four hours before one of them looked into the sky and said, "Holy jeepers!" followed by something less printable.

His neighbor looked and said, "I'll be damned!"

Once they noticed, all did. It became the most astonishing fact in the Universe.

"Look at the Shadow!"

It was spreading across the sky like an infected wound. Men looked at it, found it had doubled its size, wondered why they hadn't noticed that sooner.

Work came to a virtual halt. They besieged Ted Long.

He said, "We can't leave. We don't have the fuel to see us back to Mars and we don't have the equipment to capture another planetoid. So we've got to stay. Now the Shadow is creeping in on us because our blasting has thrown us out of orbit. We've got to change that by continuing the blasting. Since we can't blast the front end any more without endangering the ship we're building, let's try another way."

They went back to work on the jets with a furious energy that received impetus every half hour when the Shadow rose again over the horizon, bigger and more menacing than before.

Long had no assurance that it would work. Even if the jets would respond to the distant controls, even if the supply of water, which depended upon a storage chamber opening directly into the icy body of the planetoid, with built-in heat projectors steaming the propulsive fluid directly into the driving cells, were adequate, there was still no certainty that the body of the planetoid without a magnetic cable sheathing would hold together under the enormously disruptive stresses.

"Ready!" came the signal in Long's receiver.

Long called, "Ready!" and depressed the contact.

The vibration grew about him. The star field in the visiplate trembled.

In the rearview, there was a distant gleaming spume of swiftly moving ice crystals.

"It's blowing!" was the cry.

It kept on blowing. Long dared not stop. For six hours, it blew, hissing, bubbling, steaming into space; the body of the planetoid converted to vapor and hurled away.

The Shadow came closer until men did nothing but stare at the mountain in the sky, surpassing Saturn itself in spectacularity.

It's every groove and valley was a plain scar upon its face. But when it passed through the planetoid's orbit, it crossed more than half a mile behind its then position.

The steam jet ceased.

Long bent in his seat and covered his eyes. He hadn't eaten in two days. He could eat now, though. Not another planetoid was close enough to interrupt them, even if it began an approach that very moment.

Back on the planetoid's surface, Swenson said, "All the time I watched that damned rock coming down, I kept saying to myself, 'This can't happen. We can't let it happen.' "

"Hell," said Rioz, "we were all nervous. Did you see Jim Davis? He was green. I was a little jumpy myself."

"That's not it. It wasn't just—dying, you know. I was think-ing—I know it's funny, but can't help it—I was thinking that Dora warned me I'd get myself killed, she'll never let me hear the last of it. Isn't that a crummy sort of attitude at a time like that?"

"Listen," said Rioz, "you wanted to get married, so you got married. Why come to me with your troubles?"

10

The flotilla, welded into a single unit, was returning over its mighty course from Saturn to Mars. Each day it flashed over a length of space that had taken nine days outward.

Ted Long had put the entire crew on emergency. With twenty-five ships embedded in the planetoid taken out of Saturn's rings and unable to move or maneuver independently, the coordination of their power sources into unified blasts was a ticklish problem. The jarring that took place on the first day of travel nearly shook them out from under their hair.

That, at least, smoothed itself out as the velocity raced upward under the steady thrust from behind. They passed the one-hundred-thousand-mile-an-hour mark late on the second day, and climbed steadily toward the million-mile mark and beyond.

Long's ship, which formed the needle point of the frozen fleet, was the only one which possessed a five-way view of space. It was

an uncomfortable position under the circumstances. Long found himself watching tensely, imagining somehow that the stars would slowly begin to slip backward, to whizz past them, under the influence of the multiship's tremendous rate of travel.

They didn't, of course. They remained nailed to the black backdrop, their distance scorning with patient immobility any speed mere man could achieve.

The men complained bitterly after the first few days. It was not only that they were deprived of the space-float. They were burdened by much more than the ordinary pseudo-gravity field of the ships, by the effects of the fierce acceleration under which they were living. Long himself was weary to death of the relentless pressure against hydraulic cushions.

They took to shutting off the jet thrusts one hour out of every four and Long fretted.

It had been just over a year that he had last seen Mars shrinking in an observation window from this ship, which had then been an independent entity. What had happened since then? Was the colony still there?

In something like a growing panic, Long sent out radio pulses toward Mars daily, with the combined power of twenty-five ships behind it. There was no answer. He expected none. Mars and Saturn were on opposite sides of the Sun now, and until he mounted high enough above the ecliptic to get the Sun well beyond the line connecting himself and Mars, solar interference would prevent any signal from getting through.

High above the outer rim of the Asteroid Belt, they reached maximum velocity. With short spurts of power from first one side jet, then another, the huge vessel reversed itself. The composite jet in the rear began its mighty roaring once again, but now the result was deceleration.

They passed a hundred million miles over the Sun, curving down to intersect the orbit of Mars.

A week out of Mars, answering signals were heard for the first time, fragmentary, ether-torn, and incomprehensible, but they were com-

ing from Mars. Earth and Venus were at angles sufficiently different to leave no doubt of that.

Long relaxed. There were still humans on Mars, at any rate.

Two days out of Mars, the signal was strong and clear and Sankov was at the other end.

Sankov said, "Hello, son. It's three in the morning here. Seems like people have no consideration for an old man. Dragged me right out of bed."

"I'm sorry, sir."

"Don't be. They were following orders. I'm afraid to ask, son. Anyone hurt? Maybe dead?"

"No deaths, sir. Not one."

"And—and the water? Any left?"

Long said, with an effort at nonchalance, "Enough."

"In that case, get home as fast as you can. Don't take any chances, of course."

"There's trouble, then."

"Fair to middling. When will you come down?"

"Two days. Can you hold out that long?"

"I'll hold out."

Forty hours later Mars had grown to a ruddy-orange ball that filled the ports and they were in the final planet-landing spiral.

"Slowly," Long said to himself, "slowly." Under these conditions, even the thin atmosphere of Mars could do dreadful damage if they moved through it too quickly.

Since they came in from well above the ecliptic, their spiral passed from north to south. A polar cap shot whitely below them, then the much smaller one of the summer hemisphere, the large one again, the small one, at longer and longer intervals. The planet approached closer, and the landscape began to show features.

"Prepare for landing!" called Long.

11

Sankov did his best to look placid, which was difficult considering how closely the boys had shaved their return. But it had worked out well enough.

Until a few days ago, he had no sure knowledge that they had survived. It seemed more likely—inevitable, almost—that they were nothing but frozen corpses somewhere in the trackless stretches from Mars to Saturn, new planetoids that had once been alive.

The Committee had been dickering with him for weeks before the news had come. They had insisted on his signature to the paper for the sake of appearances. It would look like an agreement, voluntarily and mutually arrived at. But Sankov knew well that, given complete obstinacy on his part, they would act unilaterally and be damned with appearances. It seemed fairly certain that Hilder's election was secure now and they would take the chance of arousing a reaction of sympathy for Mars.

So he dragged out the negotiations, dangling before them always the possibility of surrender.

And then he heard from Long and concluded the deal quickly.

The papers had lain before him and he had made a last statement for the benefit of the reporters who were present.

He said, "Total imports of water from Earth are twenty million tons a year. This is declining as we develop our own piping system. If I sign this paper agreeing to an embargo, our industry will be paralyzed, any possibilities of expansion will halt. It looks to me as if that can't be what's in Earth's mind, can it?"

Their eyes met his and held only a hard glitter. Assemblyman Digby had already been replaced and they were unanimous against him.

The Committee Chairman impatiently pointed out, "You have said all this before."

"I know, but right now I'm kind of getting ready to sign and I want it clear in my head. Is Earth set and determined to bring us to an end here?"

"Of course not. Earth is interested in conserving its irreplaceable water supply, nothing else."

"You have one and a half quintillion tons of water on Earth."

The Committee Chairman said, "We cannot spare water."

And Sankov had signed.

That had been the final note he wanted. Earth had one and a half quintillion tons of water and could spare none of it.

Now, a day and a half later, the Committee and the reporters

waited in the spaceport dome. Through thick, curving windows, they could see the bare and empty grounds of Mars Spaceport.

The Committee Chairman asked with annoyance, "How much longer do we have to wait? And, if you don't mind, what are we waiting for?"

Sankov said, "Some of our boys have been out in space, out past the asteroids."

The Committee Chairman removed a pair of spectacles and cleaned them with a snowy-white handkerchief. "And they're returning?"

"They are."

The Chairman shrugged, lifted his eyebrows in the direction of the reporters.

In the smaller room adjoining, a knot of women and children clustered about another window. Sankov stepped back a bit to cast a glance toward them. He would much rather have been with them, been part of their excitement and tension. He, like them, had waited over a year now. He, like them, had thought, over and over again, that the men must be dead.

"You see that?" said Sankov, pointing.

"Hey!" cried a reporter. "It's a ship!"

A confused shouting came from the adjoining room.

It wasn't a ship so much as a bright dot obscured by a drifting white cloud. The cloud grew larger and began to have form. It was a double streak against the sky, the lower ends billowing out and upward again. As it dropped still closer, the bright dot at the upper end took on a crudely cylindrical form.

It was rough and craggy, but where the sunlight hit, brilliant high lights bounced back.

The cylinder dropped toward the ground with the ponderous slowness characteristic of space vessels. It hung suspended on those blasting jets and settled down upon the recoil of tons of matter hurling downward like a tired man dropping into his easy chair.

And as it did so, a silence fell upon all within the dome. The women and children in one room, the politicians and reporters in the other remained frozen, heads craned incredulously upward.

The cylinder's landing flanges, extending far below the two rear

jets, touched ground and sank into the pebbly morass. And then the ship was motionless and the jet action ceased.

But the silence continued in the dome. It continued for a long time.

Men came clambering down the sides of the immense vessel, inching down, down the two-mile trek to the ground, with spikes on their shoes and ice axes in their hands. They were gnats against the blinding surface.

One of the reporters croaked, "What is it?"

"That," said Sankov calmly, "happens to be a chunk of matter that spent its time scooting around Saturn as part of its rings. Our boys fitted it out with travel-head and jets and ferried it home. It just turns out the fragments in Saturn's rings are made up out of ice."

He spoke into a continuing deathlike silence. "That thing that looks like a spaceship is just a mountain of hard water. If it were standing like that on Earth, it would be melting into a puddle and maybe it would break under its own weight. Mars is colder and has less gravity, so there's no such danger.

"Of course, once we get this thing really organized, we can have water stations on the moons of Saturn and Jupiter and on the asteroids. We can scale in chunks of Saturn's rings and pick them up and send them on at the various stations. Our Scavengers are good at that sort of thing.

"We'll have all the water we need. That one chunk you see is just under a cubic mile—or about what Earth would send us in two hundred years. The boys used quite a bit of it coming back from Saturn. They made it in five weeks, they tell me, and used up about a hundred million tons. But, Lord, that didn't make any dent at all in that mountain. Are you getting all this, boys?"

He turned to the reporters. There was no doubt they were getting it.

He said, "Then get this, too. Earth is worried about its water supply. It only has one and a half quintillion tons. It can't spare us a single ton out of it. Write down that we folks on Mars are worried about Earth and don't want anything to happen to Earth people. Write down that we'll sell water to Earth. Write down that we'll

let them have million-ton lots for a reasonable fee. Write down that in ten years, we figure we can sell it in cubic-mile lots. Write down that Earth can quit worrying because Mars can sell it all the water it needs and wants."

The Committee Chairman was past hearing. He was feeling the future rushing in. Dimly he could see the reporters grinning as they wrote furiously.

Grinning.

He could hear the grin become laughter on Earth as Mars turned the tables so neatly on the anti-Wasters. He could hear the laughter thunder from every continent when word of the fiasco spread. And he could see the abyss, deep and black as space, into which would drop forever the political hopes of John Hilder and of every opponent of space flight left on Earth—his own included, of course.

In the adjoining room, Dora Swenson screamed with joy, and Peter, grown two inches, jumped up and down, calling, "Daddy! Daddy!"

Richard Swenson had just stepped off the extremity of the flange and, face showing clearly through the clear silicone of the headpiece, marched toward the dome.

"Did you ever see a guy look so happy?" asked Ted Long. "Maybe there's something in this marriage business."

"Ah, you've just been out in space too long," Rioz said.

ALFRED BESTER

1913–1987

In 1939 the magazine *Thrilling Wonder Stories* was running a contest for new writers. Alfred Bester, then in his early twenties, had just written his first short science fiction story, "The Broken Arrow." He entered it in the contest, won handily, and saw it published in the April 1939 issue of the magazine. (Interestingly, this was the same contest that another Grand Master, Robert A. Heinlein, decided at the last minute *not* to enter with his own first story, "Lifeline." It's worth a little musing to speculate on which would have won if the two stories had been in competition . . . and what would have been the effect on both writers' later careers.)

Over the next three years Bester published a dozen or so additional stories, competent journeyman science fiction for the time but of no marked distinction. They weren't particularly profitable, either. At the prevailing rates (seldom much more than a penny a word, often less), Bester's total income from three years of writing science fiction was somewhere over, but not much over, one thousand dollars. It was not a figure that impressed Bester, so around 1942 he moved his efforts to the better-paying field of writing comics, then to writing radio plays, finally to a post as a contributing editor on the travel magazine, *Holiday*.

Bester's then wife, Rollie, was a radio actress, and a good one. While I was working on Madison Avenue, not long after World War II, I used to run into them from time to time in the restaurant in the old CBS building. Alfie was always interested in the latest shoptalk about science fiction, but had, he said, no intention of ever coming back to it as a writer—well, maybe an occasional short

story now and then, just for the fun of it, but nothing *serious*.

It was Horace Gold who changed Bester's mind for him. When Gold became editor of the new science fiction magazine, *Galaxy*, in 1950, Alfie Bester was one of the first writers Horace got after to write for him. Horace Gold was a powerfully persuasive man. Alfie didn't have a chance. It took a couple of years, but it was for Horace Gold's magazine that Alfred J. Bester made his reappearance as a major science fiction writer with such powerful serials as *The Demolished Man* (notable for its semicomic view of telepathic reality as well as some fascinatingly innovative typographical tricks) and *The Stars My Destination* (*The Count of Monte Cristo* retold and set in the twenty-fifth century, as Bester himself described it, but even better than the original), as well as a flood of fine shorter pieces.

Although *Galaxy* had a lock on Bester's major works, his short stories were appearing all over the field. Many came out in *The Magazine of Fantasy and Science Fiction*, and the one called "Disappearing Act" wound up in an anthology of original stories I was editing at the time, *Star Science Fiction*. Let me give you an idea of how those stories were received by Bester's writing peers. My frequent collaborator, Cyril M. Kornbluth, was staying with me, grimly slugging his way through a commissioned story he didn't much like, when I accepted "Disappearing Act." I was so taken with Bester's story that I gave Cyril the manuscript to read. When he had finished it, he flung it down angrily, saying, "What's the matter with you, Fred? You show me this story *now*? How am I supposed to go back to writing space opera?"

The last time I saw Alfie was in Dublin, Ireland. We were both in town for an international meeting of science fiction writers. With a little free time before the meeting began, I had gone for a walk along the Liffey River; I saw Alfie walking down the street and called to him. He cut me dead. Later that night, at the con, I asked him what I had done to offend him. "Not a damn thing," he said sadly. "Fact is, I'm pretty near blind. People don't have faces for me until they're within two feet; I just didn't see you."

Blind or not, Alfie was in good form at the con, and good form still when he and I, with our spouses, then flew to Newcastle-on-

Tyne to give readings at a literary festival. Our plan was for all of us to rent a car and explore northern England together as soon as the festivities were over, but that didn't happen. The morning after our readings Alfie was too ill to get out of bed, much less to go for long touristy drives. So, regretfully, my wife and I took off for Hadrian's Wall and the Scottish border without him.

We never met again. A few years later, when Alfie was up for his Grand Master Award, his health had become so bad that it seemed unlikely that he would live long enough to accept it, as was the custom, at that year's SFWA awards banquet. For the only time in history, it was arranged to present his award to him several months early, at the annual science fiction world convention.

That didn't work out, either. Alfie's health deteriorated rapidly. He died even before the worldcon, which is why he is the only writer ever to have received the Grand Master Award posthumously.

Recommended Reading
by Alfred Bester

The Demolished Man
The Stars My Destination
$Golem_{100}$
Starburst
Starlight: The Great Short Fiction of Alfred Bester

DISAPPEARING ACT

This one wasn't the last war or a war to end war. They called it the War for the American Dream. General Carpenter struck that note and sounded it constantly.

There are fighting generals (vital to an army), political generals (vital to an administration), and public relations generals (vital to a war). General Carpenter was a master of public relations. Forthright and Four-Square, he had ideals as high and as understandable as the mottoes on money. In the mind of America he *was* the army, the administration, the nation's shield and sword and stout right arm. His ideal was the American dream.

"We are not fighting for money, for power, or for world domination," General Carpenter announced at the Press Association dinner.

"We are fighting solely for the American dream," he said to the 162nd Congress.

"Our aim is not aggression or the reduction of nations to slavery," he said at the West Point Annual Officer's Dinner.

"We are fighting for the Meaning of Civilization," he told the San Francisco Pioneers' Club.

"We are struggling for the Ideal of Civilization; for Culture, for Poetry, for the Only Things Worth Preserving," he said at the Chicago Wheat Pit Festival.

"This is a war for survival," he said. "We are not fighting for ourselves, but for our Dreams; for the Better Things in Life which must not disappear from the face of the earth."

America fought. General Carpenter asked for one hundred million men. The army was given one hundred million men. General Carpenter asked for ten thousand U-Bombs. Ten thousand U-Bombs were delivered and dropped. The enemy also dropped ten thousand U-Bombs and destroyed most of America's cities.

"We must dig in against the hordes of barbarism," General Carpenter said. "Give me a thousand engineers."

One thousand engineers were forthcoming and a hundred cities were dug and hollowed out beneath the rubble.

"Give me five hundred sanitation experts, eight hundred traffic managers, two hundred air-conditioning experts, one hundred city managers, one thousand communication chiefs, seven hundred personnel experts. . . ."

The list of General Carpenter's demand for technical experts was endless. America did not know how to supply them.

"We must become a nation of experts," General Carpenter informed the National Association of American Universities. "Every man and woman must be a specific tool for a specific job, hardened and sharpened by your training and education to win the fight for the American Dream."

"Our Dream," General Carpenter said at the Wall Street Bond Drive Breakfast, "is at one with the gentle Greeks of Athens, with the noble Romans of . . . er . . . Rome. It is a dream of the Better Things in Life. Of Music and Art and Poetry and Culture. Money is only a weapon to be used in the fight for this dream. Ambition is only a ladder to climb to this dream. Ability is only a tool to shape this dream."

Wall Street applauded. General Carpenter asked for one hundred and fifty billion dollars, fifteen hundred dedicated dollar-a-year men, three thousand experts in mineralogy, petrology, mass production, chemical warfare, and air-traffic time study. They were delivered. The country was in high gear. General Carpenter had only to press a button and an expert would be delivered.

In March of A.D. 2112 the war came to a climax and the Amer-

ican Dream was resolved, not on any one of the seven fronts where millions of men were locked in bitter combat, not in any of the staff headquarters or any of the capitals of the warring nations, not in any of the production centers spewing forth arms and supplies, but in Ward T of the United States Army Hospital buried three hundred feet below what had once been St. Albans, New York.

Ward T was something of a mystery at St. Albans. Like all army hospitals, St. Albans was organized with specific wards reserved for specific injuries. Right-arm amputees were gathered in one ward; left-arm amputees in another. Radiation burns, head injuries, eviscerations, secondary gamma poisonings, and so on were each assigned their specific location in the hospital organization. The Army Medical Corps had established nineteen classes of combat injury which included every possible kind of damage to brain and tissue. These used up letters A to S. What, then, was in Ward T?

No one knew. The doors were double-locked. No visitors were permitted to enter. No patients were permitted to leave. Physicians were seen to arrive and depart. Their perplexed expressions stimulated the wildest speculations but revealed nothing. The nurses who ministered to Ward T were questioned eagerly but they were closed mouthed.

There were dribs and drabs of information, unsatisfying and self-contradictory. A charwoman asserted that she had been in to clean up and there had been no one in the ward. Absolutely no one. Just two dozen beds and nothing else. Had the beds been slept in? Yes. They were rumpled, some of them. Were there signs of the ward being in use? Oh yes. Personal things on the tables and so on. But dusty, kind of. Like they hadn't been used in a long time.

Public opinion decided it was a ghost ward. For spooks only.

But a night orderly reported passing the locked ward and hearing singing from within. What kind of singing? Foreign language, like. What language? The orderly couldn't say. Some of the words sounded like . . . well, like: Cow dee on us eager tour . . .

Public opinion started to run a fever and decided it was an alien ward. For spies only.

St. Albans enlisted the help of the kitchen staff and checked

the food trays. Twenty-four trays went into Ward T three times a day. Twenty-four came out. Sometimes the returning trays were emptied. Most times they were untouched.

Public opinion started to run a fever and decided it was a racket. It was an informal club for goldbricks and staff grafters who caroused within. Cow dee on us eager tour indeed!

For gossip, a hospital can put a small town sewing circle to shame with ease, but sick people are easily goaded into passion by trivia. It took just three months for idle speculation to turn into downright fury. In January, 2112, St. Albans was a sound, well-run hospital. By March, 2112, St. Albans was in a ferment, and the psychological unrest found its way into the official records. The percentage of recoveries fell off. Malingering set in. Petty infractions increased. Mutinies flared. There was a staff shake-up. It did no good. Ward T was inciting the patients to riot. There was another shake-up, and another, and still the unrest fumed.

The news finally reached General Carpenter's desk through official channels.

"In our fight for the American Dream," he said, "we must not ignore those who have already given of themselves. Send me a Hospital Administration expert."

The expert was delivered. He could do nothing to heal St. Albans. General Carpenter read the reports and fired him.

"Pity," said General Carpenter, "is the first ingredient of civilization. Send me a Surgeon General."

A Surgeon General was delivered. He could not break the fury of St. Albans, and General Carpenter broke him. But by this time Ward T was being mentioned in the dispatches.

"Send me," General Carpenter said, "the expert in charge of Ward T."

St. Albans sent a doctor, Captain Edsel Dimmock. He was a stout young man, already bald, only three years out of medical school, but with a fine record as an expert in psychotherapy. General Carpenter liked experts. He liked Dimmock. Dimmock adored the general as the spokesman for a culture which he had been too specially trained to seek up to now, but which he hoped to enjoy after the war was won.

"Now look here, Dimmock," General Carpenter began. "We're

all of us tools, today—hardened and sharpened to do a specific job. You know our motto: a job for everyone and everyone on the job. Somebody's not on the job at Ward T and we've got to kick him out. Now, in the first place what the hell is Ward T?"

Dimmock stuttered and fumbled. Finally he explained that it was a special ward set up for special combat cases. Shock cases.

"Then you do have patients in the ward?"

"Yes, sir. Ten women and fourteen men."

Carpenter brandished a sheaf of reports. "Says here the St. Albans patients claim nobody's in Ward T."

Dimmock was shocked. That was untrue, he assured the general.

"All right, Dimmock. So you've got your twenty-four crocks in there. Their job's to get well. Your job's to cure them. What the hell's upsetting the hospital about that?"

"W-well, sir. Perhaps it's because we keep them locked up."

"You keep Ward T locked?"

"Yes, sir."

"Why?"

"To keep the patients in, General Carpenter."

"Keep 'em in? What d'you mean? Are they trying to get out? They violent, or something?"

"No, sir. Not violent."

"Dimmock, I don't like your attitude. You're acting damned sneaky and evasive. And I'll tell you something else I don't like. That T classification. I checked with a Filing Expert from the Medical Corps and there is no T classification. What the hell are you up to at St. Albans?"

"W-well, sir . . . We invented the T classification. It . . . They . . . They're rather special cases, sir. We don't know what to do about them or how to handle them. W-we've been trying to keep it quiet until we've worked out a modus operandi, but it's brand new, General Carpenter. Brand new!" Here the expert in Dimmock triumphed over discipline. "It's sensational. It'll make medical history, by God! It's the biggest damned thing ever."

"What is it, Dimmock? Be specific."

"Well, sir, they're shock cases. Blanked out. Almost catatonic. Very little respiration. Slow pulse. No response."

"I've seen thousands of shock cases like that," Carpenter grunted. "What's so unusual?"

"Yes, sir, so far it sounds like the standard Q or R classification. But here's something unusual. They don't eat and they don't sleep."

"Never?"

"Some of them never."

"Then why don't they die?"

"We don't know. The metabolism cycle's broken, but only on the anabolism side. Catabolism continues. In other words, sir, they're eliminating waste products, but they're not taking anything in. They're eliminating fatigue poisons and rebuilding worn tissue, but without food and sleep. God knows how. It's fantastic."

"That why you've got them locked up? Mean to say . . . D'you suspect them of stealing food and catnaps somewhere else?"

"N-No, sir." Dimmock looked shamefaced. "I don't know how to tell you this, General Carpenter. . . . We lock them up because of the real mystery. They . . . Well, they disappear."

"They what?"

"They disappear, sir. Vanish. Right before your eyes."

"The hell you say."

"I do say, sir. They'll be sitting on a bed or standing around. One minute you see them, the next minute you don't. Sometimes there's two dozen in Ward T. Other times none. They disappear and reappear without rhyme or reason. That's why we've got the ward locked, General Carpenter. In the entire history of combat and combat injury, there's never been a case like this before. We don't know how to handle it."

"Bring me three of those cases," General Carpenter said.

Nathan Riley ate French toast, eggs benedict; consumed two pints of brown ale, smoked a John Drew, belched delicately and arose from the breakfast table. He nodded quietly to Gentleman Jim Corbett, who broke off his conversation with Diamond Jim Brady to intercept him on the way to the cashier's desk.

"Who do you like for the pennant this year, Nat?" Gentleman Jim inquired.

"The Dodgers," Nathan Riley answered.

"They've got no pitching."

"They've got Snider and Furillo and Campanella. They'll take the pennant this year, Jim. I'll bet they take it earlier than any team ever did. By September 13. Make a note. See if I'm right."

"You're always right, Nat," Corbett said.

Riley smiled, paid his check, sauntered out into the street and caught a horsecar bound for Madison Square Garden.

He got off at the corner of Fiftieth Street and Eighth Avenue and walked upstairs to a handbook office over a radio repair shop. The bookie glanced at him, produced an envelope, and counted out $15,000.

"Rocky Marciano by a TKO over Roland La Starza in the eleventh," he said. "How the hell do you call them so accurate, Nat?"

"That's the way I make a living." Riley smiled. "Are you making book on the elections?"

"Eisenhower twelve to five. Stevenson—"

"Never mind Adlai." Riley placed $20,000 on the counter. "I'm backing Ike. Get this down for me."

He left the handbook office and went to his suite in the Waldorf where a tall, thin young man was waiting for him anxiously.

"Oh yes," Nathan Riley said. "You're Ford, aren't you? Harold Ford?"

"Henry Ford, Mr. Riley."

"And you need financing for that machine in your bicycle shop. What's it called?"

"I call it an Ipsimobile, Mr. Riley."

"Hmmm. Can't say I like that name. Why not call it an automobile?"

"That's a wonderful suggestion, Mr. Riley. I'll certainly take it."

"I like you, Henry. You're young, eager, adaptable. I believe in your future and I believe in your automobile. I'll invest two hundred thousand dollars in your company."

Riley wrote a check and ushered Henry Ford out. He glanced at his watch and suddenly felt impelled to go back and look around for a moment. He entered his bedroom, undressed, put on a gray shirt and gray slacks. Across the pocket of the shirt were large blue letters: U.S.A.H.

He locked the bedroom door and disappeared.

He reappeared in Ward T of the United States Army Hospital in St. Albans, standing alongside his bed which was one of twenty-four lining the walls of a long, light steel barracks. Before he could draw another breath, he was seized by three pairs of hands. Before he could struggle, he was shot by a pneumatic syringe and poleaxed by 1½ cc of sodium thiomorphate.

"We've got one," someone said.

"Hang around," someone else answered. "General Carpenter said he wanted three."

After Marcus Junius Brutus left her bed, Lela Machan clapped her hands. Her slave women entered the chamber and prepared her bath. She bathed, dressed, scented herself, and breakfasted on Smyrna figs, rose oranges, and a flagon of Lacrima Christi. Then she smoked a cigarette and ordered her litter.

The gates of her house were crowded as usual by adoring hordes from the Twentieth Legion. Two centurions removed her chair-bearers from the poles of the litter and bore her on their stout shoulders. Lela Machan smiled. A young man in a sapphire-blue cloak thrust through the mob and ran toward her. A knife flashed in his hand. Lela braced herself to meet death bravely.

"Lady!" he cried. "Lady Lela!"

He slashed his left arm with the knife and let the crimson blood stain her robe.

"This blood of mine is the least I have to give you," he cried.

Lela touched his forehead gently.

"Silly boy," she murmured. "Why?"

"For love of you, my lady."

"You will be admitted tonight at nine," Lela whispered. He stared at her until she laughed. "I promise you. What is your name, pretty boy?"

"Ben Hur."

"Tonight at nine, Ben Hur."

The litter moved on. Outside the forum, Julius Caesar passed in hot argument with Savonarola. When he saw the litter he motioned sharply to the centurions, who stopped at once. Caesar swept

back the curtains and stared at Lela, who regarded him languidly. Caesar's face twitched.

"Why?" he asked hoarsely. "I have begged, pleaded, bribed, wept, and all without forgiveness. Why, Lela? Why?"

"Do you remember Boadicea?" Lela murmured.

"Boadicea? Queen of the Britons? Good God, Lela, what can she mean to our love? I did not love Boadicea. I merely defeated her in battle."

"And killed her, Caesar."

"She poisoned herself, Lela."

"She was my mother, Caesar!" Suddenly Lela pointed her finger at Caesar. "Murderer. You will be punished. Beware the Ides of March, Caesar!"

Caesar recoiled in horror. The mob of admirers that had gathered around Lela uttered a shout of approval. Amidst a shower of rose petals and violets, she continued on her way across the Forum to the Temple of the Vestal Virgins where she abandoned her adoring suitors and entered the sacred temple.

Before the altar she genuflected, intoned a prayer, dropped a pinch of incense on the altar flame and disrobed. She examined her beautiful body reflected in a silver mirror, then experienced a momentary twinge of homesickness. She put on a gray blouse and a gray pair of slacks. Across the pocket of the blouse was lettered U.S.A.H.

She smiled once at the altar and disappeared.

She reappeared in Ward T of the United States Army Hospital where she was instantly felled by 1½ cc of sodium thiomorphate injected subcutaneously by a pneumatic syringe.

"That's two," somebody said.

"One more to go."

George Hanmer paused dramatically and stared around . . . at the opposition benches, at the Speaker on the woolsack, at the silver mace on a crimson cushion before the Speaker's chair. The entire House of Parliament, hypnotized by Hanmer's fiery oratory, waited breathlessly for him to continue.

"I can say no more," Hanmer said at last. His voice was choked with emotion. His face was blanched and grim. "I will fight for this bill at the beachheads. I will fight in the cities, the towns, the fields and the hamlets. I will fight for this bill to the death and, God willing, I will fight for it after death. Whether this be a challenge or a prayer, let the consciences of the right honorable gentlemen determine; but of one thing I am sure and determined: England must own the Suez Canal."

Hanmer sat down. The house exploded. Through the cheering and applause he made his way out into the division lobby where Gladstone, Churchill, and Pitt stopped him to shake his hand. Lord Palmerston eyed him coldly, but Pam was shouldered aside by Disraeli who limped up, all enthusiasm, all admiration.

"We'll have a bite at Tattersall's," Dizzy said. "My car's waiting."

Lady Beaconsfield was in the Rolls Royce outside the Houses of Parliament. She pinned a primrose on Dizzy's lapel and patted Hanmer's cheek affectionately.

"You've come a long way from the schoolboy who used to bully Dizzy, Georgie," she said.

Hanmer laughed. Dizzy sang: "*Gaudeamus igitur . . .*" and Hanmer chanted the ancient scholastic song until they reached Tattersall's. There Dizzy ordered Guinness and grilled bones while Hanmer went upstairs in the club to change.

For no reason at all he had the impulse to go back for a last look. Perhaps he hated to break with his past completely. He divested himself of his surtout, nankeen waistcoat, pepper and salt trousers, polished Hessians and undergarments. He put on a gray shirt and gray trousers and disappeared.

He reappeared in Ward T of the St. Albans hospital where he was rendered unconscious by 1 ½ cc of sodium thiomorphate.

"That's three," somebody said.

"Take 'em to Carpenter."

So there they sat in General Carpenter's office, PFC Nathan Riley, M/Sgt Lela Machan, and Corp/2 George Hanmer. They were in their hospital grays. They were torpid with sodium thiomorphate.

The office had been cleared and it blazed with light. Present

were experts from Espionage, Counter-Espionage, Security, and Central Intelligence. When Captain Edsel Dimmock saw the steel-faced ruthless squad awaiting the patients and himself, he started. General Carpenter smiled grimly.

"Didn't occur to you that we mightn't buy your disappearance story, eh Dimmock?"

"S-Sir?"

"I'm an expert too, Dimmock. I'll spell it out for you. The war's going badly. Very badly. There've been intelligence leaks. The St. Albans mess might point to you."

"B-But they do disappear, sir. I—"

"My experts want to talk to you and your patients about this disappearing act, Dimmock. They'll start with you."

The experts worked over Dimmock with preconscious softeners, id releases, and superego blocks. They tried every truth serum in the books and every form of physical and mental pressure. They brought Dimmock, squealing, to the breaking point three times, but there was nothing to break.

"Let him stew for now," Carpenter said. "Get on to the patients."

The experts appeared reluctant to apply pressure to the sick men and the woman.

"For God's sake, don't be squeamish," Carpenter raged. "We're fighting a war for civilization. We've got to protect our ideals no matter what the price. Get to it!"

The experts from Espionage, Counter-Espionage, Security, and Central Intelligence got to it. Like three candles, PFC Nathan Riley, M/Sgt Lela Machan and Corp/2 George Hanmer snuffed out and disappeared. One moment they were seated in chairs surrounded by violence. The next moment they were not.

The experts gasped. General Carpenter did the handsome thing. He stalked to Dimmock. "Captain Dimmock, I apologize. Colonel Dimmock, you've been promoted for making an important discovery . . . only what the hell does it mean? We've got to check ourselves first."

Carpenter snapped up the intercom. "Get me a combat-shock expert and an alienist."

The two experts entered and were briefed. They examined the witnesses. They considered.

"You're all suffering from a mild case of shock," the combat-shock expert said. "War jitters."

"You mean we didn't see them disappear?"

The shock expert shook his head and glanced at the alienist who also shook his head.

"Mass illusion," the alienist said.

At that moment PFC Riley, M/Sgt Machan, and Corp/2 Hanmer reappeared. One moment they were a mass illusion; the next, they were back sitting in their chairs surrounded by confusion.

"Dope 'em again, Dimmock," Carpenter cried. "Give 'em a gallon." He snapped up the intercom. "I want every expert we've got. Emergency meeting in my office at once."

Thirty-seven experts, hardened and sharpened tools all, inspected the unconscious shock cases and discussed them for three hours. Certain facts were obvious: This must be a new fantastic syndrome brought on by the new and fantastic horrors of the war. As combat technique develops, the response of victims of this technique must also take new roads. For every action there is an equal and opposite reaction. Agreed.

This new syndrome must involve some aspects of teleportation . . . the power of mind over space. Evidently combat shock, while destroying certain known powers of the mind must develop other latent powers hitherto unknown. Agreed.

Obviously, the patients must only be able to return to the point of departure, otherwise they would not continue to return to Ward T nor would they have returned to General Carpenter's office. Agreed.

Obviously, the patients must be able to procure food and sleep wherever they go, since neither was required in Ward T. Agreed.

"One small point," Colonel Dimmock said. "They seem to be returning to Ward T less frequently. In the beginning they would come and go every day or so. Now most of them stay away for weeks and hardly ever return."

"Never mind that," Carpenter said. "Where do they go?"

"Do they teleport behind the enemy lines?" someone asked. "There's those intelligence leaks."

"I want Intelligence to check," Carpenter snapped. "Is the enemy having similar difficulties with, say, prisoners of war who appear and disappear from their POW camps? They might be some of ours from Ward T."

"They might simply be going home," Colonel Dimmock suggested.

"I want Security to check," Carpenter ordered. "Cover the home life and associations of every one of those twenty-four disappearers. Now . . . about our operations in Ward T. Colonel Dimmock has a plan."

"We'll set up six extra beds in Ward T," Edsel Dimmock explained. "We'll send in six experts to live there and observe. Information must be picked up indirectly from the patients. They're catatonic and nonresponsive when conscious, and incapable of answering questions when drugged."

"Gentlemen," Carpenter summed it up. "This is the greatest potential weapon in the history of warfare. I don't have to tell you what it can mean to us to be able to teleport an entire army behind enemy lines. We can win the war for the American Dream in one day if we can win this secret hidden in those shattered minds. We must win!"

The experts hustled, Security checked, Intelligence probed. Six hardened and sharpened tools moved into Ward T in St. Albans Hospital and slowly got acquainted with the disappearing patients who reappeared less and less frequently. The tension increased.

Security was able to report that not one case of strange appearance had taken place in America in the past year. Intelligence reported that the enemy did not seem to be having similar difficulties with their own shock cases or with POWs.

Carpenter fretted. "This is all brand new. We've got no specialists to handle it. We've got to develop new tools." He snapped up his intercom. "Get me a college," he said.

They got him Yale.

"I want some experts in mind over matter. Develop them," Carpenter ordered. Yale at once introduced three graduate courses in Thaumaturgy, Extrasensory Perception, and Telekinesis.

The first break came when one of the Ward T experts requested the assistance of another expert. He needed a Lapidary.

"What the hell for?" Carpenter wanted to know.

"He picked up a reference to a gemstone," Colonel Dimmock explained. "He's a personnel specialist and he can't relate it to anything in his experience."

"And he's not supposed to," Carpenter said approvingly. "A job for every man and every man on the job." He flipped up the intercom. "Get me a Lapidary."

An expert Lapidary was given leave of absence from the army arsenal and asked to identify a type of diamond called Jim Brady. He could not.

"We'll try it from another angle," Carpenter said. He snapped up his intercom. "Get me a Semanticist."

The Semanticist left his desk in the War Propaganda Department but could make nothing of the words "Jim Brady." They were names to him. No more. He suggested a Genealogist.

A Genealogist was given one day's leave from his post with the Un-American Ancestors Committee, but could make nothing of the name Brady beyond the fact that it had been a common name in America for five hundred years. He suggested an Archaeologist.

An Archaeologist was released from the Cartography Division of Invasion Command and instantly identified the name Diamond Jim Brady. It was a historic personage who had been famous in the city of Little Old New York sometime between Governor Peter Stuyvesant and Governor Fiorello La Guardia.

"Christ!" Carpenter marveled. "That's ages ago. Where the hell did Nathan Riley get that? You'd better join the experts in Ward T and follow this up."

The Archaeologist followed it up, checked his references and sent in his report. Carpenter read it and was stunned. He called an emergency meeting of his staff of experts.

"Gentlemen," he announced "Ward T is something bigger than teleportation. Those shock patients are doing something far more incredible . . . far more meaningful. Gentlemen, they're traveling through time."

The staff rustled uncertainly. Carpenter nodded emphatically.

"Yes, gentlemen. Time travel is here. It has not arrived the way

we expected it . . . as a result of expert research by qualified specialists; it has come as a plague . . . an infection . . . a disease of the war . . . a result of combat injury to ordinary men. Before I continue, look through these reports for documentation."

The staff read the stenciled sheets. PFC Nathan Riley . . . disappearing into the early twentieth century in New York; M/Sgt Lela Machan . . . visiting the first century in Rome; Corp/2 George Hanmer . . . journeying into the nineteenth century in England. And all the rest of the twenty-four patients, escaping the turmoil and horrors of modern war in the twenty-second century by fleeing to Venice and the Doges, to Jamaica and the buccaneers, to China and the Han Dynasty, to Norway and Eric the Red, to any place and any time in the world.

"I needn't point out the colossal significance of this discovery," General Carpenter pointed out. "Think what it would mean to the war if we could send an army back in time a week or a month or a year. We could win the war before it started. We could protect our Dream . . . Poetry and Beauty and the Culture of America . . . from barbarism without ever endangering it."

The staff tried to grapple with the problem of winning battles before they started.

"The situation is complicated by the fact that these men and women of Ward T are *non compos*. They may or may not know how they do what they do, but in any case they're incapable of communicating with the experts who could reduce this miracle to method. It's for us to find the key. They can't help us."

The hardened and sharpened specialists looked around uncertainly.

"We'll need experts," General Carpenter said.

The staff relaxed. They were on familiar ground again.

"We'll need a Cerebral Mechanist, a Cyberneticist, a Psychiatrist, an Anatomist, an Archaeologist, and a first-rate Historian. They'll go into that ward and they won't come out until their job is done. They must learn the technique of time travel."

The first five experts were easy to draft from other war departments. All America was a tool chest of hardened and sharpened specialists. But there was trouble locating a first-class Historian until the Federal Penitentiary cooperated with the army and released Dr.

Bradley Scrim from his twenty years at hard labor. Dr. Scrim was acid and jagged. He had held the chair of Philosophic History at a Western university until he spoke his mind about the war for the American Dream. That got him the twenty years hard.

Scrim was still intransigent, but induced to play ball by the intriguing problem of Ward T.

"But I'm not an expert," he snapped. "In this benighted nation of experts, I'm the last singing grasshopper in the ant heap."

Carpenter snapped up the intercom. "Get me an Entomologist," he said.

"Don't bother," Scrim said. "I'll translate. You're a nest of ants . . . all working and toiling and specializing. For what?"

"To preserve the American Dream," Carpenter answered hotly. "We're fighting for Poetry and Culture and Education and the Finer Things in Life."

"Which means you're fighting to preserve me," Scrim said. "That's what I've devoted my life to. And what do you do with me? Put me in jail."

"You were convicted of enemy sympathizing and fellow-travelling," Carpenter said.

"I was convicted of believing in my American Dream," Scrim said. "Which is another way of saying I was jailed for having a mind of my own."

Scrim was also intransigent in Ward T. He stayed one night, enjoyed three good meals, read the reports, threw them down, and began hollering to be let out.

"There's a job for everyone and everyone must be on the job," Colonel Dimmock told him. "You don't come out until you've got the secret of time travel."

"There's no secret I can get," Scrim said.

"Do they travel in time?"

"Yes and no."

"The answer has to be one or the other. Not both. You're evading the—"

"Look," Scrim interrupted wearily. "What are you an expert in?"

"Psychotherapy."

"Then how the hell can you understand what I'm talking about? This is a philosophic concept. I tell you there's no secret

here that the army can use. There's no secret any group can use. It's a secret for individuals only."

"I don't understand you."

"I didn't think you would. Take me to Carpenter."

They took Scrim to Carpenter's office where he grinned at the general malignantly, looking for all the world like a red-headed, underfed devil.

"I'll need ten minutes," Scrim said. "Can you spare them out of your toolbox?"

Carpenter nodded.

"Now listen carefully. I'm going to give you the clues to something so vast and so strange that it will need all your fine edge to cut into it."

Carpenter looked expectant.

"Nathan Riley goes back in time to the early twentieth century. There he lives the life of his fondest dreams. He's a big-time gambler, the friend of Diamond Jim Brady and others. He wins money betting on events because he always knows the outcome in advance. He won money betting on Eisenhower to win an election. He won money betting on a prizefighter named Marciano to beat another prizefighter named La Starza. He made money investing in an automobile company owned by Henry Ford. There are the clues. They mean anything to you?"

"Not without a Sociological Analyst," Carpenter answered. He reached for the intercom.

"Don't order one, I'll explain later. Let's try some more clues. Lela Machan, for example. She escapes into the Roman Empire where she lives the life of her dreams as a *femme fatale*. Every man loves her. Julius Caesar, Savonarola, the entire Twentieth Legion, a man named Ben Hur. Do you see the fallacy?"

"No."

"She also smokes cigarettes."

"Well?" Carpenter asked after a pause.

"I continue," Scrim said, "George Hanmer escapes into England of the nineteenth century where he's a member of Parliament and the friend of Gladstone, Winston Churchill, and Disraeli, who takes him riding in his Rolls Royce. Do you know what a Rolls Royce is?"

"No."

"It was the name of an automobile."

"So?"

"You don't understand yet?"

"No."

Scrim paced the floor in exaltation. "Carpenter, this is a bigger discovery than teleportation or time travel. This can be the salvation of man. I don't think I'm exaggerating. Those two dozen shock victims in Ward T have been U-Bombed into something so gigantic that it's no wonder your specialists and experts can't understand it."

"What the hell's bigger than time travel, Scrim?"

"Listen to this, Carpenter. Eisenhower did not run for office until the middle of the twentieth century. Nathan Riley could not have been a friend of Diamond Jim Brady's and bet on Eisenhower to win an election . . . not simultaneously. Brady was dead a quarter of a century before Ike was President. Marciano defeated La Starza fifty years after Henry Ford started his automobile company. Nathan Riley's time traveling is full of similar anachronisms."

Carpenter looked puzzled.

"Lela Machan could not have had Ben Hur for a lover. Ben Hur never existed in Rome. He never existed at all. He was a character in a novel. She couldn't have smoked. They didn't have tobacco then. You see? More anachronisms. Disraeli could never have taken George Hanmer for a ride in a Rolls Royce because automobiles weren't invented until long after Disraeli's death."

"The hell you say," Carpenter exclaimed. "You mean they're all lying?"

"No. Don't forget, they don't need sleep. They don't need food. They're not lying. They're going back in time, all right. They're eating and sleeping back there."

"But you just said their stories don't stand up. They're full of anachronisms."

"Because they travel back into a time of their own imagination. Nathan Riley has his own picture of what America was like in the early twentieth century. It's faulty and anachronistic because he's no scholar, but it's real for him. He can live there. The same is true for the others."

Carpenter goggled.

"The concept is almost beyond understanding. These people have discovered how to turn dreams into reality. They know how to enter their dream realities. They can stay there, live there, perhaps forever. My God, Carpenter, *this* is your American dream. It's miracle-working, immortality, Godlike creation, mind over matter. . . . It must be explored. It must be studied. It must be given to the world."

"Can you do it, Scrim?"

"No, I cannot. I'm an historian. I'm noncreative, so it's beyond me. You need a poet . . . an artist who understands the creation of dreams. From creating dreams on paper it oughtn't be too difficult to take the step to creating dreams in actuality."

"A poet? Are you serious?"

"Certainly I'm serious. Don't you know what a poet is? You've been telling us for five years that this war is being fought to save the poets."

"Don't be facetious, Scrim, I—"

"Send a poet into Ward T. He'll learn how they do it. He's the only man who can. A poet is half doing it anyway. Once he learns, he can teach your psychologists and anatomists. Then they can teach us; but the poet is the only man who can interpret between those shock cases and your experts."

"I believe you're right, Scrim."

"Then don't delay, Carpenter. Those patients are returning to this world less and less frequently. We've got to get at that secret before they disappear forever. Send a poet to Ward T."

Carpenter snapped up his intercom. "Send me a poet," he said.

He waited, and waited . . . and waited . . . while America sorted feverishly through its two hundred and ninety millions of hardened and sharpened experts, its specialized tools to defend the American Dream of Beauty and Poetry and the Better Things in Life. He waited for them to find a poet, not understanding the endless delay, the fruitless search; not understanding why Bradley Scrim laughed and laughed and laughed at this final, fatal disappearance.

FONDLY FAHRENHEIT

He doesn't know which of us I am these days, but they know one truth. You must own nothing but yourself. You must make your own life, live your own life and die your own death . . . or else you will die another's.

The rice fields on Paragon III stretch for hundreds of miles like checkerboard tundras, a blue and brown mosaic under a burning sky of orange. In the evening, clouds whip like smoke, and the paddies rustle and murmur.

A long line of men marched across the paddies the evening we escaped from Paragon III. They were silent, armed, intent; a long rank of silhouetted statues looming against the smoking sky. Each man carried a gun. Each man wore a walkie-talkie belt pack, the speaker button in his ear, the microphone bug clipped to his throat, the glowing view-screen strapped to his wrist like a green-eyed watch. The multitude of screens showed nothing but a multitude of individual paths through the paddies. The annunciators uttered no sound but the rustle and splash of steps. The men spoke infrequently, in heavy grunts, all speaking to all.

"Nothing here."

"Where's here?"

"Jenson's fields."

"You're drifting too far west."

"Close in the line there."

"Anybody covered the Grimson paddy?"

"Yeah. Nothing."

"She couldn't have walked this far."

"Could have been carried."

"Think she's alive?"

"Why should she be dead?"

The slow refrain swept up and down the long line of beaters advancing toward the smoky sunset. The line of beaters wavered like a writhing snake, but never ceased its remorseless advance. One hundred men spaced fifty feet apart. Five thousand feet of ominous search. One mile of angry determination stretching from east to west across a compass of heat. Evening fell. Each man lit his search lamp. The writhing snake was transformed into a necklace of wavering diamonds.

"Clear here. Nothing."

"Nothing here."

"Nothing."

"What about the Allen paddies?"

"Covering them now."

"Think we missed her?"

"Maybe."

"We'll beat back and check."

"This'll be an all-night job."

"Allen paddies clear."

"God damn! We've got to find her!"

"We'll find her."

"Here she is. Sector seven. Tune in."

The line stopped. The diamonds froze in the heat. There was silence. Each man gazed into the glowing green screen on his wrist, tuning to sector seven. All tuned to one. All showed a small nude figure awash in the muddy water of a paddy. Alongside the figure an owner's stake of bronze read: VANDALEUR. The ends of the line converged toward the Vandaleur field. The necklace turned into a cluster of stars. One hundred men gathered around a small nude body, a child dead in a rice paddy. There was no water in her

mouth. There were no fingermarks on her throat. Her innocent face was battered. Her body was torn. Clotted blood on her skin was crusted and hard.

"Dead three-four hours at least."

"Her mouth is dry."

"She wasn't drowned. Beaten to death."

In the dark evening heat the men swore softly. They picked up the body. One stopped the others and pointed to the child's fingernails. She had fought her murderer. Under the nails were particles of flesh and bright drops of scarlet blood, still liquid, still uncoagulated.

"That blood ought to be clotted, too."

"Funny."

"Not so funny. What kind of blood don't clot?"

"Android."

"Looks like she was killed by one."

"Vandaleur owns an android."

"She couldn't be killed by an android."

"That's android blood under her nails."

"The police better check."

"The police'll prove I'm right."

"But andys can't kill."

"That's android blood, ain't it?"

"Androids can't kill. They're made that way."

"Looks like one android was made wrong."

"Jesus!"

And the thermometer that day registered 92.9° gloriously Fahrenheit.

So there we were aboard the *Paragon Queen* en route for Megaster V, James Vandaleur and his android. James Vandaleur counted his money and wept. In the second-class cabin with him was his android, a magnificent synthetic creature with classic features and wide blue eyes. Raised on its forehead in a cameo of flesh were the letters MA, indicating that this was one of the rare multiple-aptitude androids, worth $57,000 on the current exchange. There we were, weeping and counting and calmly watching.

"Twelve, fourteen, sixteen. Sixteen hundred dollars," Vandaleur wept. "That's all. Sixteen hundred dollars. My house was worth ten thousand. The land was worth five. There was furniture, cars, my paintings, etchings, my plane, my—And nothing to show for everything but sixteen hundred dollars. Christ!"

I leaped up from the table and turned on the android. I pulled a strap from one of the leather bags and beat the android. It didn't move.

"I must remind you," the android said, "that I am worth fifty-seven thousand dollars on the current exchange. I must warn you that you are endangering valuable property."

"You damned crazy machine," Vandaleur shouted.

"I am not a machine," the android answered. "The robot is a machine. The android is a chemical creation of synthetic tissue."

"What got into you?" Vandaleur cried. "Why did you do it? Damn you!" He beat the android savagely.

"I must remind you that I cannot be punished," I said. "The pleasure-pain syndrome is not incorporated in the android synthesis."

"Then why did you kill her?" Vandaleur shouted. "If it wasn't for kicks, why did you—"

"I must remind you," the android said, "that the second-class cabins in these ships are not soundproofed."

Vandaleur dropped the strap and stood panting, staring at the creature he owned.

"Why did you do it? Why did you kill her?" I asked.

"I don't know," I answered.

"First it was malicious mischief. Small things. Petty destruction. I should have known there was something wrong with you then. Androids can't destroy. They can't harm. They—"

"There is no pleasure-pain syndrome incorporated in the android synthesis."

"Then it got to arson. Then serious destruction. Then assault . . . that engineer on Rigel. Each time worse. Each time we had to get out faster. Now it's murder. Christ! What's the matter with you? What's happened?"

"There are no self-check relays incorporated in the android brain."

"Each time we had to get out it was a step downhill. Look at me. In a second-class cabin. Me. James Paleologue Vandaleur. There was a time when my father was the wealthiest—Now, sixteen hundred dollars in the world. That's all I've got. And you. Christ damn you!"

Vandaleur raised the strap to beat the android again, then dropped it and collapsed on a berth, sobbing. At last he pulled himself together.

"Instructions," he said.

The multiple android responded at once. It arose and awaited orders.

"My name is now Valentine. James Valentine. I stopped off on Paragon III for only one day to transfer to this ship for Megaster V. My occupation: Agent for one privately owned MA android which is for hire. Purpose of visit: To settle on Megaster V. Fix the papers."

The android removed Vandaleur's passport and papers from a bag, got pen and ink and sat down at the table. With an accurate, flawless hand—an accomplished hand that could draw, write, paint, carve, engrave, etch, photograph, design, create, and build—it meticulously forged new credentials for Vandaleur. Its owner watched me miserably.

"Create and build," I muttered, "And now destroy. Oh God! What am I going to do? Christ! If I could only get rid of you. If I didn't have to live off you. God! If only I'd inherited some guts instead of you."

Dallas Brady was Megaster's leading jewelry designer. She was short, stocky, amoral, and a nymphomaniac. She hired Vandaleur's multiple-aptitude android and put me to work in her shop. She seduced Vandaleur. In her bed one night, she asked abruptly, "Your name's Vandaleur, isn't it?"

"Yes," I murmured. Then: "No! It's Valentine. James Valentine."

"What happened on Paragon?" Dallas Brady asked. "I thought androids couldn't kill or destroy property. Prime Directives and In-

hibitions set up for them when they're synthesized. Every company guarantees they can't."

"Valentine!" Vandaleur insisted.

"Oh come off it," Dallas Brady said. "I've known for a week. I haven't hollered copper, have I?"

"The name is Valentine."

"You want to prove it? You want I should call the cops?" Dallas reached out and picked up the phone.

"For God's sake, Dallas!" Vandaleur leaped up and struggled to take the phone from her. She fended him off, laughing at him, until he collapsed and wept in shame and helplessness.

"How did you find out?" he asked at last.

"The papers are full of it. And Valentine was a little too close to Vandaleur. That wasn't smart, was it?"

"I guess not. I'm not very smart."

"Your android's got quite a record, hasn't it? Assault. Arson. Destruction. What happened on Paragon?"

"It kidnapped a child. Took her out into the rice fields and murdered her."

"Raped her?"

"I don't know."

"They're going to catch up with you."

"Don't I know it? Christ! We've been running for two years now. Seven planets in two years. I must have abandoned fifty thousand dollars' worth of property in two years."

"You better find out what's wrong with it."

"How can I? Can I walk into a repair clinic and ask for an overhaul? What am I going to say? 'My android's just turned killer. Fix it.' They'd call the police right off." I began to shake. "They'd have that android dismantled inside one day. I'd probably be booked as accessory to murder."

"Why didn't you have it repaired before it got to murder?"

"If they started fooling around with lobotomies and body chemistry and endocrine surgery, they might have destroyed its aptitudes. What would I have left to hire out? How would I live?"

"You could work yourself. People do."

"Work at what? You know I'm good for nothing. How could I

compete with specialist androids and robots? Who can, unless he's got a terrific talent for a particular job?"

"Yeah. That's true."

"I lived off my old man all my life. Damn him! He had to go bust just before he died. Left me the android and that's all. The only way I can get along is living off what it earns."

"You better sell it before the cops catch up with you. You can live off fifty grand. Invest it."

"At three percent? Fifteen hundred a year? When the android returns fifteen percent on its value? Eight thousand a year. That's what it earns. No, Dallas. I've got to go along with it."

"What are you going to do about its violence kick?"

"I can't do anything . . . except watch it and pray. What are you going to do about it?"

"Nothing. It's none of my business. Only one thing . . . I ought to get something for keeping my mouth shut."

"What?"

"The android works for me for free. Let somebody else pay you, but I get it for free."

The multiple-aptitude android worked. Vandaleur collected its fees. His expenses were taken care of. His savings began to mount. As the warm spring of Megaster V turned to hot summer, I began investigating farms and properties. It would be possible, within a year or two, for us to settle down permanently, provided Dallas Brady's demands did not become rapacious.

On the first hot day of summer, the android began singing in Dallas Brady's workshop. It hovered over the electric furnace which, along with the weather, was broiling the shop, and sang an ancient tune that had been popular half a century before.

> Oh, it's no feat to beat the heat.
> All reet! All reet!
> So jeet your seat
> Be fleet be fleet
> Cool and discreet
> Honey . . .

It sang in a strange, halting voice, and its accomplished fingers were clasped behind its back, writhing in a strange rumba all their own. Dallas Brady was surprised.

"You happy or something?" she asked.

"I must remind you that the pleasure-pain syndrome is not incorporated in the android synthesis," I answered. "All reet! All reet! Be fleet be fleet, cool and discreet, honey . . ."

Its fingers stopped their writhing and picked up a heavy pair of iron tongs. The android poked them into the glowing heart of the furnace, leaning far forward to peer into the lovely heat.

"Be careful, you damned fool!" Dallas Brady exclaimed. "You want to fall in?"

"I must remind you that I am worth fifty-seven thousand dollars on the current exchange," I said. "It is forbidden to endanger valuable property. All reet! All reet! Honey . . ."

It withdrew a crucible of glowing gold from the electric furnace, turned, capered hideously, sang crazily, and splashed a sluggish gobbet of molten gold over Dallas Brady's head. She screamed and collapsed, her hair and clothes flaming, her skin crackling. The android poured again while it capered and sang.

"Be fleet be fleet, cool and discreet, honey . . ." It sang and slowly poured and poured the molten gold. Then I left the workshop and rejoined James Vandaleur in his hotel suite. The android's charred clothes and squirming fingers warned its owner that something was very much wrong.

Vandaleur rushed to Dallas Brady's workshop, stared once, vomited, and fled. I had enough time to pack one bag and raise nine hundred dollars on portable assets. He took a third-class cabin on the *Megaster Queen*, which left that morning for Lyra Alpha. He took me with him. He wept and counted his money and I beat the android again.

And the thermometer in Dallas Brady's workshop registered 98.1° beautifully Fahrenheit.

On Lyra Alpha we holed up in a small hotel near the university. There, Vandaleur carefully bruised my forehead until the letters MA were obliterated by the swelling and the discoloration. The

letters would reappear again, but not for several months, and in the meantime Vandaleur hoped the hue and cry for an MA android would be forgotten. The android was hired out as a common laborer in the university power plant. Vandaleur, as James Venice, eked out life on the android's small earnings.

I wasn't too unhappy. Most of the other residents in the hotel were university students, equally hard up, but delightfully young and enthusiastic. There was one charming girl with sharp eyes and a quick mind. Her name was Wanda, and she and her beau, Jed Stark, took a tremendous interest in the killing android which was being mentioned in every paper in the galaxy.

"We've been studying the case," she and Jed said at one of the casual student parties which happened to be held this night in Vandaleur's room. "We think we know what's causing it. We're going to do a paper." They were in a high state of excitement.

"Causing what?" somebody wanted to know.

"The android rampage."

"Obviously out of adjustment, isn't it? Body chemistry gone haywire. Maybe a kind of synthetic cancer, yes?"

"No." Wanda gave Jed a look of suppressed triumph.

"Well, what is it?"

"Something specific."

"What?"

"That would be telling."

"Oh come on."

"Nothing doing."

"Won't you tell us?" I asked intently. "I . . . We're very much interested in what could go wrong with an android."

"No, Mr. Venice," Wanda said. "It's a unique idea and we've got to protect it. One thesis like this and we'll be set up for life. We can't take the chance of somebody stealing it."

"Can't you give us a hint?"

"No. Not a hint. Don't say a word, Jed. But I'll tell you this much, Mr. Venice. I'd hate to be the man who owns that android."

"You mean the police?" I asked.

"I mean projection, Mr. Venice. Projection! That's the danger . . . and I won't say any more. I've said too much as is."

I heard steps outside, and a hoarse voice singing softly: "Be fleet

be fleet cool and discreet, honey . . ." My android entered the room, home from its tour of duty at the university power plant. It was not introduced. I motioned to it and I immediately responded to the command and went to the beer keg and took over Vandaleur's job of serving the guests. Its accomplished fingers writhed in a private rumba of their own. Gradually they stopped their squirming, and the strange humming ended.

Androids were not unusual at the university. The wealthier students owned them along with cars and planes. Vandaleur's android provoked no comment, but young Wanda was sharp-eyed and quick-witted. She noted my bruised forehead and she was intent on the history-making thesis she and Jed Stark were going to write. After the party broke up, she consulted with Jed walking upstairs to her room.

"Jed, why'd that android have a bruised forehead?"

"Probably hurt itself, Wanda. It's working in the power plant. They fling a lot of heavy stuff around."

"That all?"

"What else?"

"It could be a convenient bruise."

"Convenient for what?"

"Hiding what's stamped on its forehead."

"No point to that, Wanda. You don't have to see marks on a forehead to recognize an android. You don't have to see a trademark on a car to know it's a car."

"I don't mean it's trying to pass as a human. I mean it's trying to pass as a lower-grade android."

"Why?"

"Suppose it had 'MA' on its forehead."

"Multiple aptitude? Then why in hell would Venice waste it stoking furnaces if it could earn more—Oh. Oh! You mean it's—?"

Wanda nodded.

"Jesus!" Stark pursed his lips. "What do we do? Call the police?"

"No. We don't know if it's an MA for a fact. If it turns out to be an MA and the killing android, our paper comes first anyway. This is our big chance, Jed. It it's *that* android we can run a series of controlled tests and—"

"How do we find out for sure?"

"Easy. Infrared film. That'll show what's under the bruise. Borrow a camera. Buy some film. We'll sneak down to the power plant tomorrow afternoon and take some pictures. Then we'll know."

They stole down into the university power plant the following afternoon. It was a vast cellar, deep under the earth. It was dark, shadowy, luminous with burning light from the furnace doors. Above the roar of the fires they could hear a strange voice shouting and chanting in the echoing vault: "All reet! All reet! So jeet your seat. Be fleet be fleet, cool and discreet, honey . . ." And they could see a capering figure dancing a lunatic rumba in time to the music it shouted. The legs twisted. The arms waved. The fingers writhed.

Jed Stark raised the camera and began shooting his spool of infrared film, aiming the camera sights at that bobbing head. Then Wanda shrieked, for I saw them and came charging down on them, brandishing a polished steel shovel. It smashed the camera. It felled the girl and then the boy. Jed fought me for a desperate hissing moment before he was bludgeoned into helplessness. Then the android dragged them to the furnace and fed them to the flames, slowly, hideously. It capered and sang. Then it returned to my hotel.

The thermometer in the power plant registered 100.9° murderously Fahrenheit. All reet! All reet!

We bought steerage on the *Lyra Queen*, and Vandaleur and the android did odd jobs for their meals. During the night watches, Vandaleur would sit alone in the steerage head with a cardboard portfolio on his lap, puzzling over its contents. That portfolio was all he had managed to bring with him from Lyra Alpha. He had stolen it from Wanda's room. It was labeled ANDROID. It contained the secret of my sickness.

And it contained nothing but newspapers. Scores of newspapers from all over the galaxy, printed, microfilmed, engraved, etched, offset, photostated . . . Rigel *Star-Banner* . . . Paragon *Picayune* . . . Megaster *Times-Leader* . . . La lande *Herald* . . . Lacaille *Journal* . . . Indi *Intelligencer* . . . Eridani *Telegram-News*. All reet! All reet!

Nothing but newspapers. Each paper contained an account of one crime in the android's ghastly career. Each paper also contained

news, domestic and foreign, sports, society, weather, shipping news, stock exchange quotations, human interest stories, features, contests, puzzles. Somewhere in that mass of uncollated facts was the secret Wanda and Jed Stark had discovered. Vandaleur pored over the papers helplessly. It was beyond him. So jeet your seat!

"I'll sell you," I told the android. "Damn you. When we land on Terra, I'll sell you. I'll settle for three percent on whatever you're worth."

"I am worth fifty-seven thousand dollars on the current exchange," I told him.

"If I can't sell you, I'll turn you in to the police," I said.

"I am valuable property," I answered. "It is forbidden to endanger valuable property. You won't have me destroyed."

"Christ damn you!" Vandaleur cried. "What? Are you arrogant? Do you know you can trust me to protect you? Is that the secret?"

The multiple-aptitude android regarded him with calm accomplished eyes. "Sometimes," it said, "it is a good thing to be property."

It was three below zero when the Lyra Queen dropped at Croydon Field. A mixture of ice and snow swept across the field, fizzing and exploding into steam under the Queen's tail jets. The passengers trotted numbly across the blackened concrete to customs inspection, and thence to the airport bus that was to take them to London. Vandaleur and the android were broke. They walked.

By midnight they reached Piccadilly Circus. The December ice storm had not slackened, and the statue of Eros was encrusted with ice. They turned right, walked down to Trafalgar Square and then along the Strand shaking with cold and wet. Just above Fleet Street, Vandaleur saw a solitary figure coming from the direction of St. Paul's. He drew the android into an alley.

"We've got to have money," he whispered. He pointed at the approaching figure. "He has money. Take it from him."

"The order cannot be obeyed," the android said.

"Take it from him," Vandaleur repeated. "By force. Do you understand? We're desperate."

"It is contrary to my prime directive," I said. "I cannot endanger life or property. The order cannot be obeyed."

"For God's sake!" Vandaleur burst out. "You've attacked, destroyed, murdered. Don't gibber about prime directives. You haven't any left. Get his money. Kill him if you have to. I tell you, we're desperate!"

"It is contrary to my prime directive," I said. "I cannot endanger life or property. The order cannot be obeyed."

I thrust the android back and leaped out at the stranger. He was tall, austere, competent. He had an air of hope curdled by cynicism. He carried a cane. I saw he was blind.

"Yes?" he said. "I hear you near me. What is it?"

"Sir . . ." Vandaleur hesitated. "I'm desperate."

"We are all desperate," the stranger replied. "Quietly desperate."

"Sir . . . I've got to have some money."

"Are you begging or stealing?" The sightless eyes passed over Vandaleur and the android.

"I'm prepared for either."

"Ah. So are we all. It is the history of our race." The stranger motioned over his shoulder. "I have been begging at St. Paul's, my friend. What I desire cannot be stolen. What is it you desire that you are lucky enough to be able to steal?"

"Money," Vandaleur said.

"Money for what? Come, my friend, let us exchange confidences. I will tell you why I beg, if you will tell me why you steal. My name is Blenheim."

"My name is . . . Vole."

"I was not begging for sight at St. Paul's, Mr. Vole. I was begging for a number."

"A number?"

"Ah yes. Numbers rational, numbers irrational, numbers imaginary. Positive integers. Negative integers. Fractions, positive and negative. Eh? You have never heard of Blenheim's immortal treatise on Twenty Zeros, or The Differences in Absence of Quantity?" Blenheim smiled bitterly. "I am the wizard of the Theory of Number, Mr. Vole, and I have exhausted the charm of number for myself. After fifty years of wizardry, senility approaches and the

appetite vanishes. I have been praying in St. Paul's for inspiration. Dear God, I prayed, if You exist, send me a number."

Vandaleur slowly lifted the cardboard portfolio and touched Blenheim's hand with it. "In here," he said, "is a number. A hidden number. A secret number. The number of a crime. Shall we exchange, Mr. Blenheim? Shelter for a number?"

"Neither begging nor stealing, eh?" Blenheim said. "But a bargain. So all life reduces itself to the banal." The sightless eyes again passed over Vandaleur and the android. "Perhaps the All-Mighty is not God but a merchant. Come home with me."

On the top floor of Blenheim's house we shared a room—two beds, two closets, two washstands, one bathroom. Vandaleur bruised my forehead again and sent me out to find work, and while the android worked, I consulted with Blenheim and read him the papers from the portfolio, one by one. All reet! All reet!

Vandaleur told him so much and no more. He was a student, I said, attempting a thesis on the murdering android. In these papers which he had collected were the facts that would explain the crimes of which Blenheim had heard nothing. There must be a correlation, a number, a statistic, something which would account for my derangement, I explained, and Blenheim was piqued by the mystery, the detective story, the human interest of number.

We examined the papers. As I read them aloud, he listed them and their contents in his blind, meticulous writing. And then I read his notes to him. He listed the papers by type, by typeface, by fact, by fancy, by article, spelling, words, theme, advertising, pictures, subject, politics, prejudices. He analyzed. He studied. He meditated. And we lived together in that top floor, always a little cold, always a little terrified, always a little closer . . . brought together by our fear of it, our hatred between us. Like a wedge driven into a living tree and splitting the trunk, only to be forever incorporated into the scar tissue, we grew together. Vandaleur and the android. Be fleet be fleet!

And one afternoon Blenheim called Vandaleur into his study and displayed his notes. "I think I've found it," he said, "but I can't understand it."

Vandaleur's heart leaped.

"Here are the correlations," Blenheim continued. "In fifty papers there are accounts of the criminal android. What is there, outside the depredations, that is also in fifty papers?"

"I don't know, Mr. Blenheim."

"It was a rhetorical question. Here is the answer. The weather."

"What?"

"The weather." Blenheim nodded. "Each crime was committed on a day when the temperature was above ninety degrees Fahrenheit."

"But that's impossible," Vandaleur exclaimed. "It was cool on Lyra Alpha."

"We have no record of any crime committed on Lyra Alpha. There is no paper."

"No. That's right, I—" Vandaleur was confused. Suddenly he exclaimed. "No. You're right. The furnace room. It was hot there. Hot! Of course. My God, yes! That's the answer. Dallas Brady's electric furnace . . . the rice deltas on Paragon. So jeet your seat. Yes. But why? Why? My God, why?"

I came into the house at that moment, and passing the study, saw Vandaleur and Blenheim. I entered, awaiting commands, my multiple aptitudes devoted to service.

"That's the android, eh?" Blenheim said after a long moment.

"Yes," Vandaleur answered, still confused by the discovery. "And that explains why it refused to attack you that night on the Strand. It wasn't hot enough to break the prime directive. Only in the heat . . . The heat, all reet!" He looked at the android. A silent lunatic command passed from man to android. I refused. It is forbidden to endanger life. Vandaleur gestured furiously, then seized Blenheim's shoulders and yanked him back out of his desk chair to the floor. Blenheim shouted once. Vandaleur leaped on him like a tiger, pinning him to the floor and sealing his mouth with one hand.

"Find a weapon," he called to the android.

"It is forbidden to endanger life."

"This is a fight for self-preservation. Bring me a weapon!" He held the squirming mathematician with all his weight. I went at once to a cupboard where I knew a revolver was kept. I checked

it. It was loaded with five cartridges. I handed it to Vandaleur. I took it, rammed the barrel against Blenheim's head and pulled the trigger. He shuddered once.

We had three hours before the cook returned from her day off. We looted the house. We took Blenheim's money and jewels. We packed a bag with clothes. We took Blenheim's notes, destroyed the newspapers; and we left, carefully locking the door behind us. In Blenheim's study we left a pile of crumpled papers under a half inch of burning candle. And we soaked the rug around it with kerosene. No, I did all that. The android refused. I am forbidden to endanger life or property.

All reet!

They took the tubes to Leicester Square, changed trains, and rode to the British Museum. There they got off and went to a small Georgian house just off Russell Square. A shingle in the window read: NAN WEBB, PSYCHOMETRIC CONSULTANT. Vandaleur had made a note of the address some weeks earlier. They went into the house. The android waited in the foyer with the bag. Vandaleur entered Nan Webb's office.

She was a tall woman with gray shingled hair, very fine English complexion, and very bad English legs. Her features were blunt, her expression acute. She nodded to Vandaleur, finished a letter, sealed it and looked up.

"My name," I said, "is Vanderbilt. James Vanderbilt."

"Quite."

"I'm an exchange student at London University."

"Quite."

"I've been researching on the killing android, and I think I've discovered something very interesting. I'd like your advice on it. What is your fee?"

"What is your college at the University?"

"Why?"

"There is a discount for students."

"Merton College."

"That will be two pounds, please."

Vandaleur placed two pounds on the desk and added to the fee

Blenheim's notes. "There is a correlation," he said, "between the crimes of the android and the weather. You will note that each crime was committed when the temperature rose above ninety degrees Fahrenheit. Is there a psychometric answer for this?"

Nan Webb nodded, studied the notes for a moment, put down the sheets of paper, and said: "Synesthesia, obviously."

"What?"

"Synesthesia," she repeated. "When a sensation, Mr. Vanderbilt, is interpreted immediately in terms of a sensation from a different sense organ from the one stimulated, it is called synesthesia. For example: A sound stimulus gives rise to a simultaneous sensation of definite color. Or color gives rise to a sensation of taste. Or a light stimulus gives rise to a sensation of sound. There can be confusion or short circuiting of any sensation of taste, smell, pain, pressure, temperature, and so on. D'you understand?"

"I think so."

"Your research has uncovered the fact that the android most probably reacts to temperature stimulus above the ninety-degree level synthetically. Most probably there is an endocrine response. Probably a temperature linkage with the android adrenal surrogate. High temperature brings about a response of fear, anger, excitement, and violent physical activity . . . all within the province of the adrenal gland."

"Yes. I see. Then if the android were to be kept in cold climates . . ."

"There would be neither stimulus nor response. There would be no crimes. Quite."

"I see. What is projection?"

"How do you mean?"

"Is there any danger of projection with regard to the owner of the android?"

"Very interesting. Projection is a throwing forward. It is the process of throwing out upon another the ideas or impulses that belong to oneself. The paranoid, for example, projects upon others his conflicts and disturbances in order to externalize them. He accuses, directly or by implication, other men of having the very sicknesses with which he is struggling himself."

"And the danger of projection?"

"It is the danger of believing what is implied. If you live with a psychotic who projects his sickness upon you, there is a danger of falling into his psychotic pattern and becoming virtually psychotic yourself. As, no doubt, is happening to you, Mr. Vandaleur."

Vandaleur leaped to his feet.

"You are an ass," Nan Webb went on crisply. She waved the sheets of notes. "This is no exchange student's writing. It's the unique cursive of the famous Blenheim. Every scholar in England knows this blind writing. There is no Merton College at London University. That was a miserable guess. Merton is one of the Oxford colleges. And you, Mr. Vandaleur, are so obviously infected by association with your deranged android . . . by projection, if you will . . . that I hesitate between calling the Metropolitan Police and the Hospital for the Criminally Insane."

I took out the gun and shot her.

Reet!

"Antares II, Alpha Aurigae, Acrux IV, Pollux IX, Rigel Centaurus," Vandaleur said. "They're all cold. Cold as a witch's kiss. Mean temperatures of forty degrees Fahrenheit. Never gets hotter than seventy. We're in business again. Watch that curve."

The multiple-aptitude android swung the wheel with its accomplished hands. The car took the curve sweetly and sped on through the northern marshes, the reeds stretching for miles, brown and dry, under the cold English sky. The sun was sinking swiftly. Overhead, a lone flight of bustards flapped clumsily eastward. High above the flight, a lone helicopter drifted toward home and warmth.

"No more warmth for us," I said. "No more heat. We're safe when we're cold. We'll hole up in Scotland, make a little money, get across to Norway, build a bankroll, and then ship out. We'll settle on Pollux. We're safe. We've licked it. We can live again."

There was a startling *bleep* from overhead, and then a ragged roar: "ATTENTION, JAMES VANDALEUR AND ANDROID. ATTENTION, JAMES VANDALEUR AND ANDROID!"

Vandaleur started and looked up. The lone helicopter was floating above them. From its belly came amplified commands: "YOU ARE SURROUNDED. THE ROAD IS BLOCKED. YOU ARE

TO STOP YOUR CAR AT ONCE AND SUBMIT TO ARREST. STOP AT ONCE!"

I looked at Vandaleur for orders.

"Keep driving," Vandaleur snapped.

The helicopter dropped lower: "ATTENTION, ANDROID. YOU ARE IN CONTROL OF THE VEHICLE. YOU ARE TO STOP AT ONCE. THIS IS A STATE DIRECTIVE SUPERSEDING ALL PRIVATE COMMANDS."

"What the hell are you doing?" I shouted.

"A state directive supersedes all private commands," the android answered. "I must point out to you that—"

"Get the hell away from the wheel," Vandaleur ordered. I clubbed the android, yanked him sideways, and squirmed over him to the wheel. The car veered off the road in that moment and went churning through the frozen mud and dry reeds. Vandaleur regained control and continued westward through the marshes toward a parallel highway five miles distant.

"We'll beat their goddamned block," he grunted.

The car pounded and surged. The helicopter dropped even lower. A searchlight blazed from the belly of the plane.

"ATTENTION, JAMES VANDALEUR AND ANDROID. SUBMIT TO ARREST. THIS IS A STATE DIRECTIVE SUPERSEDING ALL PRIVATE COMMANDS."

"He can't submit," Vandaleur shouted wildly. "There's no one to submit to. He can't and I won't."

"Christ!" I muttered. "We'll beat them yet. We'll beat the block. We'll beat the heat. We'll—"

"I must point out to you," I said, "that I am required by my prime directive to obey state directives which supersede all private commands. I must submit to arrest."

"Who says it's a state directive?" Vandaleur said. "Them? Up in that plane? They've got to show credentials. They've got to prove it's state authority before you submit. How d'you know they're not crooks trying to trick us?"

Holding the wheel with one arm, he reached into his side pocket to make sure the gun was still in place. The car skidded. The tires squealed on frost and reeds. The wheel was wrenched from his grasp and the car yawed up a small hillock and overturned.

The motor roared and the wheels screamed. Vandaleur crawled out and dragged the android with him. For the moment we were outside the circle of light boring down from the helicopter. We blundered off into the marsh, into the blackness, into concealment. . . . Vandaleur running with a pounding heart, hauling the android along.

The helicopter circled and soared over the wrecked car, searchlight peering, loudspeaker braying. On the highway we had left, lights appeared as the pursuing and blocking parties gathered and followed radio directions from the plane. Vandaleur and the android continued deeper and deeper into the marsh, working their way toward the parallel road and safety. It was night by now. The sky was a black matte. Not a star showed. The temperature was dropping. A southeast night wind knifed us to the bone.

Far behind there was a dull concussion. Vandaleur turned, gasping. The car's fuel had exploded. A geyser of flame shot up like a lurid fountain. It subsided into a low crater of burning reeds. Whipped by the wind, the distant hem of flame fanned up into a wall, ten feet high. The wall began marching down on us, cracking fiercely. Above it, a pall of oil smoke surged forward. Behind it, Vandaleur could make out the figures of men . . . a mass of beaters searching the marsh.

"Christ!" I cried and searched desperately for safety. He ran, dragging me with him, until their feet crunched through the surface ice of a pool. He trampled the ice furiously, then flung himself down in the numbing water, pulling the android with us.

The wall of flame approached. I could hear the crackle and feel the heat. He could see the searchers clearly. Vandaleur reached into his side pocket for the gun. The pocket was torn. The gun was gone. He groaned and shook with cold and terror. The light from the marsh fire was blinding. Overhead, the helicopter floated helplessly to one side, unable to fly through the smoke and flames and aid the searchers who were beating far to the right of us.

"They'll miss us," Vandaleur whispered. "Keep quiet. That's an order. They'll miss us. We'll beat them. We'll beat the fire. We'll—"

Three distinct shots sounded less than a hundred feet from the fugitives. *Blam! Blam! Blam!* They came from the last three cartridges in my gun as the marsh fire reached it where it had dropped,

and exploded the shells. The searchers turned toward the sound and began working directly toward us. Vandaleur cursed hysterically and tried to submerge even deeper to escape the intolerable heat of the fire. The android began to twitch.

The wall of flame surged up to them. Vandaleur took a deep breath and prepared to submerge until the flame passed over them. The android shuddered and burst into an earsplitting scream.

"All reet! All reet!" it shouted. "Be fleet be fleet!"

"Damn you!" I shouted. I tried to drown it.

"Damn you!" I cursed him. I smashed his face.

The android battered Vandaleur, who fought it off until it exploded out of the mud and staggered upright. Before I could return to the attack, the live flames captured it hypnotically. It danced and capered in a lunatic rumba before the wall of fire. Its legs twisted. Its arms waved. The fingers writhed in a private rumba of their own. It shrieked and sang and ran in a crooked waltz before the embrace of the heat, a muddy monster silhouetted against the brilliant sparkling flare.

The searchers shouted. There were shots. The android spun around twice and then continued its horrid dance before the face of the flames. There was a rising gust of wind. The fire swept around the capering figure and enveloped it for a roaring moment. Then the fire swept on, leaving behind it a sobbing mass of synthetic flesh oozing scarlet blood that would never coagulate.

The thermometer would have registered 1200° wondrously Fahrenheit.

Vandaleur didn't die. I got away. They missed him while they watched the android caper and die. But I don't know which of us he is these days. Projection, Wanda warned me. Projection, Nan Webb told him. If you live with a crazy man or a crazy machine long enough, I become crazy too. Reet!

But we know one truth. We know they were wrong. The new robot and Vandaleur know that because the new robot's started twitching too. Reet! Here on cold Pollux, the robot is twitching and singing. No heat, but my fingers writhe. No heat, but it's taken the little Talley girl off for a solitary walk. A cheap labor robot. A

servo-mechanism . . . all I could afford . . . but it's twitching and humming and walking alone with the child somewhere and I can't find them. Christ! Vandaleur can't find me before it's too late. Cool and discreet, honey, in the dancing frost while the thermometer registers 10° fondly Fahrenheit.

COMMENT ON
"FONDLY FAHRENHEIT"

I've always been fascinated by the way craftsmen work in their profession, and I'll spend hours with pawnbrokers, computer engineers, exterminators, anyone, in an effort to discover the backstage problems of their work. Perhaps this is a habit created by years of interviewing for the magazine for which I write and edit; perhaps it is the built-in curiosity of the writer. I don't know. But it occurred to me that readers might be interested in the backstage problems of writing "Fondly Fahrenheit."

I must describe my working methods first, otherwise this journal of the writing of the story will seem cold-blooded and mechanistic. I write out of fever. I cannot write anything until I'm so saturated with it, involved with it, bursting with it, that it must come out or I will have no rest.

Over the years I've evolved a technique for igniting this fever. It starts with outlining, first general, then increasingly detailed as the story develops. When I have what I believe to be the final outline (it never is), I begin running the story through my head over and over again; not in words, I don't tell it to myself, but in a sort of sensory cinema. I listen to the sound, visualize the scenes, feel the tempo of the characters and their conflicts.

It's at this point that the pacing begins. At home I have a good seventy-five-foot straightaway, and I walk the length of the apartment, back and forth, endlessly. In the office I have a wide corridor, the length

of a football field. The staff and the secretaries are used to my peculiarity by now and kindly clear the way for me. The pacing and the repetitions continue, the heat mounts, and, if I'm lucky, the ignition point is reached. Then I run like hell for the typewriter.

The idea for "Fondly Fahrenheit" first came to me out of a reminiscence of Mark Twain, I think in Life on the Mississippi, but I'm not sure, it was so long ago. He wrote that the first Negro slave was hanged for murder near Hannibal, Missouri. The slave had criminally assualted and killed a young girl. Twain said that the slave had been guilty of a similar crime in another state, but that his owner had smuggled him out because he was too valuable to be given up to justice and destroyed.

It seemed to me that there might be an interesting story in this conflict between master and slave; the slave aware of his value and the hold it gives him over his owner, the master constrained by greed to condone criminal acts which he abhors. It was impossible for me to set the story in antebellum days; I didn't know enough about the period or the scene. Contemporary treatment was clearly out of the question; we do have economic forms of slavery, but no chattel slavery. I decided to set the story in the future, postulating an android-slave society. The note went into my Commonplace Book, which has been the storehouse for ideas, fragments, bits of dialogue, odd situations, and gimmicks since I began my writing career. It remained there for several years.

I would think about it, off and on, but I was also thinking about dozens of other ideas which seemed to have priority. I sometimes regard story ideas as an eager crowd, jostling and elbowing each other, trying to attract your attention. The master-slave idea managed to attract my serious attention one evening, and I outlined the first three or four scenes. I could get no further, and rather than waste time struggling with it, I put it away. One of the luxuries of reaching a certain financial plateau is that the writer can take his time and give inchoate ideas a chance to sort themselves out in the unconscious. Many writers, working under the gun, are so beset by the pressure of meeting bills that they haven't the time to do their best work. I've been through it myself, and I'm deeply sympathetic.

When I looked through my outlines and notes a few months later, the unconscious had done its work. It dawned on me that what was holding me up was the fact that I hadn't thought through the android

slave's criminal behavior; I'd more or less written him off as a murderer, period. Now I asked myself why. Why does a carefully conditioned android go berserk? I remembered a note I'd made long before on the statistics of crime, relating crime rate to temperature. (This was a decade before the long, hot summer riots had become a commonplace.) "Good," I said. "The android breaks his conditioning only when the temperature rises above a certain level."

At this point it was possible to add a mystery to the chase structure. Will the owner discover what's wrong with his android? I went back, reoutlined in these terms, changing the settings to accommodate the temperature gimmick, and continued blocking forward. Then I came up against another wall. So he does discover the secret. So what? It felt like a letdown. I needed more of a climax. Once again I put the notes away to give the real writer, who lives somewhere deep down inside me, a chance to do some work.

Much later I was going through my Commonplace Book, looking for something else, when I came across a note I'd made on psychiatric projection, transcribed from one of Karen Horney's books. These are cases where disturbed people attribute their own strange behavior to others.

"That's it!" the real writer, an alert opportunist, said.

"That's what?" I asked. "I'm looking for notes on Western frontier customs."

"That's the final twist for the android story," he said. "Temperature may break the android's conditioning, but the master is really the criminal. We'll extrapolate the projection theme. The master unconsciously but actually imposes his own insanity on the slave."

We dropped everything else, worked out a detailed scene-by-scene outline, and began to pace. Suddenly an idea came, one we'd been toying with for years, that of telling a story from a multiple point of view. Here it would be the omniscient, the master's and the slave's. That was the ignition point. The fever set in, and I ran like hell for the typewriter.

What you've just read is the result of all this; years of notes, months of dovetailing ideas, weeks of outlining. Someone once asked me how long it took to write "Fondly Fahrenheit." I hedged. "Well, it took me two days to type it," I said. What else could I say?

THE FOUR-HOUR FUGUE

Fear carries a scent with it
that most humans can't detect.
Most, but not all.

By now, of course, the Northeast Corridor was the Northeast slum, stretching from Canada to the Carolinas and as far west as Pittsburgh. It was a fantastic jungle of rancid violence inhabited by a steaming, restless population with no visible means of support and no fixed residence, so vast that census takers, birth-control supervisors, and the social services had given up all hope. It was a gigantic raree-show that everyone denounced and enjoyed. Even the privileged few who could afford to live highly protected lives in highly expensive Oases and could live anywhere else they pleased never thought of leaving. The jungle grabbed you.

There were thousands of everyday survival problems but one of the most exasperating was the shortage of fresh water. Most of the available potable water had long since been impounded by progressive industries for the sake of a better tomorrow and there was very little left to go around. Rainwater tanks on the roofs, of course. A black market, naturally. That was about all. So the jungle stank. It stank worse than the court of Queen Elizabeth, which could have

bathed but didn't believe in it. The Corridor just couldn't bathe, wash clothes, or clean house, and you could smell its noxious effluvium from ten miles out at sea. Welcome to the Fun Corridor.

Sufferers near the shore would have been happy to clean up in salt water, but the Corridor beaches had been polluted by so much crude oil seepage for so many generations that they were all owned by deserving oil reclamation companies. *Keep Out! No Trespassing!* And armed guards. The rivers and lakes were electrically fenced; no need for guards, just skull and crossbones signs and if you didn't know what they were telling you, tough.

Not to believe that everybody minded stinking as they skipped merrily over the rotting corpses in the streets, but a lot did and their only remedy was perfumery. There were dozens of competing companies producing perfumes but the leader, far and away, was the Continental Can Company, which hadn't manufactured cans in two centuries. They'd switched to plastics and had the good fortune about a hundred stockholders' meetings back to make the mistake of signing a sales contract with and delivering to some cockamamie perfume brewer an enormous quantity of glowing neon containers. The corporation went bust and CCC took it over in hopes of getting some of their money back. That takeover proved to be their salvation when the perfume explosion took place: it gave them entrée to the most profitable industry of the times.

But it was neck-and-neck with the rivals until Blaise Skiaki joined CCC: then it turned into a runaway. Blaise Skiaki. Origins: French, Japanese, Black African, and Irish. Education: BA, Princeton; ME, MIT; PhD. Dow Chemical. (It was Dow that had secretly tipped CCC that Skiaki was a winner and lawsuits brought by the competition were still pending before the ethics board.) Blaise Skiaki: Age, thirty-one; unmarried, straight, genius.

His sense of scent was his genius and he was privately referred to at CCC as "The Nose." He knew everything about perfumery: the animal products, ambergris, castor, civet, musk; the essential oils distilled from plants and flowers: the balsams extruded by tree and shrub wounds, benzoin, opopanax, Peru, Talu, storax, myrrh: the synthetics created from the combination of natural and chemical scents, the latter mostly the esters of fatty acids.

He had created for CCC their most successful sellers: "Vulva,"

"Assuage," "Oxter" (a much more attractive brand name than "Armpitto"), "Preparation F," "Tongue War," et cetera. He was treasured by CCC, paid a salary generous enough to enable him to live in an Oasis and, best of all, granted unlimited supplies of fresh water. No girl in the Corridor could resist the offer of taking a shower with him.

But he paid a high price for these advantages. He could never use scented soaps, shaving creams, pomades, or depilatories. He could never eat seasoned foods. He could drink nothing but pure water. All this, you understand, to keep The Nose pure and un-contaminated so that he could smell around in his sterile laboratory and devise new creations. He was presently composing a rather promising unguent provisionally named "Correctum," but he'd been on it for six months without any positive results and CCC was alarmed by the delay. His genius had never before taken so long.

There was a meeting of the top-level executives, names with-held on the grounds of corporate privilege.

"What's the matter with him anyway?"

"Has he lost his touch?"

"It hardly seems likely."

"Maybe he needs a rest."

"Why, he had a week's holiday last month."

"What did he do?"

"Ate up a storm, he told me."

"Could that be it?"

"No. He said he purged himself before he came back to work."

"Is he having trouble here at CCC? Difficulties with middle management?"

"Absolutely not, Mr. Chairman. They wouldn't dare touch him."

"Maybe he wants a raise."

"No. He can't spend the money he makes now."

"Has our competition got to him?"

"They get to him all the time, General, and he laughs them off."

"Then it must be something personal."

"Agreed."

"Woman trouble?"

"My God! We should have such trouble."

"Family trouble?"

"He's an orphan, Mr. Chairman."

"Ambition? Incentive? Should we make him an officer of CCC?"

"I offered that to him the first of the year, sir, and he turned me down. He just wants to play in his laboratory."

"Then why isn't he playing?"

"Apparently he's got some kind of creative block."

"What the hell is the matter with him anyway?"

"Which is how you started this meeting."

"I did not."

"You did."

"Not."

"Governor, will you play back the bug."

"Gentlemen, gentlemen, please! Obviously Dr. Skiaki has personal problems which are blocking his genius. We must solve that for him. Suggestions?"

"Psychiatry?"

"That won't work without voluntary cooperation. I doubt whether he'd cooperate. He's an obstinate gook."

"Senator, I beg you! Such expressions must not be used with reference to one of our most valuable assets."

"Mr. Chairman, the problem is to discover the source of Dr. Skiaki's block."

"Agreed. Suggestions?"

"Why, the first step should be to maintain twenty-four-hour surveillance. All of the gook's—excuse me—the good doctor's activities, associates, contacts."

"By CCC?"

"I would suggest not. There are bound to be leaks which would only antagonize the good gook—doctor!"

"Outside surveillance?"

"Yes, sir."

"Very good. Agreed. Meeting adjourned."

Skip-Tracer Associates were perfectly furious. After one month they threw the case back into CCC's lap, asking for nothing more than their expenses.

"Why in hell didn't you tell us that we were assigned to a pro, Mr. Chairman, sir? Our tracers aren't trained for that."

"Wait a minute, please. What d'you mean, 'pro'?"

"A professional Rip."

"A what?"

"Rip. Gorill. Gimpster. Crook."

"Dr. Skiaki a crook? Preposterous."

"Look, Mr. Chairman. I'll frame it for you and you draw your own conclusions. Yes?"

"Go ahead."

"It's all detailed in this report anyway. We put double tails on Skiaki every day to and from your shop. When he left they followed him home. He always went home. They staked in double shifts. He had dinner sent in from the Organic Nursery every night. They checked the messengers bringing the dinners. Legit. They checked the dinners; sometimes for one, sometimes for two. They traced some of the girls who left his penthouse. All clean. So far, all clean, yes?"

"And?"

"The crunch. Couple of nights a week he leaves the house and goes into the city. He leaves around midnight and doesn't come back until four, more or less."

"Where does he go?"

"We don't know because he shakes his tails like the pro that he is. He weaves through the Corridor like a whore or a fag cruising for trade—excuse me—and he always loses our men. I'm not taking anything away from him. He's smart, shifty, quick, and a real pro. He has to be; and he's too much for Skip-Tracers to handle."

"Then you have no idea of what he does or who he meets between midnight and four?"

"No, sir. We've got nothing and you've got a problem. Not ours any more."

"Thank you. Contrary to the popular impression, corporations are not altogether idiotic. CCC understands that negatives are also results. You'll receive your expenses and the agreed-upon fee."

"Mr. Chairman, I—"

"No, no, please. You've narrowed it down to those missing four hours. Now, as you say, they're our problem."

•   •   •

CCC summoned Salem Burne. Mr. Burne always insisted that he was neither a physician nor a psychiatrist: he did not care to be associated with what he considered to be the drek of the professions. Salem Burne was a witch doctor; more precisely, a warlock. He made the most remarkable and penetrating analyses of disturbed people, not so much through his coven rituals of pentagons, incantations, incense, and the like as through his remarkable sensitivity to Body English and his acute interpretation of it. And this might be witchcraft after all.

Mr. Burne entered Blaise Skiaki's immaculate laboratory with a winning smile and Dr. Skiaki let out a rending howl of anguish.

"I told you to sterilize before you came."

"But I did, Doctor. Faithfully."

"You did not. You reek of anise, ilang-ilang, and methyl anthranilate. You've polluted my day. Why?"

"Dr. Skiaki, I assure you that I—" Suddenly Salem Burne stopped. "Oh my God!" he groaned. "I used my wife's towel this morning."

Skiaki laughed and turned up the ventilators to full force. "I understand. No hard feelings. Now let's get your wife out of here. I have an office about half a mile down the hall. We can talk there."

They sat down in the vacant office and looked at each other. Mr. Burne saw a pleasant, youngish man with cropped black hair, small expressive ears, high telltale cheekbones, slitty eyes that would need careful watching and graceful hands that would be a dead giveaway.

"Now, Mr. Burne, how can I help you?" Skiaki said while his hands asked. "Why the hell have you come pestering me?"

"Dr. Skiaki, I'm a colleague in a sense: I'm a professional witch doctor. One crucial part of my ceremonies is the burning of various forms of incense, but they're all rather conventional. I was hoping that your expertise might suggest something different with which I could experiment."

"I see. Interesting. You've been burning stacte, onycha, galbanum, frankincense . . . that sort of thing?"

"Yes. All quite conventional."

"Most interesting. I could, of course, make many suggestions for new experiments and yet—" Here Skiaki stopped and stared into space.

After a long pause the warlock asked, "Is anything wrong, Doctor?"

"Look here," Skiaki burst out. "You're on the wrong track. It's the burning of incense that's conventional and old-fashioned, and trying different scents won't solve your problem. Why not experiment with an altogether different approach?"

"And what would that be?"

"The Odophone principle."

"Odophone?"

"Yes. There's a scale that exists among scents as among sounds. Sharp smells correspond to high notes and heavy smells with low notes. For example, ambergris is in the treble clef while violet is in the bass. I could draw up a scent scale for you, running perhaps two octaves. Then it would be up to you to compose the music."

"This is positively brilliant, Dr. Skiaki."

"Isn't it?" Skiaki beamed. "But in all honesty I should point out that we're collaborators in brilliance. I could never have come up with the idea if you hadn't presented me with a most original challenge."

They made contact on this friendly note and talked shop enthusiastically, lunched together, told each other about themselves, and made plans for the witchcraft experiments in which Skiaki volunteered to participate despite the fact that he was no believer in diabolism.

"And yet the irony lies in the fact that he is indeed devil-ridden," Salem Burne reported.

The Chairman could make nothing of this.

"Psychiatry and diabolism use different terms for the same phenomenon," Burne explained. "So perhaps I'd better translate. Those missing four hours are fugues."

The Chairman was not enlightened. "Do you mean the musical expression, Mr. Burne?"

"No, sir. A fugue is also the psychiatric description of a more advanced form of somnambulism . . . sleepwalking."

"Blaise Skiaki walks in his sleep?"

"Yes, sir, but it's more complicated than that. The sleepwalker is a comparatively simple case. He is never in touch with his surroundings. You can speak to him, shout at him, address him by name, and he remains totally oblivious."

"And the fugue?"

"In the fugue the subject is in touch with his surroundings. He can converse with you. He has awareness and memory for the events that take place within the fugue, but while he is within his fugue he is a totally different person from the man he is in real life. And—and this is most important, sir—after the fugue he remembers nothing of it."

"Then in your opinion Dr. Skiaki has these fugues two or three times a week."

"That is my diagnosis, sir."

"And he can tell us nothing of what transpires during the fugue?"

"Nothing."

"Can you?"

"I'm afraid not, sir. There's a limit to my powers."

"Have you any idea what is causing these fugues?"

"Only that he is driven by something. I would say that he is possessed by the devil, but that is the cant of my profession. Others may use different terms—compulsion or obsession. The terminology is unimportant. The basic fact is that something possessing him is compelling him to go out nights to do—what? I don't know. All I do know is that this diabolical drive most probably is what is blocking his creative work for you."

One does not summon Gretchen Nunn, not even if you're CCC whose common stock has split twenty-five times. You work your way up through the echelons of her staff until you are finally admitted to the Presence. This involves a good deal of backing and forthing between your staff and hers, and ignites a good deal of exasperation, so the Chairman was understandably put out when at last he was ushered into Miss Nunn's workshop, which was cluttered with the books and apparatus she used for her various investigations.

Gretchen Nunn's business was working miracles; not in the sense of the extraordinary, anomalous or abnormal brought about by a superhuman agency, but rather in the sense of the extraordinary and/or abnormal perception and manipulation of reality. In any situation she could and did achieve the impossible begged by her desperate clients, and her fees were so enormous that she was thinking of going public.

Naturally the Chairman had anticipated Miss Nunn as looking like Merlin in drag. He was flabbergasted to discover that she was a Watusi princess with velvety black skin, aquiline features, great black eyes, tall, slender, twentyish, ravishing in red.

She dazzled him with a smile, indicated a chair, sat in one opposite and said, "My fee is one hundred thousand. Can you afford it?"

"I can. Agreed."

"And your difficulty—is it worth it?"

"It is."

"Then we understand each other so far. Yes, Alex?"

The young secretary who had bounced into the workshop said, "Excuse me. LeClerque insists on knowing how you made the positive identification of the mold as extraterrestrial."

Miss Nunn clicked her tongue impatiently. "He knows that I never give reasons. I only give results."

"Yes'N."

"Has he paid?"

"Yes'N."

"All right, I'll make an exception in his case. Tell him that it was based on the levo and dextro probability in amino acids and tell him to have a qualified exobiologist carry on from there. He won't regret the cost."

"Yes'N. Thank you."

She turned to the Chairman as the secretary left. "You heard that. I only give results."

"Agreed, Miss Nunn."

"Now your difficulty. I'm not committed yet. Understood?"

"Yes. Miss Nunn."

"Go ahead. Everything. Stream of consciousness, if necessary."

An hour later she dazzled him with another smile and said,

"Thank you. This one is really unique. A welcome change. It's a contract, if you're still willing."

"Agreed, Miss Nunn. Would you like a deposit or an advance?"

"Not from CCC."

"What about expenses? Should that be arranged?"

"No. My responsibility."

"But what if you have to—if you're required to—if—"

She laughed. "My responsibility. I never give reasons and I never reveal methods. How can I charge for them? Now don't forget; I want that Skip-Trace report."

A week later Gretchen Nunn took the unusual step of visiting the Chairman in his office at CCC. "I'm calling on you, sir, to give you the opportunity of withdrawing from our contract."

"Withdraw? But why?"

"Because I believe you're involved in something far more serious than you anticipated."

"But what?"

"You won't take my word for it?"

"I must know."

Miss Nunn compressed her lips. After a moment she sighed. "Since this is an unusual case I'll have to break my rules. Look at this, sir." She unrolled a large map of a segment of the Corridor and flattened it on the Chairman's desk. There was a star in the center of the map. "Skiaki's residence," Miss Nunn said. There was a large circle scribed around the star. "The limits to which a man can walk in two hours." Miss Nunn said. The circle was crisscrossed by twisting trails all emanating from the star. "I got this from the Skip-Trace report. This is how the tails traced Skiaki."

"Very ingenious, but I see nothing serious in this, Miss Nunn."

"Look closely at the trails. What do you see?"

"Why . . . each ends in a red cross."

"And what happens to each trail before it reaches the red cross?"

"Nothing. Nothing at all, except—except that the dots change to dashes."

"And that's what makes it serious."

"I don't understand, Miss Nunn."

"I'll explain. Each cross represents the scene of a murder. The

dashes represent the backtracking of the actions and whereabouts of each murder victim just prior to death."

"Murder!"

"They could trace their actions just so far back and no further. Skip-Trace could tail Skiaki just so far forward and no further. Those are the dots. The dates join up. What's your conclusion?"

"It must be coincidence," the Chairman shouted. "This brilliant charming young man. Murder? Impossible!"

"Do you want the factual data I've drawn up?"

"No, I don't. I want the truth. Proof positive without any inferences from dots, dashes and dates."

"Very well, Mr. Chairman. You'll get it."

She rented the professional beggar's pitch alongside the entrance to Skiaki's Oasis for a week. No success. She hired a Revival Band and sang hymns with it before the Oasis. No success. She finally made the contact after she promoted a job with the Organic Nursery. The first three dinners she delivered to the penthouse she came and went unnoticed; Skiaki was entertaining a series of girls, all scrubbed and sparkling with gratitude. When she made the fourth delivery he was alone and noticed her for the first time.

"Hey," he grinned. "How long has this been going on?"

"Sir?"

"Since when has Organic been using girls for delivery boys?"

"I am a delivery person, sir," Miss Nunn answered with dignity. "I have been working for the Organic Nursery since the first of the month."

"Knock off the sir bit."

"Thank you, s—Dr. Skiaki."

"How the devil do you know that I've got a doctorate?"

She'd slipped. He was listed at the Oasis and the Nursery merely as B. Skiaki, and she should have remembered. As usual, she turned her mistake into an advantage. "I know all about you, sir. Dr. Blaise Skiaki, Princeton, MIT, Dow Chemical. Chief Scent Chemist at CCC."

"You sound like 'Who's Who.'"

"That's where I read it, Dr. Skiaki."

"You read me up in 'Who's Who'? Why on earth?"

"You're the first famous man I've ever met."

"Whatever gave you the idea that I'm famous, which I'm not."

She gestured around. "I knew you had to be famous to live like this."

"Very flattering. What's your name, love?"

"Gretchen, sir."

"What's your last name?"

"People from my class don't have last names, sir."

"Will you be the delivery b—person tomorrow, Gretchen?"

"Tomorrow is my day off, Doctor."

"Perfect. Bring dinner for two."

So the affair began and Gretchen discovered, much to her aston-ishment, that she was enjoying it very much. Blaise was indeed a brilliant, charming young man, always entertaining, always consid-erate, always generous. In gratitude he gave her (remember he be-lieved she came from the lowest Corridor class) one of his most prized possessions, a five-carat diamond he had synthesized at Dow. She responded with equal style; she wore it in her navel and prom-ised that it was for his eyes only.

Of course he always insisted on her scrubbing up each time she visited, which was a bit of a bore; in her income bracket she prob-ably had more fresh water than he did. However, one convenience was that she could quit her job at the Organic Nursery and attend to other contracts while she was attending to Skiaki.

She always left his penthouse around eleven-thirty but stayed outside until one. She finally picked him up one night just as he was leaving the Oasis. She'd memorized the Salem Burne report and knew what to expect. She overtook him quickly and spoke in an agitated voice, "Mistuh. Mistuh."

He stopped and looked at her kindly without recognition. "Yes, my dear?"

"If yuh gone this way kin I come too. I scared."

"Certainly, my dear."

"Thanks, mistuh. I gone home. You gone home?"

"Well, not exactly."

"Where you gone? Y'ain't up to nothin' bad, is you? I don't want no part."

"Nothing bad, my dear. Don't worry."

"Then what you up to?"

He smiled secretly. "I'm following something."

"Somebody?"

"No, something."

"What kine something?"

"My, you're curious, aren't you. What's your name?"

"Gretchen. How 'bout you?"

"Me?"

"What's your name?"

"Wish. Call me Mr. Wish." He hesitated for a moment and then said, "I have to turn left here."

"Thas OK, Mistuh Wish. I go left, too."

She could see that all his senses were prickling, and reduced her prattle to a background of unobtrusive sound. She stayed with him as he twisted, turned, sometimes doubling back, through streets, alleys, lanes and lots, always assuring him that this was her way home too. At a rather dangerous-looking refuse dump he gave her a fatherly pat and cautioned her to wait while he explored its safety. He explored, disappeared and never reappeared.

"I replicated this experience with Skiaki six times," Miss Nunn reported to CCC. "They were all significant. Each time he revealed a little more without realizing it and without recognizing me. Burne was right. It is fugue."

"And the cause, Miss Nunn?"

"Pheromone trails."

"What?"

"I thought you gentlemen would know the term, being in the chemistry business. I see I'll have to explain. It will take some time so I insist that you do not require me to describe the induction and deduction that led me to my conclusion. Understood?"

"Agreed, Miss Nunn."

"Thank you, Mr. Chairman. Surely you all know hormones, from the Greek *hormaein*, meaning 'to excite'. They're internal secretions which excite other parts of the body into action. Pheromones are external secretions which excite other creatures into action. It's a mute chemical language.

"The best example of the pheromone language is the ant. Put

a lump of sugar somewhere outside an ant hill. A forager will come across it, feed, and return to the nest. Within an hour the entire commune will be single-filing to and from the sugar, following the pheromone trail first laid down quite undeliberately by the first discoverer. It's an unconscious but compelling stimulant."

"Fascinating. And Dr. Skiaki?"

"He follows human pheromone trails. They compel him; he goes into fugue and follows them."

"Ah! An outré aspect of The Nose. It makes sense, Miss Nunn. It really does. But what trails is he compelled to follow?"

"The death-wish."

"Miss Nunn!"

"Surely you're aware of this aspect of the human psyche. Many people suffer from an unconscious but powerful death-wish, especially in these despairing times. Apparently this leaves a pheromone trail which Dr. Skiaki senses, and he is compelled to follow it."

"And then?"

"Apparently he grants the wish."

"Apparently! Apparently!" the Chairman shouted. "I ask you for proof positive of this monstrous accusation."

"You'll get it, sir. I'm not finished with Blaise Skiaki yet. There are one or two things I have to wrap up with him, and in the course of that I'm afraid he's in for a shock. You'll have your proof pos—"

That was a half-lie from a woman half in love. She knew she had to see Blaise again but her motives were confused. To find out whether she really loved him, despite what she knew? To find out whether he loved her? To tell him the truth about herself? To warn him or save him or run away with him? To fulfill her contract in a cool, professional style? She didn't know. Certainly she didn't know that she was in for a shock from Skiaki.

"Were you born blind?" he murmured that night.

She sat bolt upright in the bed. "What? Blind? What?"

"You heard me."

"I've had perfect sight all my life."

"Ah. Then you don't know, darling. I rather suspected that might be it."

"I certainly don't know what you're talking about, Blaise."

"Oh, you're blind all right," he said calmly. "But you've never

known because you're blessed with a fantastic freak facility. You have extrasensory perception of other people's senses. You see through other people's eyes. For all I know you may be deaf and hear through their ears. You may feel with their skin. We must explore it some time."

"I never heard of anything more absurd in all my life," she said angrily.

"I can prove it to you, if you like, Gretchen."

"Go ahead, Blaise. Prove the impossible."

"Come into the lounge."

In the living room he pointed to a vase. "What color is that?"

"Brown, of course."

"What color is that?" A tapestry.

"Gray."

"And that lamp?"

"Black."

"QED," Skiaki said. "It has been demonstrated."

"What's been demonstrated?"

"That you're seeing through my eyes."

"How can you say that?"

"Because I'm color-blind. That's what gave me the clue in the first place."

"What?"

He took her in his arms to quiet her trembling. "Darling Gretchen, the vase is green. The tapestry is amber and gold. The lamp is crimson. I can't see the colors but the decorator told me and I remember. Now why the terror? You're blind, yes, but you're blessed with something far more miraculous than mere sight: you see through the eyes of the world. I'd change places with you any time."

"It can't be true," she cried.

"It's true, love."

"What about when I'm alone?"

"When are you alone? When is anybody in the Corridor ever alone?"

She snatched up a shift and ran out of the penthouse, sobbing hysterically. She ran back to her own Oasis nearly crazed with terror. And yet she kept looking around and there were all the colors:

red, orange, yellow, green, indigo, blue, violet. But there were also people swarming through the labyrinths of the Corridor as they always were, twenty-four hours a day.

Back in her apartment she was determined to put the disaster to the test. She dismissed her entire staff with stern orders to get the hell out and spend the night somewhere else. She stood at the door and counted them out, all amazed and unhappy. She slammed the door and looked around. She could still see.

"The lying son-of-a-bitch." she muttered and began to pace furiously. She raged through the apartment, swearing venomously. It proved one thing: never get into personal relationships. They'll betray you, they'll try to destroy you, and she'd made a fool of herself. But why, in God's name, did Blaise use this sort of dirty trick to destroy her? Then she smashed into something and was thrown back. She recovered her balance and looked to see what she had blundered into. It was a harpsichord.

"But . . . but I don't own a harpsichord," she whispered in bewilderment. She started forward to touch it and assure herself of its reality. She smashed into the something again, grabbed it, and felt it. It was the back of a couch. She looked around frantically. This was not one of her rooms. The harpsichord. Vivid Brueghels hanging on the walls. Jacobean furniture. Linenfold paneled doors. Crewel drapes.

"But . . . this is the . . . the Raxon apartment downstairs. I must be seeing through their eyes. I must . . . he was right. I . . ." She closed her eyes and looked. She saw a mélange of apartments, streets, crowds, people, events. She had always seen this sort of montage on occasion but had always thought it was merely the total visual recall which was a major factor in her extraordinary abilities and success. Now she knew the truth.

She began to sob again. She felt her way around the couch and sat down, despairing. When at last the convulsion spent itself she wiped her eyes courageously, determined to face reality. She was no coward. But when she opened her eyes she was shocked by another bombshell. She saw her familiar room in tones of gray. She saw Blaise Skiaki standing in the open door smiling at her.

"Blaise?" she whispered.

"The name is Wish, my dear. Mr. Wish. What's yours?"

"Blaise, for God's sake, not me! Not me. I left no death-wish trail."

"What's your name my dear? We've met before?"

"Gretchen," she screamed. "I'm Gretchen Nunn and I have no death-wish."

"Nice meeting you again, Gretchen," he said in glassy tones, smiling the glassy smile of Mr. Wish. He took two steps toward her. She jumped up and ran behind the couch.

"Blaise, listen to me. You are not Mr. Wish. There is no Mr. Wish. You are Dr. Blaise Skiaki, a famous scientist. You are chief chemist at CCC and have created many wonderful perfumes."

He took another step toward her, unwinding the scarf he wore around his neck.

"Blaise, I'm Gretchen. We've been lovers for two months. You must remember. Try to remember. You told me about my eyes tonight . . . being blind. You must remember that."

He smiled and whirled the scarf into a cord.

"Blaise, you're suffering from fugue. A blackout. A change of psyche. This isn't the real you. It's another creature driven by a pheromone. But I left no pheromone trail. I couldn't. I've never wanted to die."

"Yes, you do, my dear. Only happy to grant your wish. That's why I'm called Mr. Wish."

She squealed like a trapped rat and began darting and dodging while he closed in on her. She feinted him to one side, twisted to the other with a clear chance of getting out the door ahead of him, only to crash into three grinning goons standing shoulder to shoulder. They grabbed and held her.

Mr. Wish did not know that he also left a pheromone trail. It was a pheromone trail of murder.

"Oh, it's you again." Mr. Wish sniffed.

"Hey, old buddy-boy, got a looker this time, huh?"

"And loaded. Dig this layout."

"Great. Makes up for the last three which was nothin'. Thanks buddy-boy. You can go home now."

"Why don't I ever get to kill one?" Mr. Wish exclaimed petulantly.

"Now, now. No sulks. We got to protect our bird dog. You lead. We follow and do the rest."

"And if anything goes wrong, you're the setup," one of the goons giggled.

"Go home, buddy-boy. The rest is ours. No arguments. We already explained the standoff to you. We know who you are but you don't know who we are."

"I know who I am," Mr. Wish said with dignity. "I am Mr. Wish and I still think I have the right to kill at least one."

"All right, all right. Next time. That's a promise. Now blow."

As Mr. Wish exited resentfully, they ripped Gretchen naked and let out a huge wow when they saw the five-carat diamond in her navel. Mr. Wish turned and saw its scintillation too.

"But that's mine," he said in a confused voice. "That's only for my eyes. I—Gretchen said she would never—" Abruptly Dr. Blaise Skiaki spoke in a tone accustomed to command: "Gretchen, what the hell are you doing here? What's this place? Who are these creatures? What's going on?"

When the police arrived they found three dead bodies and a composed Gretchen Nunn sitting with a laser pistol in her lap. She told a perfectly coherent story of forcible entry, an attempt at armed rape and robbery, and how she was constrained to meet force with force. There were a few loopholes in her account. The bodies were not armed, but if the men had said they were armed Miss Nunn, of course, would have believed them. The three were somewhat battered, but goons were always fighting. Miss Nunn was commended for her courage and cooperation.

After her final report to the Chairman (which was not the truth, the whole truth and nothing but the truth) Miss Nunn received her check and went directly to the perfume laboratory, which she entered without warning. Dr. Skiaki was doing strange mysterious things with pipettes, flasks, and reagent bottles. Without turning he ordered. "Out. Out. Out."

"Good morning, Dr. Skiaki."

He turned, displaying a mauled face and black eyes, and smiled. "Well, well, well. The famous Gretchen Nunn, I presume. Voted Person of the Year three times in succession."

"No, sir. People from my class don't have last names."

"Knock off the sir bit."

"Yes s—Mr. Wish."

"Oi!" He winced. "Don't remind me of that incredible insanity. How did everything go with the Chairman?"

"I snowed him. You're off the hook."

"Maybe I'm off his hook but not my own. I was seriously thinking of having myself committed this morning."

"What stopped you?"

"Well, I got involved in this patchouli synthesis and sort of forgot."

She laughed. "You don't have to worry. You're saved."

"You mean cured?"

"No, Blaise. Not any more than I'm cured of my blindness. But we're both saved because we're aware. We can cope now."

He nodded slowly but not happily.

"So what are you going to do today?" she asked cheerfully. "Struggle with patchouli?"

"No," he said gloomily. "I'm still in one hell of a shock. I think I'll take the day off."

"Perfect. Bring two dinners."

HOBSON'S CHOICE

This is a warning to accomplices like you, and me, and Addyer.

Can you spare price of one cup coffee, honorable sir? I am indigent organism which are hungering.

By day, Addyer was a statistician. He concerned himself with such matters as statistical tables, averages and dispersions, groups that are not homogeneous, and random sampling. At night, Addyer plunged into an elaborate escape fantasy divided into two parts. Either he imagined himself moved back in time a hundred years with a double armful of the *Encyclopaedia Britannica*, best-sellers, hit plays, and gambling records; or else he imagined himself transported forward in time a thousand years to the Golden Age of perfection.

There were other fantasies which Addyer entertained on odd Thursdays, such as (by a fluke) becoming the only man left on earth with a world of passionate beauties to fecundate; such as acquiring the power of invisibility which would enable him to rob banks and right wrongs with impunity; such as possessing the mysterious power of working miracles.

Up to this point you and I and Addyer are identical. Where we part company is in the fact that Addyer was a statistician.

Can you spare cost of one cup coffee, honorable miss?
For blessed charitability? I am beholden.

On Monday, Addyer rushed into his chief's office, waving a sheaf of papers. "Look here, Mr. Grande," Addyer sputtered. "I've found something fishy. Extremely fishy . . . In the statistical sense, that is."

"Oh, hell," Grande answered. "You're not supposed to be finding anything. We're in between statistics until the war's over."

"I was leafing through the Interior Department's reports. D'you know our population's up?"

"Not after the atom bomb it isn't," said Grande. "We've lost double what our birthrate can replace." He pointed out the window to the twenty-five-foot stub of the Washington Monument. "There's your documentation."

"But our population's up 3.0915 percent." Addyer displayed his figures. "What about that, Mr. Grande?"

"Must be a mistake somewhere," Grande muttered after a moment's inspection. "You'd better check."

"Yes, sir," said Addyer scurrying out of the office. "I knew you'd be interested, sir. You're the ideal statistician, sir." He was gone.

"Poop," said Grande and once again began computing the quantity of bored respirations left to him. It was his personalized anesthesia.

On Tuesday, Addyer discovered that there was no correlation between the mortality/birthrate ratio and the population increase. The war was multiplying mortality and reducing births; yet the population was minutely increasing. Addyer displayed his discovery to Grande, received a pat on the back, and went home to a new fantasy in which he woke up a million years in the future, learned the answer to the enigma, and decided to remain amid snow-capped mountains and snow-capped bosoms, safe under the aegis of a culture saner than Aureomycin.

On Wednesday, Addyer requisitioned the comptometer and file and ran a test check on Washington, D.C. To his dismay he discovered that the population of the former capital was down 0.0029 percent. This was distressing, and Addyer went home to escape into

a dream about Queen Victoria's Golden Age where he amazed and confounded the world with his brilliant output of novels, plays, and poetry, all cribbed from Shaw, Galsworthy, and Wilde.

> *Can you spare price of one coffee, honorable sir? I am*
> *distressed individual needful of chariting.*

On Thursday, Addyer tried another check, this time on the city of Philadelphia. He discovered that Philadelphia's population was up 0.0959 percent. Very encouraging. He tried a rundown on Little Rock. Population up 1.1329 percent. He tested St. Louis. Population up 2.0924 percent . . . and this despite the complete extinction of Jefferson County owing to one of those military mistakes of an excessive nature.

"My God!" Addyer exclaimed, trembling with excitement. "The closer I get to the center of the country, the greater the increase. But it was the center of the country that took the heaviest punishment in the buz-raid. What's the answer?"

That night he shuttled back and forth between the future and the past in his ferment, and he was down at the shop by 7 A.M. He put a twenty-four-hour claim on the compo and files. He followed up his hunch and he came up with a fantastic discovery which he graphed in approved form. On the map of the remains of the United States he drew concentric circles in colors illustrating the areas of population increase. The red, orange, yellow, green, and blue circles formed a perfect target around Finney County, Kansas.

"Mr. Grande," Addyer shouted in a high statistical passion, "Finney County has got to explain this."

"You go out there and get that explanation," Grande replied, and Addyer departed.

"Poop," muttered Grande and began integrating his pulse rate with his eye-blink.

> *Can you spare price of one coffee, dearly madam? I am*
> *starveling organism requiring nutritiousment.*

Now, travel in those days was hazardous. Addyer took ship to Charleston (there were no rail connections remaining in the North Atlantic states) and was wrecked off Hatteras by a rogue mine. He drifted in the icy waters for seventeen hours, muttering through his teeth: "Oh, Christ! If only I'd been born a hundred years ago."

Apparently this form of prayer was potent. He was picked up by a navy sweeper and shipped to Charleston where he arrived just in time to acquire a subcritical radiation burn from a raid which fortunately left the railroad unharmed. He was treated for the burn from Charleston to Macon (change) from Birmingham to Memphis (bubonic plague) to Little Rock (polluted water) to Tulsa (fallout quarantine) to Kansas City (the O.K. Bus Co. Accepts No Liability for Lives Lost through Acts of War) to Lyonesse, Finney County, Kansas.

And there he was in Finney County with its great magma pits and scars and radiation streaks; whole farms blackened and razed; whole highways so blasted they looked like dotted lines; whole population 4-F. Clouds of soot and fallout neutralizers hung over Finney County by day, turning it into a Pittsburgh on a still afternoon. Auras of radiation glowed at night, highlighted by the blinking red warning beacons, turning the county into one of those overexposed night photographs, all blurred and cross-hatched by deadly slashes of light.

After a restless night in the Lyonesse Hotel, Addyer went over to the county seat for a check on their birth records. He was armed with the proper credentials, but the county seat was not armed with the statistics. That excessive military mistake again. It had extinguished the seat.

A little annoyed, Addyer marched off to the County Medical Association office. His idea was to poll the local doctors on births. There was an office and one attendant who had been a practical nurse. He informed Addyer that Finney County had lost its last doctor to the army eight months previous. Midwives might be the answer to the birth enigma but there was no record of midwives. Addyer would simply have to canvass from door to door, asking if any lady within practiced that ancient profession.

Further piqued, Addyer returned to the Lyonesse Hotel and wrote on a slip of tissue paper: HAVING DATA DIFFICULTIES. WILL

REPORT AS SOON AS INFORMATION AVAILABLE. He slipped the message into an aluminum capsule, attached it to his sole surviving carrier pigeon, and dispatched it to Washington with a prayer. Then he sat down at his window and brooded.

He was aroused by a curious sight. In the street below, the O.K. Bus Co. had just arrived from Kansas City. The old coach wheezed to a stop, opened its door with some difficulty and permitted a one-legged farmer to emerge. His burned face was freshly bandaged. Evidently this was a well-to-do burgess who could afford to travel for medical treatment. The bus backed up for the return trip to Kansas City and honked a warning horn. That was when the curious sight began.

From nowhere . . . absolutely nowhere . . . a horde of people appeared. They skipped from back alleys, from behind rubble piles; they popped out of stores, they filled the street. They were all jolly, healthy, brisk, happy. They laughed and chatted as they climbed into the bus. They looked like hikers and tourists, carrying knapsacks, carpetbags, box lunches, and even babies. In two minutes the bus was filled. It lurched off down the road, and as it disappeared Addyer heard happy singing break out and echo from the walls of rubble.

"I'll be damned," he said.

He hadn't heard spontaneous singing in over two years. He hadn't seen a carefree smile in over three years. He felt like a color-blind man who was seeing the full spectrum for the first time. It was uncanny. It was also a little blasphemous.

"Don't those people know there's a war on?" he asked himself.

And a little later: "They looked too healthy. Why aren't they in uniform?"

And last of all: "Who *were* they anyway?"

That night Addyer's fantasy was confused.

Can you spare price of one cup coffee, kindly sir? I am estrangered and faintly from hungering.

The next morning Addyer arose early, hired a car at an exorbitant fee, found he could not buy any fuel at any price, and ultimately settled for a lame horse. He was allergic to horse dander

and suffered asthmatic tortures as he began his house-to-house canvass. He was discouraged when he returned to the Lyonesse Hotel that afternoon. He was just in time to witness the departure of the O.K. Bus Co.

Once again a horde of happy people appeared and boarded the bus. Once again the bus hirpled off down the broken road. Once again the joyous singing broke out.

"I *will* be damned," Addyer wheezed.

He dropped into the county surveyor's office for a large-scale map of Finney County. It was his intent to plot the midwife coverage in accepted statistical manner. There was a little difficulty with the surveyor who was deaf, blind in one eye, and spectacleless in the other. He could not read Addyer's credentials with any faculty or facility. As Addyer finally departed with the map, he said to himself, "I think the old idiot thought I was a spy."

And later he muttered, "Spies?"

And just before bedtime: "Holy Moses! Maybe *that's* the answer to *them*."

That night he was Lincoln's secret agent, anticipating Lee's every move, outwitting Jackson, Johnston, and Beauregard, foiling John Wilkes Booth, and being elected President of the United States by 1968.

The next day the O.K. Bus Co. carried off yet another load of happy people.

And the next.

And the next.

"Four hundred tourists in five days," Addyer computed. "The country's filled with espionage."

He began loafing around the streets trying to investigate these joyous travelers. It was difficult. They were elusive before the bus arrived. They had a friendly way of refusing to pass the time. The locals of Lyonesse knew nothing about them and were not interested. Nobody was interested in much more than painful survival these days. That was what made the singing obscene.

After seven days of cloak-and-dagger and seven days of counting, Addyer suddenly did the big take. "It adds up," he said. "Eighty people a day leaving Lyonesse. Five hundred a week. Twenty-five thousand a year. Maybe that's the answer to the population in-

crease." He spent fifty-five dollars on a telegram to Grande with no more than a hope of delivery. The telegram read: "EUREKA: I HAVE FOUND (IT)."

Can you spare price of lone cup coffee, honorable madam? I am not tramp-handler but destitute life form.

Addyer's opportunity came the next day. The O.K. Bus Co. pulled in as usual. Another crowd assembled to board the bus, but this time there were too many. Three people were refused passage. They weren't in the least annoyed. They stepped back, waved energetically as the bus started, shouted instructions for future reunions and then quietly turned and started off down the street.

Addyer was out of his hotel room like a shot. He followed the trio down the main street, turned left after them onto Fourth Avenue, passed the ruined schoolhouse, passed the demolished telephone building, passed the gutted library, railroad station, Protestant church, Catholic church . . . and finally reached the outskirts of Lyonesse and then open country.

Here he had to be more cautious. It was difficult stalking the spies with so much of the dusky road illuminated by warning lights. He wasn't suicidal enough to think of hiding in radiation pits. He hung back in an agony of indecision and was at last relieved to see them turn off the broken road and enter the old Baker farmhouse.

"Ah-ha!" said Addyer.

He sat down at the edge of the road on the remnants of a missile and asked himself: "Ah-ha what?" He could not answer, but he knew where to find the answer. He waited until dusk deepened to darkness and then slowly wormed his way forward toward the farmhouse.

It was while he was creeping between the deadly radiation glows and only occasionally butting his head against grave markers that he first became aware of two figures in the night. They were in the barnyard of the Baker place and were performing most peculiarly. One was tall and thin. A man. He stood stock-still, like a lighthouse. Upon occasion he took a slow, stately step with infinite caution and waved an arm in slow motion to the other figure. The

second was also a man. He was stocky and trotted jerkily back and forth.

As Addyer approached, he heard the tall man say: "Rooo booo fooo mooo hwaaa looo fooo."

Whereupon the trotter chattered, "Wd-nk-kd-ik-md-pd-ld-nk."

Then they both laughed: the tall man like a locomotive, the trotter like a chipmunk. They turned. The trotter rocketed into the house. The tall man drifted in. And that was amazingly that.

"Oh-ho," said Addyer.

At that moment a pair of hands seized him and lifted him from the ground. Addyer's heart constricted. He had time for one convulsive spasm before something vague was pressed against his face. As he lost consciousness his last idiotic thought was of telescopes.

Can you spare price of solitary coffee for no-loafing unfortunate, honorable sir? Charity will blessings.

When Addyer awoke he was lying on a couch in a small whitewashed room. A gray-haired gentleman with heavy features was seated at a desk alongside the couch, busily ciphering on bits of paper. The desk was cluttered with what appeared to be intricate timetables. There was a small radio perched on one side.

"L-Listen . . ." Addyer began faintly.

"Just a minute, Mr. Addyer," the gentleman said pleasantly. He fiddled with the radio. A glow germinated in the middle of the room over a circular copper plate and coalesced into a girl. She was extremely nude and extremely attractive. She scurried to the desk, patted the gentleman's head with the speed of a pneumatic hammer. She laughed and chattered, "Wd-nk-tk-ik-lt-nk."

The gray-haired man smiled and pointed to the door. "Go outside and walk it off," he said. She turned and streaked through the door.

"It has something to do with temporal rates," the gentleman said to Addyer. "I don't understand it. When they come forward they've got accumulated momentum." He began ciphering again. "Why in the world did you have to come snooping, Mr. Addyer?"

"You're spies," Addyer said. "She was talking Chinese."

"Hardly. I'd say it was French. Early French. Middle fifteenth century."

"Middle fifteenth century!" Addyer exclaimed.

"That's what I'd say. You begin to acquire an ear for those stepped-up tempos. Just a minute, please."

He switched the radio on again. Another glow appeared and solidified into a nude man. He was stout, hairy, and lugubrious. With exasperating slowness he said, "Mooo fooo blooo wawww hawww pooo."

The gray-haired man pointed to the door. The stout man departed in slow motion.

"The way I see it," the gray-haired man continued conversationally, "when they come back they're swimming against the time current. That slows 'em down. When they come forward, they're swimming with the current. That speeds 'em up. Of course, in any case it doesn't last longer than a few minutes. It wears off."

"What?" Addyer said. "Time travel?"

"Yes. Of course."

"That thing . . ." Addyer pointed to the radio. "A time machine?"

"That's the idea. Roughly."

"But it's too small."

The gray-haired man laughed.

"What is this place anyway? What are you up to?"

"It's a funny thing," the gray-haired man said. "Everybody used to speculate about time travel. How it would be used for exploration, archaeology, historical, and social research, and so on. Nobody ever guessed what the real use would be. . . . Therapy."

"Therapy? You mean medical therapy?"

"That's right. Psychological therapy for the misfits who won't respond to any other cure. We let them emigrate. Escape. We've set up stations every quarter century. Stations like this."

"I don't understand."

"This is an immigration office."

"Oh, my God!" Addyer shot up from the couch. "Then you're the answer to the population increase. Yes? That's how I happened to notice it. Mortality's up so high and birth's down so low these days that your time-addition becomes significant. Yes?"

"Yes, Mr. Addyer."

"Thousands of you coming here. From where?"

"From the future, of course. Time travel wasn't developed until c/h 127. That's . . . oh, say, A.D. 2505 your chronology. We didn't set up our chain of stations until c/h 189."

"But those fast-moving ones. You said they came forward from the past."

"Oh, yes, but they're all from the future originally. They just decided they went too far back."

"Too far?"

The gray-haired man nodded and reflected. "It's amusing, the mistakes people will make. They become unrealistic when they read history. Lose contact with facts. Chap I knew . . . wouldn't be satisfied with anything less than Elizabethan times. 'Shakespeare,' he said. 'Good Queen Bess. Spanish Armada. Drake and Hawkins and Raleigh. Most virile period in history. The Golden Age. That's for me.' I couldn't talk sense into him, so we sent him back. Too bad."

"Well?" Addyer asked.

"Oh, he died in three weeks. Drank a glass of water. Typhoid."

"You didn't inoculate him? I mean, the army when it sends men overseas always . . ."

"Of course we did. Gave him all the immunization we could. But diseases evolve and change too. New strains develop. Old strains disappear. That's what causes pandemics. Evidently our shots wouldn't take against the Elizabethan typhoid. Excuse me. . . ."

Again the glow appeared. Another nude man appeared, chattered briefly and then whipped through the door. He almost collided with the nude girl who poked her head in, smiled and called in a curious accent, "le vous prie de me pardonner. Quy estoit cette gentilhomme?"

"I was right," the gray-haired man said. "That's Medieval French. They haven't spoken like that since Rabelais." To the girl he said, "Middle English, please. The American dialect."

"Oh, I'm sorry, Mr. Jelling. I get so damned fouled up with my linguistics. Fouled? Is that right? Or do they say . . ."

"Hey!" Addyer cried in anguish.

"They say it, but only in private these years. Not before strangers."

"Oh, yes. I remember. Who was that gentleman who just left?"

"Peters."

"From Athens?"

"That's right."

"Didn't like it, eh?"

"Not much. Seems the Peripatetics didn't have plumbing."

"Yes. You begin to hanker for a modern bathroom after a while. Where do I get some clothes . . . or don't they wear clothes this century?"

"No, that's a hundred years forward. Go see my wife. She's in the outfitting room in the barn. That's the big red building."

The tall lighthouse-man Addyer had first seen in the farmyard suddenly manifested himself behind the girl. He was now dressed and moving at normal speed. He stared at the girl; she stared at him. "Splem!" they both cried. They embraced and kissed shoulders.

"St'u my rock-ribbering rib-rockery to heart the hearts two," the man said.

"Heart's too, argal, too heart," the girl laughed.

"Eh? Then you st'u too."

They embraced again and left.

"What was that? Future talk?" Addyer asked. "Shorthand?"

"Shorthand?" Jelling exclaimed in a surprised tone. "Don't you know rhetoric when you hear it? That was thirtieth-century rhetoric, man. We don't talk anything else up there. Prosthesis, Diastole, Epergesis, Metabasis, Hendiadys . . . And we're all born scanning."

"You don't have to sound so stuck up," Addyer muttered enviously. "I could scan too if I tried."

"You'd find it damned inconvenient trying at your time of life."

"What difference would that make?"

"It would make a big difference," Jelling said, "because you'd find that living is the sum of conveniences. You might think plumbing is pretty unimportant compared to ancient Greek philosophers. Lots of people do. But the fact is, we already know the philosophy. After a while you get tired of seeing the great men and listening to them expound the material you already know. You begin to miss

the conveniences and familiar patterns you used to take for granted."

"That," said Addyer, "is a superficial attitude."

"You think so? Try living in the past by candlelight, without central heating, without refrigeration, canned foods, elementary drugs . . . Or, futurewise, try living with Berganlicks, the Twenty-Two Commandments, duodecimal calendars and currency, or try speaking in meter, planning and scanning each sentence before you talk . . . and damned for a contemptible illiterate if you forget yourself and speak spontaneously in your own tongue."

"You're exaggerating," Addyer said. "I'll bet there are times where I could be very happy. I've thought about it for years, and I . . ."

"Tcha!" Jelling snorted. "The great illusion. Name one."

"The American Revolution."

"Pfui! No sanitation. No medicine. Cholera in Philadelphia. Malaria in New York. No anesthesia. The death penalty for hundreds of small crimes and petty infractions. None of the books and music you like best. None of the jobs or professions for which you've been trained. Try again."

"The Victorian Age."

"How are your teeth and eyes? In good shape? They'd better be. We can't send your inlays and spectacles back with you. How are your ethics? In bad shape? They'd better be or you'd starve in that cutthroat era. How do you feel about class distinctions? They were pretty strong in those days. What's your religion? You'd better not be a Jew or Catholic or Quaker or Moravian or any minority. What's your politics? If you're a reactionary today the same opinions would make you a dangerous radical a hundred years ago. I don't think you'd be happy."

"I'd be safe."

"Not unless you were rich; and we can't send money back. Only the flesh. No, Addyer, the poor died at the average age of forty in those days . . . worked out, worn out. Only the privileged survived, and you wouldn't be one of the privileged."

"Not with my superior knowledge?"

Jelling nodded wearily. "I knew *that* would come up sooner or

later. What superior knowledge? Your hazy recollection of science and invention? Don't be a damned fool, Addyer. You enjoy your technology without the faintest idea of how it works."

"It wouldn't have to be hazy recollection. I could prepare."

"What, for instance?"

"Oh . . . say, the radio. I could make a fortune inventing the radio."

Jelling smiled. "You couldn't invent radio until you'd first invented the hundred allied technical discoveries that went into it. You'd have to create an entire new industrial world. You'd have to discover the vacuum rectifier and create an industry to manufacture it; the self-heterodyne circuit, the nonradiating neutrodyne receiver and so forth. You'd have to develop electric power production and transmission and alternating current. You'd have to—but why belabor the obvious? Could you invent internal combustion before the development of fuel oils?"

"My God!" Addyer groaned.

"And another thing," Jelling went on grimly. "I've been talking about technological tools, but language is a tool too; the tool of communication. Did you ever realize that all the studying you might do could never teach you how a language was really used centuries ago? Do you know how the Romans pronounced Latin? Do you know the Greek dialects? Could you learn to speak and think in Gaelic, seventeenth-century Flemish, Old Low German? Never. You'd be a deaf-mute."

"I never thought about it that way," Addyer said slowly.

"Escapists never do. All they're looking for is a vague excuse to run away."

"What about books? I could memorize a great book and . . ."

"And what? Go back far enough into the past to anticipate the real author? You'd be anticipating the public too. A book doesn't become great until the public's ready to understand it. It doesn't become profitable until the public's ready to buy it."

"What about going forward into the future?" Addyer asked.

"I've already told you. It's the same problem only in reverse. Could a medieval man survive in the twentieth century? Could he stay alive in street traffic? Drive cars? Speak the language? Think

in the language? Adapt to the tempo, ideas, and coordinations you take for granted? Never. Could someone from the twenty-fifth century adapt to the thirtieth? Never."

"Well, then," Addyer said angrily, "if the past and future are so uncomfortable, what are those people traveling around for?"

"They're not traveling," Jelling said. "They're running."

"From what?"

"Their own time."

"Why?"

"They don't like it."

"Why not?"

"Do you like yours? Does any neurotic?"

"Where are they going?"

"Any place but where they belong. They keep looking for the Golden Age. Tramps! Time stiffs! Never satisfied. Always searching, shifting . . . bumming through the centuries. Pfui! Half the panhandlers you meet are probably time bums stuck in the wrong century."

"And those people coming here . . . they think *this* is a Golden Age?"

"They do."

"They're crazy," Addyer protested. "Have they seen the ruins? The radiation? The war? The anxiety? The hysteria?"

"Sure. That's what appeals to them. Don't ask me why. Think of it this way: you like the American Colonial period, yes?"

"Among others."

"Well, if you told Mr. George Washington the reasons why you liked his time, you'd probably be naming everything he hated about it."

"But that's not a fair comparison. This is the worst age in all history."

Jelling waved his hand. "That's how it looks to you. Everybody says that in every generation; but take my word for it, no matter when you live and how you live, there's always somebody else somewhere else who thinks you live in the Golden Age."

"Well, I'll be damned," Addyer said.

Jelling looked at him steadily for a moment. "You will be," he

said sorrowfully. "I've got bad news for you, Addyer. We can't let you remain. You'll talk and make trouble, and our secret's got to be kept. We'll have to send you out one-way."

"I can talk wherever I go."

"But nobody'll pay attention to you outside your own time. You won't make sense. You'll be an eccentric . . . a lunatic . . . a foreigner . . . safe."

"What if I come back?"

"You won't be able to get back without a visa, and I'm not tattooing any visa on you. You won't be the first we've had to transport if that's any consolation to you. There was a Japanese, I remember . . ."

"Then you're going to send me somewhere in time? Permanently?"

"That's right. I'm really very sorry."

"To the future or the past?"

"You can take your choice. Think it over while you're getting undressed."

"You don't have to act so mournful," Addyer said. "It's a great adventure. A high adventure. It's something I've always dreamed."

"That's right. It's going to be wonderful."

"I could refuse," Addyer said nervously.

Jelling shook his head. "We'd only drug you and send you anyway. It might as well be your choice."

"It's a choice I'm delighted to make."

"Sure. That's the spirit, Addyer."

"Everybody says I was born a hundred years too soon."

"Everybody generally says that . . . unless they say you were born a hundred years too late."

"Some people say that too."

"Well, think it over. It's a permanent move. Which would you prefer . . . the phonetic future or the poetic past?"

Very slowly Addyer began to undress as he undressed each night when he began the prelude to his customary fantasy. But now his dreams were faced with fulfillment and the moment of decision terrified him. He was a little blue and rather unsteady on his legs when he stepped to the copper disk in the center of the floor. In answer to Jelling's inquiry he muttered his choice. Then he turned

argent in the aura of an incandescent glow and disappeared from his time forever.

Where did he go? You know. I know. Addyer knows. Addyer traveled to the land of our pet fantasy. He escaped into the refuge that is our refuge, to the time of our dreams; and in practically no time at all he realized that he had in truth departed from the only time for himself.

Through the vistas of the years every age but our own seems glamorous and golden. We yearn for the yesterdays and tomorrows, never realizing that we are faced with Hobson's choice . . . that to-day, bitter or sweet, anxious or calm, is the only day for us. The dream of time is the traitor, and we are all accomplices to the betrayal of ourselves.

Can you spare price of one coffee, honorable sir? No, sir, I am not panhandling organism. I am starveling Japanese transient stranded in this somiserable year. Honorable sir! I beg in tears for holy charity. Will you donate to this destitute person one ticket to township of Lyonesse? I want to beg on knees for visa. I want to go back to year 1945 again. I want to be in Hiroshima again. I want to go home.

RAY BRADBURY

b. 1920

Ray Bradbury was born in Waukegan, Illinois, a town which also gave the world Jack Benny (and both these men have left their names on bits of the city's geography). When Bradbury was fourteen, the Great Depression sat heavily on the land. Jobs were scarce in the Midwest, and so Bradbury's father took the family to California in the hope of brighter prospects. Employment wasn't markedly easier in California, but there young Ray Bradbury found something that changed his life. He discovered, and entered, the world of science fiction fandom.

The people—mostly youngsters—who went out of their way to read science fiction in those days were a special breed, unlike the readers of any other kind of literature. They were a lot less passive. They habitually wrote letters to the editors of their magazines (every sf magazine contained a letter column, often the first thing those readers turned to when a new issue appeared). They sought out other like-minded readers, and they formed clubs—correspondence clubs for those in out of the way parts of the world, regular get-togethers in the flesh for those in communities large enough to support a fan population. The center of fannish activities in Los Angeles was the Los Angeles Science Fantasy Society (and still is; LASFS is still meeting regularly more than sixty years later). Young Ray immersed himself in the group. He joined it at seventeen, at nineteen began publishing his own science fiction fan magazine, *Futuria Fantasia*. He filled the fanzine with his own stories, but before long began sending them off to the professional magazines, collected his share of rejections and, in 1941, made his first sale. It

was a collaboration with Henry Hasse, "Pendulum," and with it Ray was on his way.

Unusually for his generation of science fiction writers, Ray Bradbury was not a part of John Campbell's "Golden Age" of *Astounding*; Bradbury's poetic brand of sf was not to Campbell's taste. It was to everyone else's, though. His stories appeared in *Planet Stories*, *Thrilling Wonder Stories*, *Weird Tales*, and nearly every other magazine of science fiction or fantasy for the next half-dozen years. They were workmanlike shorts, appreciated by editors and enjoyed by readers, but it wasn't until 1946 that Bradbury published the story that lifted him out of the pack. The piece was called "The Million Year Picnic," and it turned out to be the first installment of his most famous work, *The Martian Chronicles*.

The Mars of Bradbury's *Chronicles* is not much like the one currently being explored by the real world's telescopes and space probes. Physically Bradbury's Mars is a lot like the American Midwest of his childhood, plus canals. Unlike the real Mars, it is inhabited, and its people have the capacity to change shape—conveniently making themselves look like the human colonists when they chose. As a book, *The Martian Chronicles* is indestructible. It has been continuously in print for forty years, has been filmed for TV, and translated into dozens of foreign languages.

By the time the book appeared Bradbury had begun to move out of the science fiction magazines, with his work appearing in such mass circulation slicks as *Collier's* and *The Saturday Evening Post*, big glossy weeklies which were the prestige markets of the time—with correspondingly fatter paychecks. In 1951 he returned to the science fiction magazine *Galaxy* with a novella called "The Fireman," a sort of tangential response to the flamboyant witch-hunts of Senator McCarthy; in the story, books have become forbidden, and the "Fireman," charged with the duty of seeking out and burning libraries, is himself a secret reader. Expanded to book length and published (and filmed) as *Fahrenheit 451*, it became Bradbury's other masterwork.

There is a curious subtext to Bradbury's work, evident in both *The Martian Chronicles* and *Fahrenheit 451*. By and large, science fiction

writers celebrate technology. Ray Bradbury does not. In his stories the gadgets and machines of the future are dehumanizing. Virtue lies in the simpler, gentler times of his midwestern childhood. Bradbury himself is sufficiently hostile to technology that for many years (like that other Grand Master, Isaac Asimov) he refused to fly. Even more unusual, he may be the only Californian alive who declines to drive a car, for most of his life biking or taking taxis around the sprawling city of Los Angeles. (When he and I were walking along the streets of Century City some years ago, a sizable fraction of the cab drivers who drove past us waved greetings to Ray.)

Ray Bradbury was, however, Californian enough to become active in the film industry from early on, writing (or sharing the writing of) such sci-fi films of the early 1950s as *The Beast from 20,000 Fathoms* and *It came from Outer Space*. In 1956 he collaborated with John Huston on a major project, the filming of one of the great classics of American literature, Herman Melville's *Moby Dick*. More recently he has had his own television series and has been deeply involved in creating images for the Walt Disney theme parks.

Almost from the beginning Bradbury's work explored areas of writing outside of science fiction, as shown in such collections and novels as *Dandelion Wine*, *Something Wicked This Way Comes*, and *The Illustrated Man*. After the 1950s he wrote little that was purely science fiction. Nevertheless for generations of Americans, who were learning the pleasures of reading from the flood of schoolbook texts which nearly unanimously included Bradbury stories, he represented their first encounter with science fiction.

Ray Bradbury is a unique voice, in science fiction and in the world, and he is indeed a Grand Master.

Recommended Reading
by Ray Bradbury

Fahrenheit 451
The Martian Chronicles
The Illustrated Man
Something Wicked This Way Comes
Dandelion Wine

THE CITY

The city waited twenty thousand years.

The planet moved through space and the flowers of the fields grew up and fell away, and still the city waited; and the rivers of the planet rose and waned and turned to dust. Still the city waited. The winds that had been young and wild grew old and serene, and the clouds of the sky that had been ripped and torn were left alone to drift in idle whitenesses. Still the city waited.

The city waited with its windows and its black obsidian walls and its sky towers and its unpennanted turrets, with its untrod streets and its untouched doorknobs, with not a scrap of paper or a fingerprint upon it. The city waited while the planet arced in space, following its orbit about a blue-white sun, and the seasons passed from ice to fire and back to ice and then to green fields and yellow summer meadows.

It was on a summer afternoon in the middle of the twenty-thousandth year that the city ceased waiting.

In the sky a rocket appeared.

The rocket soared over, turned, came back, and landed in the shale meadow fifty yards from the obsidian wall.

There were booted footsteps in the thin grass and calling voices from men within the rocket to men without.

"Ready?"

"All right, men. Careful! Into the city. Jensen, you and Hutch-inson patrol ahead. Keep a sharp eye."

The city opened secret nostrils in its black walls and a steady suction vent deep in the body of the city drew storms of air back through channels, through thistle filters and dust collectors, to a fine and tremblingly delicate series of coils and webs which glowed with silver light. Again and again the immense suctions occurred; again and again the odors from the meadow were borne upon warm winds into the city.

"Fire odor, the scent of a fallen meteor, hot metal. A ship has come from another world. The brass smell, the dusty fire smell of burned powder, sulphur and rocket brimstone."

This information, stamped on tapes which sprocketed into slots, slid down through yellow cogs into further machines.

Click-chakk-chakk-chakk.

A calculator made the sound of a metronome. Five, six, seven, eight, nine. Nine men! An instantaneous typewriter inked this message on tape which slithered and vanished.

Clickety-click-chakk-chakk.

The city awaited the soft tread of their rubberoid boots.

The great city nostrils dilated again.

The smell of butter. In the city air, from the stalking men, faintly, the aura which wafted to the great Nose broke down into memories of milk, cheese, ice cream, butter, the effluvia of a dairy economy.

Click-click.

"Careful, men!"

"Jones, get your gun out. Don't be a fool!"

"The city's dead; why worry?"

"You can't tell."

Now, at the barking talk, the Ears awoke. After centuries of listening to winds that blew small and faint, of hearing leaves strip from trees and grass grow softly in the time of melting snows, now the Ears oiled themselves in a self-lubrication, drew taut, great drums upon which the heartbeat of the invaders might pummel and thud delicately as the tremor of a gnat's wing. The Ears listened and the Nose siphoned up great chambers of odor.

The perspiration of frightened men arose. There were islands

of sweat under their arms, and sweat in their hands as they held their guns.

The Nose sifted and worried this air, like a connoisseur busy with an ancient vintage.

Chikk-chikk-chakk-click.

Information rotated down on parallel check tapes. Perspiration; chlorides such-and-such percent; sulphates so-and-so; urea nitrogen, ammonia nitrogen. *thus:* creatinine, sugar, lactic acid, *there!*

Bells rang. Small totals jumped up.

The Nose whispered, expelling the tested air. The great Ears listened:

"I think we should go back to the rocket, Captain."

"I give the orders, Mr. Smith!"

"Yes, sir."

"You, up there! Patrol! *See* anything?"

"Nothing, sir. Looks like it's been dead a long time!"

"You see, Smith? Nothing to fear."

"I don't like it. I don't know why. You ever feel you've seen a place before? Well, this city's too familiar."

"Nonsense. This planetary system's billions of miles from Earth; we couldn't possibly've been here ever before. Ours is the only light-year rocket in existence."

"That's how I feel, anyway, sir. I think we should get out."

The footsteps faltered. There was only the sound of the intruder's breath on the still air.

The Ear heard and quickened. Rotors glided, liquids glittered in small creeks through valves and blowers. A formula and a concoction—one followed another. Moments later, responding to the summons of the Ear and Nose, through giant holes in the city walls a fresh vapor blew out over the invaders.

"Smell *that,* Smith? Ahh. Green grass. Ever smell anything better? By God, I just like to stand here and smell it."

Invisible chlorophyll blew among the standing men.

"*Ahh!*"

The footsteps continued.

"Nothing wrong with *that,* eh, Smith? Come on!"

The Ear and Nose relaxed a billionth of a fraction. The countermove had succeeded. The pawns were proceeding forward.

•   •   •

Now the cloudy Eyes of the city moved out of fog and mist.

"Captain, the windows!"

"What?"

"Those house windows, there! I saw them move!"

"*I* didn't see it."

"They shifted. They changed color. From dark to light."

"Look like ordinary square windows to me."

Blurred objects focused. In the mechanical ravines of the city oiled shafts plunged, balance wheels dipped over into green oil pools. The window frames flexed. The windows gleamed.

Below, in the street, walked two men, a patrol, followed, at a safe interval, by seven more. Their uniforms were white, their faces as pink as if they had been slapped; their eyes were blue. They walked upright, upon hind legs, carrying metal weapons. Their feet were booted. They were males, with eyes, ears, mouths, noses.

The windows trembled. The windows thinned. They dilated imperceptibly, like the irises of numberless eyes.

"I tell you, Captain, it's the windows!"

"Get along."

"I'm going back, sir."

"What?"

"I'm going back to the rocket."

"Mr. Smith!"

"I'm not falling into any trap!"

"Afraid of an empty city?"

The others laughed, uneasily.

"Go on, laugh!"

The street was stone-cobbled, each stone three inches wide, six inches long. With a move unrecognizable as such, the street settled. It weighed the invaders.

In a machine cellar a red wand touched a numeral: 178 pounds . . . 210, 154, 201, 198—each man weighed, registered, and the record spooled down into a correlative darkness.

Now the city was fully awake!

Now the vents sucked and blew air, the tobacco odor from the invaders mouths, the green soap scent from their hands. Even their

eyeballs had a delicate odor. The city detected it, and this information formed totals which scurried down to total other totals. The crystal windows glittered, the Ear tautened and skinned the drum of its hearing tight, tighter—all of the senses of the city swarming like a fall of unseen snow, counting the respiration and the dim hidden heartbeats of the men, listening, watching, tasting.

For the streets were like tongues, and where the men passed, the taste of their heels ebbed down through stone pores to be calculated on litmus. This chemical totality, so subtly collected, was appended to the now increasing sums waiting the final calculation among the whirling wheels and whispering spokes.

Footsteps. Running.

"Come back! Smith!"

"No, blast you!"

"Get him, men!"

Footsteps rushing.

A final test. The city, having listened, watched, tasted, felt, weighed, and balanced, must perform a final task.

A trap flung wide in the street. The captain, unseen by the others, running vanished.

Hung by his feet, a razor drawn across his throat, another down his chest, his carcass instantly emptied of its entrails, exposed upon a table under the street, in a hidden cell, the captain died. Great crystal microscopes stared at the red twines of muscle; bodiless fingers probed the still-pulsing heart. The flaps of his sliced skin were pinned to the table while hands shifted parts of his body like a quick and curious player of chess, using the red pawns and the red pieces.

Above on the street the men ran. Smith ran, men shouted. Smith shouted and below in this curious room blood flowed into capsules, was shaken, spun, shoved on smear slides under further microscopes, counts made, temperatures taken, heart cut in seventeen sections, liver and kidneys expertly halved. Brain was drilled and scooped from bone socket, nerves pulled forth like the dead wires of a switchboard, muscles plucked for elasticity, while in the electric subterrene of the city the Mind at last totaled out its grandest total and all of the machinery ground to a monstrous and momentary halt.

The total.

These are men. These are men from a far world, a certain planet, and they have certain eyes, certain ears, and they walk upon legs in a specified way and carry weapons and think and fight, and they have particular hearts and all such organs as are recorded from long ago.

Above, men ran down the street toward the rocket.

Smith ran.

The total.

These are our enemies. These are the ones we have waited for twenty thousand years to see again. These are the men upon whom we waited to visit revenge. Everything totals. These are the men of a planet called Earth, who declared war upon Taollan twenty thousand years ago, who kept us in slavery and ruined us and destroyed us with a great disease. Then they went off to live in another galaxy to escape that disease which they visited upon us after ransacking our world. They have forgotten that war and that time, and they have forgotten us. But we have not forgotten them. These are our enemies. This is certain. Our waiting is done.

"Smith, come back!"

Quickly. Upon the red table, with the spread-eagled captain's body empty, new hands began a flight of motion. Into the wet interior were placed organs of copper, brass, silver, aluminum, rubber, and silk; spiders spun gold web which was stung into the skin; a heart was attached, and into the skull case was fitted a platinum brain which hummed and fluttered small sparkles of blue fire, and the wires led down through the body to the arms and legs. In a moment the body was sewn tight, the incisions waxed, healed at neck and throat and about the skull—perfect, fresh, new.

The captain sat up and flexed his arms.

"Stop!"

On the street the captain reappeared, raised his gun, and fired.

Smith fell, a bullet in his heart.

The other men turned.

The captain ran to them.

"That fool! Afraid of a city!"

They looked at the body of Smith at their feet.

They looked at their captain, and their eyes widened and narrowed.

"Listen to me," said the captain. "I have something important to tell you."

Now the city, which had weighed and tasted and smelled them, which had used all its powers save one, prepared to use its final ability, the power of speech. It did not speak with the rage and hostility of its massed walls or towers, nor with the bulk of its cobbled avenues and fortresses of machinery. It spoke with the quiet voice of one man.

"I am no longer your captain," he said. "Nor am I a man."

The men moved back.

"I am the city," he said, and smiled.

"I've waited two hundred centuries," he said. "I've waited for the sons of the sons of the sons to return."

"Captain, sir!"

"Let me continue. Who built me? The city. The men who died built me. The old race who once lived here. The people whom the Earth Men left to die of a terrible disease, a form of leprosy with no cure. And the men of that old race, dreaming of the day when Earth Men might return, built this city, and the name of this city was and is Revenge, upon the Planet of Darkness, near the shore of the Sea of Centuries, by the Mountains of the Dead; all very poetic. This city was to be a balancing machine, a litmus, an antenna to test all future space travelers. In twenty thousand years only two other rockets landed here. One from a distant galaxy called Ennt, and the inhabitants of that craft were tested, weighed, found wanting, and let free, unscathed, from the city. As were the visitors in the second ship. But today! At long last, you've come! The revenge will be carried out to the last detail. Those men have been dead two hundred centuries, but they left a city here to welcome you."

"Captain, sir, you're not feeling well. Perhaps you'd better come back to the ship, sir."

The city trembled.

The pavements opened and the men fell, screaming. Falling, they saw bright razors flash to meet them!

Time passed. Soon came the call:

"Smith?"

"Here!"

"Jensen?"

"Here!"

"Jones, Hutchinson, Springer?"

"Here!" "Here!" "Here!"

They stood by the door of the rocket.

"We return to Earth immediately."

"Yes, sir!"

The incisions on their necks were invisible, as were their hidden brass hearts and silver organs and the fine golden wire of their nerves. There was a faint electric hum from their heads.

"On the double!"

Nine men hurried the golden bombs of disease culture into the rocket.

"These are to be dropped on Earth."

"Right, sir!"

The rocket valve slammed. The rocket jumped into the sky.

As the thunder faded, the city lay upon the summer meadow. Its glass eyes were dulled over. The Ear relaxed, the great nostril vents stopped, the streets no longer weighed or balanced, and the hidden machinery paused in its bath of oil.

In the sky the rocket dwindled.

Slowly, pleasurably, the city enjoyed the luxury of dying.

THE MILLION-YEAR PICNIC

Somehow the idea was brought up by Mom that perhaps the whole family would enjoy a fishing trip. But they weren't Mom's words; Timothy knew that. They were Dad's words, and Mom used them for him somehow.

Dad shuffled his feet in a clutter of Martian pebbles and agreed. So immediately there was a tumult and a shouting, and very quickly the camp was tucked into capsules and containers, Mom slipped into traveling jumpers and blouse, Dad stuffed his pipe full with trembling hands, his eyes on the Martian sky, and the three boys piled yelling into the motorboat, none of them really keeping an eye on Mom and Dad, except Timothy.

Dad pushed a stud. The water boat sent a humming sound up into the sky. The water shook back and the boat nosed ahead, and the family cried, "Hurrah!"

Timothy sat in the back of the boat with Dad, his small fingers atop Dad's hairy ones, watching the canal twist, leaving the crumbled place behind where they had landed in their small family rocket all the way from Earth. He remembered the night before they left Earth, the hustling and hurrying, the rocket that Dad had found somewhere, somehow, and the talk of a vacation on Mars. A long way to go for a vacation, but Timothy said nothing because

of his younger brothers. They came to Mars and now, first thing, or so they said, they were going fishing.

Dad had a funny look in his eyes as the boat went up-canal. A look that Timothy couldn't figure. It was made of strong light and maybe a sort of relief. It made the deep wrinkles laugh instead of worry or cry.

So there went the cooling rocket, around a bend, gone.

"How far are we going?" Robert splashed his hand. It looked like a small crab jumping in the violent water.

Dad exhaled. "A million years."

"Gee," said Robert.

"Look, kids." Mother pointed one soft long arm. "There's a dead city."

They looked with fervent anticipation, and the dead city lay dead for them alone, drowsing in a hot silence of summer made on Mars by a Martian weatherman.

And Dad looked as if he was pleased that it was dead.

It was a futile spread of pink rocks sleeping on a rise of sand, a few tumbled pillars, one lonely shrine, and then the sweep of sand again. Nothing else for miles. A white desert around the canal and a blue desert over it.

Just then a bird flew up. Like a stone thrown across a blue pond, hitting, falling deep, and vanishing.

Dad got a frightened look when he saw it. "I thought it was a rocket."

Timothy looked at the deep ocean sky, trying to see Earth and the war and the ruined cities and the men killing each other since the day he was born. But he saw nothing. The war was as removed and far off as two flies battling to the death in the arch of a great high and silent cathedral. And just as senseless.

William Thomas wiped his forehead and felt the touch of his son's hand on his arm, like a young tarantula, thrilled. He beamed at his son. "How goes it, Timmy?"

"Fine, Dad."

Timothy hadn't quite figured out what was ticking inside the vast adult mechanism beside him. The man with the immense hawk nose, sunburnt, peeling—and the hot blue eyes like agate marbles

you play with after school in summer back on Earth, and the long thick columnar legs in the loose riding breeches.

"What are you looking at so hard, Dad?"

"I was looking for Earthian logic, common sense, good government, peace, and responsibility."

"All that up there?"

"No. I didn't find it. It's not there any more. Maybe it'll never be there again. Maybe we fooled ourselves that it was ever there."

"Huh?"

"See the fish," said Dad, pointing.

There rose a soprano clamor from all three boys as they rocked the boat in arching their tender necks to see. They *oobed* and *abed*. A silver ring fish floated by them, undulating, and closing like an iris, instantly, around food particles, to assimilate them.

Dad looked at it. His voice was deep and quiet.

"Just like war. War swims along, sees food, contracts. A moment later—Earth is gone."

"William," said Mom.

"Sorry," said Dad.

They sat still and felt the canal water rush cool, swift, and glassy. The only sound was the motor hum, the glide of water, the sun expanding the air.

"When do we see the Martians?" cried Michael.

"Quite soon, perhaps," said Father. "Maybe tonight."

"Oh, but the Martians are a dead race now," said Mom.

"No, they're not. I'll show you some Martians, all right," Dad said presently.

Timothy scowled at that but said nothing. Everything was odd now. Vacations and fishing and looks between people.

The other boys were already engaged making shelves of their small hands and peering under them toward the seven-foot stone banks of the canal, watching for Martians.

"What do they look like?" demanded Michael.

"You'll know them when you see them." Dad sort of laughed, and Timothy saw a pulse beating time in his cheek.

Mother was slender and soft, with a woven plait of spun-gold hair over her head in a tiara, and eyes the color of the deep cool canal water where it ran in shadow, almost purple, with flecks of amber caught in it. You could see her thoughts swimming around in her eyes, like fish—some bright, some dark, some fast, quick, some slow and easy, and sometimes, like when she looked up where Earth was, being nothing but color and nothing else. She sat in the boat's prow, one hand resting on the side lip, the other on the lap of her dark blue breeches, and a line of sunburnt soft neck showing where her blouse opened like a white flower.

She kept looking ahead to see what was there, and, not being able to see it clearly enough, she looked backward toward her husband, and through his eyes, reflected then, she saw what was ahead; and since he added part of himself to this reflection, a determined firmness, her face relaxed and she accepted it and she turned back, knowing suddenly what to look for.

Timothy looked too. But all he saw was a straight pencil line of canal going violent through a wide shallow valley penned by low, eroded hills, and on until it fell over the sky's edge. And this canal went on and on, through cities that would have rattled like beetles in a dry skull if you shook them. A hundred or two hundred cities dreaming hot summer-day dreams and cool summer-night dreams . . .

They had come millions of miles for this outing—to fish. But there had been a gun on the rocket. This was a vacation. But why all the food, more than enough to last them years and years, left hidden back there near the rocket? Vacation. Just behind the veil of the vacation was not a soft face of laughter, but something hard and bony and perhaps terrifying. Timothy could not lift the veil, and the two other boys were busy being ten and eight years old, respectively.

"No Martians yet. Nuts." Robert put his V-shaped chin on his hands and glared at the canal.

Dad had brought an atomic radio along, strapped to his wrist. It functioned on an old-fashioned principle: you held it against the bones near your ear and it vibrated singing or talking to you. Dad listened to it now. His face looked like one of those fallen Martian cities, caved in, sucked dry, almost dead.

Then he gave it to Mom to listen. Her lips dropped open.

"What—" Timothy started to question, but never finished what he wished to say.

For at that moment there were two titanic, marrow-jolting explosions that grew upon themselves, followed by a half-dozen minor concussions.

Jerking his head up, Dad notched the boat speed higher immediately. The boat leaped and jounced and spanked. This shook Robert out of his funk and elicited yelps of frightened but ecstatic joy from Michael, who clung to Mom's legs and watched the water pour by his nose in a wet torrent.

Dad swerved the boat, cut speed, and ducked the craft into a little branch canal and under an ancient, crumbling stone wharf that smelled of crab flesh. The boat rammed the wharf hard enough to throw them all forward, but no one was hurt, and Dad was already twisted to see if the ripples on the canal were enough to map their route into hiding. Water lines went across, lapped the stones, and rippled back to meet each other, settling, to be dappled by the sun. It all went away.

Dad listened. So did everybody.

Dad's breathing echoed like fists beating against the cold wet wharf stones. In the shadow, Mom's cat eyes just watched Father for some clue to what next.

Dad relaxed and blew out a breath, laughing at himself.

"The rocket, of course. I'm getting jumpy. The rocket."

Michael said, "What happened, Dad, what happened?"

"Oh, we just blew up our rocket, is all," said Timothy, trying to sound matter-of-fact. "I've heard rockets blown up before. Ours just blew."

"Why did we blow up our rocket?" asked Michael. "Huh, Dad?"

"It's part of the game, silly!" said Timothy.

"A game!" Michael and Robert loved the word.

"Dad fixed it so it would blow up and no one'd know where we landed or went! In case they ever came looking, see?"

"Oh boy, a secret!"

"Scared by my own rocket," admitted Dad to Mom. "I am nervous. It's silly to think there'll ever *be* any more rockets. Except *one*, perhaps, if Edwards and his wife get through with *their* ship."

He put his tiny radio to his ear again. After two minutes he dropped his hand as you would drop a rag.

"It's over at last," he said to Mom. "The radio just went off the atomic beam. Every other world station's gone. They dwindled down to a couple in the last few years. Now the air's completely silent. It'll probably remain silent."

"For how long?" asked Robert.

"Maybe—your great-grandchildren will hear it again," said Dad. He just sat there, and the children were caught in the center of his awe and defeat and resignation and acceptance.

Finally he put the boat out into the canal again, and they continued in the direction in which they had originally started.

It was getting late. Already the sun was down the sky, and a series of dead cities lay ahead of them.

Dad talked very quietly and gently to his sons. Many times in the past he had been brisk, distant, removed from them, but now he patted them on the head with just a word and they felt it.

"Mike, pick a city."

"What, Dad?"

"Pick a city, Son. Any one of these cities we pass."

"All right," said Michael. "How do I pick?"

"Pick the one you like the most. You, too, Robert and Tim. Pick the city you like best."

"I want a city with Martians in it," said Michael.

"You'll have that," said Dad. "I promise." His lips were for the children, but his eyes were for Mom.

They passed six cities in twenty minutes. Dad didn't say anything more about the explosions; he seemed much more interested in having fun with his sons, keeping them happy, than anything else.

Michael liked the first city they passed, but this was vetoed because everyone doubted quick first judgments. The second city nobody liked. It was an Earth Man's settlement, built of wood and already rotting into sawdust. Timothy liked the third city because it was large. The fourth and fifth were too small and the sixth brought acclaim from everyone, including Mother, who joined in the Gees, Goshes, and Look-at-thats!

There were fifty or sixty huge structures still standing, streets

were dusty but paved, and you could see one or two old centrifugal fountains still pulsing wetly in the plazas. That was the only life— water leaping in the late sunlight.

"This is the city," said everybody.

Steering the boat to a wharf, Dad jumped out.

"Here we are. This is ours. This is where we live from now on!"

"From now on?" Michael was incredulous. He stood up, look- ing, and then turned to blink back at where the rocket used to be. "What about the rocket? What about Minnesota?"

"Here," said Dad.

He touched the small radio to Michael's blond head. "Listen."

Michael listened.

"Nothing," he said.

"That's right. Nothing. Nothing at all any more. No more Min- neapolis, no more rockets, no more Earth."

Michael considered the lethal revelation and began to sob little dry sobs.

"Wait a moment," said Dad the next instant. "I'm giving you a lot more in exchange, Mike!"

"What?" Michael held off the tears, curious, but quite ready to continue in case Dad's further revelation was as disconcerting as the original.

"I'm giving you this city, Mike. It's yours."

"Mine?"

"For you and Robert and Timothy, all three of you, to own for yourselves."

Timothy bounded from the boat. "Look, guys, all for *us*! All of *that*!" He was playing the game with Dad, playing it large and playing it well. Later, after it was all over and things had settled, he could go off by himself and cry for ten minutes. But now it was still a game, still a family outing, and the other kids must be kept playing.

Mike jumped out with Robert. They helped Mom.

"Be careful of your sister," said Dad, and nobody knew what he meant until later.

They hurried into the great pink-stoned city, whispering among themselves, because dead cities have a way of making you want to whisper, to watch the sun go down.

"In about five days," said Dad quietly, "I'll go back down to

where our rocket was and collect the food hidden in the ruins there and bring it here; and I'll hunt for Bert Edwards and his wife and daughters there."

"Daughters?" asked Timothy. "How many?"

"Four."

"I can see that'll cause trouble later." Mom nodded slowly.

"Girls." Michael made a face like an ancient Martian stone image. "Girls."

"Are they coming in a rocket, too?"

"Yes. If they make it. Family rockets are made for travel to the Moon, not Mars. We were lucky we got through."

"Where did you get the rocket?" whispered Timothy, for the other boys were running ahead.

"I saved it. I saved it for twenty years, Tim. I had it hidden away, hoping I'd never have to use it. I suppose I should have given it to the government for the war, but I kept thinking about Mars. . . ."

"And a picnic!"

"Right. This is between you and me. When I saw everything was finishing on Earth, after I'd waited until the last moment, I packed us up. Bert Edwards had a ship hidden, too, but we decided it would be safer to take off separately, in case anyone tried to shoot us down."

"Why'd you blow up the rocket, Dad?"

"So we can't go back, ever. And so if any of those evil men ever come to Mars they won't know we're here."

"Is that why you look up all the time?"

"Yes, it's silly. They won't follow us, ever. They haven't anything to follow with. I'm being too careful, is all."

Michael came running back. "Is this really *our* city, Dad?"

"The whole darn planet belongs to us, kids. The whole darn planet."

They stood there, King of the Hill, Top of the Heap, Ruler of All They Surveyed, Unimpeachable Monarchs and Presidents, trying to understand what it meant to own a world and how big a world really was.

Night came quickly in the thin atmosphere, and Dad left them

in the square by the pulsing fountain, went down to the boat, and came walking back carrying a stack of paper in his big hands.

He laid the papers in a clutter in an old courtyard and set them afire. To keep warm, they crouched around the blaze and laughed, and Timothy saw the little letters leap like frightened animals when the flames touched and engulfed them. The papers crinkled like an old man's skin, and the cremation surrounded innumerable words: "GOVERNMENT BONDS; Business Graph, 1999; Religious Prejudice: An Essay; The Science of Logistics; Problems of the Pan-American Unity; Stock Report for July 3, 1998; The War Digest . . ."

Dad had insisted on bringing these papers for this purpose. He sat there and fed them into the fire, one by one, with satisfaction, and told his children what it all meant.

"It's time I told you a few things. I don't suppose it was fair, keeping so much from you. I don't know if you'll understand, but I have to talk, even if only part of it gets over to you."

He dropped a leaf in the fire.

"I'm burning a way of life, just like that way of life is being burned clean of Earth right now. Forgive me if I talk like a politician. I am, after all, a former state governor, and I was honest and they hated me for it. Life on Earth never settled down to doing anything very good. Science ran too far ahead of us too quickly, and the people got lost in a mechanical wilderness, like children making over pretty things, gadgets, helicopters, rockets; emphasizing the wrong items, emphasizing machines instead of how to run the machines. Wars got bigger and bigger and finally killed Earth. That's what the silent radio means. That's what we ran away from.

"We were lucky. There aren't any more rockets left. It's time you knew this isn't a fishing trip at all. I put off telling you. Earth is gone. Interplanetary travel won't be back for centuries, maybe never. But that way of life proved itself wrong and strangled itself with its own hands. You're young. I'll tell you this again every day until it sinks in."

He paused to feed more papers to the fire.

"Now we're alone. We and a handful of others who'll land in a few days. Enough to start over. Enough to turn away from all that back on Earth and strike out on a new line—"

The fire leaped up to emphasize his talking. And then all the papers were gone except one. All the laws and beliefs of Earth were burnt into small hot ashes which soon would be carried off in a wind.

Timothy looked at the last thing that Dad tossed in the fire. It was a map of the World, and it wrinkled and distorted itself hotly and went—flimpf—and was gone like a warm, black butterfly. Timothy turned away.

"Now I'm going to show you the Martians," said Dad. "Come on, all of you. Here, Alice." He took her hand.

Michael was crying loudly, and Dad picked him up and carried him, and they walked down through the ruins toward the canal.

The canal. Where tomorrow or the next day their future wives would come up in a boat, small laughing girls now, with their father and mother.

The night came down around them, and there were stars. But Timothy couldn't find Earth. It had already set. That was something to think about.

A night bird called among the ruins as they walked. Dad said, "Your mother and I will try to teach you. Perhaps we'll fail. I hope not. We've had a good lot to see and learn from. We planned this trip years ago, before you were born. Even if there hadn't been a war we would have come to Mars, I think, to live and form our own standard of living. It would have been another century before Mars would have been really poisoned by the Earth civilization. Now, of course—"

They reached the canal. It was long and straight and cool and wet and reflective in the night.

"I've always wanted to see a Martian," said Michael. "Where are they, Dad? You promised."

"There they are," said Dad, and he shifted Michael on his shoulder and pointed straight down.

The Martians were there. Timothy began to shiver.

The Martians were there—in the canal—reflected in the water. Timothy and Michael and Robert and Mom and Dad.

The Martians stared back up at them for a long, long silent time from the rippling water. . . .

ALL SUMMER IN A DAY

Ready?"

"Ready."

"Now?"

"Soon."

"Do the scientists really know? Will it happen today, will it?"

"Look, look; see for yourself!"

The children pressed to each other like so many roses, so many weeds, intermixed, peering out for a look at the hidden sun.

It rained.

It had been raining for seven years; thousands upon thousands of days compounded and filled from one end to the other with rain, with the drum and gush of water, with the sweet crystal fall of showers and the concussion of storms so heavy they were tidal waves come over the islands. A thousand forests had been crushed under the rain and grown up a thousand times to be crushed again. And this was the way life was forever on the planet Venus, and this was the schoolroom of the children of the rocket men and women who had come to a raining world to set up civilization and live out their lives.

"It's stopping, it's stopping!'

"Yes, yes!"

Margot stood apart from them, from these children who could

never remember a time when there wasn't rain and rain and rain. They were all nine years old, and if there had been a day, seven years ago, when the sun came out for an hour and showed its face to the stunned world, they could not recall. Sometimes, at night, she heard them stir, in remembrance, and she knew they were dreaming and remembering gold or yellow crayon or a coin large enough to buy the world with. She knew they thought they remembered a warmness, like a blushing in the face, in the body, in the arms and legs and trembling hands. But then they always awoke to the tatting drum, the endless shaking down of clear bead necklaces upon the roof, the walk, the gardens, the forests, and their dreams were gone.

All day yesterday they had read in class about the sun. About how like a lemon it was, and how hot. And they had written small stories or essays or poems about it:

> *I think the sun is a flower,*
> *That blooms for just one hour.*

That was Margot's poem, read in a quiet voice in the still classroom while the rain was falling outside.

"Aw, you didn't write that!" protested one of the boys.

"I did," said Margot. "I *did*."

"William!" said the teacher.

But that was yesterday. Now the rain was slackening, and the children were crushed in the great thick windows.

"Where's teacher?"

"She'll be back."

"She'd better hurry, we'll miss it!"

They turned on themselves, like a feverish wheel, all tumbling spokes.

Margot stood alone. She was a very frail girl who looked as if she had been lost in the rain for years and the rain had washed out the blue from her eyes and the red from her mouth and the yellow from her hair. She was an old photograph dusted from an album, whitened away, and if she spoke at all her voice would be a ghost. Now she stood, separate, staring at the rain and the loud wet world beyond the huge glass.

"What're *you* looking at?" said William.

Margot said nothing.

"Speak when you're spoken to." He gave her a shove. But she did not move; rather she let herself be moved only by him and nothing else.

They edged away from her, they would not look at her. She felt them go away. And this was because she would play no games with them in the echoing tunnels of the underground city. If they tagged her and ran, she stood blinking after them and did not follow. When the class sang songs about happiness and life and games her lips barely moved. Only when they sang about the sun and the summer did her lips move as she watched the drenched windows.

And then, of course, the biggest crime of all was that she had come here only five years ago from Earth, and she remembered the sun and the way the sun was and the sky was when she was four in Ohio. And they, they had been on Venus all their lives, and they had been only two years old when last the sun came out and had long since forgotten the color and heat of it and the way it really was. But Margot remembered.

"It's like a penny," she said once, eyes closed.

"No, it's not!" the children cried.

"It's like a fire," she said, "in the stove."

"You're lying, you don't remember!" cried the children.

But she remembered and stood quietly apart from all of them and watched the patterning windows. And once, a month ago, she had refused to shower in the school shower rooms, had clutched her hands to her ears and over her head, screaming the water mustn't touch her head. So after that, dimly, dimly, she sensed it, she was different and they knew her difference and kept away.

There was talk that her father and mother were taking her back to Earth next year; it seemed vital to her that they do so, though it would mean the loss of thousands of dollars to her family. And so, the children hated her for all these reasons of big and little consequence. They hated her pale snow face, her waiting silence, her thinness, and her possible future.

"Get away!" The boy gave her another push. "What're you waiting for?"

Then, for the first time, she turned and looked at him. And what she was waiting for was in her eyes.

"Well, don't wait around here!" cried the boy savagely. "You won't see nothing!"

Her lips moved.

"Nothing!" he cried. "It was all a joke, wasn't it?" He turned to the other children. "Nothing's happening today. *Is* it?"

They all blinked at him and then, understanding, laughed and shook their heads. "Nothing, nothing!"

"Oh, but," Margot whispered, her eyes helpless. "But this is the day, the scientists predict, they say, they *know*, the sun . . ."

"All a joke!" said the boy, and seized her roughly. "Hey, everyone, let's put her in a closet before teacher comes!"

"No," said Margot, falling back.

They surged about her, caught her up and bore her, protesting, and then pleading, and then crying, back into a tunnel, a room, a closet, where they slammed and locked the door. They stood looking at the door and saw it tremble from her beating and throwing herself against it. They heard her muffled cries. Then, smiling, they turned and went out and back down the tunnel, just as the teacher arrived.

"Ready, children?" She glanced at her watch.

"Yes!" said everyone.

"Are we all here?"

"Yes!"

The rain slackened still more.

They crowded to the huge door.

The rain stopped.

It was as if, in the midst of a film concerning an avalanche, a tornado, a hurricane, a volcanic eruption, something had, first, gone wrong with the sound apparatus, thus muffling and finally cutting off all noise, all of the blasts and repercussions and thunders, and then, second, ripped the film from the projector and inserted in its place a peaceful tropical slide which did not move or tremor. The world ground to a standstill. The silence was so immense and unbelievable that you felt your ears had been stuffed or you had lost your hearing altogether. The children put their hands to their ears. They stood apart. The door slid back and the smell of the silent, waiting world came in to them.

The sun came out.

It was the color of flaming bronze and it was very large. And the sky around it was a blazing blue tile color. And the jungle burned with sunlight as the children, released from their spell, rushed out, yelling, into the springtime.

"Now, don't go too far," called the teacher after them. "You've only two hours, you know. You wouldn't want to get caught out!"

But they were running and turning their faces up to the sky and feeling the sun on their cheeks like a warm iron; they were taking off their jackets and letting the sun burn their arms.

"Oh, it's better than the sun lamps, isn't it?"

"Much, much better!"

They stopped running and stood in the great jungle that covered Venus, that grew and never stopped growing, tumultuously, even as you watched it. It was a nest of octopi, clustering up great arms of fleshlike weed, wavering, flowering in this brief spring. It was the color of rubber and ash, this jungle, from the many years without sun. It was the color of stones and white cheeses and ink, and it was the color of the moon.

The children lay out, laughing, on the jungle mattress, and heard it sigh and squeak under them, resilient and alive. They ran among the trees, they slipped and fell, they pushed each other, they played hide-and-seek and tag, but most of all they squinted at the sun until tears ran down their faces, they put their hands up to that yellowness and that amazing blueness and they breathed of the fresh, fresh air and listened and listened to the silence which suspended them in a blessed sea of no sound and no motion. They looked at everything and savored everything. Then, wildly, like animals escaped from their caves, they ran and ran in shouting circles. They ran for an hour and did not stop running.

And then—

In the midst of their running one of the girls wailed.

Everyone stopped.

The girl, standing in the open, held out her hand.

"Oh, look, look," she said, trembling.

They came slowly to look at her opened palm.

In the center of it, cupped and huge, was a single raindrop.

She began to cry, looking at it.

They glanced quietly at the sky.

"Oh. Oh."

A few cold drops fell on their noses and their cheeks and their mouths. The sun faded behind a stir of mist. A wind blew cool around them. They turned and started to walk back toward the underground house, their hands at their sides, their smiles vanishing away.

A boom of thunder startled them and like leaves before a new hurricane, they tumbled upon each other and ran. Lightning struck ten miles away, five miles away, a mile, a half mile. The sky darkened into midnight in a flash.

They stood in the doorway of the underground for a moment until it was raining hard. Then they closed the door and heard the gigantic sound of the rain falling in tons and avalanches, everywhere and forever.

"Will it be seven more years?"

"Yes. Seven."

Then one of them gave a little cry.

"Margot!"

"What?"

"She's still in the closet where we locked her."

"Margot."

They stood as if someone had driven them, like so many stakes, into the floor. They looked at each other and then looked away. They glanced out at the world that was raining now and raining and raining steadily. They could not meet each other's glances. Their faces were solemn and pale. They looked at their hands and feet, their faces down.

"Margot."

One of the girls said, "Well . . . ?"

No one moved.

"Go on," whispered the girl.

They walked slowly down the hall in the sound of cold rain. They turned through the doorway to the room in the sound of the storm and thunder, lightning on their faces, blue and terrible. They walked over to the closet door slowly and stood by it.

Behind the closet door was only silence.

They unlocked the door, even more slowly, and let Margot out.

THERE WILL COME SOFT RAINS

In the living room the voice-clock sang, *Tick-tock, seven o'clock, time to get up, time to get up, seven o'clock!* as if it were afraid that nobody would. The morning house lay empty. The clock ticked on, repeating and repeating its sounds into the emptiness. *Seven-nine, breakfast time, seven-nine!*

In the kitchen the breakfast stove gave a hissing sigh and ejected from its warm interior eight pieces of perfectly browned toast, eight eggs sunnyside up, sixteen slices of bacon, two coffees, and two cool glasses of milk.

"Today is August 4, 2026," said a second voice from the kitchen ceiling, "in the city of Allendale, California." It repeated the date three times for memory's sake. "Today is Mr. Featherstone's birthday. Today is the anniversary of Tilita's marriage. Insurance is payable, as are the water, gas, and light bills."

Somewhere in the walls, relays clicked, memory tapes glided under electric eyes.

Eight-one, tick-tock, eight-one o'clock, off to school, off to work, run, run, eight-one! But no doors slammed, no carpets took the soft tread of rubber heels. It was raining outside. The weather box on the front door sang quietly: "Rain, rain, go away; rubbers, raincoats for today . . ." And the rain tapped on the empty house, echoing.

Outside, the garage chimed and lifted its door to reveal the

waiting car. After a long wait the door swung down again.

At eight-thirty the eggs were shriveled and the toast was like stone. An aluminum wedge scraped them into the sink, where hot water whirled them down a metal throat which digested and flushed them away to the distant sea. The dirty dishes were dropped into a hot washer and emerged twinkling dry.

Nine-fifteen, sang the clock, *time to clean.*

Out of warrens in the wall, tiny robot mice darted. The rooms were acrawl with the small cleaning animals, all rubber and metal. They thudded against chairs, whirling their mustached runners, kneading the rug nap, sucking gently at hidden dust. Then, like mysterious invaders, they popped into their burrows. Their pink electric eyes faded. The house was clean.

Ten o'clock. The sun came out from behind the rain. The house stood alone in a city of rubble and ashes. This was the one house left standing. At night the ruined city gave off a radioactive glow which could be seen for miles.

Ten-fifteen. The garden sprinklers whirled up in golden founts, filling the soft morning air with scatterings of brightness. The water pelted windowpanes, running down the charred west side where the house had been burned evenly free of its white paint. The entire west face of the house was black, save for five places. Here the silhouette in paint of a man mowing a lawn. Here, as in a photograph, a woman bent to pick flowers. Still farther over, their images burned on wood in one titanic instant, a small boy, hands flung into the air; higher up, the image of a thrown ball, and opposite him a girl, hands raised to catch a ball which never came down.

The five spots of paint—the man, the woman, the children, the ball—remained. The rest was a thin charcoaled layer.

The gentle sprinkler rain filled the garden with falling light.

Until this day, how well the house had kept its peace. How carefully it had inquired, "Who goes there? What's the password?" and, getting no answer from lonely foxes and whining cats, it had shut up its windows and drawn shades in an old-maidenly preoccupation with self-protection which bordered on a mechanical paranoia.

It quivered at each sound, the house did. If a sparrow brushed

a window, the shade snapped up. The bird, startled, flew off! No, not even a bird must touch the house!

The house was an altar with ten thousand attendants, big, small, servicing, attending, in choirs. But the gods had gone away, and the ritual of the religion continued senselessly, uselessly.

Twelve noon.

A dog whined, shivering, on the front porch.

The front door recognized the dog voice and opened. The dog, once huge and fleshy, but now gone to bone and covered with sores, moved in and through the house, tracking mud. Behind it whirred angry mice, angry at having to pick up mud, angry at inconvenience.

For not a leaf fragment blew under the door but what the wall panels flipped open and the copper scrap rats flashed swiftly out. The offending dust, hair, or paper, seized in miniature steel jaws, was raced back to the burrows. There, down tubes which fed into the cellar, it was dropped into the sighing vent of an incinerator which sat like evil Baal in a dark corner.

The dog ran upstairs, hysterically yelping to each door, at last realizing, as the house realized, that only silence was here.

It sniffed the air and scratched the kitchen door. Behind the door, the stove was making pancakes which filled the house with a rich baked odor and the scent of maple syrup.

The dog frothed at the mouth, lying at the door, sniffing, its eyes turned to fire. It ran wildly in circles, biting at its tail, spun in a frenzy, and died. It lay in the parlor for an hour.

Two o'clock, sang a voice.

Delicately sensing decay at last, the regiments of mice hummed out as softly as blown gray leaves in an electrical wind.

Two-fifteen.

The dog was gone.

In the cellar, the incinerator glowed suddenly and a whirl of sparks leaped up the chimney.

Two thirty-five.

Bridge tables sprouted from patio walls. Playing cards fluttered onto pads in a shower of pips. Martinis manifested on an oaken bench with egg-salad sandwiches. Music played.

But the tables were silent and the cards untouched.

At four o'clock the tables folded like great butterflies back through the paneled walls.

Four-thirty.

The nursery walls glowed.

Animals took shape: yellow giraffes, blue lions, pink antelopes, lilac panthers cavorting in crystal substance. The walls were glass. They looked out upon color and fantasy. Hidden films clocked through well-oiled sprockets, and the walls lived. The nursery floor was woven to resemble a crisp, cereal meadow. Over this ran aluminum roaches and iron crickets, and in the hot still air butterflies of delicate red tissue wavered among the sharp aromas of animal spoors! There was the sound like a great matted yellow hive of bees within a dark bellows, the lazy bumble of a purring lion. And there was the patter of okapi feet and the murmur of a fresh jungle rain, like other hoofs, falling upon the summer-starched grass. Now the walls dissolved into distances of parched weed, mile on mile, and warm endless sky. The animals drew away into thorn brakes and water holes.

It was the children's hour.

Five o'clock. The bath filled with clear hot water.

Six, seven, eight o'clock. The dinner dishes manipulated like magic tricks, and in the study a *click*. In the metal stand opposite the hearth where a fire now blazed up warmly, a cigar popped out, half an inch of soft gray ash on it, smoking, waiting.

Nine o'clock. The beds warmed their hidden circuits, for nights were cool here.

Nine-five. A voice spoke from the study ceiling:

"Mrs. McClellan, which poem would you like this evening?"

The house was silent.

The voice said at last, "Since you express no preference, I shall select a poem at random." Quiet music rose to back the voice. "Sara Teasdale. As I recall, your favorite. . . ."

There will come soft rains and the smell of the ground,
And swallows circling with their shimmering sound;

And frogs in the pools singing at night,
And wild plum trees in tremulous white;

Robins will wear their feathery fire,
Whistling their whims on a low fence-wire;

And not one will know of the war, not one
Will care at last when it is done.

Not one would mind, neither bird nor tree,
If mankind perished utterly;

And Spring herself, when she woke at dawn
Would scarcely know that we were gone.

The fire burned on the stone hearth and the cigar fell away into a mound of quiet ash on its tray. The empty chairs faced each other between the silent walls, and the music played.

At ten o'clock the house began to die.

The wind blew. A falling tree bough crashed through the kitchen window. Cleaning solvent, bottled, shattered over the stove. The room was ablaze in an instant!

"Fire!" screamed a voice. The house lights flashed, water pumps shot water from the ceilings. But the solvent spread on the linoleum, licking, eating, under the kitchen door, while the voices took it up in chorus: "Fire, fire, fire!"

The house tried to save itself. Doors sprang tightly shut, but the windows were broken by the heat and the wind blew and sucked upon the fire.

The house gave ground as the fire in ten billion angry sparks moved with flaming ease from room to room and then up the stairs. While scurrying water rats squeaked from the walls, pistoled their water, and ran for more. And the wall sprays let down showers of mechanical rain.

But too late. Somewhere, sighing, a pump shrugged to a stop. The quenching rain ceased. The reserve water supply which had filled baths and washed dishes for many quiet days was gone.

The fire crackled up the stairs. It fed upon Picassos and Matisses in the upper halls, like delicacies, baking off the oily flesh, tenderly crisping the canvases into black shavings.

Now the fire lay in beds, stood in windows, changed the colors of drapes!

And then, reinforcements.

From attic trapdoors, blind robot faces peered down with faucet mouths gushing green chemical.

The fire backed off, as even an elephant must at the sight of a dead snake. Now there were twenty snakes whipping over the floor, killing the fire with a clear cold venom of green froth.

But the fire was clever. It had sent flame outside the house, up through the attic to the pumps there. An explosion! The attic brain which directed the pumps was shattered into bronze shrapnel on the beams.

The fire rushed back into every closet and felt of the clothes hung there.

The house shuddered, oak bone on bone, its bared skeleton cringing from the heat, its wire, its nerves revealed as if a surgeon had torn the skin off to let the red veins and capillaries quiver in the scalded air. Help, help! Fire! Run, run! Heat snapped mirrors like the first brittle winter ice. And the voices wailed, Fire, fire, run, run, like a tragic nursery rhyme, a dozen voices, high, low, like children dying in a forest, alone, alone. And the voices fading as the wires popped their sheathings like hot chestnuts. One, two, three, four, five voices died.

In the nursery the jungle burned. Blue lions roared, purple giraffes bounded off. The panthers ran in circles, changing color, and ten million animals, running before the fire, vanished off toward a distant steaming river. . . .

Ten more voices died. In the last instant under the fire avalanche, other choruses, oblivious, could be heard announcing the time, playing music, cutting the lawn by remote-control mower, or setting an umbrella frantically out and in, the slamming and opening front door, a thousand things happening, like a clock shop when

each clock strikes the hour insanely before or after the other, a scene of maniac confusion, yet unity; singing, screaming, a few last cleaning mice darting bravely out to carry the horrid ashes away! And one voice, with sublime disregard for the situation, read poetry aloud in the fiery study, until all the films spools burned, until all the wires withered and the circuits cracked.

The fire burst the house and let it slam flat down, puffing out skirts of spark and smoke.

In the kitchen, an instant before the rain of fire and timber, the stove could be seen making breakfasts at a psychopathic rate, ten dozen eggs, six loaves of toast, twenty dozen bacon strips, which, eaten by fire, started the stove working again, hysterically hissing!

The crash. The attic smashing into kitchen and parlor. The parlor into cellar, cellar into subcellar. Deep freeze, armchair, film tapes, circuits, beds, and all like skeletons thrown in a cluttered mound deep under.

Smoke and silence. A great quantity of smoke.

Dawn showed faintly in the east. Among the ruins, one wall stood alone. Within the wall, a last voice said, over and over again and again, even as the sun rose to shine upon the heaped rubble and steam:

"Today is August 5, 2026, today is August 5, 2026, today is . . ."

THE AFFLUENCE OF DESPAIR

H ow come? How come we're one of the greatest nations in the world . . . and yet, there is this feeling of Doom? How come, while our president walks wounded, we ourselves jog along nicely, but . . . under a dark cloud that says something awful is about to happen? How come, with 500,000 immigrants a year yammering to flood in . . . we enjoy what could be described as The Affluence of Despair?

America today: We wonder how we look at this hour, what we feel this minute, what we're imagining now. So we switch the television on. How do we look in the 80 million-lensed TV eye on America the beautiful? Did you catch me last night confessing what I caught and what caught me?

Recall Starbuck's advice to mad Ahab? "Do not fear me, old man. Beware of thy self, my captain." America should beware of itself. Today, we are everywhere loving to be watched. My God, look, I am on Channel Nine! We do not suffer from totalitarian lunatics, but from the astonishing proliferation of our images. We perform for ourselves, not Big Brother. We have fallen in love with mirrors. Flash a camera and your merest broccoli-headed citizen morphs into Travolta or Madonna.

And all of it on local TV news, in 15-second disaster updates.

Breaking bones, breaking news, at 11. "Tell us, Mrs. Guiterrez, how's it feel with your son shotgunned minutes ago?"

We do not go to the theater, we *are* the theater. We have invaded the TV studios and run the country to mania on talking-head shows. We display our brilliance on "Jeopardy," forgetting that its factoids are 90% useless once you kill the set. We don't ask who Napoleon was but where he was buried. Or why he invaded Russia, but when.

A friend of mine bragged he had bought a dish that could cup, cull, and catch 200 channels raining across a moron sky. Hell, I said, you've just got a bigger windmill to catch more of nothing: O. J. blood here, House of Usher AIDS there, the Killing Fields of America's high roads, each car a glorious pyre to mindless speed. And in every front yard a Mrs. Guiterrez being questioned but watching the TV mirror to see how she plays.

Those epileptic souls at football, baseball, hockey matches, who frenzy for the TV camera—how to end their pantomimes? We the judges and jurors trying, damning or freeing the guilty, weighing topics we're unqualified to answer—how to cork this motor-mouth?

The problem is not necessarily with our national full-coverage news, which can be only mildly depressing. It is with the assault of the local TV paparazzi, who machine-gun you with decapitations, sexual harassments, gangster executions in 15-second explosions for the full half-hour. No attack army could survive that fusillade. Bullets, real and psychological, wound and kill.

So we must stand alert, ward off a central core despair, target our Panic of the Week Syndrome, guard against the local TV news séance. Every week, 52 weeks a year, they need a prime disaster focus to spin the garbage and glue the potato people to the tube.

Remember the Alar-poisoned apples that the dinner time news-bites claimed would destroy us, so they destroyed some part of the apple industry? Recall the poison cellar gas rising to asphyxiate your kids? Or those arsenic Peruvian grapes promising to strip our gears? Or the Three Mile Island nuclear meltdown where nothing melted, no injuries, no deaths? Panic for two weeks, make it three. Ratings up. Morale down.

What to do? Leave a message on your local station's machine,

describing their stupidity. If you meet their news readers, tell them that they are overpaid and underbrained. Ask them if it would be too much trouble to air 20-second newsbites instead of 15-second flashes. Think of the extra enrichment!

Stop saying that these TV hookers are high-class thinkers. Ask them to give back their fortunes and hand us real news. Instead of treating them as Cinderellas, tell them they are ugly sisters whose lips spew not diamonds and emeralds but spiders, frogs and toads: Each time they open their mouths, they spoil the ecology.

We must speak to these confessors of our dark souls and tell them that their awful truths in awesome repetition end with the Big Lie. We are not as bad as they say we are, but we feel this despair because they have somehow won us over.

The bottom line is that if you stare like stunned deer in mid-road, blinded by the lights that rush to run you down, you must expect that 1,000 such nights will convince you that the end of the world is at hand, that America is bestial, and that suicide, murder, rape, and AIDS are our lot.

We have condemned ourselves. Now we must save ourselves. No one else can. Shut off the set. Write your local TV news people. Tell them to go to hell. Go sit on the lawn with friends.

LaVergne, TN USA
19 August 2010
193870LV00001B/44/A

NOTES

NOTES